Sixth Edition

Manual of Rheumatology

Editors of Previous Editions

1st and 2nd Editions

Editor-in-chief

Prakash K Pispati

Associate editors

Nirupa E. Borges, SS Uppal

3rd Edition

Editor-in-chief

URK Rao

Editors

KM Mahendranath, Ramnath Misra, SJ Gupta, Rohini Handa, Annil Mahajan

Associate editor

Firdaus Fatima

4th Edition

Editor-in-chief

URK Rao

Editors

KM Mahendranath, Ramnath Misra, SJ Gupta, Rohini Handa, Annil Mahajan, Ved Chaturvedi, V Krishnamurthy, Binoy Paul, S Shankar, Firdaus Fatima

5th Edition

Editor-in-chief

Ved Chaturvedi

Editors

Molly M Thabah, Debashish Danda, Rajiva Gupta, Durga Prasanna Misra, Vir Singh Negi, Vinod Ravindran, Vivek Vasdev

Sixth Edition

Manual of Rheumatology

Editor-in-Chief

Ramnath Misra MD FRCP FAMS Masters (APLAR)
Professor and Head
Department of Clinical Immunology and Rheumatology
Kalinga Institute of Medical Sciences
KIIT University, Bhubaneswar
Formerly Professor and Head
Department of Clinical Immunology and Rheumatology
SGPGIMS, Lucknow

Associate and Section Editors

Molly Mary Thabah MD FRCP (Edin)
Professor of Medicine
Head, Department of Clinical Immunology
Jawaharlal Institute of Postgraduate Medical Education and Research, Puducherry

Sakir Ahmed MD DM MAMS
Associate Professor
Department of Clinical Immunology and Rheumatology
Kalinga Institute of Medical Sciences, Bhubaneswar

Prasanta Padhan MD PDF
Professor
Department of Clinical Immunology and Rheumatology
Kalinga Institute of Medical Sciences
KIIT University, Bhubaneswar

Section Editors

BG Dharmanand MD DM
Consultant Rheumatologist, Manipal Hospital
Bengaluru

Bidyut Das MD PhD
Professor and Head, Department of Clinical Immunology and Rheumatology
SCB Medical College, Cuttack

Sapan Pandya MD DM
Rheumatologist, Vedanta Institute of Medical Sciences
Assistant Professor, Rheumatology, Smt NHL Municipal Medical College linked with SVP Hospital, Ahmedabad

K Shanmuganandan MD
Professor of Rheumatology and Medicine
Sree Balaji Medical College and Hospital
Chromepet, Chennai

Aman Sharma MD FRCP (London)
Professor
Department of Internal Medicine
Post Graduate Institute of Medical Education and Research, Chandigarh

Amita Aggarwal MD DM FAMS FNASc FNA
Professor and Head
Department of Clinical Immunology and Rheumatology
Sanjay Gandhi Post Graduate Institute of Medical Sciences, Lucknow

Arghya Chattopadhya MD DM
Assistant Professor of Rheumatology
North Bengal Medical College
Darjeeling

Subramanian Shankar MD DNB MNAMS FICP FRCP (Glasgow)
Senior Consultant, Rheumatology and Clinical Immunology
Commandant, Command Hospital (Air Force)
Bengaluru

CBSPD

CBS Publishers & Distributors Pvt Ltd

New Delhi • Bengaluru • Chennai • Kochi • Kolkata • Lucknow • Mumbai
Hyderabad • Jharkhand • Nagpur • Patna • Pune • Uttarakhand

Disclaimer
Science and technology are constantly changing fields. New research and experience broaden the scope of information and knowledge. The editors have tried their best in giving information available to them while preparing the material for this book. Although all efforts have been made to ensure optimum accuracy of the material, yet it is quite possible some errors might have been left uncorrected. The publisher, the printer and the editors will not be held responsible for any inadvertent errors, omissions or inaccuracies.

Sixth Edition

Manual of

Rheumatology

ISBN: 978-93-5466-802-9

Sixth Edition: 2024
First Edition: 1999
Second Edition: 2002
Third Edition: 2009
Fourth Edition: 2014
Fifth Edition: 2018
Reprint: 2022

Published by Satish Kumar Jain and produced by Varun Jain for
CBS Publishers & Distributors Pvt Ltd
4819/XI Prahlad Street, 24 Ansari Road, Daryaganj, New Delhi 110 002, India
Ph: 011-23289259, 23266861 Website: www.cbspd.com
e-mail: delhi@cbspd.com

Corporate Office: 204 FIE, Industrial Area, Patparganj, Delhi 110 092, India
Ph: 011-4934 4934 Fax: 011-4934 4935 e-mail: publishing@cbspd.com; publicity@cbspd.com

Branches

- **Bengaluru:** Seema House 2975, 17th Cross, KR Road, Banasankari 2nd Stage, Bengaluru 560 070, Karnataka, India
  Ph: +91-80-26771678/79 Fax: +91-80-26771680 e-mail: bangalore@cbspd.com
- **Chennai:** 7, Subbaraya Street, Shenoy Nagar, Chennai 600 030, Tamil Nadu, India
  Ph: +91-44-26680620, 26681266 Fax: +91-44-42032115 e-mail: chennai@cbspd.com
- **Kochi:** 42/1325, 1326, Power House Road, Opp KSEB, Power House, Ernakulum Kochi 682 018, Kerala, India
  Ph: +91-484-4059061-65,67 Fax: +91-484-4059065 e-mail: kochi@cbspd.com
- **Kolkata:** 147, Hind Ceramics Compound, 1st Floor, Nilgunj Road, Belghoria, Kolkata 700 056, West Bengal, India
  Ph: +91-33-25633055/56 e-mail: kolkata@cbspd.com
- **Lucknow:** Basement, Khushnuma Complex, 7 Meerabai Marg (behind Jawahar Bhawan), Lucknow 226 001, UP, India
  Ph: +910522-4000032 e-mail: tiwari.lucknow@cbspd.com
- **Mumbai:** PWD Shed, Gala no 25/26, Ramchandra Bhatt Marg, Next to JJ Hospital Gate no. 2, Opp. Union Bank of India, Noorbaug, Mumbai 400 009, Maharashtra, India
  Ph: +91-22-66661880/89 e-mail: mumbai@cbspd.com

Representatives

- **Hyderabad** 0-9885175004
- **Patna** 0-9334159340
- **Jharkhand** 0-9811541605
- **Pune** 0-9664372571
- **Nagpur** 0-8692091830
- **Uttarakhand** 0-9716462459

Printed at: Nutech Print Services – India

Preface to the Sixth Edition

Rheumatology is gaining increasing importance as a superspecialty of medicine and pediatrics. The awareness to seek consultations by a rheumatologists/clinical immunologists has increased both by patients and their general physicians. Probably no other branches of medicine have witnessed a revolutionary changes as rheumatology and clinical immunology. These have been primarily due to advances in our understanding of pathogenesis of diseases caused by progress in immunology, molecular biology and technological development in radiological investigations.

Five editions of the *Manual of Rheumatology* have been published, the first appeared in 1999 and subsequently 2nd (2002), 3rd (2009), 4th (2014) and 5th (2018) by the Indian Rheumatology Association. The first edition was meant for use by general practitioners, trainee rheumatologists and orthropedic surgeons; subsequently, the contents of the manual have undergone changes to capture the needs of trainee rheumatologists and clinical immunologist keeping in the mind the developments in field. The present edition of the manual has been further revised to be exclusively used as a handbook for managing patients with rheumatic diseases. Almost all the chapters have been rewritten to exclude theoretical background, pathogenesis, controversies so that the users will be familiarized with the standard of care.

The present edition consists of XII sections having 116 chapters written by rheumatologists, internists, radiologists of national and international repute. In true sense, it is a manual and not a substitute for textbooks. It deals with salient features in clinical examination, investigations and treatment for each rheumatological disease, leaving out epidemiology, pathogenesis, controversies and treatment modalities that are yet to be cleared by the regulatory authorities. This will facilitate treatment decisions and set a platform for uniform standard care. Several chapters are new with extensive coverage of laboratory and imaging investigations. This captures the recent advances in the field. We hope this will be a handy book for all rheumatologists, internists, pediatricians who provide care to patients with rheumatic diseases.

All contributors are to be complimented for this edition, but it is with pride to put on records the untiring efforts of Associate and Section Editor, Molly Mary Thabah, without whom this project was not possible. The editorial efforts of Dr Sakir Ahmed and Prof Prasanta Padhan are gratefully acknowledged.

Ramnath Misra
Editor-in-Chief

Preface to the First Edition

Perhaps nowhere in the world as in India that the arthritic patient is vulnerable to influences and counter-influences of modem medicine, homoeopathy, ayurveda and unani systems of medicine, not to speak of acupuncture, copper bangles, magnetic therapy and what have you. In an ancient land such as India, a rheumatologist is competing with these modalities of alternate medicine all the time. Alternate medicine, if practiced in a scientific way may be justifiable, but under this garb outright quackery is practiced as well. Steroids are mixed on the sly with ayurvedic and homoeopathic preparations. Branding of joints with hot iron rods in the hope of curing arthritis still goes on rampantly. Some arthritic patients have lost teeth under the false belief that removal of "septic focus" would cure arthritis. Not surprisingly, even practitioners of modem medicine at times prescribe drugs of alternate medicine without necessarily understanding their role. The stark reality of the Indian situation is that there is such little understanding of rheumatic diseases in the minds of average practitioners. This is attributed to the fact that rheumatology is not taught in medical schools. Perhaps a few orthopaedic surgeons may refer to rheumatic diseases during their interaction with students. But is this enough?

There is thus a paramount need for a *Manual of Rheumatology* intended for practitioners, postgraduates in medicine and orthopaedics, orthopaedic surgeons who mainly treat rheumatic diseases day in and day out. Rheumatologists are so few in India that much of the arthritis care is delivered by these practitioners. Hence, this manual is mainly addressed to this target audience.

No doubt, the Indian Rheumatism Association (IRA) conducts CME programmes for practitioners throughout the country from time to time, but its reach is restricted. The Manual of Rheumatology aims at bringing recent diagnostic and therapeutic skills available in modem medicine to the practitioner. For example, there are few practitioners who realize that there are a hundred different types of arthritis. The manual aims at building their confidence in at least making a tentative diagnosis on clinical grounds. It sets out guidelines on laboratory investigations for arthritis, which to order and how to interpret the results. Radiology of arthritis is well illustrated. The reader should be able to discern between rheumatoid arthritis and seronegative spondyloarthropathies. The practitioner should be able to treat successfully a case of infective arthritis with cure as the outcome. The book emphasizes the wide prevalence of tuberculous arthritis in our country. It brings into focus the new diseases like HIV in arthritis. Complexities of vasculitis and antiphospholipid syndrome are explained in simple terms. Therapeutic modalities are described in a way that the practitioner should be able to choose a rational NSAID and not be afraid to prescribe DMARDs. Finally, the manual raises the challenge of patient education in the management of chronic diseases such as arthritis.

This Manual is a dream come true. It is a labor of love of us rheumatologists in India. It was indeed a privilege to write for this manual and to edit the various chapters and finally publish it within the stipulated time, for the new millennium. Initially, the print run is a modest five thousand. We hope that the sponsors M/s. Pfizer Ltd. will take up the challenge of reaching the practising community at large and multiply the print run several times. We pray that the manual will be received and read by the practitioners with enthusiasm in the hope of better care and treatment for the arthritic patient to whom the book is dedicated.

Prakash K Pispati
Editor-in-Chief

Nirupa E Borges
Associate Editor

SS Uppal
Associate Editor

Contributors

Manjari Agarwal MD
Consultant
Division of Pediatric Rheumatology, Institute of Child Health
Sir Ganga Ram Hospital
New Delhi

Vikas Agarwal MD DM FRCP (Edin)
Professor
Department of Clinical Immunology and Rheumatology
Sanjay Gandhi Postgraduate Institute of Medical Sciences
Lucknow

Vishal Agarwal MD
Senior Resident
Department of Medicine
Assam Medical College and Hospital
Dibrugarh, Assam

Amita Aggarwal MD DM FAMS FNASc FNA
Professor and Head
Department of Clinical Immunology and Rheumatology
Sanjay Gandhi Post Graduate Institute of Medical Sciences
Lucknow

Parshant Aggarwal MD DM
Consultant Rheumatologist
Punjab Rheumatology and Immunology Centre
Ludhiana

Sumeet Agrawal MD DM
Senior Consultant
Department of Rheumatology and Clinical Immunology
Artemis Hospitals
Gurugram

Sakir Ahmed MD DM MAMS
Associate Professor
Department of Clinical Immunology and Rheumatology
Kalinga Institute of Medical Sciences
Bhubaneshwar

Sajal Ajmani MD DM
Consultant
Arthritis and Rheumatology Clinic
New Delhi

Paul T Antony MD DM
Associate Professor
Department of Clinical Immunology and Rheumatology
Amala Institute of Medical Sciences, Thrissur

Neha Arora DNB (Medicine)
Consultant Rheumatologist
Holy Family Hospital, Bandra West
Mumbai

Kalpana Babu MD
Department of Uveitis and Ocular Inflammation
Prabha Eye Clinic and Research Centre
Vittala International Institute of Ophthalmology
Bengaluru

C Balakrishnan MD
Consultant Rheumatologist
PD Hinduja Hospital and Medical Research Centre
Mumbai

Suma Balan MD MRCP Pediatrics CCT UK
Professor of Rheumatology, School of Medicine, Amrita Vishwa Vidyapeetham
Consultant Pediatric Rheumatologist
Amrita Institute of Medical Sciences
Kochi

Aaqib Zaffar Banday MD
Senior Resident
Allergy Immunology Unit, Department of Pediatrics
Advanced Pediatric Center
Post Graduate Institute of Medical Education and Research
Chandigarh

Pooja Belani MD DM
Consultant Rheumatologist
Divine Life Hospital, Kutch, Gujarat

Darshan Singh Bhakuni MD
Director
Max Institute of Musculoskeletal Sciences
Ghaziabad

Dharmagat Bhattarai MD DM
Senior Resident
Allergy Immunology Unit, Department of Pediatrics
Advanced Pediatrics Centre
Post Graduate Institute of Medical Education and Research
Chandigarh

Satyam Bhatt MD DNB (Rheumatology)
Assistant Professor
Department of Clinical Immunology and Rheumatology
Geetanjali Medical College and Hospital, Udaipur

Vinod Chandran MD DM PhD FRCPC
Division of Rheumatology, Department of Medicine
University of Toronto
Schroeder Arthritis Institute, Krembil Research Institute
Toronto, Canada

Laxmisha Chandrashekar MD
Professor
Department of Dermatology
Jawaharlal Institute of Postgraduate Medical Education and Research
Puducherry

Chandrashekara S MD DM
Managing Director
ChanRe Rheumatology and Immunology Center and Research
Bengaluru

Ved Chaturvedi MD DM
Professor of Rheumatology
Gangaram Institute of Postgraduate Medical Education and Research
Senior Consultant Rheumatologist
Sir Ganga Ram Hospital
New Delhi

Arghya Chattopadhya MD DM
Assistant Professor of Rheumatology
North Bengal Medical College
Darjeeling

Chengappa KG MD DM
Associate Professor
Department of Clinical Immunology
Jawaharlal Institute of Postgraduate Medical Education and Research
Puducherry

Bhavya Chintala MD, DNB (Rheumatology)
Senior Resident
Department of Clinical Immunology and Rheumatology
Sir Ganga Ram Hospital
New Delhi

Arvind Chopra MD DNB FRCP (London), ACR Master
Director and Chief Rheumatologist
Centre for Rheumatic Diseases
Pune

Gautam Dhar Choudhury MD FICP
Professor of Medicine
Rheumatologist and Clinical Immunologist
Command Hospital
Kolkata

Vaidehi Chowdhary MD DM
Associate Professor
Clinical Chief Section of Rheumatology, Allergy and immunology
Yale School of Medicine
New Haven, Connecticut, USA

Abhra Chandra Chowdhury MD DM
Consultant Rheumatologist
Joint and Tooth Clinic
Kolkata

Debashish Danda MD DM FRCP FACR FAMS FICP
Professor and Founder Head
Department of Clinical Immunology and Rheumatology
Christian Medical College, Vellore

P Damodaram MD DM
Consultant Clinical Immunologist and Rheumatologist
Subodaya Rheumatology hospital
Tirupati

Anna C Das MD DM
Assistant Professor
Department of Clinical Immunology and Rheumatology
St. John's National Academy of Health Sciences
Bengaluru

Bidyut Das MD PhD
Professor and Head
Department of Clinical Immunology and Rheumatology
SCB Medical College
Cuttack

Siddharth Kumar Das MD
Professor and Head
Department of Rheumatology
Era's Medical College, Era University
Lucknow

Prajakta Dekate MD
Senior Resident
Hyderabad Rheumatology Center
Hyderabad

Anu Mohan Desai DNB (Medicine) MRCP MMed
Southend University Hospital, Southend-On-Sea, United Kingdom

Phani Kumar Devarasetti MD DM
Associate Professor
Department of Clinical Immunology and Rheumatology
Nizam's Institute of Medical Sciences
Hyderabad

Pooja Dhaon MD
Professor of Medicine
Hind Medical College
Barabanki, Uttar Pradesh

BG Dharmanand MD DM
Consultant Rheumatologist
Manipal Hospital
Bengaluru

Varun Dhir MD DM
Professor
Department of Internal Medicine (Rheumatology Unit)
Postgraduate Institute of Postgraduate Medical Education and Research
Chandigarh

Aadhaar Dhooria MD DM
Honorary Consultant, Rheumatology
Santokba Durlabhji Memorial Hospital cum Medical Research Institute
Jaipur

Rajkiran Dudam MD
Consultant and Director
Hyderabad Rheumatology Center
Begumpet, Hyderabad

Lalit Duggal MD FRCP
Head of Department of Rheumatology and Clinical Immunology
Sir Ganga Ram Hospital
New Delhi

Alakendu Ghosh DNB
Former Professor and Head, Department of Clinical Immunology and Rheumatology,
Institute of Post Graduate Medical Education and Research
Kolkata

Dipendra Nath Ghosh MD DM
Department of Clinical Immunology and Rheumatology
Institute of Post Graduate Medical Education and Research
Kolkata

Parasar Ghosh MD DM
Professor and Head
Department of Clinical Immunology and Rheumatology
Institute of Post Graduate Medical Education and Research
Kolkata.

Shounak Ghosh MD, DNB (Rheumatology)
Consultant Rheumatologist
CMRI Hospital
Kolkata

Aishwarya Gopal MD DM
Assistant Professor
Department of Clinical Immunology
Jawaharlal Institute of Postgraduate Medical Education and Research, Puducherry

Sundeep Grover MD DM
Consultant Rheumatology
Arthritis and Immunology Clinic, Meerut

Anju Gupta MD
Professor
Allergy Immunology Unit, Department of Pediatrics
Advanced Pediatrics Centre
Postgraduate Institute of Postgraduate Medical Education and Research
Chandigarh

Latika Gupta MD DM
Ex-Assistant Professor
Department of Clinical Immunology and Rheumatology
Sanjay Gandhi Post Graduate Institute of Medical Sciences
Lucknow

Rajiva Gupta MD DNB MRCP FRCP (Glasgow)
Director and Head
Department of Clinical Immunology and Rheumatology
Medanta – the Medicity, Gurugram

Ranjan Gupta MD DM
Associate Professor
Department of Rheumatology
AIIMS, New Delhi

SJ Gupta FRCP (Glasgow) FRCP (Edin) FICP
Senior Consultant Rheumatologist
Apollo Indraprastha and Sant Parmanand Hospitals
New Delhi

Vikas Gupta MD DM
Assistant Professor
Department of Rheumatology and Immunology
Dayanand Medical College and Hospital
Ludhiana

Rohini Handa MD DNB FAMS FICP FACR FRCP (Glasgow)
Professor and Senior Consultant
Department of Rheumatology
Apollo Hospitals, New Delhi

BV Harish MD
Senior Resident
Department of Clinical Immunology and Rheumatology
Institute of Medical Sciences and SUM Hospital
Bhubaneswar

Roopa Hathwar MRCP
Consultant Rheumatologist
Aster RV Hospital
Bengaluru

Arun Hegde MD, DNB (Rheumatology)
Senior advisor (Medicine) and Rheumatologist
Command Hospital (Central command)
Lucknow

Pravin Hissaria MD DM MRCPath (Australia)
Professor
Department of Clinical Immunology and Immunopathology
Royal Adelaide Hospital /SA pathology
Adelaide, South Australia

Ankit Jain MD DM
Consultant
Dr DK Jain Memorial Multispeciality Clinic
Meerut

Avinash Jain MD DM
Assistant Professor
Department of Rheumatology
SMS College and Hospital
Jaipur

Siddharth Jain MD DM
Assistant Professor
Department of Medicine
AIIMS, New Delhi

Reeta James MD
Associate Professor of Medicine
KMCT Medical College
Calicut, Kerala

Ramya Janardana MD PDF
Associate Professor
Department of Clinical Immunology and Rheumatology
St John's National Academy of Medical Sciences
Bengaluru

Saket Jha MD DM
Assistant professor of Rheumatology
Department of Internal Medicine
Tribhhuvan University Teaching Hospital
Kathmandu, Nepal

Ramesh Jois MD MRCP CCST (Rheumatology, UK)
Consultant Rheumatologist
Department of Rheumatology
Vikram Hospital
Bengaluru

Gurjit S Kaeley MRCP RhMSUS
Professor, Division of Rheumatology
University of Florida College of Medicine,
Jacksonville, FL, USA

Sanjeeb Kakati MD
Professor
Department of Medicine, In-charge of Rheumatology Clinic
Assam Medical College and Hospital
Dibrugarh, Assam

Nutan Kamath MD
Professor
Department of Pediatrics
Kasturba Medical College, Mangaluru

Madhavi Kandagaddala MD
Department of Radiodiagnosis
Christian Medical College, Vellore

Sanjiv Kapoor MD DM
Senior Consultant Rheumatologist
Indian Spinal Injuries Centre
New Delhi

S Kartik MD DNB (Rheumatology)
Professor and Head
Department of Rheumatology
Army Hospital (Research and Referral)
New Delhi

Jani Ami Kaushik MD
Fellow Musculoskeletal Imaging
Max Superspeciality Hospital, Saket
New Delhi

V Krishnamurthy MD DM FRCP
Consultant Rheumatologist
Apollo Speciality Hospital & Chennai Meenakshi Speciality Hospital, Chennai

Abhishek Kumar MD
Classified Specialist
Department of Rheumatology
Army Hospital Research and Referral
New Delhi

Ashok Kumar MD FRCP (London)
Director and Head of Rheumatology
Fortis Flt. Lt. Rajan Dhall Hospital, Vasant Kunj
New Delhi

Sachin Kumar MD
Consultant Radiologist
Ruban Memorial Hospital, Patna

Sathish Kumar MD DCH
Professor
Department of Pediatrics
Christian Medical College, Vellore

Uma Kumar MD
Professor and Head
Department of Rheumatology
All India Institute of Medical Sciences
New Delhi

Arup Kumar Kundu MD FICP MNAS
Ex-Professor of Medicine
Visiting Faculty & Senior Consultant Rheumatologist
IQ City Medical College, West Bengal

Able Lawrence MD DM
Professor
Department of Clinical Immunology & Rheumatology
Sanjay Gandhi Postgraduate Institute of Medical Sciences
Lucknow

Abhichandra Madineni DNB (Medicine)
Senior Resident
Department of Clinical Immunology and Rheumatology
Institute of Medical Sciences and SUM Hospital
Bhubaneswar

Challa Madhuri MD
Senior Resident
Department of Clinical Immunology and Rheumatology
Nizam's Institute of Medical Sciences
Hyderabad

Akhil Mahajan MD
Senior Resident
Post Graduate Department of General Medicine
Government Medical College
Jammu

Annil Mahajan MD FRCP FICP MAMS
Former Professor and Head
Post Graduate Department of General Medicine
Government Medical College
Jammu

KM Mahendranath MD FRCP ACR Master APLAR Master
Senior Consultant Rheumatologist
Samarpan Arthritis and Rheumatology Center
Bengaluru

Debashis Maikap MD PDF
Assistant Professor
Kalinga Institute of Medical Sciences
KIIT University, Bhubaneswar

Anand N Malaviya MD FRCP (London) ACR Master APLAR Master FACP FICP FAMS FNASc
Consultant Rheumatologist, A&R Clinic
Visiting Senior Consultant, Indian Spinal Injuries Center
Vasant Kunj, New Delhi

Manesh Manoj MD DM
Department of Clinical Immunology and Rheumatology
A.K.G. Memorial Co-operative Hospital
Dr. Shenoy's Centre for Arthritis and Rheumatism Excellence
Kannur, Kerala

Abhilasha Manwatkar MD
Registrar
Department of Clinical Immunology and Rheumatology
Christian Medical College, Vellore

Christina Mary Mariaselvam PhD
Assistant Professor (Lab Services)
Department of Clinical Immunology
Jawaharlal Institute of Postgraduate Medical Education and Research
Puducherry

Ashish J Mathew DNB DM PhD
Professor
Department of Clinical Immunology and Rheumatology
Christian Medical College
Vellore

John Mathew MD DM
Professor and Head
Department of Clinical Immunology and Rheumatology
Christian Medical College
Vellore

Bhowmik Meghnathi MD DNB (Rheumatology)
Consultant Rheumatologist and Clinical Immunologist
CIMS Hospital
Ahmedabad

Sonal Mehra MD DM
Senior Consultant Rheumatologist
Apollo Hospitals
Noida

Pankti Mehta MD DM
Assistant Professor
Department of Clinical Immunology and Rheumatology
KGMU
Lucknow

Debashish Mishra MD DM
Consultant Rheumatologist
Lifecare Hospital, Abu Dhabi

Durga Prasanna Misra MD DM MSc (Epidemiology) FRCP (Edin)
Associate Professor
Department of Clinical Immunology and Rheumatology
Sanjay Gandhi Post Graduate Institute of Medical Sciences
Lucknow

Ramnath Misra MD FRCP FAMS Masters (APLAR)
Professor and Head
Department of Clinical Immunology and Rheumatology
Kalinga Institute of Medical Sciences
KIIT University
Bhubaneswar

Rutviz Mistry MD DM
Consultant, GMERS Hospital
Sola and KD Hospitals
Ahmedabad

Kavitha Mohanasundaram MD DM
Associate Professor
Department of Rheumatology
Saveetha Medical College and Hospital
Chennai, Tamil Nadu

Sumantro Mondal MD DM
Assistant Professor
Department of Clinical Immunology and Rheumatology,
Institute of Post Graduate Medical Education and Research
Kolkata

Ritambra Nada MD
Professor
Department of Histopathology
Post Graduate Institute of Medical Education and Research
Chandigarh

GSRSNK Naidu MD DM
Associate Professor
Department of Internal Medicine
Post Graduate Institute of Medical Education and Research
Chandigarh

Kaveri K Nalianda MD, MRCP (UK) PDF
Consultant Rheumatologist
CARE, Kochi

G Narsimulu MD
Consultant Rheumatologist
GVN Medical Center, Hyderabad

Vir Singh Negi MD DM FAMS
Executive Director
All India Institute of Medical Sciences
Bilaspur, Himachal Pradesh

Nilesh Nolkha MD DM
Consultant Rheumatologist
Wockhardt Hospitals, Mumbai

Jyotsna Oak MD
Consultant Rheumatologist and Physician
Kokilaben Dhirubhai Ambani Hospital,
Mumbai

Prasanta Padhan MD PDF
Professor
Department of Clinical Immunology and Rheumatology
Kalinga Institute of Medical Sciences, KIIT University
Bhubaneswar

Sapan Pandya MD DM
Rheumatologist
Vedanta Institute of Medical Sciences
Assistant Professor of Rheumatology
Smt NHL Municipal Medical College linked with SVP Hospital, Ahmedabad

Ghan Shyam Pangtey MD
Professor of Medicine
In-charge Rheumatology Clinic
Lady Hardinge Medical College
New Delhi

Jyoti Ranjan Parida MD DM PG Dip (UCAMS)
Medical Director
Odisha Arthritis & Rheumatology Center
Bhubaneswar

Taral Parikh MD DNB (Rheumatology)
Zydus Hospital and Vedanta Hospital of Medical Sciences
Ahmedabad

Namisha Patel MD
Senior Consultant Rheumatologist
City Clinic, Vadodara
Bhailal Amin General Hospital
Vadodara

Himanshu Pathak MD MRCP (UK)
Consultant Rheumatologist
Tricolour Hospitals, Vadodara
Pramukhswami Medical College and Shri Krishna Hospital
Bhaikaka University
Karamsad, Anand

Pradeepta Sekhar Patro MD DM
Professor
Department of Clinical Immunology and Rheumatology,
Institute of Medical Sciences and SUM Hospital
Bhubaneswar

Binoy J Paul MD PhD DNB FRCP(Edin)
Professor of Medicine & Chief of Rheumatology
KMCT Medical College, Calicut

Sanat Phatak MD DM
Associate Consultant, Rheumatology
DBT/Wellcome India Alliance Fellow
KEM Hospital and Research Centre, Pune

Rakesh Kumar Pilania MD DM MAMS
Assistant Professor
Allergy and Immunology Unit, Department of Pediatrics
Advanced Pediatric Center
Post Graduate Institute of Medical Education and Research
Chandigarh

Benzeeta Pinto MD DM
Associate Professor
Department of Clinical Immunology and Rheumatology
St. John's National Academy of Health Sciences
Bengaluru

Prita Pradhan MD
Associate Professor
Department of Pathology
Kalinga Institute of Medical Sciences
Bhubaneswar

Anu Punnen MD
Associate Professor
Department of Pediatrics
Christian Medical College
Vellore

Abshishek Rai MD
Senior Resident
Department of Medicine
Jawaharlal Institute of Postgraduate Medical Education and Research, Puducherry

Liza Rajasekhar MD
Professor and Head
Department of Clinical Immunology and Rheumatology
Nizam's Institute of Medical Sciences
Hyderabad, Telangana

S Rajeswari MD DM
Professor and Head
Department of Rheumatology
Sri Ramachandra Medical Centre, Porur
Chennai, Tamil Nadu

Ramakant MD DNB (Rheumatology)
Consultant Rheumatologist
INHS Asvini, Mumbai

Logamoorthy Ramamoorthy MD
Senior Resident
Department of Dermatology
Jawaharlal Institute of Postgraduate Medical Education and Research, Puducherry

Kodali Ramya MD
Senior Resident
Department of Clinical Immunology and Rheumatology
St. John's National Academy of Health Sciences
Bengaluru

PD Rath MD FACR FRCP (Edin) FRCP (Glasgow) Grad Cert Paed Rheum (Aus), Diploma MSK USG (UCAM, Spain)
Director and Head of Department of Rheumatology
Max Super Speciality Hospital, Saket
New Delhi

Vinod Ravindran MD MRCP MSc (Rheumatology) MRCP (Rheumatology) FRCP (Edin)
Director, Centre for Rheumatology Calicut
Department of Rheumatology
National Hospital, Calicut

Claire Reynolds MBBS
Department of Clinical Immunology and Immunopathology
Royal Adelaide Hospital / SA pathology
Adelaide, South Australia

Rashmi Roongta MD DM
Senior Resident
Department of Clinical Immunology and Rheumatology
Institute of Post Graduate Medical Education and Research
Kolkata

Rasmi Ranjan Sahoo MD DM
Associate Professor
Department of Clinical Immunology and Rheumatology,
Institute of Medical Sciences and SUM Hospital
Bhubaneswar

Amit Kumar Sahu MD
Consultant Musculoskeletal Radiologist
Max Super Speciality Hospital, Saket
New Delhi

Rohini Samant MD
Consultant Rheumatologist
PD Hinduja Hospital and Medical Research Center
Mumbai

Pulukool Sandhya MD PDF
Senior Consultant
Department of Rheumatology
St Stephen's Hospital, New Delhi

Pradip Kumar Sarma MD DM
Consultant Rheumatologist
Excel Care Hospitals
Guwahati

Sujata Sawhney MD
Senior Consultant in Pediatric Rheumatology
Institute of Child Health
Sir Ganga Ram Hospital
New Delhi

Banwari Sharma MD DM
Consultant Clinical Immunologist and Rheumatologist,
Niramaya Health Care
Jaipur

Ankit B Shah DNB (Radiology) PG Dip (UCAMS)
Consultant Radiologist
Division of Musculoskeletal Imaging
Eclat Imaging Center
Mumbai

Bipin R Shah MD (Radiology)
Consultant Radiologist
Eclat Imaging Center
Mumbai

Sanket Shah MD DM
Assistant Professor
Department of Medicine
CU Shah Medical College and Hospital
Surendranagar
Gujarat

Subramanian Shankar MD DNB MNAMS FICP FRCP (Glasgow)
Senior Consultant, Rheumatology and Clinical Immunology
Commandant, Command Hospital (Air Force)
Bengaluru

K Shanmuganandan MD
Professor of Rheumatology and Medicine
Sree Balaji Medical College and Hospital, Chromepet
Chennai

Aman Sharma MD FRCP (London)
Professor
Department of Internal Medicine
Post Graduate Institute of Medical Education and Research
Chandigarh

Anuj Sharma MD
Pathologist
Aanavik Diagnostics
Jaipur

Shefali K Sharma MD
Professor
Department of Internal Medicine
Unit of Clinical Immunology and Rheumatology
Post Graduate Institute of Medical Education and Research
Chandigarh

Padmanabha Shenoy MD DM
Consultant Rheumatologist
Medical Director, CARE, Kochi

Vineeta Shobha MD DM
Professor and Head
Department of Clinical Immunology and Rheumatology
St John's National Academy of Health Sciences
Bengaluru

Hima Shreekumar DNB (Medicine)
Consultant Physician
Institute for Rheumatology and Immunology Sciences
Thiruvananthapuram

Anuj Shukla MD DM
Consultant Rheumatologist
Niruj Rheumatology Clinic, Ahmedabad

Surjit Singh MD DCH (London) FRCP (London) FRCPCH (London) FAMS
Professor and Head, Department of Pediatrics
In-charge Allergy Immunology Unit
Advanced Pediatrics Centre
Post Graduate Institute of Medical Education and Research
Chandigarh

Anuj Singhal MD DNB PDCC (Rheumatology) FRCP
Professor and Senior Advisor Medicine
Army Hospital Research and Referral
New Delhi

Debanjali Sinha MD DM
Senior Resident
Department of Clinical Immunology and Rheumatology
Institute of Post Graduate Medical Education and Research
Kolkata

Geetabali Sircar MD DM
Associate Professor
Department of Clinical Immunology and Rheumatology
Institute of Post Graduate Medical Education and Research
Kolkata

Isha Sood MD DNB (Rheumatology)
Consultant Rheumatologist
Kiara's Clinic and Nanavati Superspecialty Hospital
Mumbai

Puja Srivastava MD DM
Consultant Rheumatologist, STAR Rheumatology Clinics
Division of Rheumatology, NHL Medical College
Ahmedabad

N Subramanian MD MRCP (UK) MRCP CCT (Rheumatology) FRCP (Edin)
Consultant Rheumatologist Tirunelveli
Assistant Professor of Rheumatology
Velammal Medical College Hospital and Research Institute
Madurai

Gadde Sudhish MD
Senior Resident
Department of Clinical Immunology and Rheumatology
Institute of Medical Sciences and SUM Hospital
Bhubaneswar

Keerthi Talari MD DM
Consultant Rheumatologist
Yashoda Hospitals
Secunderabad

Vishal R Tandon MD FIMSA MAMS
Professor
Post Graduate Department of Pharmacology and Therapeutics
Government Medical College
Jammu

Molly Mary Thabah MD FRCP (Edin)
Professor of Medicine
Head, Department of Clinical Immunology
Jawaharlal Institute of Postgraduate Medical Education and Research, Puducherry

U Ravi Theja DMRD DNB (Radiology)
Krishna Institute of Medical Sciences
Secunderabad

Joe Thomas MD DNB (Rheumatology)
Consultant Rheumatologist
Aster Medcity
Kochi

Koshy Nithin Thomas MD DM
Assistant Professor
Department of Clinical Immunology and Rheumatology
Sanjay Gandhi Postgraduate Institute of Medical Sciences
Lucknow

Saumya Ranjan Tripathy MD DM
Assistant Professor
Department of Clinical Immunology and Rheumatology
SCB Medical College, Cuttack

Sundeep Kumar Upadhyaya MD DM
Senior Consultant Rheumatology-Immunology
Indraprastha Apollo Hospitals
New Delhi
Professor adjunct Apollo Health and Education Research Foundation (AHERF)

Ramakrishna Rao Uppuluri MD FRCP (London)
Consultant Rheumatologist
Sri Deepti Rheumatology Centre, Hyderabad

Harikrishnan V MD DM
Assistant professor
Department of Clinical immunology & Rheumatology
Amala institute of medical sciences
Thrissur

Rajendra Varaprasad MD DM
Consultant Rheumatologist
Yashoda Hospitals, Somajiguda
Hyderabad

Vivek Vasdev MD DNB (Rheumatology)
Consultant Rheumatologist
Professor and Head, Department of Geriatrics
Armed Forces Medical College, Pune

Anuradha Venugopalan PhD
In-charge Laboratory and Microbiologist
Centre for Rheumatic Diseases
Pune

Vishad Viswanath MD DM
Consultant Rheumatologist and Medical Director
Institute for Rheumatology and Immunology Sciences
Thiruvananthapuram

Anupam Wakhlu MD DM
Chief Consultant, Clinical Immunology and Rheumatology
Apollomedics Superspeciality Hospitals
Lucknow

Ajay Wanchu MD DM
Rheumatologist
Adventist Medical Center
Portland, OR, USA

Sandeep Yadav MD DNB (Rheumatology)
Rheumatologist
PD Hinduja Hospital and Medical Research Centre
Mumbai

Abhishek Zanwar MD DM
Consultant Rheumatologist
Poona Superspeciality Clinic, Pune

Contents

SECTION IV: DRUGS

SECTION V: DISEASE OUTCOME MEASURES

SECTION VI: IMAGING INVESTIGATIONS AND JOINT INJECTIONS

SECTION VII: LABORATORY INVESTIGATIONS

SECTION VIII: RHEUMATOID ARTHRITIS, SPONDYLOARTHRITIS, LUPUS, APS, AND SJÖGREN'S SYNDROME

SECTION IX: SYSTEMIC SCLEROSIS, MYOSITIS, MCTD, AND VASCULITIS

SECTION X: CRYSTAL ARTHRITIDES, SARCOIDOSIS, OSTEOARTHRITIS, OSTEOPOROSIS, JIA, AOSD, MACROPHAGE ACTIVATION SYNDROME, AND SEPTIC ARTHRITIS

SECTION XI: ARTHRITIS IN SYSTEMIC DISEASES AND INFECTIONS, RELAPSING POLYCHONDRITIS, OPTICOSPINAL SYNDROME, IPAF, AND PAH IN CTDs

SECTION XII: KAWASAKI DISEASE, PRIMARY IMMUNODEFICIENCY DISEASES, AUTOINFLAMMATORY SYNDROMES, AMYLOIDOSIS, PANNICULITIS, AND SOFT TISSUE RHEUMATISM

Section

I

GENERAL

Chapter 1.1

History Taking for Patients with Rheumatic Complaints

Ramnath Misra

INTRODUCTION

Eliciting history is the most important part of the clinical evaluation to arrive at a diagnosis. Studies have shown that approximately 60–80% of the information towards making a diagnosis comes from clinical history; approximately 7–12% of additional information is gathered from the physical examination and laboratory investigations including imaging add only approximately 5–11%.

This is particularly pertinent in rheumatology, as the majority of rheumatic diseases are chronic, physicians need to be patient while eliciting history and spend time with the patient. History taking requires skill and considerable knowledge regarding prevalence of rheumatic diseases. As always, communication with patients in his or her local language is ideal and rheumatologists have to be familiar with the socioeconomic condition and educational status of the patient. The aim of the history taking is to answer the following:

- Which organ system is involved?
- Is it life/organ threatening?
- What are the likely diagnostic possibilities?
- What is the impact of the illness in daily activities?
- Is it hereditary in nature?
- What is the socioeconomic background of the patients?

History taking includes history of present illness, past illness including an account of all medications (drugs) taken and their untoward effects, personal history, family history, and social background.

HISTORY OF PRESENT ILLNESS

This is to be noted chronologically starting with the initial symptoms and subsequent evolution of symptoms. The duration of illness is the most important component. If the duration of illness is within 6 weeks it is acute, 6–12 weeks is subacute, and beyond 3 months is chronic. Acute or subacute illness involving joints with or without other system involvement could be due to infections, drug hypersensitivity, or even malignancy.

In the presence of long-standing history, the initial event and subsequent progress is often difficult to recall, and in this situation symptoms related to vital organs should be elicited. For joint related symptoms it is frequently observed that patients would mention from the time when the pain was severe or difficulty in performing a task rather than actually when it first occurred. Another confounding factor is that the patient is keen to share earlier consultation reports or results of investigations rather than reporting his/her complaints.

It is important to determine whether the illness is monophasic or with recurring episodes or chronic. In rheumatology practice while eliciting the history, it will be evident that the patients' symptoms suggest involvement of one of the categories mentioned as follows.

1. Sole or predominant involvement of joints.
2. Pain in low back, neck and shoulders.
3. Joints with other system involvement or multisystem involvement.

4. Systemic features such as fever or weight loss.
5. Generalized aches and pain without any localizing system.

1. **Predominant involvement of joints:** One must try to categorize joint involvement as single joint involvement (monoarticular), 2–4 joint involvement (oligoarticular), or >5 joint involvement (polyarticular) as their differential diagnosis varies. The presence of morning stiffness is suggestive of inflammatory arthritis, whereas pain increasing with physical activity and subsiding with rest suggest degenerative disease. Acute attacks of single joint affliction suggest septic, crystal, or reactive arthritis. Chronic oligoarthritis in children and adolescents is suggestive of juvenile idiopathic arthritis (JIA) enthesitis related arthritis (ERA) subtype, in young adults it suggests reactive arthritis and seronegative spondyloarthropathy. Chronic inflammatory polyarthritis of the small joints of hands and feet in a symmetrical fashion is highly suggestive of rheumatoid arthritis (RA). This is particularly so if history suggests presence of deformity. The chapters on approach to monoarthritis and polyarthritis further details points to be elicited in the history.
2. **Pain in the back, neck, and shoulder:** (Also see chapter on approach to low back pain neck and shoulder pain for more comprehensive information). Low back pain is a common complaint in history, and association with morning stiffness suggests inflammatory nature symptoms that improve upon physical activity. More than 90% of patients with a history of low back are due to mechanical reasons such as degenerative spinal disease. Radiation to lower limbs suggests radiculopathy and pain on walking suggests lumbar canal stenosis. If associated with neurological symptoms, bladder and bowel involvement, or systemic features it suggests serious illness like tuberculosis or malignancy.

   Acute presentations are more likely mechanical rather than due to inflammatory disease like spondyloarthropathy. History of shoulder pain could be due to shoulder joint involvement or cervical disc radiculopathy. History of neck pain needs to be ascertained whether it is associated with movement of neck or radiation of pain into the shoulder or beyond. Burning and tingling sensations with neck pain suggest cervical radiculopathy. To resolve the underlying cause, examination is essential.
3. **History suggestive of multisystem involvement with joint involvement:** Requires symptoms to be directly enquired for each system involvement. This is dealt in a later chapter on approach to multisystem involvement.

   Symptoms of redness of eyes, or dryness suggest episcleritis (seen in RA), uveitis (suggests spondyloarthropathy, Behçet's disease), and visual impairment suggests SLE or systemic vasculitis, while proptosis suggests granulomatosis with polyangiitis (GPA).

   Skin rash over the face and other parts of the body is usually brought out by the patients. Whereas symptoms of photosensitivity, location of the rash, blackening or ulcerations need to be probed by the physician. Presence of Raynaud's and tightness of skin suggest systemic sclerosis. Examination of the skin is mandatory to confirm the nature and pathology of the lesions. Oral mucosal lesions provide clues to SLE, Behçet's disease, reactive arthritis, or due to cytotoxic drugs.

   History of chronic cough, dyspnea indicative of lung involvement is seen in several connective tissue diseases. Pain in the chest needs to be asked for and if present relation to breathing and exertion noted.

   Occurrence of edema or of hypertension could provide hints of renal involvement.

   Difficulty in getting up from sitting posture or climbing steps or combing the hair indicate proximal muscle weakness and detailed muscle examination.

   Further details on abdominal system and neurological systems are given in the chapter on approach to multisystem examination.
4. **Complaints of fever and weight loss:** Fever and weight loss of more than 3 to 4 weeks that are not due to infective causes could be presenting features of SLE, inflammatory myositis, and systemic vasculitis. Approach to fever is covered elsewhere.

5. **Generalized aches and pain with no localizing clue:** Could suggest fibromyalgia and history needs to be elicited about the difficulty in sleep. Evaluation of such a patient could be challenging.

PAST, FAMILY, AND PERSONAL HISTORY

Past history is relevant particularly for infections such as tuberculosis or similar illness in the childhood or of any hospitalization or surgery. History in the recent past of a febrile episode, genitourinary infection, gastrointestinal infection preceding joint disease may lead to a diagnosis of reactive arthritis, gonococcal arthritis, or peripheral spondyloarthritis. In India it is not uncommon to see patients with hip arthritis due to spondyloarthritis or JIA being treated with antitubercular drugs.

A history of recurrent infections in the past could be a pointer toward primary immunodeficiency diseases.

Family history is revealing of illnesses that are hereditary. Patients having low back pain or psoriasis or uveitis need to be probed for similar illness in family members. This is so because ankylosing spondylitis is associated with strong family history (Table 1.1.1).

Personal history of smoking, alcoholic intake are important considerations for management of inflammatory arthritis. There is a strong link between smoking and inflammatory arthritis.

Obstetric history in women needs to be taken. Presence of spontaneous abortions or stillbirths need to be determined as they may suggest antiphospholipid syndrome. Any adverse maternal outcome during pregnancy such as preeclampsia needs to be probed.

In summary, history is the most important part in the diagnostic evaluation of a patient with rheumatic diseases. Very often the presence of 'typical history' gives vital clues in clinching a diagnosis (Tables 1.1.2 and 1.1.3), these can be supplemented with examination and relevant investigation.

Table 1.1.1: Rheumatic diseases that are associated with a positive family history

Condition	*Association*
Rheumatoid arthritis (RA)	Patients with RA often have other family members that have other autoimmune rheumatic diseases. A recent large study (Kronzer et al.) found that the presence of another autoimmune condition in the family is a risk factor for early-onset RA. Non-autoimmune conditions in other family members such as pulmonary fibrosis, and inflammatory bowel disease also confers a risk for the development of RA.
Ankylosing spondylitis (AS)	It is known that children of women with AS are at risk of AS much more than children of men with AS. Further, it is also shown (Baudoin et al.) that in AS, firstborn children are more at risk of AS than later-born children, and in many cases the maternal age at delivery is younger (as compared to the general population).
Psoriatic arthritis (PsA)	The presence of a blood relative with psoriasis is considered a strong risk for PsA.
Systemic lupus erythematosus (SLE)	A Danish study had shown that presence of a family member with SLE increased the risk for SLE. About 11% of SLE patients often have another family member with another autoimmune disease.
Hand osteoarthritis (OA)	In this non-autoimmune disease there is greater concordance for hand OA in monozygotic than in dizygotic twins. There is also evidence of increased risk of hand OA in siblings, parents, and offspring (first-degree relatives) of subjects with hand OA.

Table 1.1.2: Typical features in history favoring a diagnosis

Symptoms of joint involvement		*Symptoms of joint with other organ involvement*	
History	**Likely diagnosis**	**History**	**Likely diagnosis**
Acute arthritis of single joint	Septic arthritis	Facial rash, oral ulcers, with polyarthritis	SLE
Acute arthritis of the knee or the first MTP in an elderly male	Gout/ pseudogout	Rash, proximal muscle weakness, and arthritis	Dermatomyositis
Chronic pain and swelling of knee in middle aged female	Osteoarthritis	Fever, arthritis, dry cough, and breathlessness	Antisynthetase syndrome
Acute or subacute arthritis of lower limb joints with or without a preceding GIT or genitourinary infections	Reactive arthritis	Chronic oligoarthritis/ polyarthritis associated with a scaly skin rash	Psoriatic arthritis
Chronic arthritis involving multiple finger joints and wrists in a female	Rheumatoid arthritis	Episodes of monoarthritis or oligoarthritis in a patient with CKD	Gout
Chronic low back pain associated with early morning stiffness in a young male	Ankylosing spondylitis	Asymmetrical oligoarthritis with painful oral/genital ulcers	Behçet's disease (rare in India)

SLE: Systemic lupus erythematosus; *MTP:* Metatarsophalangeal joint; *GI:* Gastrointestinal tract; *CKD:* Chronic kidney disease

Table 1.1.3: Examples of typical history (other than joint symptoms) that clinches a diagnosis

History	*Likely diagnosis*
Tingling and numbness of thumb and index finger	Carpal tunnel syndrome
Foot drop or wrist drop	Vasculitis primary or secondary
Recurrent oral and genital ulcerations	Behçet's disease
Proximal muscle weakness	Inflammatory myositis
Persistent generalized pruritus in elderly females	Primary biliary cirrhosis
Chronic dry cough and dyspnea	Interstitial lung disease (ILD)
Dryness of eyes and mouth	Sjögren's syndrome
Non-healing ulcer	Vasculitis
Sudden onset of unilateral headache with or without visual loss	Giant cell arteritis
Intermittent fever with evanescent skin rash	Systemic onset JIA
Abdominal pain following food	Abdominal angina—systemic vasculitis
Raynaud's phenomenon or digital gangrene	Systemic sclerosis
Blackening of the digits (gangrene)	Polyarteritis nodosa (PAN)
Tender erythematous nodules with ankle swelling	Sarcoidosis
Sudden onset of pain in the hip joint that persists	Avascular necrosis of the hip
Intermittent swelling of ear	Relapsing polychondritis
Collapse of bridge of nose	Granulomatosis with polyangiitis (GPA)

LEARNING POINTS

- The history should be sought from patient in his/her own words.
- Chronological recording of evolution of events is needed.
- Physicians should try to identify the organs affected.
- Duration of illness provides important information on reversibility of manifestations.
- Certain typical history clinches the diagnosis in many diseases.

FURTHER READING

1. Baudoin P, van der Horst-Bruinsma IE, Dekker-Saeys AJ, et al. Increased risk of developing ankylosing spondylitis among first-born children. Arthritis Rheum. 2000; 43:2818–22.
2. Hampton JR, Harrison MJG, Mitchell JRA, et al. Relative contributions of history-taking, physical examination, and laboratory investigation to diagnosis and management of medical outpatients. Br Med J 1975;2:486–9.
3. Kronzer VL, Crowson CS, Sparks JA, et al. Family History of Rheumatic, Autoimmune, and Nonautoimmune Diseases and Risk of Rheumatoid Arthritis. Arthritis Care Res (Hoboken). 2021;73:180–7.
4. Liang MH, Sturrock RD. Evaluation of musculoskeletal symptoms. In: Klippel JH, Dieppe PA, editors. Practical Rheumatology. London: Mosby; 1995. p. 3–20.
5. Markert RJ, Rich EC, Sakowski HA, et al. Medscape General Medicine. 2004;6(2):64 (online).
6. Peterson MC, Holbrook JH, Von Hales D, et al. Contributions of the history, physical examination, and laboratory investigation in making medical diagnoses. West J Med. 1992;156:163–5.

Chapter 1.2

Communication with Patients of Rheumatic Diseases

KM Mahendranath, Roopa Hathwar

INTRODUCTION

A successful outcome of any disease management including chronic rheumatic diseases requires a correct diagnosis, appropriate treatment, and good compliance by the patient. Patient education and awareness forms the basis of successful outcome of treatment. Patient education is as important as the treatment itself. Good communication between the physician and the patient plays a pivotal role to achieve this. It is an integral part of clinical care and studies have shown that the quality of a physician's communicative behaviour has a positive impact on patient health outcomes. More emphasis needs to be given to develop good communication skills during the medical training period.

PURPOSE OF INTERACTION

The purpose of interaction between a physician and the patient is to provide information and support on the diagnosis and its prognosis, trust building and implementation of appropriate treatment strategies and medication side effects. The patients' education level and cultural background need to be taken into consideration during physician–patient interaction. The preferred language should be the patient's mother tongue as much as possible. The language must be simple and easily understandable. Whenever possible they can be reinforced by giving printed leaflets, booklets, and audiovisual materials. Patient education is a lifelong commitment which begins with the first consultation and continues. A physician's communicative abilities and attitude help to build a good rapport with the patient which influences trust building. The behaviour of the physician validates the patient's concerns and empathy for them can alleviate anxiety and fear. Developing effective and strong communication skills is integral to becoming an efficient healthcare provider.

Medication adherence: This is crucial in controlling disease activity and preventing complications such as cardiovascular risk and organ damage. It comes from a better understanding of the illness, medication and its side effects. A longitudinal study by Viller et al. showed that medication adherence can be improved with quality of communication with the professionals and the amount of available patient information. Trust in physicians will encourage drug adherence and fewer drug side effects.

Active and positive patient participation: It helps achieve low disease activity, feeling of being understood, fewer drug side effects, greater treatment satisfaction, positive beliefs about health and improved disclosure of information. Patients are more satisfied with the treatment experience with shared decision-making strategy. This can lead to reduced incidences of malpractice lawsuits against the physician. Due to a shortage of rheumatologists, shortage of supporting staff and huge number of cases, the time we spend with patients is unfortunately little. So effective communication in the available time is a skilful art. Most of our obese patients do not accept they are overeating. They will say to me even before I begin to talk about a diet that "they hardly eat". I always tell them "I never said you are overeating but what I am telling is that you are not spending whatever little you are eating" This is one way of convincing them to do physical activities and exercises.

Patient-reported outcome (PRO) measures: These measures are useful in the improvement of the quality of healthcare and for both physician and the patient in making better decisions. A prospective cohort study by Bartlett et al., have shown that using PRO during RA visits is feasible and helps in communication, shared decision making, a better understanding of disease effects on patient quality of life, improved satisfaction and confidence in the treatment. Modern technology can be used in aiding communication with patients. A qualitative study by Navarro-Millán et al., on the perspectives of RA patients on electronic communication and PRO data collection between clinical encounters helps the communication with the healthcare providers and acquiring appropriate information on RA.

Personalized risk tools: The tools have been developed to be used for various diseases such as diabetes, heart disease, osteoporosis, cancers, etc. These are designed to educate at-risk individuals about early symptoms and signs, address high-risk behavioural factors and encourage screening for early detection of the disease. These tools are available in many formats ranging from web-based information, and counselling to motivational interviewing techniques. For rheumatic diseases such as RA and SLE, various factors such as demographics, family history, lifestyle, genetics and biomarkers can be used to provide personalized risk information on disease development. A randomized controlled trial by Marshall et al. showed that the effect of web-based personalized RA risk information on concern for the development of RA provided reassurance even in the absence of a health educator. These personalized risk tools can help to alleviate psychological distress and educate patients on modifiable behavioural risks, to recognize early symptoms and signs and seek medical help.

LEARNING POINTS

- Communication plays a key role in the clinical care of patients with rheumatic diseases.
- There should be an emphasis to include communication skills as a part of the medical training curriculum.
- A good rapport and trust between physician and patient has a positive impact on treatment outcomes.
- Effective physician–patient communication and trust improve medical adherence.
- Active patient participation and shared decision-making strategy lead to better treatment satisfaction.
- Patient-reported outcome measures can improve the quality of healthcare provision.

FURTHER READING

1. Arora NK. Interacting with cancer patients: the significance of physicians' communication behavior. Soc Sci Med. 2003; 57:791–806.
2. Bartlett SJ, De Leon E, Orbai AM, et al. Patient-reported outcomes in RA care improve patient communication, decision-making, satisfaction and confidence: qualitative results. Rheumatology (Oxford). 2020;59:1662–70.
3. Marshall AA, Zaccardelli A, Yu Z, et al. Effect of communicating personalized rheumatoid arthritis risk on concern for developing RA: A randomized controlled trial. Patient Educ Couns. 2019;102:976–83.
4. Navarro-Millán I, Zinski A, Shurbaji S, et al. Perspectives of Rheumatoid Arthritis Patients on Electronic Communication and Patient-Reported Outcome Data Collection: A Qualitative Study. Arthritis Care Res (Hoboken). 2019;71:80–7.
5. Viller F, Guillemin F, Briançon S, et al. Compliance to drug treatment of patients with rheumatoid arthritis: a 3-year longitudinal study. J Rheumatol. 1999; 26:2114–22.

Chapter 1.3

Epidemiology of Rheumatic Diseases in India

Arvind Chopra

INTRODUCTION

Much of the current information on the epidemiology of rheumatic diseases in India is derived from population surveys at multiple sites in India conducted as part of the WHO International League of Rheumatology (ILAR) and community-oriented program for control of rheumatic diseases (COPCORD) programs.

COPCORD was launched by the WHO and ILAR in 1981 to fill the void created by lack of epidemiological data on musculoskeletal (MSK) disorders from developing countries. Over 21 countries have completed COPCORD and in several instances with multiple surveys. In India, the maiden WHO-ILAR COPCORD India was launched in Bhigwan village of Pune district, Pune in 1996. The Bhigwan survey had the unique distinction of evolving a fast-track COPCORD model (Fig. 1.3.1) that was adopted by several sites in India (Fig. 1.3.2) and several countries.

PREVALENCE

Musculoskeletal (MSK) Pain

Of several key messages that emerged from these population surveys was that the burden of rheumatic diseases in rural and urban India is huge. The clinical spectrum varies from benign non-specific MSK aches and pains to infrequent life-threatening disorders such as lupus and systemic vasculitis. In the author's community-based rheumatology practice at Centre for Rheumatic Diseases (CRD) Pune, inflammatory arthritis was frequently encountered

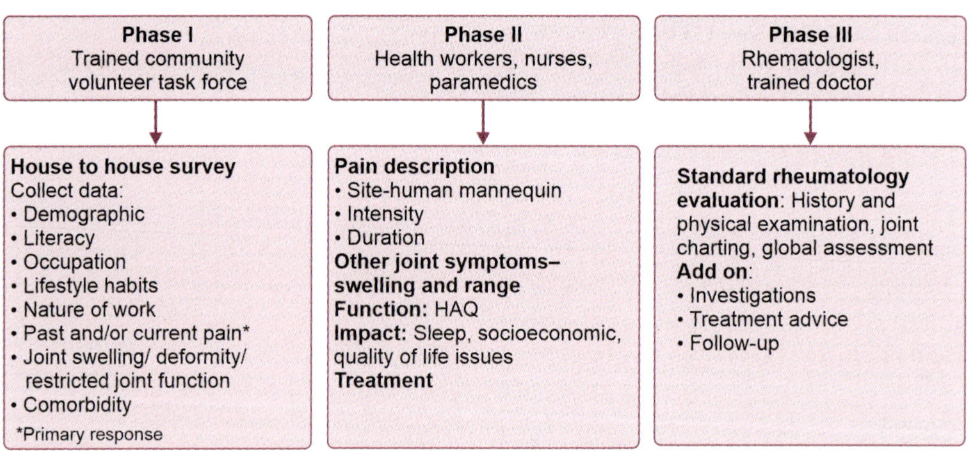

Fig. 1.3.1: WHO-ILAR COPCORD Bhigwan Pune India Model (Community Oriented Program for Control of Rheumatic Diseases). (*Adapted from COPCORD Bhigwan India 1996*) (*Note:* All phases were carried out in parallel).

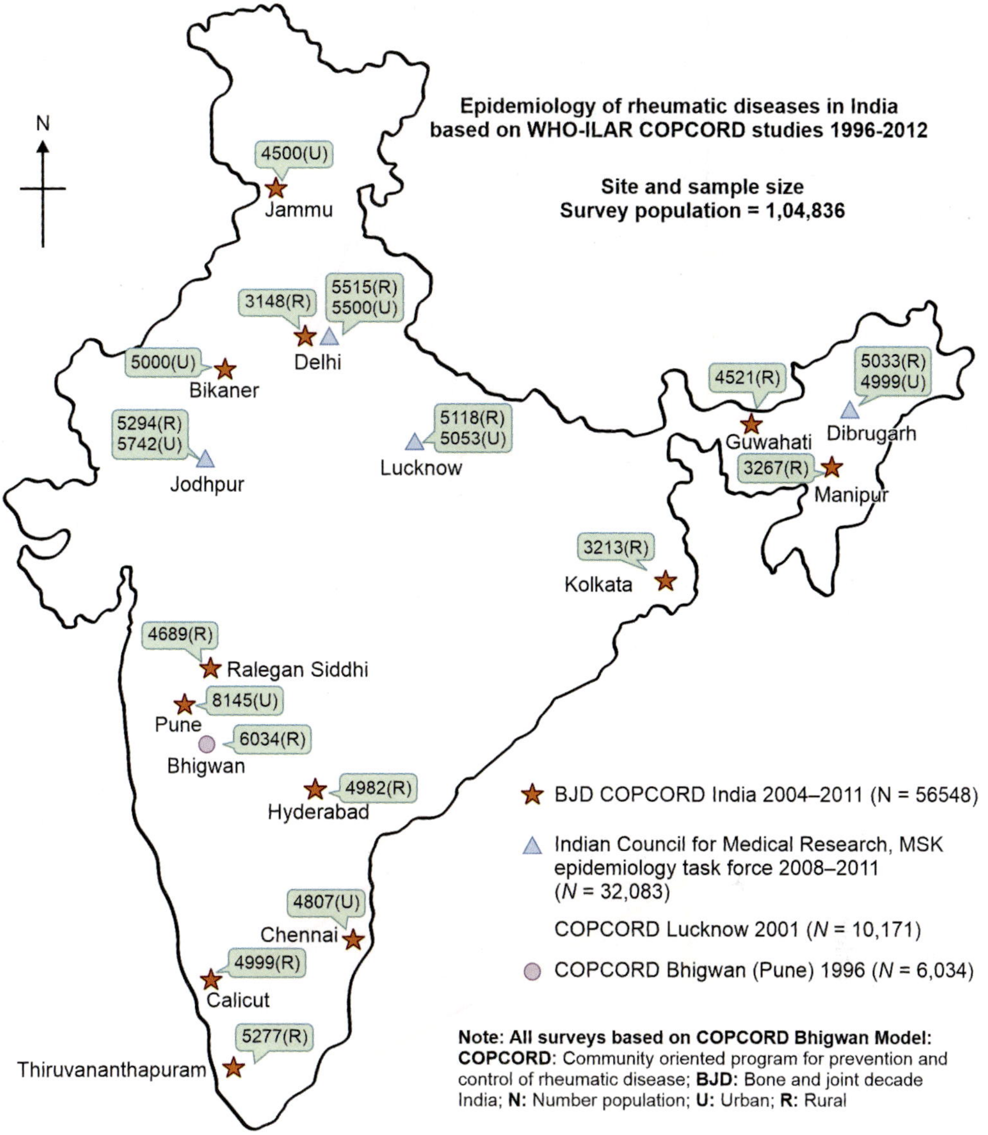

Fig. 1.3.2: WHO-ILAR COPCORD (Community Oriented Program for Control of Rheumatic Diseases) population survey sites in India (Stage I) 1996–2015 (sample size at each site is shown).

(Fig. 1.3.3a). But though inflammatory arthritis is the predominant condition seen in tertiary settings it constituted <10% of the total MSK disorders load in the community (Fig. 1.3.3b) where degenerative arthritis, ill-defined MSK symptoms and nonspecific arthralgia, and soft tissue rheumatism (STR) formed the bulk of MSK disorders and are much more common.

The prevalence of MSK pain in surveys conducted by the COPCORD Bone and Joint Decade (BJD) India in about 56,500 individuals screened was 20%, 10% and 16% in the rural, urban and overall population, respectively (Table 1.3.1). These data highlight the huge burden of MSK pain in the general population. The most common site of MSK pain is the knee followed by back pain. What was also found in the rural Bhigwan COPCORD project was that nonspecific MSK symptoms may not be totally benign because 14% of individuals with nonspecific MSK aches and pains, and 11% with soft

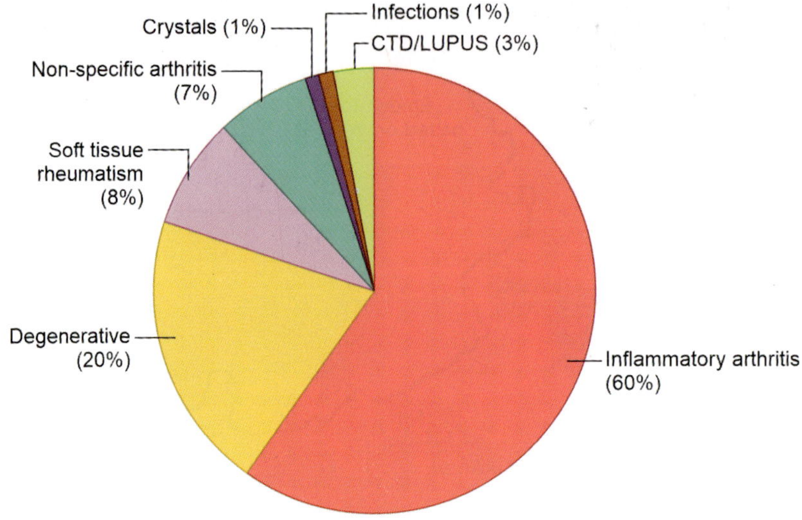

Fig. 1.3.3a: Frequency of rheumatic musculoskeletal (MSK) disorders in a community-based rheumatology practise: Centre Rheumatic Diseases, Pune e-Database 2001–2012 (n = 39,756).

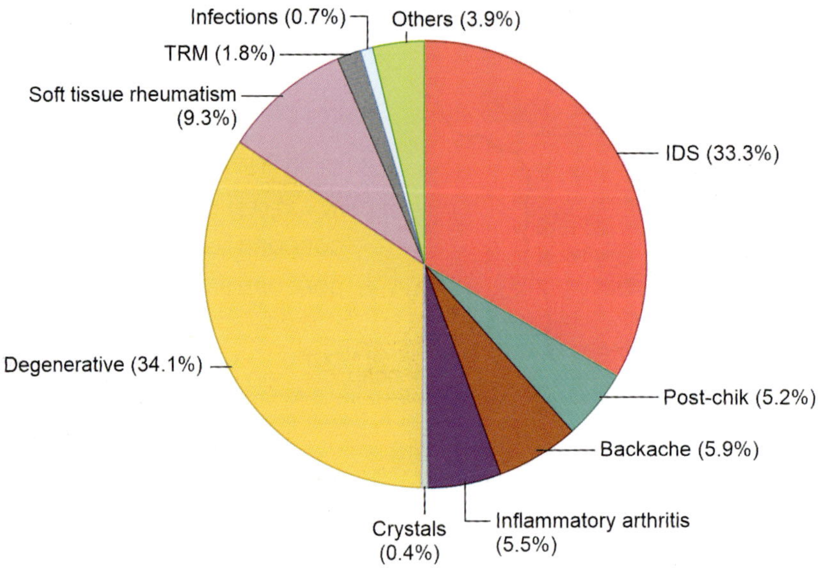

Fig. 1.3.3b: Frequency (%) of rheumatic musculoskeletal disorders in pooled data from all India BJD-India COPCORD population surveys (n = 56,548) [n: number population]

BJD: The bone and joint decade national action network; *COPCORD:* Community oriented program for control of rheumatic diseases; *CTD:* Connective tissue disorders; *TRM:* Trauma related arthritis; *post-CHIK:* post-chikungunya arthritis and rheumatism; *IDS:* Ill-defined musculoskeletal symptoms/non-specific arthralgias; 6 patients had CTD and clubbed with inflammatory arthritis.

tissue rheumatism had moderate to severe functional disability as measured by the Indian version of the health assessment questionnaire (iHAQ).

The important modifiable risk factors of MSK pains and rheumatic diseases include injury, occupational overuse and misuse, obesity, psychological stress, deficient nutritional status, tobacco (any form), infections, overzealous treatment (including physiotherapy and yoga, local massage and applications), and lifestyle.

Table 1.3.1: Frequency (%) of musculoskeletal pain in BJD-COPCORD India population surveys 2005–2012

Pain site	*Rural* *n = 34,096*	*Urban* *n = 22,452*	*Total* *n = 56,548*
Pain any site	20.04 (17.86, 22.37)	10.34 (8.79, 12.07)	16.14 (14.19, 18.29)
Neck	1.70 (1.04, 2.55)	1.08 (0.61, 1.78)	1.45 (0.89, 2.30)
Shoulder	4.41 (3.33, 5.68)	1.53 (0.94, 2.31)	3.24 (2.36, 4.38)
Elbow	4.40 (3.33, 5.68)	0.81 (0.40, 1.42)	2.93 (2.09, 4.03)
Hand/wrist	3.83 (2.84, 5.05)	1.49 (0.94, 2.31)	2.87 (2.03, 3.94)
Knee	10.11 (8.53, 11.95)	6.20 (5.01, 7.63)	8.51 (7.00, 10.13)
Ankle/feet	5.28 (4.10, 6.66)	1.72 (1.12, 2.57)	3.83 (2.90, 5.09)
Back any site	7.97 (6.55, 9.63)	3.67 (2.76, 4.82)	6.23 (4.95, 7.67)

COPCORD: WHO-ILAR Community oriented program for control of rheumatic disease; *BJD:* The bone and joint decade india national action network; *n:* Number of population

Inflammatory and Non-inflammatory Rheumatic MSK Disorders

The prevalence of inflammatory rheumatic diseases and non-inflammatory rheumatic diseases is depicted in Table 1.3.2.

Rheumatoid Arthritis

The pooled prevalence of rheumatoid arthritis (RA) was 0.34%, this may translate to a prevalence of >7 million RA patients in India. The often quoted 1% prevalence of RA was not reported by any Indian COPCORD site.

Table 1.3.2: Adjusted standardized prevalence of rheumatic musculoskeletal disorders in India: BJD-COPCORD population surveys 2005–2012

Category	*Rural India* *n = 34,096*	*Urban India* *n = 17,645*	*All India* *n = 51,741*
RA	0.29 (0.09, 0.82)	0.42 (0.01, 0.94)	0.34 (0.08, 0.79)
IA-U	0.22 (0.05, 0.70)	0.22 (0.04, 0.63)	0.22 (0.05, 0.68)
SpA	0.28 (0.09, 0.82)	0.12 (0.02, 0.52)	0.23 (0.05, 0.68)
AS	0.04 (0.00, 0.44)	0.03 (0.02, 0.04)	0.03 (0.02, 0.05)
Psoriatic arthritis	0.01 (0.00, 0.02)	0.02 (0.01, 0.03)	0.01 (0.00, 0.02)
OA	4.66 (3.54, 5.95)	3.83 (2.89, 4.99)	4.39 (3.30, 5.61)
OA knee	3.43 (2.50, 4.60)	3.09 (2.26, 4.17)	3.34 (2.43, 4.47)
OA cervical spine	0.45 (0.18, 1.04)	0.30 (0.08, 0.74)	0.39 (0.13, 0.90)
OA lumbar spine	0.77 (0.38, 1.46)	0.97 (0.50, 1.60)	0.86 (0.43, 1.52)
PGOA	0.10 (0.00, 0.44)	0.14 (0.02, 0.52)	0.12 (0.02, 0.56)
OA hip	0.05 (0.04, 0.07)	0.17 (0.02, 0.52)	0.09 (0.00, 0.43)
STR	1.63 (0.98, 2.46)	0.72 (0.35, 1.33)	1.31 (0.77, 2.11)
SR/IDS	4.79 (3.68, 6.13)	3.36 (2.45, 4.42)	4.25 (3.23, 5.53)
GOUT	0.07 (0.00, 0.44)	0.02 (0.02, 0.03)	0.05 (0.04, 0.07)
CTD	0.03 (0.02, 0.04)	0.01 (0.00, 0.01)	0.02 (0.01, 0.03)
SLE	0.01 (0.00, 0.02)	–	0.01 (0.00, 0.02)

n = Number of population; *COPCORD:* WHO-ILAR Community oriented program for control of rheumatic diseases; *BJD:* The bone and joint decade india national action network; *RA:* Rheumatoid arthritis; *IA-U:* Undifferentiated inflammatory arthritis; *SpA:* Spondyloarthritis; *AS:* Ankylosing spondylitis; *OA:* Osteoarthritis; *PGOA:* Primary generalized osteoarthritis; *STR:* Soft tissue rheumatism; *SR/IDS:* Symptom related and ill-defined symptoms; *CTD:* Connective tissue disorders; 95% confidence intervals shown in parenthesis.

RA was predominant among young women (Table 1.3.3). Almost 33% of women with RA had the onset of disease at 20–40 years. This finding merits intervention as it imposes adverse effects on life, livelihood and longevity of women. In COPCORD studies, 40–50% of clinical RA was reported seronegative for rheumatoid factor (RF). In analysis of causes of mortality using data from CRD Pune, cardiac and infections were leading causes of mortality in RA, but there are several other causes and contributory factors including drugs (Fig. 1.3.4).

Salient features on immunogenetics in RA are shown in Table 1.3.4. The seropositivity for rheumatoid factor (RF) and anti-cyclic citrullinated peptide antibodies (anti-CCP) in COPCORD Bhigwan was low compared to referral and hospital practice (Table 1.3.4). In the neighbouring Pune COPCORD urban survey, the seropositivity for RF was 60% and anti-CCP was 100% in RA patients.

Almost 54% of all RA cases in Bhigwan COPCORD showed radiological erosions in the small joints of hands and wrists. Eleven subjects (seropositive 29% for RF and 65% for anti-CCP) from Bhigwan were identified as incident RA during the period 1996–2008 (Incidence rate 44/100,000). None of the HLA DRB1* alleles were significantly associated with RA in the Bhigwan RA survey 1996 cohort (Table 1.3.4).

Table 1.3.3: Prevalence of rheumatoid arthritis (RA) per 100,000 population in COPCORD Bhigwan survey 1996 (India) to represent South East Asia Region (WHO)

Age bands (years)	15–29	30–44	45–59	60–74	75+
Males	–	479	–	1136	–
Females	113	1639	1775	1914	3846

Note: Diagnosis as per ACR 1988 classification criteria; Rates for 30–44 age band in other countries: USA 300, Norway 150, South Africa 1042, Indonesia 279, Iraq 742, China 237; *Source:* Reproduced with permission from WHO-Publication Technical Research Series (2003),919.

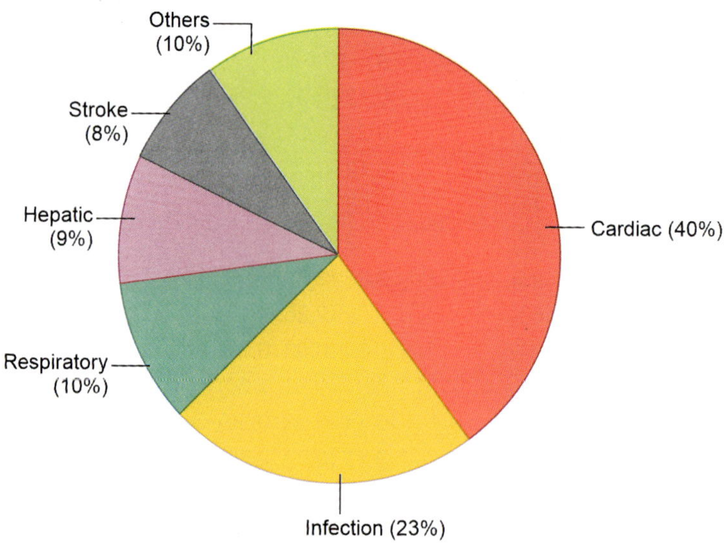

Fig. 1.3.4: Mortality in rheumatoid arthritis: Based on retrospective case series (n = 60) from Centre for Rheumatic Diseases, Pune (*Note: n:* Number of deaths; Others include multi-organ failure, disseminated intravascular coagulation; Cardiac includes ischemic heart disease, hypertension, cardiomyopathy; infections include pneumonia, post-joint replacement septic arthritis, dental sepsis, pancreatitis, fracture femur, septicaemia (3 cases of methotrexate-induced pancytopenia and severe hepatic dysfunction; hepatitis may include drug induced; respiratory was dominantly respiratory failure and interstitial lung disease; Other clinically important contributory factors—5 diabetes, 5 hypertension, 1 cerebrovascular disease, 1 coronary artery bypass surgery, 2 gastrointestinal bleed, 2 peptic ulcer (probably related to non-steroidal anti-inflammatory drugs), and 1 chronic renal failure.

Table 1.3.4: Immunogenetics of rheumatoid arthritis in COPCORD Bhigwan India Survey 1996

*DRB1**	*CONTROL(n = 70)**	*REFERRAL (n = 30)**			*BHIGWAN (n = 24)**		
	%	%	OR	CI	%	OR	CI
01	11.7	15.4	1.38	0.5, 3.7	–	–	–
04	10.4	17.3	1.78	0.7, 4.9	8.0	1.05	0.2, 5.2
10	18.2	32.7	2.16	1.1, 4.8	32	1.85	0.7, 5.2
1/4/10	33.8	55.8	2.44	1.2, 4.9	40	1.13	0.4, 2.9
RF**	4%	75	–	–	48	–	–
Anti-CCP***	–	76.9%	–	–	60	–	–

n: Number of subjects; *These were sample sizes for HLA typing only; **RF was by nephelometry, and values >40 IU/mL was considered positive; ***Anti-CCP was tested by second generation ELISA, and values >5 RU/mL was considered positive; *OR:* Odds ratio; *CI:* 95% confidence interval; *RF:* Rheumatoid factor; *anti-CCP:* Anti-cyclic citrullinated peptide antibody; *CONTROL:* Healthy subjects in village Bhigwan; *REFERRAL:* Referral practise in Centre Rheumatic Diseases, Pune; Sample sizes for RF and anti-CCP for control and referral >500 except in case of Bhigwan sample size was 24.

Intriguingly, a significant association was reported between MSK pain and oral tobacco use in Bhigwan (odds ratio 1.71) and Pune (odds ratio 3.16) but the same could not be shown for RA (possibly a larger sample size was required).

Spondyloarthritis

Ankylosing spondylitis (AS) and psoriatic arthritis formed a sizable number in clinical rheumatology practice but are comparatively less frequent as compared to RA, this trend appeared to be similar in the community (Table 1.3.2).

Though an inciting infectious trigger is often not obvious, several cases of seronegative undifferentiated inflammatory arthritis (IA-U) are probable reactive arthritis or post-infective. There may be a clinical overlap between spondyloarthritis and RA which is often missed. The frequency of HLA B27 in Indian patients is shown in Table 1.3.5.

Hyperuricemia and Gout

The diagnosis of acute gout is based on history in population surveys. The crude incidence rate for acute gout in COPCORD Bhigwan was 9/100000 person years during 1996–2008 (unpublished). The prevalence data of 0.05% of gout (Table 1.3.2) during 2005–2012 may be an underestimate of crystal deposition disorders. Tophaceous gout seems uncommon in the community. The co-occurrence of RA and gout is very unusual and a case series was reported from CRD, Pune.

Chikungunya Arthritis and Rheumatism

A substantial burden of post-Chikungunya arthritis and rheumatism (PCAR) has emerged following the 2006 epidemic (Fig. 1.3.3b). A comprehensive description on 'Chikungunya arthritis and rheumatism' is provided in a separate chapter.

Table 1.3.5: Frequency and relative risk of B27 locus antigen in Indian spondyloarthritis patients reported from Indian studies

Subset	*Pune (Chopra et al.)*		*Delhi (Malaviya et al.)*		*Chennai (Mahadevan et al.)*		*Caucasians*	
Disease	f	RR	f	RR	f	RR	f	RR
AS	73	26	92	193	83	1091	90–100	90–118
RS	67	20	80	66	57	307	65–100	17–40
SSA-U	41	7	84	83	21.4	70	60–70	18
Healthy	9	–	6	–	0–2.5	–	9+	–

f: Frequency percent; *RR:* Relative risk; *AS:* Ankylosing spondylitis; *RS:* Reiter's syndrome; *SpA-U:* Undifferentiated spondyloarthritis.

Source: Malaviya AN, et al. J Assoc Physicians India 1979; 27:487–92; Mahadevan R, et al. J Indian Rheumatol Assoc 1996; V4; 3:91–5; Chopra A, et al. J Assoc Physicians India 1990; 38:351–5

Several self-limited arthralgias/arthritis in the community is presumably due to viral infections which are often erroneously diagnosed as rheumatic disorders causing needless investigation and mental stress. Though infrequent, pyogenic arthritis, tuberculosis and leprosy should be remembered in atypical arthritis and unusual clinical settings.

Soft Tissue Rheumatism (STR)

STR encompasses a broad range of diverse conditions affecting different tissues such as tendon, fascia and bursae. Focal or regional forms of STR (fasciitis, bursitis, enthesitis, tendonitis, epicondylitis) are commonly encountered in clinical practice. As shown in Table 1.3.2, the prevalence of STR is more in rural compared to urban areas, and it is more prevalent in the community than RA. Though causality is often difficult to establish, COPCORD studies speculated several risk factors—occupation misuse and overuse, mental stress and trauma. Patients suffering from other rheumatic diseases such as RA and OA were also found to have STR which was often neglected by the doctor; painful heels and feet were common complaints in surveys and often considered to be due to improper footwear. A substantial extent of STR disorders were reported as a sequel to Chikungunya by COPCORD sites in Kerala.

Fibromyalgia

Fibromyalgia (FM) is characterized by more widespread and diffuse musculoskeletal pain, well-defined tender points, and patients often complain of fatigue, sleep and psychological disturbances. FM can coexist with other rheumatic diseases. A high prevalence of FM was reported by COPCORD Lucknow (urban 3.8%, rural 4.5%).

Connective Tissue Disorders (CTDs)

There is a lack of population based prevalence studies of CTDs. As per COPCORD surveys, systemic lupus erythematosus (SLE), Sjögren's syndrome, vasculitis, etc. are infrequent in the community (Table 1.3.2).

Only 21 cases (0.03%) of CTDs were diagnosed amongst 68,273 inpatients (civilians and services) during 1982–1986 in a large Armed Forces referral-teaching hospital in Pune. A landmark study (Malaviya et al.) carried out in Delhi reported a point prevalence of 3 per 100,000. Only one case of neuropsychiatric lupus with coexistent RA (Rhupus) was diagnosed in the Bhigwan COPCORD population during the period 1996–2008. Danda et all. in 2015 reported the clinical characteristics of 323 patients with confirmed primary Sjögren's syndrome.

Table 1.3.6: Frequency (percent) distribution of juvenile idiopathic arthritis (JIA) in published Indian studies

JIA subsets	*Lucknow* (n = 89)*	*Delhi* (n = 361)*	*Pune** (n = 272)*		
			Subset	*RF (%)*	*ANA (%)*
Systemic onset	14	24	9	0	27
Oligoarthritis	34	30	26	0	19
Persistent	–	–	20	0	19
Extended	–	–	6	0	0
Polyarthritis	52	46	31	29	26
Seronegative	–	–	22	0	16
Seropositive	–	–	9	100	10
Psoriatic arthritis	–	–	1	0	0
Enthesitis	–	–	27	0	7
Undifferentiated arthritis	–	–	6	88	41

Note: *JRA subsets; **ILAR-JIA subsets.

Source: Agarwal A, et al. Rheumatol Int 1994; 15: 53–56; Seth V, et al. Indian J Pediatr 1996; 63: 293–300; Kunjir V, et al. J Rheumatol 2010; 37: 1756–62.

Vasculitis

In a retrospective analysis of rheumatology outpatient data from 1979 to 1994 in Mumbai, 100 patients (1.3%) were diagnosed as vasculitis; interestingly there were no cases of necrotizing vasculitis (Samanth et al.). Only 5 patients of Takayasu arteritis were reported in a retrospective analysis of 8600 rheumatology patients between 1992–1996 in a large referral hospital in southern India (Chandrasekaran et al.).

Infections

The prevalence of infections in 1236 rheumatology patients in a tertiary center in Hyderabad is 20%. A retrospective study from rheumatology outpatients in a large medical teaching institute in Lucknow reported a spectrum of infections that included septic arthritis, tropical pyomyositis, tuberculosis, and leprosy associated arthritis.

However, only 0.35% cases of tuberculosis (TB) was found amongst the e-records of 23,651 patients attending CRD Pune from 2005 to 2009; TB complicated 0.4% RA. In this report, 12 of the 16 cases with MSK TB suffered from Poncet's disease; 2 cases showed multifocal lesions which also included non-contiguous spine involvement.

Though infrequent, leprous arthritis is an interesting clinical challenge in rheumatology practice and several reports from India are published. Rarely, leprous arthritis may be an acute onset painful polyarticular presentation and mimic RA.

Childhood-onset Arthritis

Juvenile idiopathic arthritis (JIA) in a community setting is uncommon, most data on prevalence are hospital-based. COPCORD Bhigwan survey (which included children as well) reported an unusually high crude point prevalence of JIA 0.26%, rheumatic fever is 0.09%.

Table 1.3.6 depicts data on JIA from three Indian centers: Lucknow, Delhi, and CRD, Pune. In a report from a pediatric rheumatology center (2003 and 2011) by Khubchandani et al. from Mumbai, of 1365 children 32% were JIA, 11% CTD, 10% vasculitis, 5% pain syndromes, 1% was auto-inflammatory; several children also suffered from mechanical problems.

Miscellaneous Disorders

There are case series of uncommon rheumatic disorders, namely: Sarcoidosis, brucellosis, Behçet disease, multicentric reticulohistiocytosis, Handi-Godu disease, endemic fluorosis, vitamin D deficiency, etc. Though osteoporosis is an important and common public health hazard, population-based studies of osteoporosis are scarce.

Coronavirus disease-2019 (COVID-19) pandemic led to increased focus on rheumatology for several reasons including repurposing of drugs used for rheumatic diseases for COVID-19. Moderate to severe body aches and arthralgias were commonly reported in acute infection. Many rheumatic diseases were triggered by COVID-19 including inflammatory arthritis. Post-COVID syndrome or long COVID has predominant MSK manifestations.

FURTHER NOTES ON THE WHO-ILAR COPCORD INDIA

The purpose of population and community-based epidemiological surveys is to provide robust estimates of disease prevalence. Such surveys are logistically and socioeconomically challenging. The sample size should be sufficient based on the primary objective. Rare diseases will require a large sample. The principal objective of COPCORD was to measure pain and disability (MSK) in developing countries. However, the design and methodology was suitable to provide prevalence estimates only for common MSK rheumatic diseases. Randomized sampling is recommended but cumbersome. COPCORD surveys have generally used convenience to measure burden of disease.

Though the current data is believed to be robust (Table 1.3.1, Fig. 1.3.1), India is a large country with a diverse population. Thus many more population surveys are required. The maiden India COPCORD in village Bhigwan surveyed 7000 people in five weeks-time with a concerted and systematic team effort and this fast-track model was replicated several times in India at different sites (Fig. 1.3.2) and the world (*www.copcord.org*). COPCORD Bhigwan is the only project of its kind in the world that has completed over 25 years of community service with a pre-planned follow-up. The community has availed free of cost rheumatology services till date.

LEARNING POINTS

- The WHO-ILAR COPCORD India population studies have demonstrated the huge burden and spectrum of rheumatic disorders in the Indian population. However, longitudinal and prospective cohort studies are required.
- Thus control of rheumatic diseases can impact life and livelihood positively.
- Degenerative arthritis, ill-defined MSK symptoms and nonspecific arthralgia, and soft tissue rheumatism (STR) formed the bulk of MSK disorders in the community.
- Rheumatology needs much more visibility in the public health domain.
- India needs to include rheumatic diseases in National Health Programs.

FURTHER READING

1. Centre for Rheumatic Diseases, Pune. Available at *http://www.rheumatologyindia.org.*
2. Chopra A, Anuradha V, Ghorpade R, et al. Acute Chikungunya and persistent musculoskeletal pain following the 2006 Indian epidemic: a 2-year prospective rural community study. Epidemiol Infect. 2012;140:842–50.
3. Chopra A. Community rheumatology in India. COPCORD driven perspective. Indian J Rheumatol 2009;4:119–26.
4. Chopra A. Epidemiology of rheumatoid arthritis. In: Mukherjee S, Ghosh A, editors. Monograph on Rheumatoid Arthritis. Indian College of Physicians. Academic Wing of API. Kolkata: Marksman Media Service;2012.pp.1–9.
5. Chopra A, Saluja M, Patil J, Tandle H. Pain and disability, perceptions and beliefs of a rural Indian population: A WHO-ILAR COPCORD study. J Rheumatol 2002;29:614–21.
6. Chopra A. The COPCORD world of musculoskeletal pain and arthritis. Rheumatology (Oxford) 2013;52:1925–8.
7. Ghodke Y, Joshi K, Chopra A, Patwardhan B. HLA and disease. Eur J Epidemiol. 2005;20(6):475–88.
8. Joshi VL, Chopra A. Is there an urban rural divide? Population surveys of rheumatic musculoskeletal disorders in the Pune region of India using the COPCORD Bhigwan model. J Rheumatol 2009;36:614–22.
9. Malaviya AN, Singh RR, Kapoor SK, et al. Prevalence of rheumatic diseases in India: Results of a population survey. J Indian Rheumatol Assoc. 1994;2:13–7.
10. Report of a WHO scientific group. The burden of musculoskeletal conditions at the start of the new millennium. Geneva (Switzerland): World Health Organization 2003. WHO Technical Report Series 919.

Chapter 1.4

Health Economics in Rheumatology

Subramanian Shankar, Satyam Bhatt

INTRODUCTION

Besides clinical effectiveness and adverse effects, understanding healthcare costs is a key dimension during therapeutic decision-making in rheumatologic practice. India unenviably has one of the lowest public healthcare expenditures (~1% of GDP) worldwide with over two-thirds of healthcare costs being borne out of pocket by the individual (Table 1.4.1). In a nation where the mean monthly income is ₹12,000 (median ₹8,000 due to skewed income distribution), passionate adherence to western guidelines (originating in an entirely different economic milieu) translates to millions of Indians being pushed below the poverty line annually due to healthcare expenses.

The whole principle of health economics lies in effective allocation of finite resources between alternate courses of action. A sound understanding of health economics is a mandatory skill to possess in a doctor's armamentarium and translates to prudent therapeutic decisions.

COSTS, EFFICACY AND EFFECTIVENESS

Costs include both direct and indirect costs. While the former is easily quantifiable and measurable, the latter includes many that are not apparently linked to patient care (Table 1.4.2). Cost estimation is a complex procedure and varies depending on the stakeholder perspective.

'Efficacy' outcomes are often measured with randomised controlled trials (RCTs) or meta-analysis. They often overestimate the treatment effect and may not be suitable for economic analysis. 'Effectiveness' is the benefit that accrues from intervention in a real-life setting. Both costs and effectiveness are time-dependent and their effects may not be immediate. The future cost is estimated by a method called discounting based on present-day

Table 1.4.1: Comparing healthcare costs between USA and India

Factors	*USA*	*India*	*Ratio*
Population	330 Million	1.3 Billion	1:4
Economy (Annual GDP)	$ 20 Trillion	₹ 2.6 Trillion	8:1
Per capita annual income	$ 60,000	₹ 2,000	30:1
Per capita income (adjusted for purchase power parity)	$ 60,000	₹ 7,200	8.3:1
Per capita expenditure by Govt on health (adjusted for purchase power parity)	$ 5,355	₹ 72	74:1
Percentage of health expenditure covered by Govt/Insurance	90%	30%	3:1
Out of pocket expenditure	10%	70%	1:7

Table 1.4.2: Costs included in health analysis	
Direct (medical)	*Diagnostic tests, hospitalization costs, medicines, devices, procedural costs*
Direct (non-medical)	Transportation, accommodation, food, utilities
Indirect	Loss of productivity
Intangible	Pain, suffering, worry, stress

Table 1.4.3: Perspectives of health costs	
Perspective	*Costs included*
Patient	Out-of-pocket costs for medical expenses not covered by insurance (co-payments for drugs, expendables and over-the-counter medications, etc.) and indirect costs for patient transportation, time off from work and pay loss, etc.
Hospital	Direct medical and direct nonmedical costs during a hospitalization
Payer	Covered medical services excluding patient out-of-pocket costs and indirect costs
Societal	All healthcare, social service, and patient out-of-pocket medical expenses and indirect costs

value. Usually, a discounting rate of 3% per annum is applied. The benefits and the costs of using an intervention to prevent or treat a disease comprise its value. It varies between patients, physicians, healthcare payers, and policymakers perspective (Table 1.4.3). The societal perspective is the most comprehensive assessment with all others being its subsets.

TYPES OF ECONOMIC ANALYSIS

In healthcare, one usually does four types of cost analysis (Table 1.4.4). In most of the cost analysis studies (except cost-minimisation analysis), a single metric, combining costs and outcome measures, is used for interpretation and analysis. The metric used in cost-benefit analyses is a unit of currency (USD/INR), while cost-effectiveness ratio is used in cost-effectiveness and cost-utility analyses. Incremental cost-effectiveness ratio (ICER), defined as the ratio of change in cost to the change in effectiveness (Δ Cost/Δ Effectiveness), is the key outcome variable of a cost-effectiveness analysis. The lower the ratio, the better is the gain derived per unit of expenditure.

Economic analysis is done in comparison to the existing strategy/intervention and assessed based on benefits accrued for the cost expended. This might be best understood by the cost-effectiveness plane (Fig. 1.4.1). The existing/comparator strategy is located at the intersection of the X and Y axis against which other strategies/interventions are compared. A strategy with the high cost and low efficacy (Quadrant A) is rejected while a low cost with good effectiveness becomes the dominant strategy (Quadrant D). When a new intervention/strategy is introduced that is not only more effective but also more expensive (Quadrant B) one needs to do various forms of cost analysis. Clinicians often compare the incremental costs and outcomes (Δ Costs/Δ Outcome) for a new intervention with the current standard.

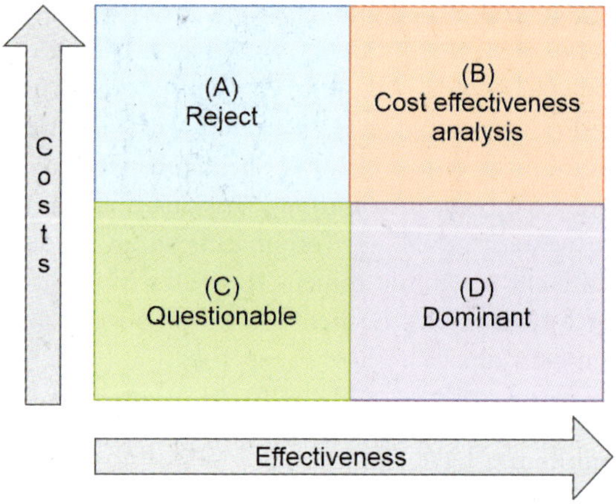

Fig. 1.4.1: Cost effectiveness plane

Table 1.4.4: Types of health economic analysis

Type	*Cost measurement*	*Benefits measurement*	*Remarks*
Cost minimization analysis	Rupees/Dollars	None	Identifies the least costly option. Assumes equal effectiveness of all interventions.
Cost-benefit analysis (CBA)	Rupees/Dollars	Rupees/Dollars	All costs and benefits converted into a single monetary value. If sum of all benefits > sum of all costs, an intervention is adopted. Indicates economic benefit of single intervention. Does not measure health outcome
Cost effectiveness analysis (CEA)	Rupees/Dollars	Predefined units of health outcome (e.g. lives saved/Illness avoided)	How much additional cost to gain an additional unit of benefit? No value needs to be put on life unlike CBA. Most useful when comparing 2 strategies for same outcome; Limitation: No numerical value of health outcome, e.g. Cost per death averted.
Cost utility analysis (CUA) special form of CEA	Rupees/Dollars	Health related quality of life/Quality adjusted life years (HRQoL/QALY). Disability adjusted life years (DALY)	How much additional cost to gain an additional unit of benefit measured in HRQoL/QALY? Costs compared on utility-based scales like QALY/DALY (net cost per QALY gained or DALY gained)

ECONOMIC APPLICATIONS IN RHEUMATIC DISEASES

Biological response modifiers and small molecule inhibitors have revolutionized the treatment of various rheumatological disorders over the last two decades. Biosimilars and generic small molecule inhibitors have reduced the costs significantly making it seemingly affordable to many more. Does it actually make it a cost-effective alternative?

An illustrative example would be the role of TNF blockers in NSAID failure in patients with spondyloarthropathy (SpA). The guidelines advise shifting to a TNF blocker within 4 weeks of failing two consequent NSAIDs. Since almost 30% of patients would fail therapy, they are automatic candidates for anti-TNF. In SpA, most patients would eventually need biologics and guidelines remain silent on when to stop therapy. Considering that 85% of the Indian population cannot afford anti-TNF, this leaves the rheumatologist in a dilemma as to how to proceed further. Also, the annual costs of even the cheapest biosimilar would be over ₹ 2 lakh per annum, precluding 85% of Indians automatically. A rheumatologist with a grounding in health economics will appreciate the problem instinctively and search for innovative strategies (Fig. 1.4.2).

CONCLUSION

Health economic analyses in medicine includes cost-minimisation, cost-benefit, cost-effectiveness, and cost-utility analyses. Cost utility analysis is used most commonly to determine the most effective allocation of resources. In clinical practice, these economic analyses not only inform cost-effective care, such as in assessing treatment strategies in RA, osteoarthritis, and osteoporosis but also summarize evidence of harms and benefits of the options and thereby promote evidence-based effective and efficient care.

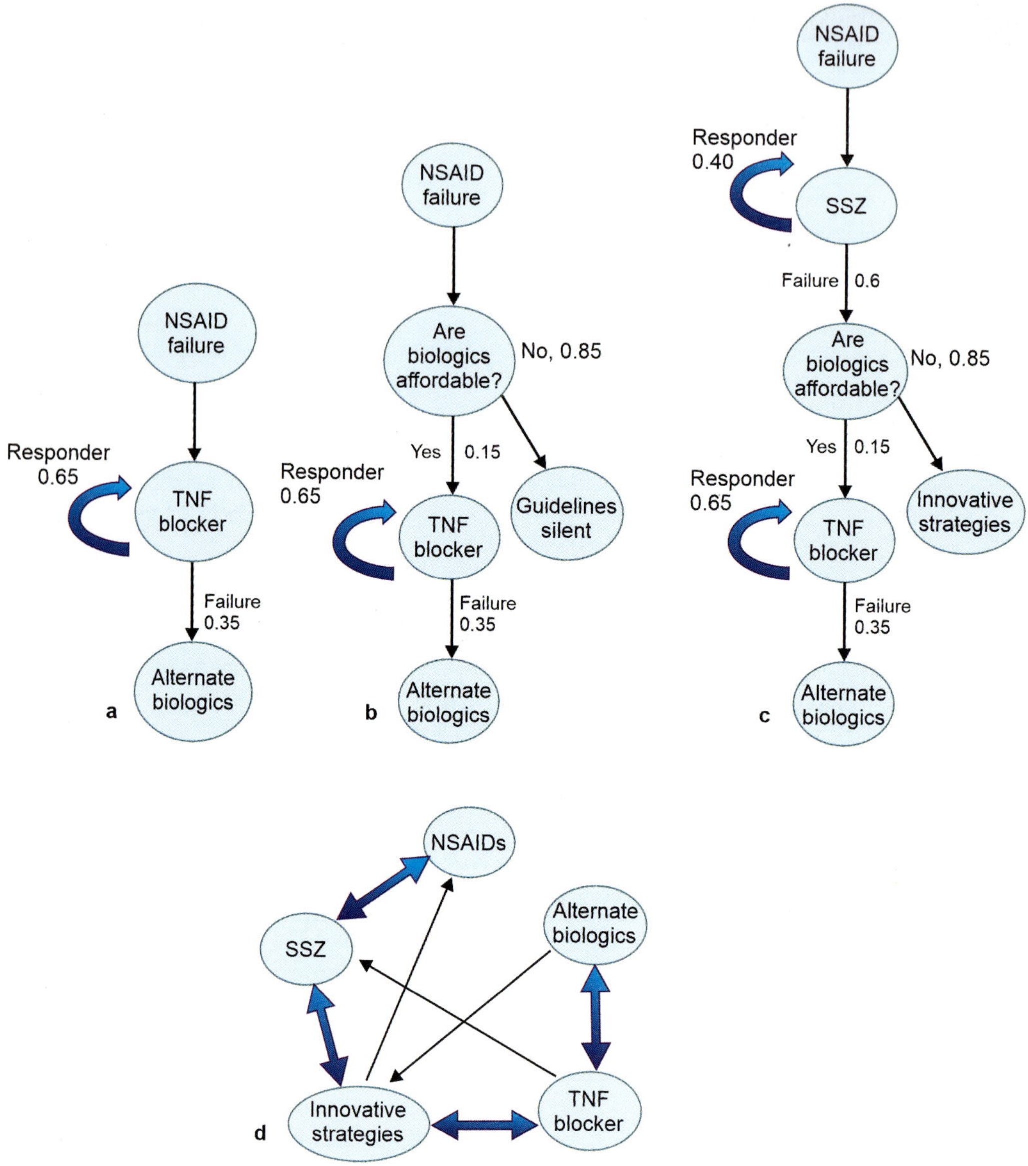

Fig. 1.4.2: Algorithms for management of axial spondyloarthropathy: (a) As per ACR/EULAR that can be applicable in just 15% Indians, (b) Algorithm modified including economic reality in India, (c) Suggested alternative algorithm being explored, (d) Algorithms needing further research

LEARNING POINTS

1. Besides clinical efficiency and adverse effects, understanding healthcare costs is a key axis in therapeutic decision-making.
2. The Indian and Western healthcare milieu are entirely different.
3. Translating western guidelines on Indian patients can have disastrous economic consequences.
4. The principle of health economics lies in effective allocation of finite resources between alternative courses of action, both at policy maker level and individual doctor level.
5. Multiple perspectives exist while assessing costs and effectiveness of an intervention. The societal perspective is the optimal one.
6. Cost-utility and cost-effectiveness analyses are the most appropriate health economic analysis.

FURTHER READING

1. Detsky AS, Naglie G, Krahn MD, et al. Primer on medical decision analysis: Part 1–Getting started. Med Decis Making. 1997;17:123–25.
2. Detsky AS, Naglie G, Krahn MD, et al. Primer on medical decision analysis: Part 2–Building a tree. Med Decis Making. 1997;17:126–35.
4. Krahn MD, Naglie G, Naimark D, et al. Primer on medical decision analysis: Part 4–Analyzing the model and interpreting the results. Med Decis Making. 1997; 17:142–51.
3. Naglie G, Krahn MD, Naimark D, et al. Primer on medical decision analysis: Part 3–Estimating probabilities and utilities. Med Decis Making. 1997;17:136–41.
5. Naimark D, Krahn MD, Naglie G, et al. Primer on medical decision analysis: Part 5–Working with Markov processes. Med Decis Making. 1997;17:152–59.
7. Shankar S, Hegde A. Sulfasalazine in the management of pure axial spondyloarthritis: Need to have a relook! Indian J Rheumatol 2020;15:S57–63.
6. Tan MC, Regier DA, Esdaile JM, et al. Health economic evaluation: a primer for the practicing rheumatologist. Arthritis Rheum. 2006;55:648–56.

Section

II

EXAMINATION

Chapter 2.1

Examination of Large Joints

Rohini Samant, Sandeep Yadav

INTRODUCTION

The shoulder, hip and knee are large joints and can be affected by inflammatory, non-inflammatory, and mechanical conditions (Table 2.1.1). The purpose of clinical examination is to ascertain the degree of abnormality both structural and functional and if present, whether it is due to an inflammatory or degenerative condition. Further, it is important to distinguish whether pain and limitation of the joint is articular in origin and not periarticular, neurological or vascular in origin.

SHOULDER JOINT

The shoulder joint is complex and consists of the glenohumeral joint which is a multiaxial spheroidal synovial joint and the acromioclavicular joint. The stability of the shoulder joint depends on the rotator cuff that comprises tendons of the subscapularis, infraspinatus, supraspinatus and teres minor muscles.

Inspection

With the patient seated, inspect the shoulder from the front, behind, and from the side. The shoulder normally appears rounded and symmetrical bilaterally. Subluxation of the acromioclavicular joint is manifested with a step deformity whereby the acromion lies below the clavicle. Inferior subluxation of the glenohumeral joint leads to a sulcus just below the acromion (sulcus sign).

Table 2.1.1: Disease conditions that involve shoulder, hip and knee joint

Shoulder	Rotator cuff tendinopathy or tear Periarthritis or frozen shoulder Arthritis of the glenohumeral joint occurs in rheumatoid arthritis (RA), spondyloarthritis (SpA), juvenile idiopathic arthritis (JIA), and crystal arthritis Acromioclavicular arthritis occurs in RA, degenerative arthritis
Hip	JIA SpA RA Avascular necrosis (AVN) of head of femur Perthes' disease, slipped upper capital epiphysis, hemarthrosis
Knee	Osteoarthritis RA JIA SpA Crystal deposition disease: Gout and CPPD Bursitis—prepatellar and anserine bursitis

Palpation

The glenohumeral joint is palpated lateral to the coracoid process. The acromioclavicular joint is palpated 2–3 cm medial to the 'tip' of the shoulder. Assess the joints for warmth, tenderness, swelling, and crepitus.

Movements

The normal range of movement of the shoulder is wider than any other joint (Table 2.1.2). The patient is instructed to perform two movements: (a) Putting both hands behind the head and (b) putting both hands behind the back. If the patient can perform both movements (Fig. 2.1.1) comfortably the glenohumeral and rotator cuff apparatus is probably normal.

Table 2.1.2: Normal range of motion of the shoulder
Abduction is 180°, flexion 180°, and extension 60°.
With shoulder abducted to 90° and elbow flexed the normal range of internal and external rotation is 90º each.
With the elbow at the side of the waist normal external rotation is 45–90° and internal rotation is 55–80°.
Internal rotation is 120° if the patient can reach an inferior angle of the opposite scapula from behind.

The patient is then asked to actively abduct the arm from the side of the body to complete overhead abduction to form an arc (Fig. 2.1.2) and any painful movement is noted. Early involvement of glenohumeral movement is elicited by limitation of external or internal rotation. In glenohumeral joint disease, active and passive abduction of the shoulder will elicit pain throughout the range of motion whereas if active abduction is more painful than passive movement a muscle, tendon or nerve lesion is more likely. Painful arc syndrome or impingement syndrome is a condition whereby the patient lifting the arm above the head experiences pain between 30 and 60° of abduction. This is caused by impingement of the rotator cuff in the subacromial space or by subacromial bursitis. Pain that is elicited at the extreme 20° "superior painful arc" suggests acromioclavicular pathology.

HIP JOINT

Hip joint pathology presents as the anterior thigh or groin pain, limp, or limb length discrepancy. The inability of the patient to sit on the floor crossed legs is a good screening test that indicates hip joint pathology. The examination aims to distinguish primary hip joint pathology from pain originating in periarticular bursae or entheses or distant anatomical structures like sacroiliac joint or spine (Fig. 2.1.3).

Inspection

A limp indicates hip joint synovitis or hip joint damage due to long-standing arthritis. A waddling gait may be due to weakness of the abductor muscles or due to hamstring weakness in knee

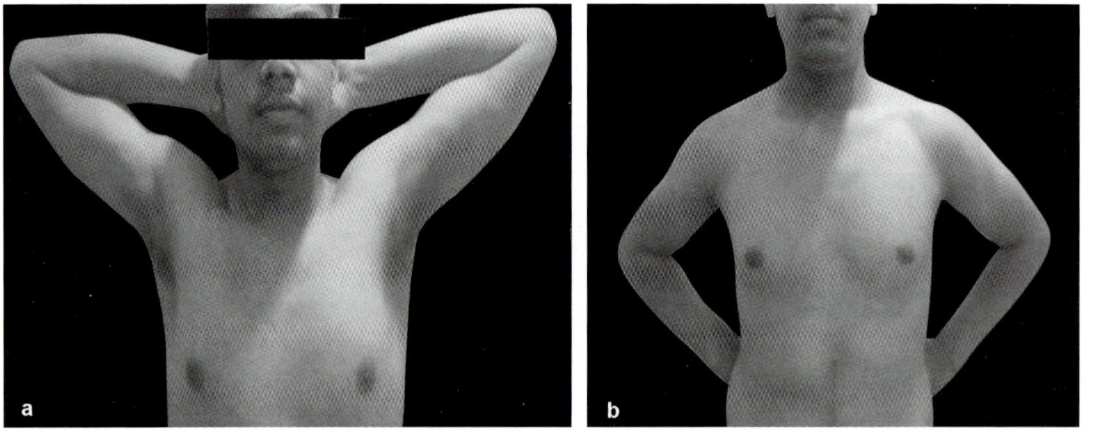

Fig. 2.1.1: Test for composite movement of the shoulder joint: (a) Hands behind the head; (b) Hands behind the back

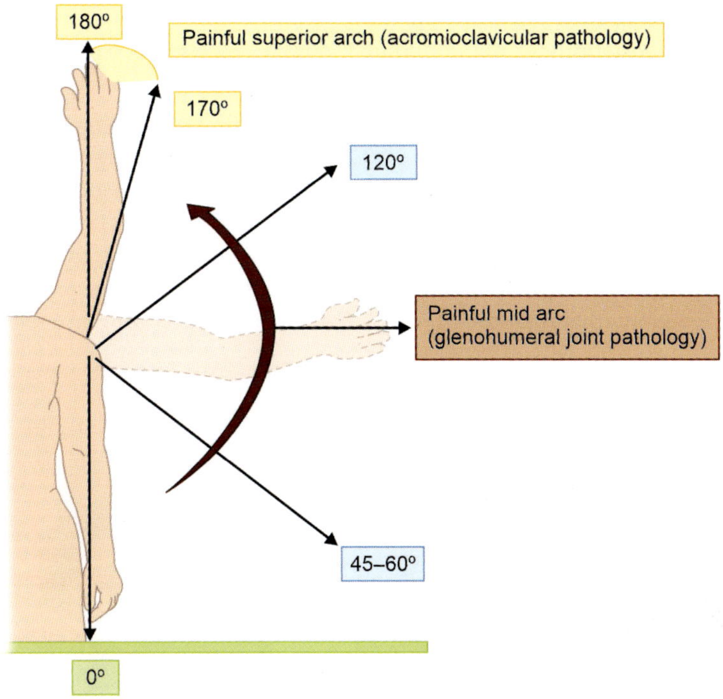

Fig. 2.1.2: Ask the patient to actively abduct the arm from the side of the body to complete overhead abduction and check whether there is a painful mid arc/superior end of arc or pain during the entire arc of movement

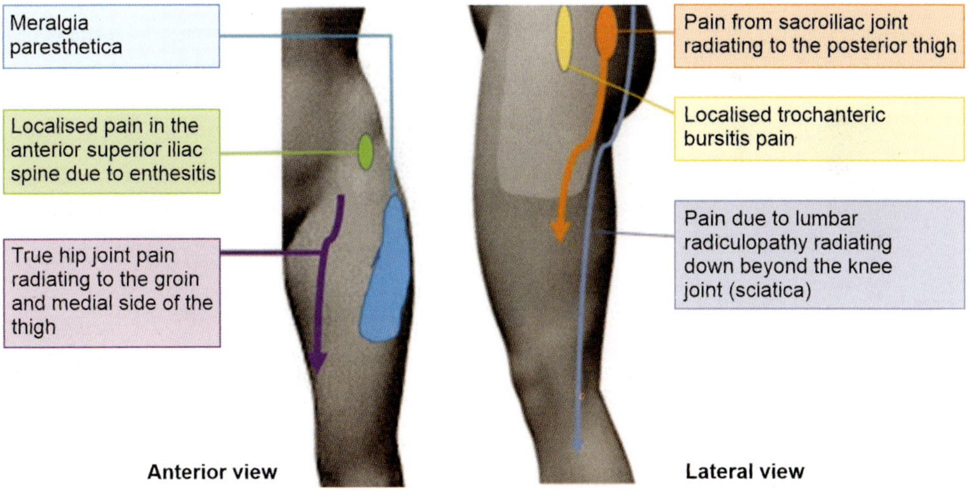

Fig. 2.1.3: Illustration of the site of pain in the hip region and likely cause thereof

osteoarthritis. Exaggerated lumbar lordosis may indicate fixed flexion deformity of the hip. Disuse atrophy of proximal quadriceps muscle is a pointer for hip arthritis. Limb length discrepancy should be suspected if the patient needs to flex one knee to keep the pelvis level or if the pelvis is tilted to one side when the knees are fully extended.

Palpation

Palpation should begin by feeling the bony landmarks that include the iliac crest, greater trochanter, adductor tendon, ischial tuberosity, pubic symphysis, posterior superior iliac spine (PSIS), and anterior superior iliac spine (ASIS) which also are sites of enthesitis in spondyloarthritis.

Hip joint tenderness is elicited anteriorly in the Scarpa's triangle, and posteriorly at the midpoint between the greater trochanter and ischial tuberosity.

Movements

Figures 2.1.4 to 2.1.6 demonstrate flexion and extension, abduction and adduction, internal rotation and external rotation, repectively at the hip. Hip movements that are lost early in hip joint disease are external and internal rotation.

Special Tests

Thomas test is used to test for the presence of flexed deformity of the hip. In this test, the patient lies supine with legs hanging off the examination table. The examiner passively brings the uninvolved flexed hip and knee up toward the patient's chest, while feeling for flattening of the lumbar lordosis with the other hand behind the lower back. In case of fixed flexion deformity, the patient will bring the opposite thigh upwards creating an angle with the examining

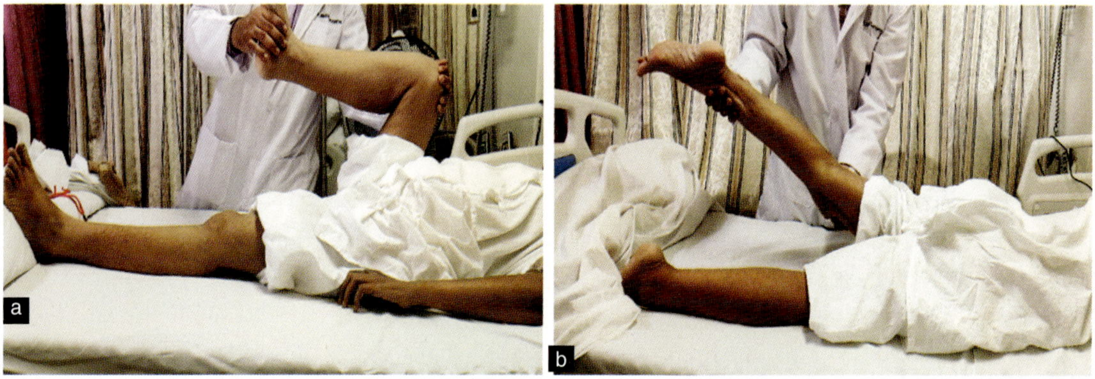

Fig. 2.1.4: (a) Examination for hip flexion and (b) extension. To examine hip flexion the patient lies supine, on the side being examined the knee is flexed, and examiner holds the flexed knee with one hand and the foot with the other hand and passively flexes the hip joint (a). To examine hip extension, with the patient lying prone, support the knee with one hand with the knee extended passively lift the entire leg as to extend the hip (b). Normal hip flexion is 100–135° and hip extension is 15–30°.

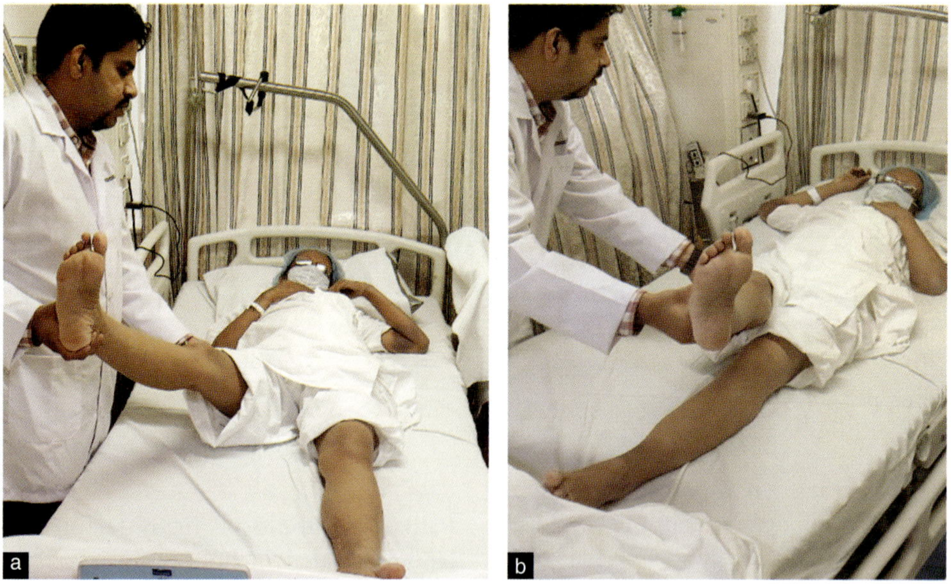

Fig. 2.1.5: (a) Examination for hip abduction and (b) adduction. To examine abduction, with patient lying supine and knee extended, passively move leg away from midline (a). To examine adduction, with patient lying supine and knee extended, passively move leg towards the midline (b). Normal range of hip abduction is 40° and hip adduction is up to 30°

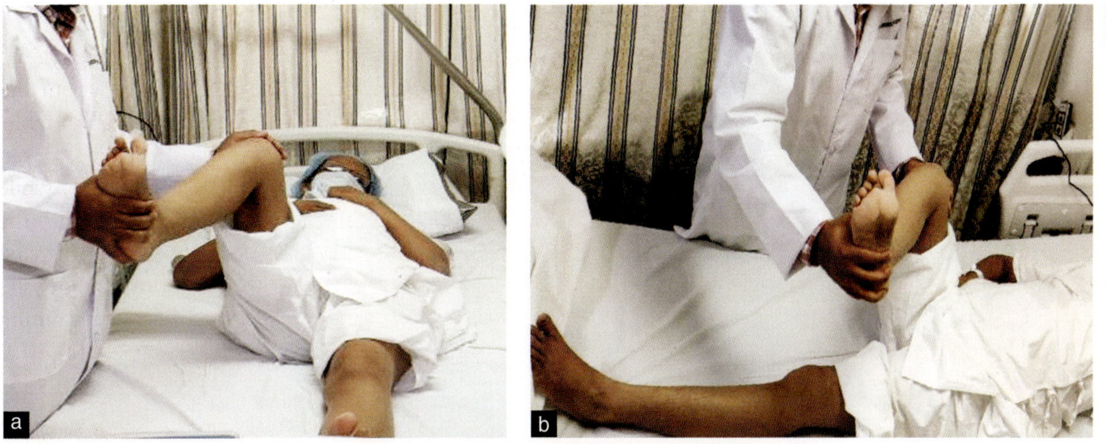

Fig. 2.1.6: (a) Examination for hip internal rotation and (b) external rotation. Normal hip internal rotation is 30–40°. To examine hip joint rotation movements, with patient lying supine, knee and hip both flexed, support knee with one hand and ankle with the other, now move ankle away from midline for internal rotation (a) and towards midline for external rotation (b)

table that indicates the presence of fixed flexion deformity in that hip joint.

Ely test is used to indicate a tight rectus femoris.

Tests for lateral compartment pathology are the *Ober test* (iliotibial pathology) and *Young's test* (tight tensor fascia lata). Tests for posterior compartment pathology are the *PACE test*, *FAIR test*, *piriformis test*, and *tripod sign* (for tight hamstrings). Tests for labrum pathology are the *apprehension test*, and the *McCarthy test*. The *FABER test* also helps to indicate the hip joint disease is described in the section on examination of the sacroiliac joint.

KNEE JOINT

The knee is the largest synovial joint and contains three compartments: The medial tibiofemoral, lateral tibiofemoral, and the patellofemoral compartment that share a common synovial cavity.

Inspection

In standing position: From the front, we can see genu varus or genu valgum. Laterally, we can see genu recurvatum and from behind, we can observe popliteal cysts or Bakers' cysts. A ruptured Baker's cyst will produce swelling of the calf. Swelling of the joint, flexion deformity, and quadriceps wasting are noted. A diffuse knee swelling indicates effusion or synovitis, whereas an asymmetric, localized swelling indicates bursitis or tendon lesion. Mild knee effusion fills in the medial dimple at the side of the patella. While moderate-to-severe knee effusion expands the suprapatellar pouch, giving a horseshoe swelling above and to either side of the patella.

Palpation

Normally, the medial and lateral joint lines are clearly palpable (Fig. 2.1.7). Synovitis of the knee causes synovial thickening and diffuse joint line tenderness along medial and lateral compartments. In chronic synovitis, synovial swelling can be palpated along the joint line with the knee flexed at 90°.

Tests to Detect Effusion in the Knee Joint

Patellar tap test is used when there is moderate fluid. The examiner uses one hand to empty the suprapatellar pouch and presses down sharply on the patella with the other hand to demonstrate the tap (Fig. 2.1.8).

In order to detect minimal fluid in the knee, fluid is milked sequentially from the medial gutter to the suprapatellar pouch with one hand and then swept along the lateral gutter, from proximal to distal with the other hand (Fig. 2.1.8). A fluid shift indicates the presence of an effusion.

Periarticular Structures

Tenderness of insertion of the medial collateral ligament at medial tibial condyle and lateral

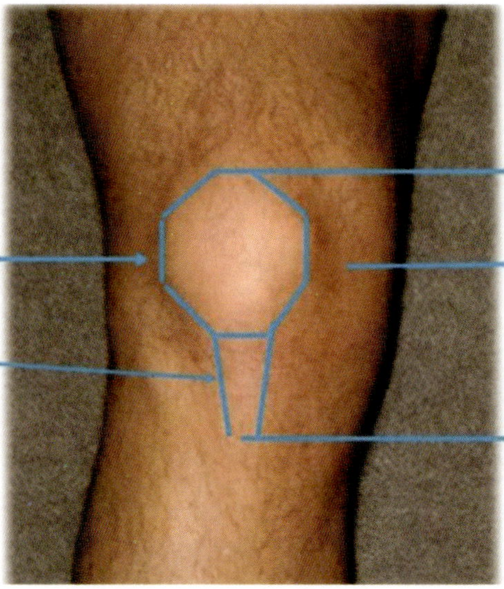

Fig. 2.1.7: Surface marking of the knee

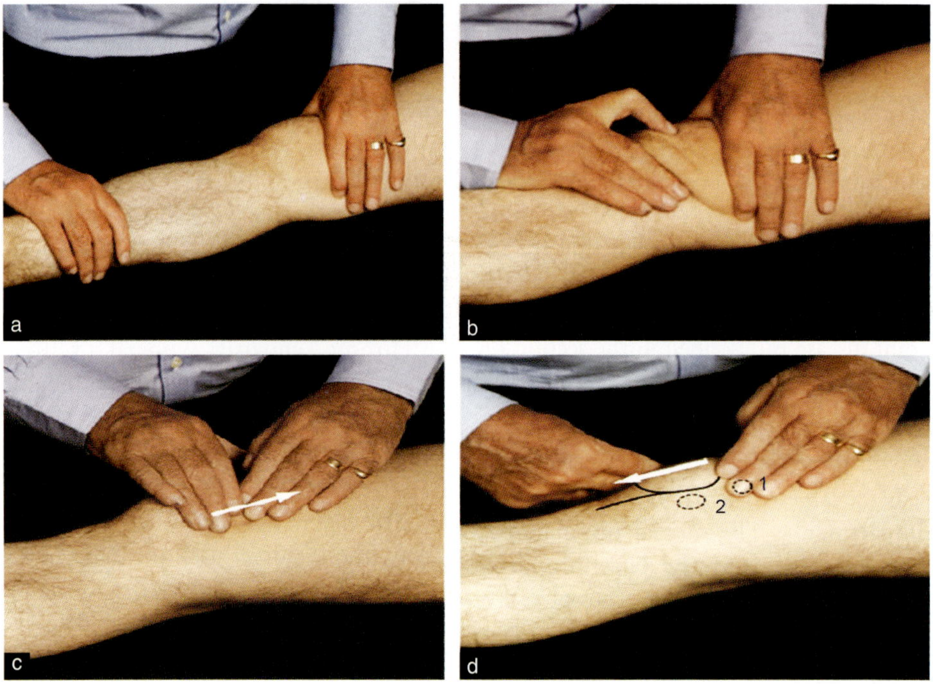

Fig. 2.1.8: In the patellar tap test the examiner uses one hand to empty the suprapatellar pouch (a) and presses down sharply on the patella with the other hand to demonstrate the tap (b). To examine for minimal fluid in knee joint, fluid is milked sequentially from the medial gutter to the suprapatellar pouch with one hand (c) and then swept along the lateral gutter, from proximal to distal with the other hand (d). A fluid shift indicates the presence of an effusion

collateral ligament at the head of the fibula indicates varus/valgus strain due to osteoarthritis (OA). In anserine bursitis, the area of tenderness is inferior to the medial joint line. Prepatellar bursitis or housemaids' knees classically cause swelling and tenderness superficial to the patella.

Patellar tendon attachment at the upper and lower border of the patella and at the tibial tubercle, and biceps femoris insertion on the head of the fibula are common sites of enthesitis which should be looked for.

Range of Motion

Normal knee moves within the range from 0 to 135°. A grating sound (crepitus) while flexing and extending the knee is suggestive of osteoarthritis and/or loose bodies. Fixed flexion deformity (inability to completely extend the knee) indicates damage to the articular surfaces, cartilage and surrounding soft tissues commonly seen in primary or secondary OA.

Special Tests for Internal Injury

Tests to determine meniscal injury and joint stability (Lachman test, MacMurray test) should be done when patients with RA or OA present with an acute onset of pain or swelling in the knee joint after a trivial or major injury.

CONCLUSION

Knowledge of physical examination of the shoulder, hip, and knee (and of course other joints) are essential for the physician practicing rheumatology. Because it helps narrow down the differential diagnosis and obviates unnecessary tests such as MRI.

LEARNING POINTS

- The shoulder joints consist of the glenohumeral joint and the acromiclavicular joint. If the patient is able to easily perform two movements, i.e. "putting both hands behind the head" and "hands behind the back" comfortably, then the glenohumeral and rotator cuff apparatus is likely normal.
- Inability of the patient to sit cross-legged is a simple screening test indicating hip pathology.
- The knee being a large joint and accessible can be palpated, and effusions are detectable by clinical examination.

FURTHER READING

1. Doherty M, Hazleman B, Hutton C, et al. Rheumatology Examination and Injection Techniques. 2nd edition. W.B. Saunders, 1999.
2. Doherty M, Doherty P. Clinical Examination in Rheumatology. Wolfe Publication Ltd. 1992.
3. Gross JM, Fetto J, Rosen E. Examination of Joints. Musculoskeletal Examination, 4th edition. Wiley, 2015; pp. 229–86.
4. Swartz MH, Chen D, Chan J. The Musculoskeletal System. Textbook of Physical Diagnosis: History and Examination. 8th edition. Elsevier, 2021; pp.429–72.

Examination of Lumbar Spine and Sacroiliac Joint

Jyotsna Oak

INTRODUCTION

The sacroiliac (SI) joint is a true synovial joint and therefore subjected to the same inflammatory and infectious processes that affect other synovial joints. Examination of the lumbar spine and SI joint is performed through a combination of maneuvers and observations; no single test is truly diagnostic of SI joint dysfunction.

EXAMINATION OF THE LUMBAR SPINE

Examination of the lumbar spine involves inspection, palpation and assessing the range of movements followed by certain special tests.

Inspection

Inspection is performed with the patient standing. Posture, alignment, and curvatures are carefully observed. Normally the anterior superior iliac spine (ASIS), the iliac crest, and the greater trochanter are symmetrically positioned on both sides. Carefully inspect the entire spinal column for the normal curvatures of the spine. Look for any scoliosis or kyphosis. Loss of normal lumbar lordosis can be seen with increasing age, ankylosing spondylitis or other structural abnormalities.

Palpation

Palpate the spinous processes for any tenderness

Range of Motion

Movements observed at the lumbar spine include flexion, extension and lateral movement.

- **Lumbar flexion:** Ask the patient to bend forward and attempt to touch the toes with knees in extension. Normally this results in a reversal of the lumbar lordosis.
- **Lumbar extension:** Ask the patient to bend backwards while supporting his lower back with one hand of the examiner and the other hand on his shoulder to provide stability.
- **Lateral flexion:** Ask the patient to bend laterally on either side while the examiner supports their shoulder.

Tests for dorsolumbar spine mobility are listed in Table 2.2.1.

Table 2.2.1: Tests for dorsolumbar spine mobility

Dorsolumbar spine	Measurement of chest wall expansion
Lumbar anterior flexion	Fingertips to floor distance Schober test Modified Schober test Modified-modified Schober test
Lumbar lateral flexion	Domjan method BASMI method INSPIRE method

Chest Expansion

Chest expansion (Fig. 2.2.1) is measured placing a measuring tape at the level of the fourth intercostal space in males and just below the breasts at the xiphisternal level in females. The difference in measurement on maximal inspiration and after forced maximal expiration are taken. Values below 5 cm in young people are pathological and could suggest the presence of ankylosing spondylitis in a person with an insidious onset of chronic, inflammatory low back pain.

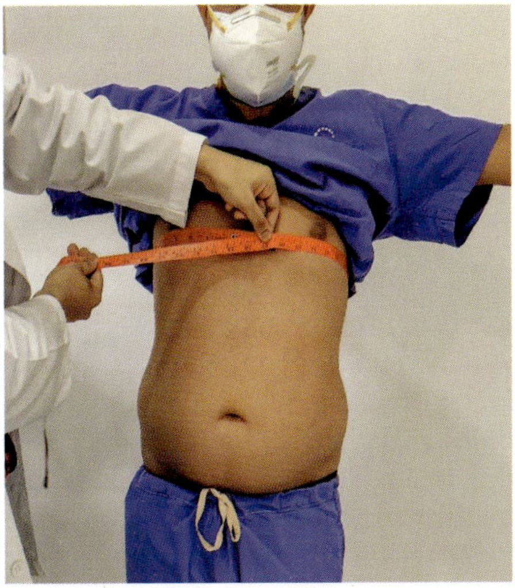

Fig. 2.2.1: Chest expansion

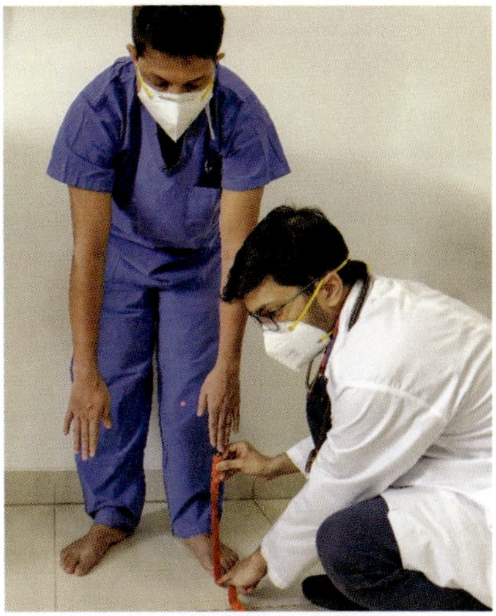

Fig. 2.2.2: Fingertips to floor

Fingertips-to-floor Distance

Measurement of the distance from the fingertips to the floor (Fig. 2.2.2) is a test for anterior flexion of the lumbar spine. The patient stands straight with the knees fully extended and heels on the floor, and is asked to bend forward as far as possible. The distance between the tip of the middle finger and the floor is measured.

Schober Test, Modified Schober Test and Modified-modified Schober Test

Schober test: It was first described by Schober in 1937 to assess the lumbar spine movement. As shown in Figures. 2.2.3 and 2.2.4, the examiner puts a mark on the lumbosacral joint and another mark 10 cm above that. The patient is asked to bend forward as far as possible with the knees in extension. The distance between the two marks is measured. Normally, the distance should increase by 4–5 cm.

Modified Schober test: The Schober test was modified by Moll and Wright in 1969. In the modified test the examiner draws a horizontal line between the posterior superior iliac spines, next a vertical line 10 cm above and 5 cm below the horizontal line is measured. Then the patient is asked to flex forward as far as possible. The distance between the two marks is re-measured (Fig. 2.2.5). Normal values are consistent with a greater than

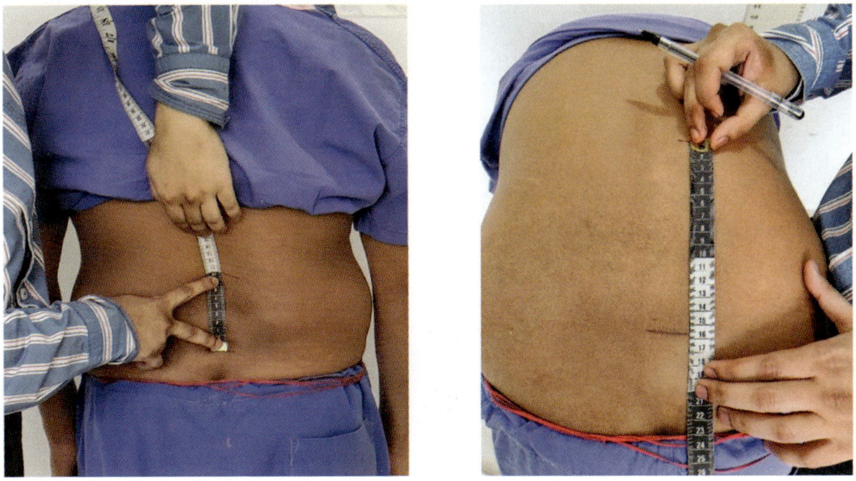

Figs. 2.2.3 and 2.2.4: Schober test

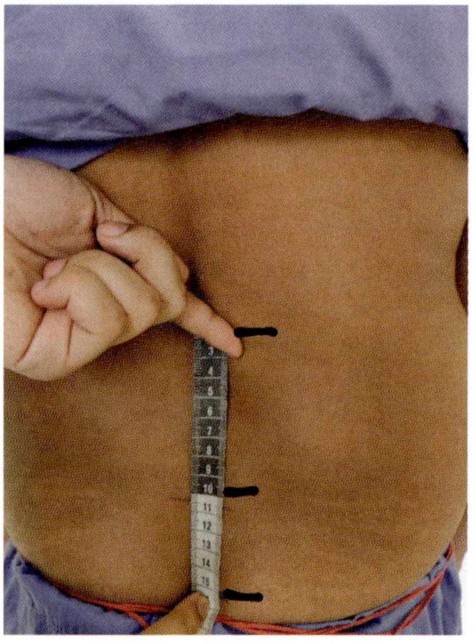

Figs. 2.2.5: Modified Schober test

5 cm increase in distance between the two marks. It is specific but not sensitive when comparing patients with and without low back pain.

Modified-modified Schober Test: This is similar to modified Schober, except that the first line is marked at the dimple of Venus corresponding to the posterior superior iliac spine and another mark 10 cm above that. The patient is asked to bend forward as far as possible with the knees in extension. The distance between the two marks is measured. Normally, the distance should increase by 4–5 cm.

Tests for Lateral Flexion

Domjan Method (1990)

In this method, the patient stands straight with both hands by the side. A mark is made on the thigh adjacent to the tip of the middle finger. A second mark is made adjacent to the tip of the middle finger on the thigh or leg at maximum lateral flexion with knees in full extension. The difference between the 2 marks is measured using a tape measure. The same is repeated on the other side and the average is taken.

BASMI Method (1994)

In this method, the patient stands straight with both hands by the side and the distance from the tip of the middle finger to the floor is measured. Next the distance between the middle finger to the floor at maximum lateral flexion is measured. The difference between the two measurements before and after maximal lateral bending is measured. The same is repeated on the other side. A distance of ≥10 cm is considered normal.

INSPIRE Method (2007)

In this method, a mark is made on the right side when the patient is bending maximally to the left and a mark is made on the left when the patient is bending maximally to the right. The distance between lateral flexion to the left and right is recorded as the distance between the 2 marks on the right side. This reflects both right and left lateral bending. It correlates well with the other two methods.

Straight Leg Raising Test

The straight leg raising (SLR) also known as the Lasègue sign is a passive test used to reproduce pain arising from irritation of sciatic nerve roots, commonly due to a prolapsed intervertebral disc. To perform the SLR test (Fig. 2.2.6), the patient lies supine. The clinician standing on the side to be tested places one hand around the patient's heel and the other hand on the patient's thigh then lifts the patient's leg to flex the hip while keeping the knee in a fully extended position. The clinician continues to lift the patient's leg until the patient experiences pain.

The SLR test is considered positive when pain radiating to the posterior thigh and below the knee is reproduced when the limb is elevated to between

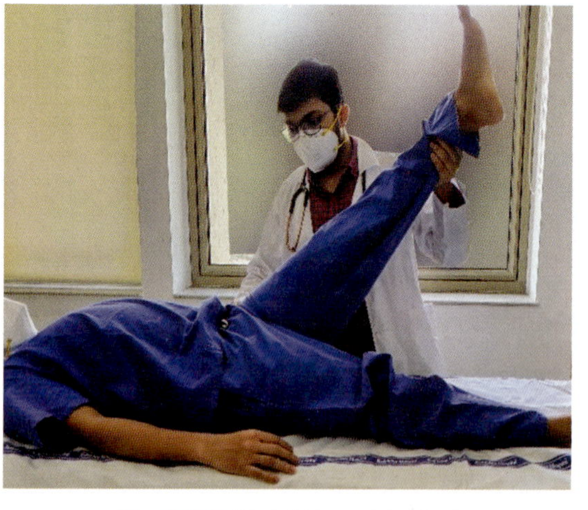

Fig. 2.2.6: Straight leg raising test

30° and 70°. The occurrence of pain when the limb is lifted to less than 30° is not considered to be related to nerve root irritation; while pain induced beyond 70° of leg elevation is likely to be related to tightness within the hamstrings or gluteal muscles.

EXAMINATION OF SACROILIAC (SI) JOINT

No single test is diagnostic of SI joint dysfunction. But a combination of the tests (SI joint provocation tests) listed in Table 2.2.2 is useful to make a clinical diagnosis of SI joint pathology.

Fortin Finger Test

The patient points to the area of pain with one finger. The result is positive if the site of pain is within 1 cm of the PSIS, generally inferomedially.

Distraction Test or Anterior Gapping Test

This test is performed with the patient in the supine position. As shown in Figure 2.2.7, the examiner places his/her hands on either anterior superior iliac spine (ASIS) pressing firmly downward and laterally. This maneuver stretches (gaps) the SI joint's anterior ligaments and capsule, and compresses the posterior part of the joint. The test is considered positive if it reproduces the patient's symptoms.

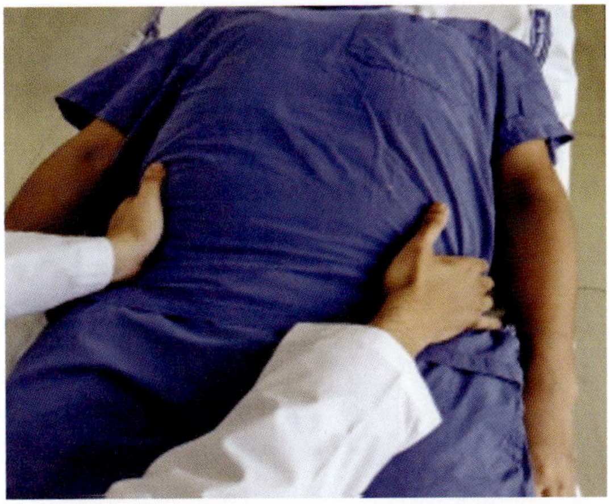

Fig. 2.2.7: Distraction or anterior gapping

Compression Test or Posterior Gapping Test

As shown in Figure 2.2.8, the posterior gapping or compression test is performed with the patient lying on his/her painless side. The examiner stands behind the patient, places both hands (elbows extended and palms interlocked) over the patient's anterolateral iliac crest and applies firm pressure directed towards the opposite iliac crest. The test is considered positive if pain is elicited in the back over the SI joint or gluteal region.

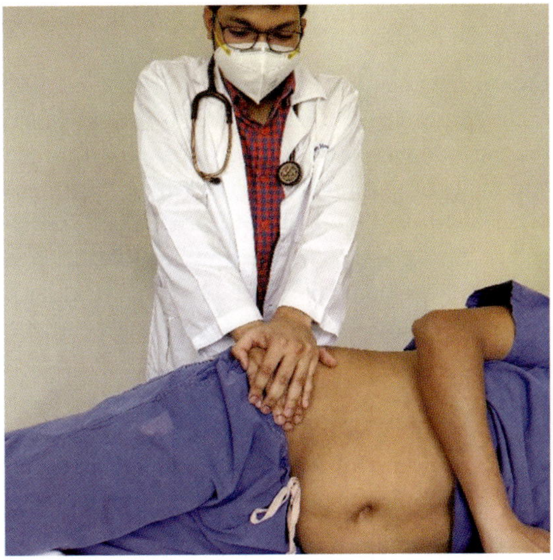

Fig. 2.2.8: Posterior gapping or compression test

Table 2.2.2: Sacroiliac (SI) joint pain provocation tests

Tests for SI joint anterior ligaments are: • Distraction or anterior gapping test • Patrick's test (FABER)
Tests for SI joint posterior ligaments are: • Compression or posterior gapping test
Tests for SI joint anterior and posterior ligaments are: • Sacral thrust or downward pressure test • Posterior shear or thigh thrust test • Pelvic torsion test (Gaenslen's) • Yeoman's test • Newton's test

Patrick (FABER) Test

FABER is an acronym for Flexion, Abduction, External Rotation. This test was first described in 1917 by Hugh Patrick and is used to stress the ipsilateral sacroiliac joint. As shown in Figure 2.2.9 the patient lies supine on the examination table and the tested leg is placed in a figure of 4, i.e. the hip is flexed and abducted with the ankle resting on

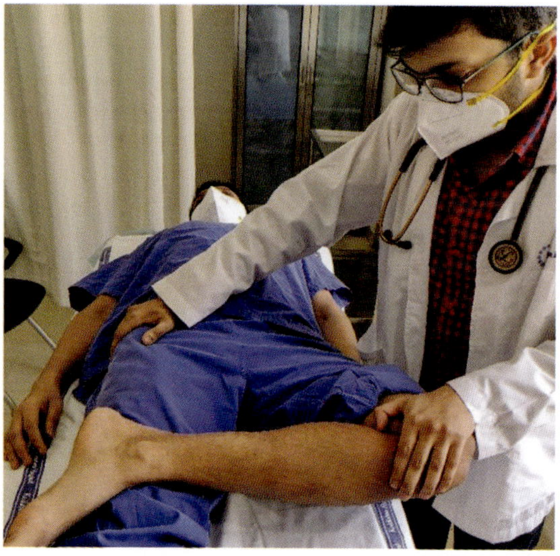

Fig. 2.2.9: Patrick (FABER) test

the contralateral thigh proximal to the knee. The examiner applies gentle pressure to the ipsilateral knee in a downward direction to the table until the end range of motion is achieved while putting his other hand on the opposite ASIS to stabilize the pelvis. This pressure stresses the hip joint as well as the SI joint on the ipsilateral tested side. If back pain is reproduced, the test is considered positive.

Gaenslen Test or Pelvic Torsion Test

This test (Fig. 2.2.10) is performed with the patient lying supine with one leg hanging down the examination table. On the opposite leg, the hip is passively flexed as far as possible to the chest. The examiner applies firm pressure on the knee of the flexed leg, and on the knee of the leg hanging on the edge of the examination table. The test is considered positive if the patient's pain is reproduced on the leg hanging down.

Yeoman's Test

This test is performed with the patient lying prone (Fig. 2.2.11). The examiner stands at the painful side and puts one hand on the sacrum. The other hand extends the hip. A positive test produces pain over the sacroiliac joint. Paresthesia over the anterior thigh may indicate a femoral nerve stretch.

Posterior Shear or Thigh Thrust Test

The patient lies supine and the examiner stands on the (normal) asymptomatic side. With one hand the examiner flexes the patient's hip (with slight adduction) on the symptomatic side to 90°, then places the other hand on the patient's sacrum, then applies a longitudinal pressure "thrust" through the femur that will cause pressure on the SI joint. The test is considered positive when there is reproduction of the patient's pain.

Newton's Test

The patient lies supine on the examination couch. The examiner then fully flexes and presses the tested-side hip and knee joints toward the abdomen. The test is considered positive if the patient experienced increased pain in the SIJ.

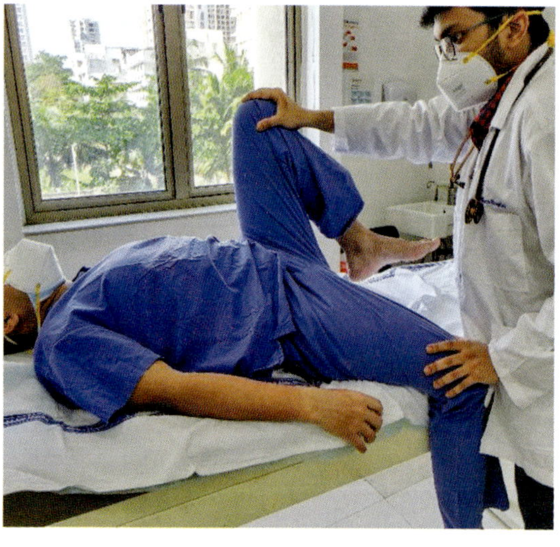

Fig. 2.2.10: Gaenslen test

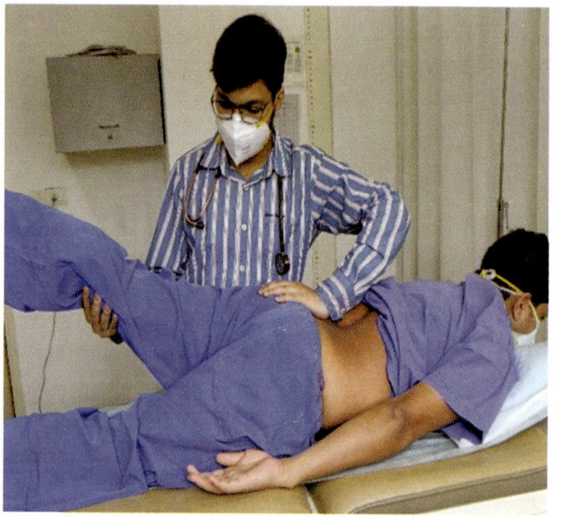

Fig. 2.2.11: Yeoman's test

Performance of SI Joint Provocative Tests

According to Laslett et al. a positive of two of four tests (distraction, compression, thigh thrust, and sacral thrust) gives a positive predictive value and negative predictive value of 67% and 93% to detect SI joint involvement.

To conclude, examination of the lumbar spine is relatively straightforward, but it is difficult to accurately examine the SI joint being a deep seated joint with many ligaments and muscles around it.

LEARNING POINTS

- A sound knowledge of how to examine the lumbar spine is important both at the initial clinical assessment of ankylosing spondylitis and for the follow-up to know functional impairment.
- Tests for eliciting SI joint involvement are many, but not one test is diagnostic. A combination of tests gives a better negative predictive value.

FURTHER READING

1. Gladman DD, Inman RD, Cook RJ, et al. International spondyloarthritis interobserver reliability exercise-the INSPIRE study: I. Assessment of spinal measures. J Rheumat. 2007;34:1733–9.
2. Líška D, Zelník R, Hegedüšová N. Clinical examination of the sacroiliac joint. J Orthop Trauma Rehabil. January 2021. doi:10.1177/22104917211000755
3. Laslett M, Aprill CN, McDonald B, et al. Diagnosis of sacroiliac joint pain: validity of individual provocation tests and composites of tests. Man Ther. 2005; 10:207–18.
4. Nejati P, Sartaj E, Imani F, et al. Accuracy of the Diagnostic Tests of Sacroiliac Joint Dysfunction. J Chiropr Med. 2020;19:28–37.
5. Stuber KJ. Specificity, sensitivity, and predictive values of clinical tests of the sacroiliac joint: a systematic review of the literature. J Can Chiropr Assoc. 2007; 51:30–41.
6. Telli H, Telli S, Topal M. The Validity and Reliability of Provocation Tests in the Diagnosis of Sacroiliac Joint Dysfunction. Pain Physician. 2018;21:E367–76.

Chapter 2.3

Examination of Hands in Rheumatology

C Balakrishnan

INTRODUCTION

Hands are often the 'doorway' to the diagnosis of rheumatological diseases. Examination of the hand gives a wealth of information and has to be done quickly, yet thoroughly. This chapter gives a practical outline on hand examination and also gives a pictorial depiction of clinical signs of various rheumatic diseases that are typically seen on examination of the hands.

CLINICAL EXAMINATION OF THE HANDS

Inspection of the skin, nails, pulp of the fingers, dorsum of the hand and volar aspect of the hand gives crucial pointers to the eventual diagnosis.

Examination of the joints of the hands includes inspection and palpation of the distal interphalangeal (DIP), proximal interphalangeal (PIP), metacarpophalangeal (MCP), inter-phalangeal (IP) joint of the thumb and the wrist joints. Each finger joint is palpated by placing the thumb and index finger on the lateral and medial aspects at the level of the joint line. Palpation of the tendons on the volar aspect and dorsal aspect is also vital. The presence of deformities should be noted and described.

The ability to make a fist, full fist, half fist and quarter fist, gives information as to which joint has been predominantly affected. Further important grips have been described, e.g. pinch grip and power grip which gives us an assessment of the functional aspect of the joints which is important especially prior to planning surgery. The examination of the hand is incomplete if one does not palpate for the pulses and test the peripheral nerves, especially in those with neuro-vascular symptoms.

Hands in Various Rheumatic Diseases

Rheumatoid Arthritis (RA)

Although all the joints of the hands can be involved in RA, involvement of the DIPs is distinctly uncommon but can be seen in a few patients late in the disease. A subset of patients start as palindromic RA characterised by episodic, short-lived pain, swelling and erythema around the affected joints (Fig. 2.3.1).

In early RA there is a combination of synovitis and tenosynovitis which affects the grip of the hands (Fig. 2.3.2). Over a period of time, if left untreated, the patient develops reduced joint movements and deformities. Ulnar deviation of the fingers called wind-swept deformity (Fig. 2.3.3) is typical of advanced RA, as are boutonniére deformity, swan-neck deformity and Z deformity of the thumbs (Fig. 2.3.4a and b).

Dropped fingers (especially the medial three fingers) due to attrition rupture of the extensor tendon over the ulnar styloid is a late but preventable

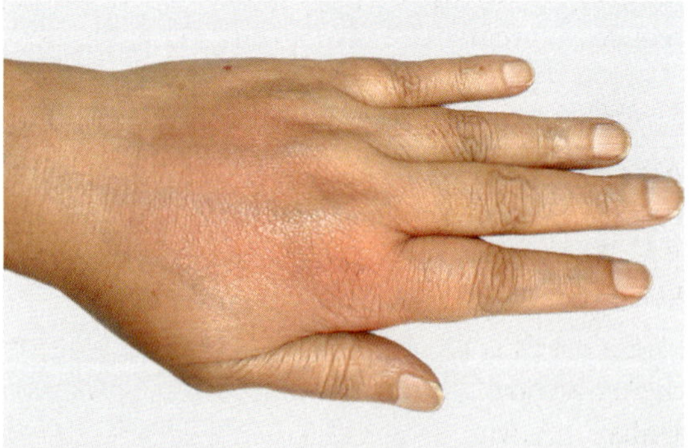

Fig. 2.3.1: Typical swelling and peri-articular erythema of the left index and middle finger MCPs in palindromic RA

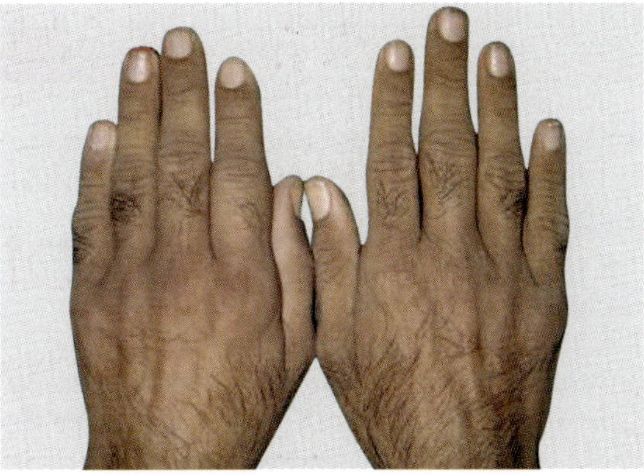

Fig. 2.3.2: Early RA: Left hand is more involved. There is swelling of the PIPs of the index, middle, ring fingers on the left and right index and middle fingers. There is also synovitis of left index and middle MCPs and right little finger MCPs

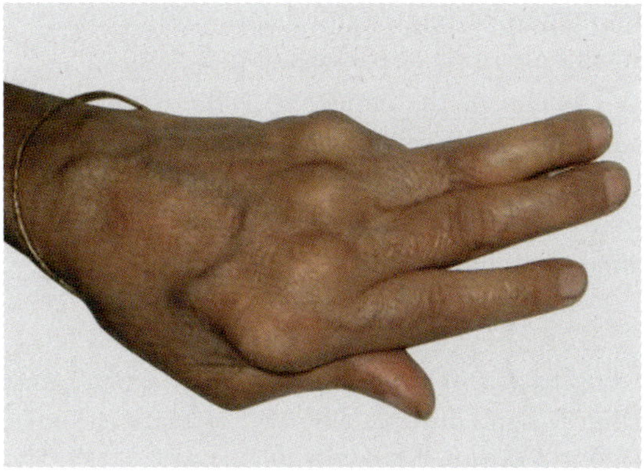

Fig. 2.3.3: Left hand showing ulnar deformities (wind swept appearance), 'Z' deformity of the thumb and over-riding deformity of the little finger

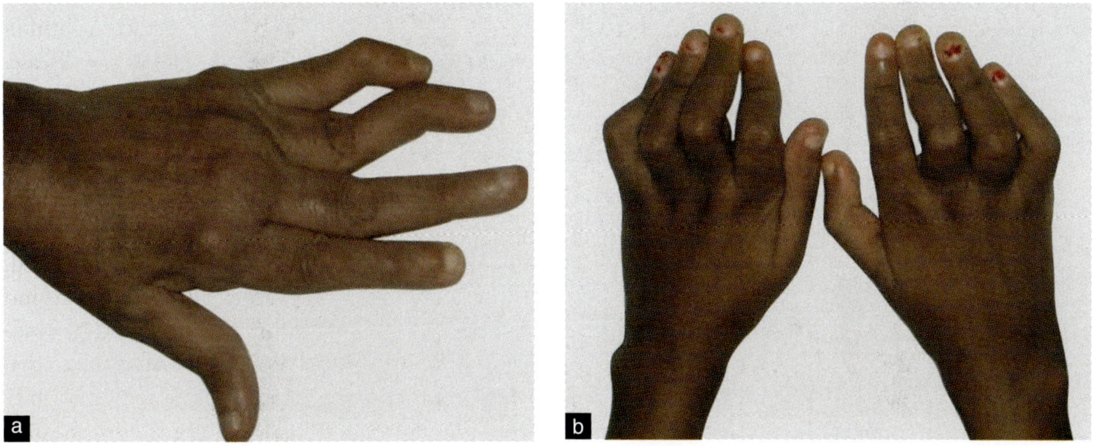

Fig. 2.3.4: (a) Showing the classical 'swan neck' in the left ring and little finger. (b) Showing the typical boutonniére's deformities in fingers of both hands

complication (Fig. 2.3.5). At the wrist as the disease progresses one sees prominence of the ulnar styloid, reduced movement and later fusion.

Psoriatic Arthritis (PsA)

All the joints of the hands can be involved in PsA, and DIPs involvement distinguishes it from RA. Typical dactylitis with post-inflammatory hyperpigmentation is shown in Figure 2.3.6a.

Dactylitis is due to combined inflammation of the tenosynovium, synovium and the periosteum. Unlike RA wind-swept deformities are rare with a deviation of fingers occurring both towards the ulnar side and radial side in the same patient. Arthritis mutilans where there is complete damage,

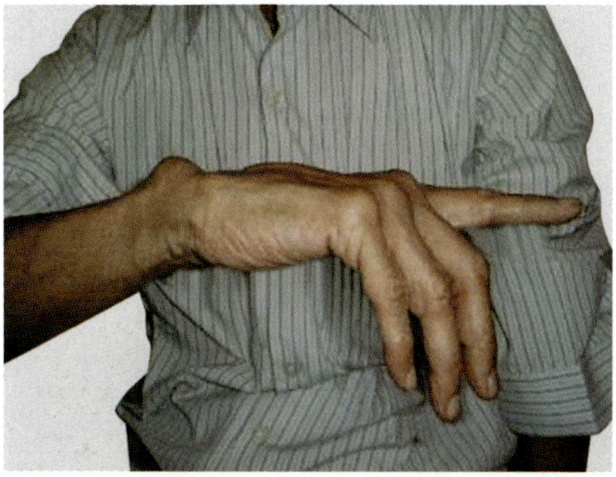

Fig. 2.3.5: Dropped fingers due to attrition rupture of the medial three finger extensor tendons causing the ulnar styloid to appear prominent

telescoping of fingers and deformities occurs in a small proportion of patients (Fig. 2.3.6b).

Dorsum of the hands especially the knuckles and at times the palms (palmoplantar psoriasis) are typical sites for psoriasis. Examination of the nails may show the characteristic nail pits, onycholysis and subungual hyperkeratosis (Fig. 2.3.6a).

Systemic Sclerosis (SSc)

Examination of the hands can elicit a myriad of clinical signs in a patient with systemic sclerosis (SSc). Raynaud's phenomenon (Fig. 2.3.7a), digital gangrene, sclerodactyly, pulp atrophy, telangiectasia and pitted scars are visible in many patients (Fig. 2.3.7b).

Acute ischemia leads to gangrene (Fig. 2.3.8a) while repeated episodes of fingertip ischemia lead to acro-osteolysis, shortening of fingers and pseudo-clubbing (Fig. 2.3.8b).

Periungual vascular changes are visible in early disease and can prognosticate the future outcome. These changes are seen on nail-fold capillaroscopy or even by an ophthalmoscope with oil immersion. Tendon friction rubs can be palpated over the flexor tendons in the palm and around the wrist joint.

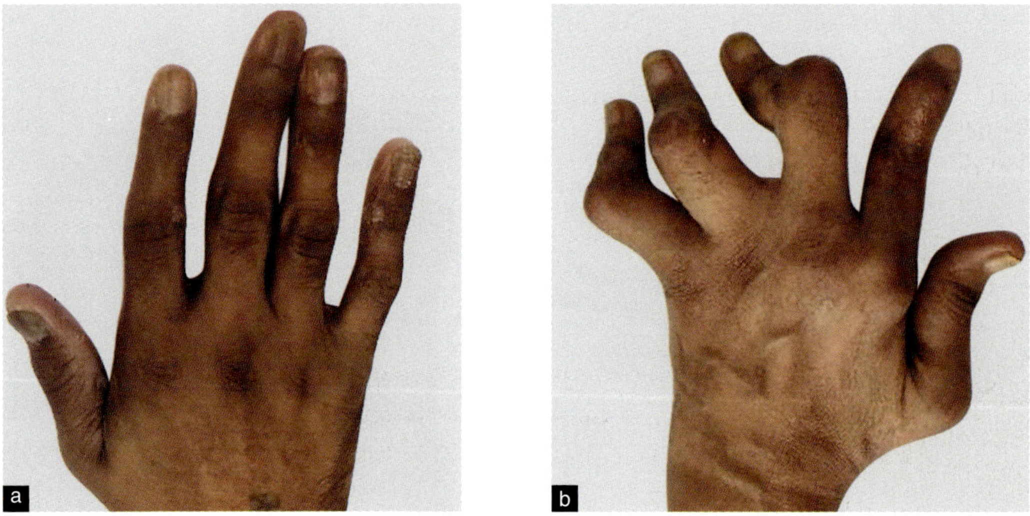

Fig. 2.3.6: (a) Typical nail onycholysis, pitting and post-inflammatory hyperpigmentation of knuckles in PsA. (b) Severe deforming arthritis (arthritis mutilans) in long-standing PsA

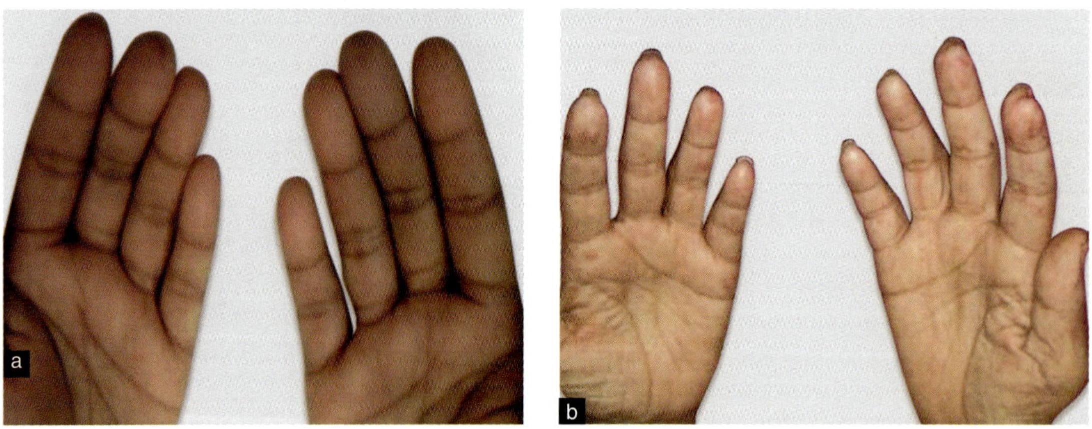

Fig. 2.3.7: (a) Raynaud's phenomenon in right and left index and middle fingers. (b) Typical scars seen in right index finger and telangiectasias seen in the fingers and palms

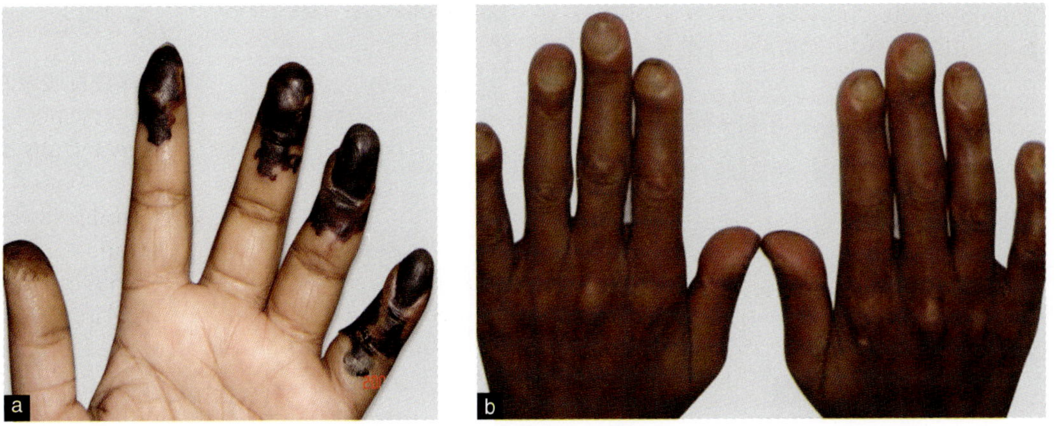

Fig. 2.3.8: (a) Gangrene fingers. (b) Pseudo-clubbing due to acro-osteolysis. Calcinosis on the knuckles

Mixed Connective Tissue Disease (MCTD)

MCTD is characterised by Raynaud's phenomenon, puffy fingers (Fig. 2.3.9), interstitial lung disease, myositis and esophageal reflux.

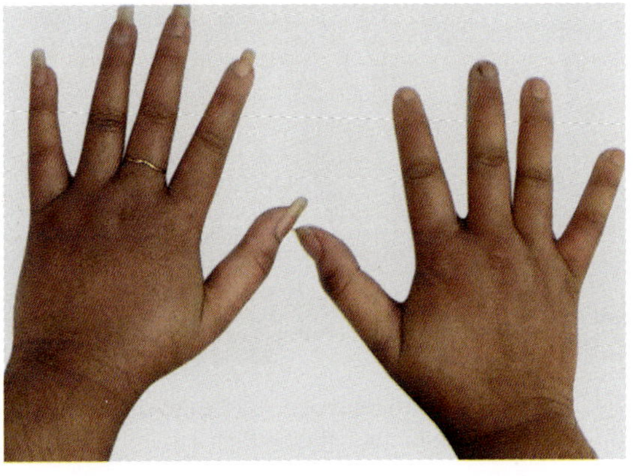

Fig. 2.3.9: Puffy hands and fingers typical of MCTD

Systemic Lupus Erythematosus (SLE)

All skin lesions described in SLE can be found on the hands. Unlike dermatomyositis (DM), the erythematous rash of SLE typically spares the knuckles and affects the intervening areas. The arthritis of SLE is non-erosive. As shown in Figure 2.3.10, the finger joints may show reversible deformities called "Jaccoud's arthritis".

Dermatomyositis

The typical findings on the hands of patients with dermatomyositis (DM) are Gottron's papules which occur on the knuckles (Fig. 2.3.11a). The periungual changes seen in SSc are also seen in DM. Another typical finding in DM is mechanic's hands which is a hyperpigmented, hyperkeratotic rash on palms, radial borders of the fingers and hands

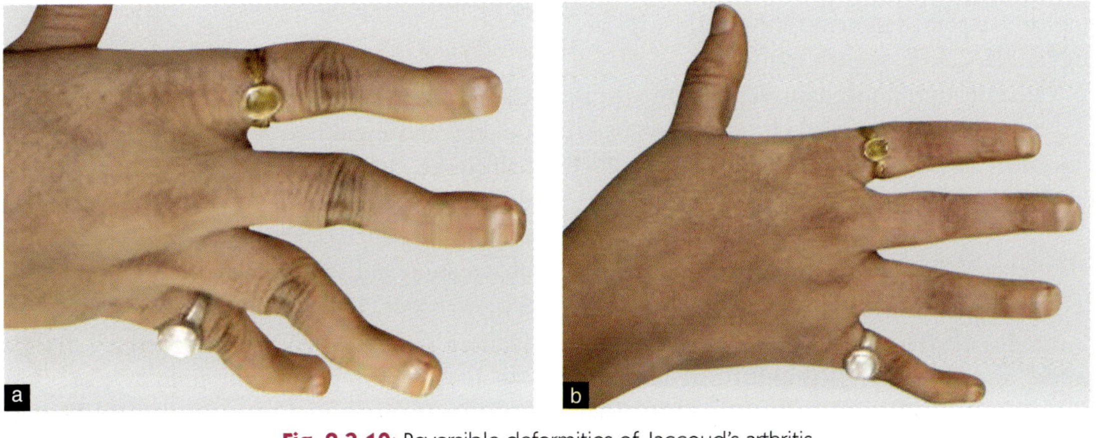

Fig. 2.3.10: Reversible deformities of Jaccoud's arthritis

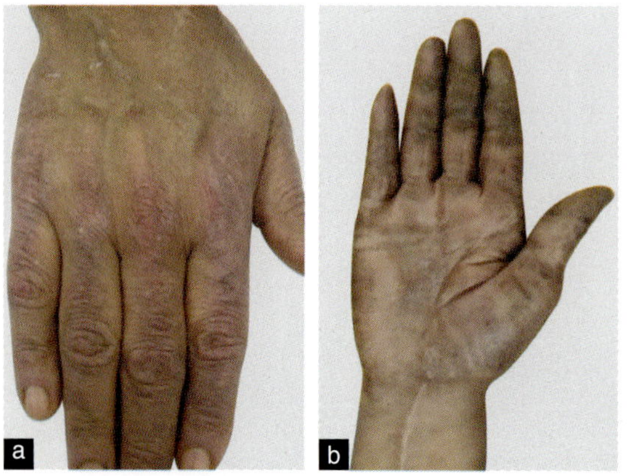

Fig. 2.3.11: (a) Gottron's lesion on the knuckles in DM. (b) Typical mechanic's hands

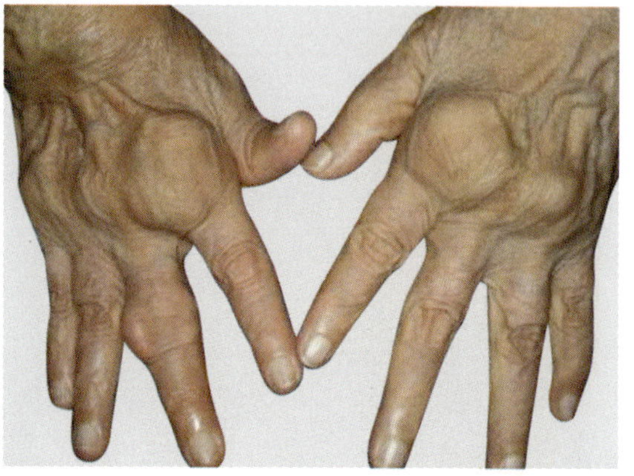

Fig. 2.3.12: Chronic tophaceous gout of the hands, showing large tophi on the MCPs and right middle finger PIPsv

(Fig. 2.3.11b). It is commonly associated with the antisynthetase syndrome.

Vasculitis

Large vessel vasculitis especially Takayasu's arteritis can present with ischemia and digital infarcts when upper limb arteries are involved. Similar infarcts can also be seen in those with polyarteritis nodosa. Mononeuritis multiplex often involves median or ulnar nerves and its clinical signs include sensory loss, motor loss, muscle wasting and many times autonomic dysfunction can be seen.

Crystal-induced Arthritis

Though gout classically involves the distal joints of the lower limbs, it can in advanced cases involve the hand joints. Typical attacks of acute gouty arthritis can be seen in the hand joints. In chronic tophaceous gout, destructive arthropathy with large tophi (Fig. 2.3.12) is often seen.

Calcium pyrophosphate deposition disease (CPPD) can typically attack the hand joints, especially the wrists. A plain radiograph taken at the appropriate moment can document the chondrocalcinosis.

Primary Osteoarthritis (OA)

This is a genetic disorder with pain and swelling involving DIPs (Heberden's node), PIPs (Bouchard's node) and first CMC (thumb) osteoarthritis. Figure 2.3.13 demonstrates the typical Heberden's nodes and Bouchard's nodes. In contradistinction

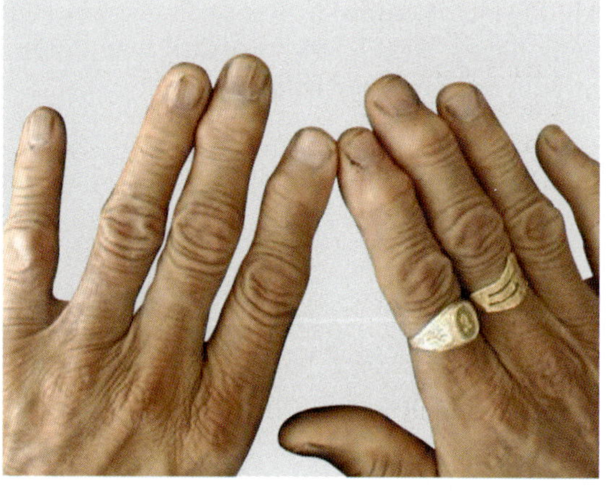

Fig. 2.3.13: Typical Heberden's nodes in the DIPs and Bouchard's node in the left little PIPs

to PsA which can also involve the DIPs in OA, the swellings are bony.

Miscellaneous Conditions

Carpal tunnel syndrome: Usually presents with tingling and numbness of the radial three and a half fingers. Initially there is no persistent neuro-deficit. However, over a period of time when the pressure neuropraxia becomes severe, persistent loss of sensation and typical thenar muscle wasting is seen as shown in Figure 2.3.14.

Hansen's disease: Although Hansen's disease can involve any part of the body, typical skin and nerve changes are often found in the hands (Fig. 2.3.15).

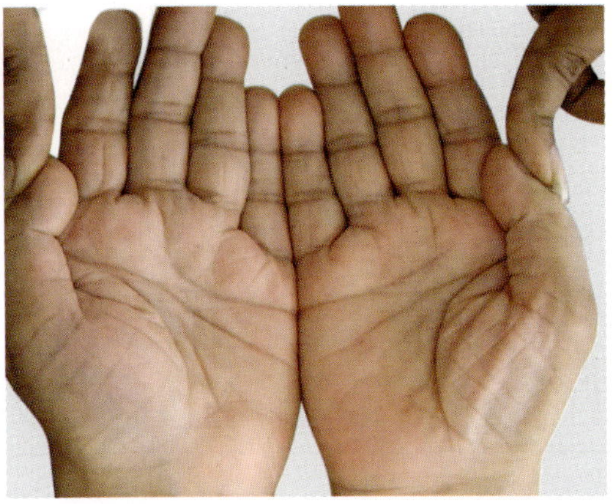

Fig. 2.3.14: Wasted right thenar eminence due to long-standing carpal tunnel syndrome

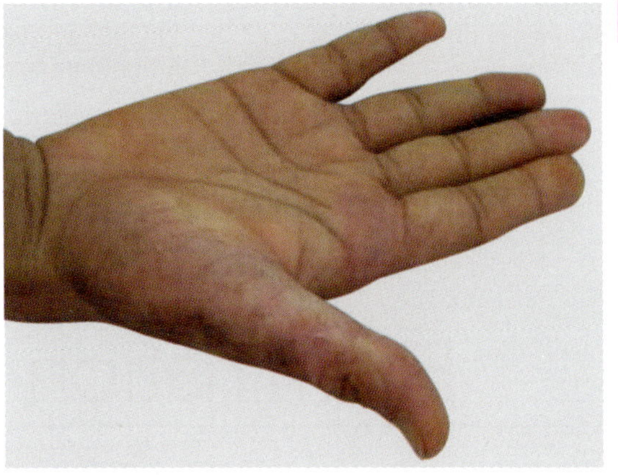

Fig. 2.3.15: Erythematous scaly plaques of Hansen's disease seen on the thenar eminence, thumb and index finger of the right hand

LEARNING POINTS

- Examination of the hands gives plenty of information related to the diagnosis of inflammatory rheumatic diseases. This is especially true for the diagnosis of RA, PsA, SSc, inflammatory myositis, SLE, and vasculitis.
- Many of the skin findings that establish the diagnosis of inflammatory myositis are visible on the hands.
- When examining the hands do not forget to systematically inspect the skin, nails, pulp of the fingers, dorsum of the hands, and volar aspect of the hands.
- Inspect the hands for swollen joints, namely the MCPs, PIPs, and DIPs. Do not forget to also inspect the first carpometacarpal joint and the thumb interphalangeal joint.
- After inspection, palpate the above-mentioned joints of the hands for joint line tenderness. Note that an accurate examination of the number of swollen joints, and the number of tender joints help in the assessment of disease activity in RA and PsA.

FURTHER READING

1. Day CS, Wu WK, Smith CC. Examination of the Hand and Wrist. N Engl J Med. 2019;380:e15
2. Fitnat D, Samut G. Physical Examination of the Hand. In: Duruöz MT, editor. Hand Function. New York: Springer; 2014. p. 23–40.
3. Gross JM, Fetto J, Rosen E. Wrist and Hand. In: Gross JM, Fetto J, Rosen E, editors. Musculoskeletal Examination. 4th edition. New York: Wiley; 2015. p. 229–86.

Examination of Ankle and Foot

Namisha Patel

INTRODUCTION

The ankle and foot are weight-bearing joints and can be involved by inflammatory arthritis, mechanical problems, fractures, as well as systemic medical and neurological conditions. This chapter gives an overview from a rheumatology perspective as to how to examine the ankle and foot.

ANATOMY OF THE ANKLE AND FOOT

The foot can be divided anatomically into the forefoot, midfoot and hindfoot. The lower ends of the tibia and fibula, talus, and calcaneus form the hindfoot. The cuboid, navicular, and cuneiform bones form the midfoot. The metatarsals and phalanges form the forefoot. Strong ligaments give stability to the ankle and foot. The tendons crossing the ankle joint lie outside the joint and are covered by tendon sheaths, and are held down anteriorly by the extensor retinaculum, medially by the flexor retinaculum, and laterally by the peroneal retinaculum.

The ankle is a saddle-shaped hinge joint between the distal ends of the tibia and fibula and the trochlea of the talus.

- The tibiotalar joint is the weight-bearing part of the ankle joint, while the fibula articulates with the inferior end of the tibia. The malleoli of the tibia and fibula extend inferiorly to articulate with the talus, providing more stability. Dorsiflexion and plantar flexion are two movements occurring at this joint (Table 2.4.1).
- The subtalar joint is formed when the talus articulates inferiorly with the calcaneum to form the talocalcaneal joint. Inversion and eversion occur at this joint (Table 2.4.1).
- The midtarsal (transverse tarsal) joint comprises the combined talonavicular and calcaneocuboid joints. Movements here include inversion and eversion movements at the subtalar joint, including 20° of adduction (foot turned toward the midline), and 10° of abduction (foot turned away from the midline). The axis of rotation of the subtalar and midtarsal joints is such that inversion is invariably accompanied by adduction of the forefoot called supination, and eversion by abduction of the forefoot called pronation.

Table 2.4.1: Movements at the ankle joint

Ankle	*Movement*	*Range of motion*	*Muscle*	*Nerve root value*
Tibiotalar joint	Plantarflexion	0–45°	Gastrocnemius and soleus	S1, S2
	Dorsiflexion	0–20°	Tibialis anterior	L4, L5, S1
Talocalcaneal joint (subtalar joint)	Inversion	0–30°	Tibialis posterior	L5, S1
	Eversion	0–15°	Peroneus longus, peroneus brevis	L4, L5, S1

EXAMINATION OF THE ANKLE AND FOOT

Before the examination, ask the patient to point to the exact site of pain, and try to identify the anatomical location of pain so that a focused examination can be done. Usually, pain only during weight bearing is due to degenerative disease, stress fracture, and sometimes due to plantar fasciitis. Inflammatory pain is more during activity and disturbs sleep. Sometimes ankle and foot pain is pain referred from the spine, or due to bad footwear. Start by observing the gait of the patient as he/she enters the room. A painful ankle or foot causes a decrease in the stance phase of gait on the affected side with a tendency to transfer weight to the non-affected foot.

Inspection

- Check the position of the foot in the standing position. From the side observe whether the arch of the foot is normal or the patient has pes cavus or pes planus.
- On the dorsal surface look for the presence of swelling whether it is localised over the ankles or diffusely present over both feet and ankle as in pedal edema due to heart failure. Swelling of feet due to heart failure or other volume overload states is non-tender. Look for the presence of joint synovial swelling, tendon swelling, or tophi or nodules.
- Observe the toes for sausage digits. Common deformities of the big toe are hallux valgus, and hammer toes. Deformities of the smaller toes are mallet toe, hammer toes, and claw toes.
- If the patient does not have overt ankle arthritis, ask the patient to stand on tiptoe, normally the heels/ankles go in varus positions on tiptoes, indicating normal subtalar movement.
- Ventrally, on the soles of the foot, you may see a rash of psoriasis or keratoderma blenorrhagicum. Callosities and corns are characterized by thickened skin and can be painful, and are commonly seen over areas of increased pressure. Sesamoid bones are common in the foot and can be visible.
- Posteriorly observe whether the Achilles tendon is thickened or normal as compared to the other leg.
- Observe the nails for pitting or dystrophy.
- Other things to look for are the presence of muscle wasting that could be due to neurogenic foot. Varicose veins can give rise to skin discoloration and ulcers. Lower limb ulcers can be vasculitic, traumatic and rarely, pyoderma gangrenosum.

Palpation

Before touching, ask the patient if there is any particular area that is painful so that you can avoid causing more pain during the examination.

- *Synovitis and/or tenosynovitis:* Palpate along the joint lines and tendon insertions for tenderness and swelling to conclude whether it is synovitis or tenosynovitis. Ankle synovitis is seen and palpated anteriorly. Palpate also for a point or diffuse tenderness in the midfoot, metatarsals, metatarsophalangeal (MTP) joints, and the toes. Tenderness of the forefoot can be elicited by metatarsal squeeze: Hold the forefoot horizontally and give a squeeze.
- *Exquisite tenderness of the great toe* with localized or diffuse swelling and erythema almost resembling cellulitis is present during acute gout.
- Inter-metatarsal tenderness is seen in Morton's metatarsalgia. Stress fractures usually give rise to severe localized tenderness.
- *Enthesitis* particularly the heel at the insertion of the Achilles tendon, and insertion of the plantar fascia. Deep palpation of the calcaneum from the sole medially can elicit pain of plantar fasciitis.
- *Retrocalcaneal* bursitis gives rise to tenderness just below the Achilles tendon with or without swelling.

Testing for Movements

Pain, synovitis, and deformed or fused joints will affect passive and active movements at the hindfoot, midfoot, and forefoot. Neurological disease will result in weakness and loss of active movements.

Ask the patient to perform active dorsiflexion, plantar flexion, inversion and eversion. Next, perform a check for passive movement. With the patient in the supine position, hold the lower end of the leg with one hand and test movements at the ankle with the other hand. Check for dorsiflexion, plantar flexion, inversion and eversion. Foot drop is characterized by loss of dorsiflexion at the ankle and is due to mononeuritis multiplex as a result of vasculitis, or nerve root compression, or leprosy.

Table 2.4.2: Causes of foot and ankle pain

Cause	*Site of pain*		
	Ankle and hindfoot	**Midfoot**	**Forefoot**
Mechanical	Fracture, corns or callosities, pes planus, pes cavus, osteonecrosis of os trigonum	Pes planus, pes cavus, exostosis	Hallux valgus
Non-inflammatory	OA, drug induced	OA, navicular osteochondritis, L5 root pain	OA, Morton's metatarsalgia, stress fracture, drug induced
Inflammatory	RA, SpA, PsA, crystal arthritis, sarcoidosis, drug induced	RA, SpA, gout	RA, SpA, gout
Tendinitis	Achilles tendinitis, plantar fasciitis, peroneal/posterior tibialis tendinitis, drug induced		Drug induced

OA: Osteoarthritis; *RA:* Rheumatoid arthritis; *SpA:* Spondyloarthritis; *PsA:* Psoriatic arthritis.
Drug-induced non-inflammatory swelling of the ankle and feet is not uncommon (calcium channel blockers). Many drugs have been implicated in causing arthritis/arthralgias/tendinitis. These drugs are quinolones, pyrazinamide, ethambutol, statins, diuretics, cyclosporine, risedronate, aromatase inhibitors—letrozole, anastrozole, etc.

Pronation and supination midfoot movements are tested by holding the back of the leg with one hand, grasping the calcaneum between the other index finger and thumb, and rotating the foot inwards and outwards at the calcaneum. Test for MTP joint movements of flexion and extension.

Neurological Examination

Neurological examination and test for muscle function should accompany examination of the foot and ankle. A positive straight leg raising test and femoral stretch test indicate involvement of the sciatic and femoral nerves respectively (usually disc or other compressive lesions). Look for muscle weakness and loss of ankle tendon jerks. L5 nerve root lesions result in weakness of flexion of toes and dorsiflexion of the foot; sensory loss may be seen on the medial aspect of the dorsum of the foot. S1 root lesions cause weakness of plantar flexion and sensory changes on the sole. Tibial nerve entrapment medially can give rise to a positive Tinnel's sign and sensory symptoms on the sole.

CAUSES OF ANKLE AND FOOT PAIN

The pain of the ankle and foot could arise due to various causes. The origin of pain could be mechanical, inflammatory, non-inflammatory, or tendinitis (Table 2.4.2). Although not listed in Table 2.4.2, lumbosacral disc lesions, peripheral neuropathy, mononeuritis due to vasculitis, or SLE or Sjögren's syndrome or leprosy are important causes of foot problems that result in sensory changes and at times motor weakness.

LEARNING POINTS

- Good history should precede clinical examination so that we know where to focus when doing the examination.
- When performing an examination of the foot and ankle, it is always advisable to include a neurological examination so as not to miss foot drop or leprosy or referred pain from the lower back.
- There are different causes for pain of the hindfoot/ankle, midfoot, and forefoot.

FURTHER READING

1. Alazzawi S, Sukeik M, King D, et al. Foot and ankle history and clinical examination: A guide to everyday practice. World J Orthop. 2017;8:21–9.
2. Papaliodis DN, Vanushkina MA, Richardson NG, et al. The foot and ankle examination. Med Clin North Am. 2014;98:181–204.
3. Young CC, Niedfeldt MW, Morris GA, et al. Clinical examination of the foot and ankle. Prim Care. 2005; 32:105–32.

Chapter 2.5

Muscle Examination

Manesh Manoj, Latika Gupta

INTRODUCTION

Muscle examination is an integral component of musculoskeletal assessment. A demonstration of true muscle weakness, as opposed to a limitation of movement due to pain, muscle spasm, or fibrous or bony changes, is a prerequisite for the diagnosis of idiopathic inflammatory myopathy (IIM). IIMs are a clinically, histopathologically, and pathophysiologically heterogenous group of disorders and are characterized by gradual progressive, non-neurological, muscle weakness affecting the proximal musculature, truncal, and respiratory muscles. Dermatomyositis (DM), polymyositis (PM), cancer-associated myositis (CAM), and overlap myositis (OM) all manifest with symmetric muscle weakness. Inclusion body myositis (IBM), on the other hand, presents with asymmetric weakness and predominant quadriceps and finger flexor weakness.

Though long-standing arthritis can also lead to disuse atrophy which can manifest as significant muscle weakness, IIMs are associated with more remarkable muscle weakness in a proximal, symmetrical distribution. Neurological involvement in rheumatic diseases due to vasculitis may also present with muscle weakness and tends to have distal and asymmetrical distribution. Various muscular dystrophies and storage disorders can present with muscle weakness and may be difficult to distinguish clinically from the above disorders.

Fortunately, key aspects of examination and disparity in muscle weakness between various muscle groups, symmetry, and onset of weakness may all be important pointers towards the differential diagnosis. The inclusion of relative weakness of flexor versus extensor and distal versus proximal muscles in the new EULAR/ACR classification criteria for adult and juvenile IIM further reiterates the importance of diligent muscle strength testing for the classification of IIM. Moreover, documenting the severity of muscle weakness plays a central role in the objective assessment and monitoring improvement with treatment.

MUSCLE EXAMINATION

Muscle examination consists mainly of inspection and muscle strength testing.

Inspection

Observing a patient walking into the clinic gives a clue to the pattern and severity of neuromuscular weakness. Inspection of symmetry, bulk, gait, and involuntary movements are pointers to the underlying etiology.

- The inability of the patient to lift their hands above shoulder level and to get up from a squatting position, but with retained ability to walk over or grip small objects, point towards IIM or muscular dystrophy as the underlying cause for weakness. Inherited myopathies may be associated with differential involvement of agonists and antagonists performing the same type of movement.
- A prominent distal involvement suggests either IBM or a neuropathy that may present with foot drop or wrist drop.

- Long-standing, inadequately treated polymyositis may present with only generalized muscular atrophy. In the presence of localized weakness, joints proximal and distal to the affected area should always be examined.
- Inability to hold the limb in a certain position may be due to mild weakness (e.g. pronator drift) and should be examined.
- The presence of fasciculations suggests a lower motor neuron involvement or motor neuron disease should prompt a neurology referral.
- Any skin lesion should be thoroughly sought for and may be associated with dermatomyositis (either *de-novo* or cancer-related). Subtle clues in the presentation may suggest the diagnosis and are elaborated in Table 2.5.1.

Palpation

Palpation is not routinely required to diagnose muscle disorders but may offer clues to diagnosis. An inflamed muscle in IIMs is usually non-tender. Muscle girth comparison on both sides may reveal subtle asymmetrical atrophy and suggests a neurogenic disorder or IBM. Increased tone of the muscle suggests upper motor neuron lesions. Patterns of muscle weakness and corresponding etiologies are shown in Figure 2.5.1.

Assessment of Muscle Strength

Objective assessment of muscle strength is imperative for clinical diagnosis, treatment, and follow-up. The recorded strength of a muscle is an essential part of communication between different doctors and aids in the assessment of improvement or deterioration of functional status. Several tools have been devised to measure muscle strength objectively. However, all of them are prone to biases and interobserver variability.

Medical Research Council (MRC) scale: The strength of different muscles/muscle groups is graded most commonly using the Medical Research Council (MRC) scale (Table 2.5.2). A system of subgrades (4^+, 4^-, etc.) is used by many clinicians.

Table 2.5.1: Clinical clues to underlying etiology of muscle weakness

Facial involvement, orbital muscle involvement	FSHD, myasthenia gravis, mitochondrial myopathy
Skin involvement	Dermatomyositis, sarcoidosis.
Distal more than proximal muscles	IBM, hereditary distal myopathies.
Proximal more than distal, symmetrical	IIMs (except IBM), hereditary myopathies, metabolic myopathies (some glycolytic and lipid pathway defects).
Distal arm, proximal leg	IBM, myotonic dystrophy (uncommon presentation).
Proximal arm and distal leg (scapuloperoneal)	FSHD, acid maltase deficiency, LGMD, nemaline myopathy, Emery-Dreifuss dystrophy.
Prominent neck extensor weakness ("dropped head")	IIMs, FSHD, carnitine deficiency, myotonic dystrophy, hyperparathyroidism.
Presenting with predominant bulbar weakness	Oculopharyngeal muscular dystrophy.
Episodic weakness	Myasthenia gravis, glycogenoses, lipid disorders, channelopathies.
Stiff muscles, inability to relax	Hypertonia in UMN lesions, myotonic dystrophy, paramyotonia, stiff person syndrome.
Enlarged calf muscles	Bilateral–Duchenne and Becker's muscular dystrophies (pseudo-hypertrophy). Unilateral—occasionally seen with intervertebral disc prolapse.

FSHD: Fascioscapulohumeral muscular dystrophy; *IBM:* Inclusion body myositis; *IIMs:* Idiopathic inflammatory myopathies; *LGMD:* Limb-girdle muscular dystrophies; *UMN:* Upper motor neuron.

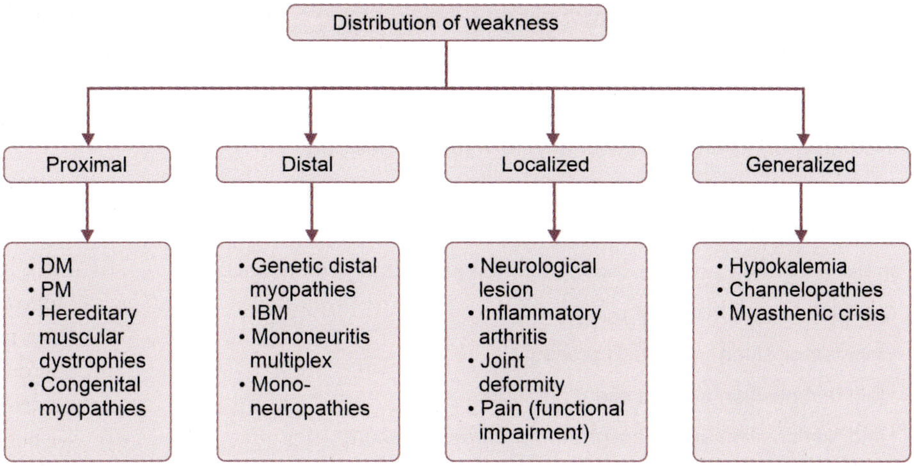

Fig. 2.5.1: Patterns of muscle weakness and their corresponding etiologies. *DM*: Dermatomyositis; *PM*: Polymyositis; *IBM*: Inclusion body myositis

Table 2.5.2: MRC system for grading muscle strength

MRC grade	*Description*
0	No contraction
1	A flicker or trace of contraction
2	Active movement with gravity eliminated
3	Active movement against gravity
4	Active movement against gravity and resistance
5	Normal power

Table 2.5.3: Muscles tested in manual muscle testing (MMT)

Muscles tested in MMT–8	*Additional muscles tested in MMT–26*
Neck flexors	Neck extensors
Deltoid	Trapezius
Biceps	Iliopsoas
Gluteus maximus	Hamstrings
Gluteus medius	Wrist flexors
Quadriceps	Ankle plantar flexors
Wrist extensors	
Ankle dorsiflexors	

MMT-8 is easier to use in the clinic and is done on muscles on one side usually the right. Potential scores: MMT8–(0–80); MMT26–(0–260).

This scale is nonlinear and heavily weighted towards the evaluation of weaker muscles. It is not sensitive to detect mild weakness, therefore, not optimal for monitoring myositis patients, and it also has considerable interobserver and intraobserver variability. Consequently, a number of tools have been developed and validated to examine muscle function in these disorders. This attempt to standardize the grading of muscle strength and technique to grade muscle strength has led to the development of manual muscle testing (MMT).

Manual muscle testing: MMT-8 is the manual muscle testing in 8 designated muscles (Table 2.5.3) tested unilaterally generally on the right. This tool has been specifically developed and validated for the monitoring of disease activity of IIMs. Each of the muscles is graded on a scale of 0–10 to a maximum score of 80 (Table 2.5.4). MMT-26 similarly tests 12 muscle groups (Table 2.5.3). Both MMT-8 and MMT-26 have excellent inter and intra-rater reliability. Examination techniques used in MMT-8 are shown in (Fig. 2.5.2). Examination of severe muscle weakness requires gravity to be eliminated by adopting positions facilitated by the examiner supporting the patient's limb. This is also depicted in Figure 2.5.2.

The International Myositis Assessment and Clinical Studies (IMACS) Group: Disease Activity Core Set Measures (CSM) are the current gold standard of IIM disease activity assessment and

Table 2.5.4: Grading muscle power in manual muscle testing (MMT)

Grade	*Function of muscle*
0	No contraction felt in the muscle
T	Tendon contraction felt without any movement of the part
1	In the horizontal plane, moves through partial range of motion
2	In the horizontal plane, moves through complete range of motion
3	In the antigravity position, moves through partial range of motion
4	Gradual release from test position
5	Hold test position (no added pressure)
6	Hold test position against slight pressure
7	Hold test position against slight-to-moderate pressure
8	Hold test position against moderate pressure
9	Hold test position against moderate-to-strong pressure
10	Hold test position against strong pressure

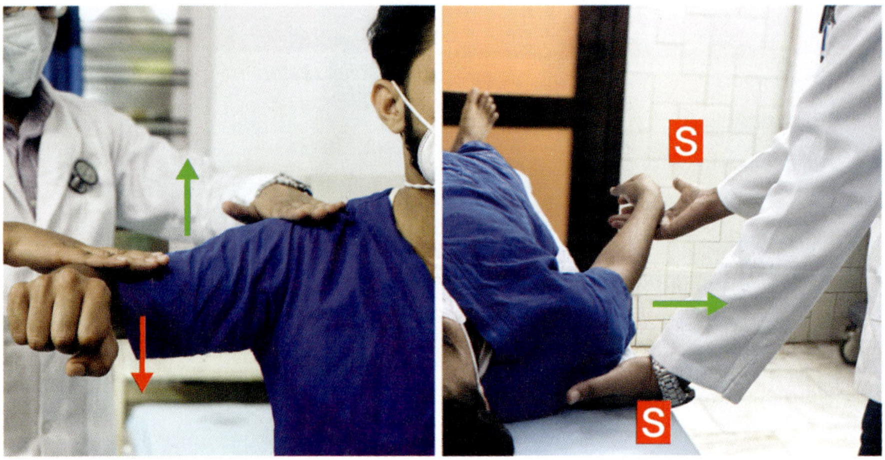

Fig. 2.5.2a: Testing the deltoid muscle against gravity (left) and with gravity eliminated (right)

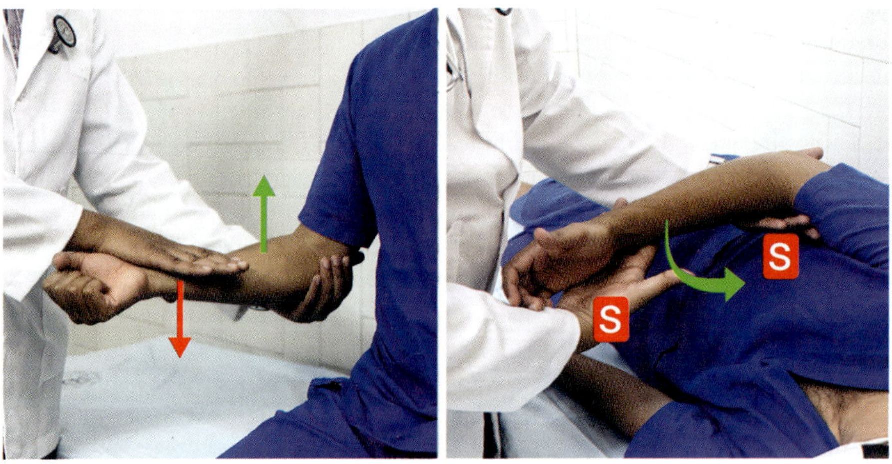

Fig. 2.5.2b: Testing the biceps muscle against gravity (left) and with gravity eliminated (right)

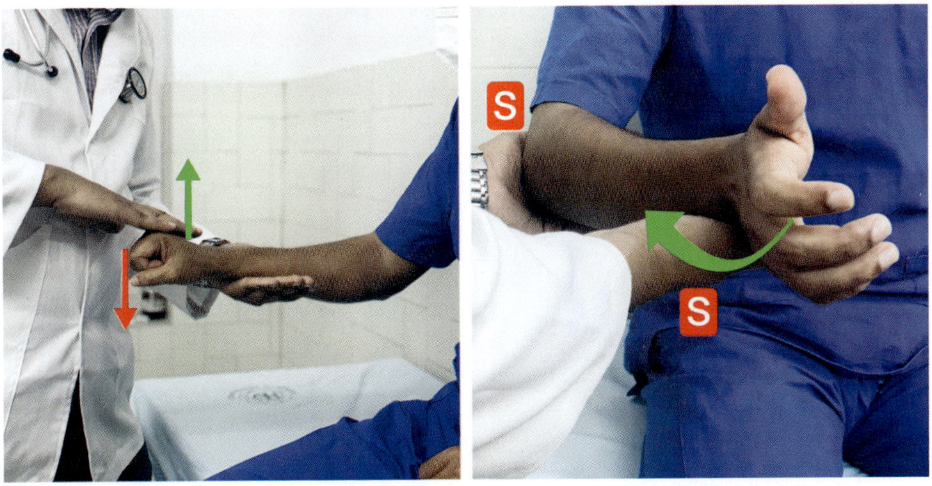

Fig. 2.5.2c: Testing the wrist extensors against gravity (left) and with gravity eliminated (right)

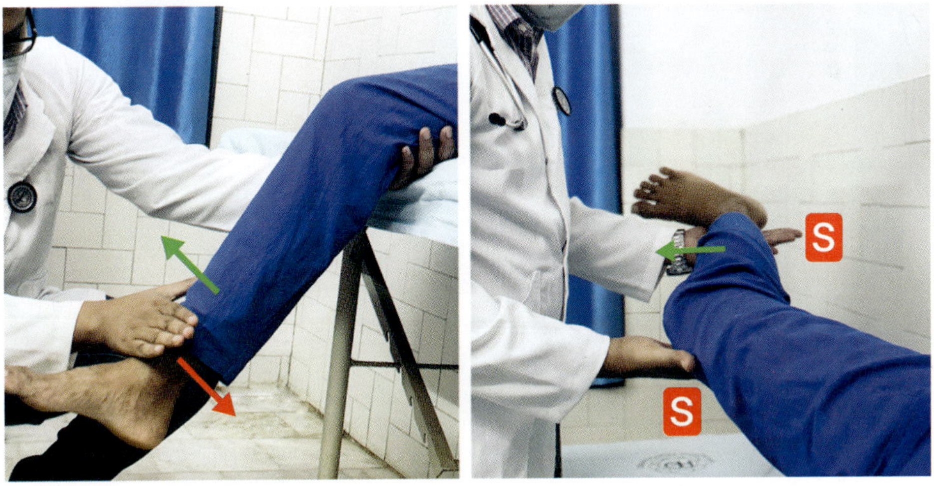

Fig. 2.5.2d: Testing the quadriceps muscle against gravity (left) and with gravity eliminated (right)

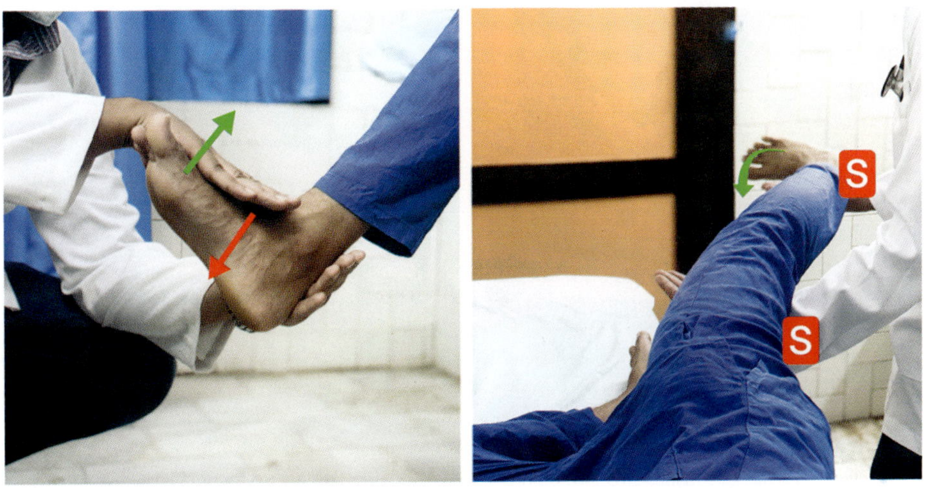

Fig. 2.5.2e: Testing the ankle dorsiflexors against gravity (left) and with gravity eliminated (right)

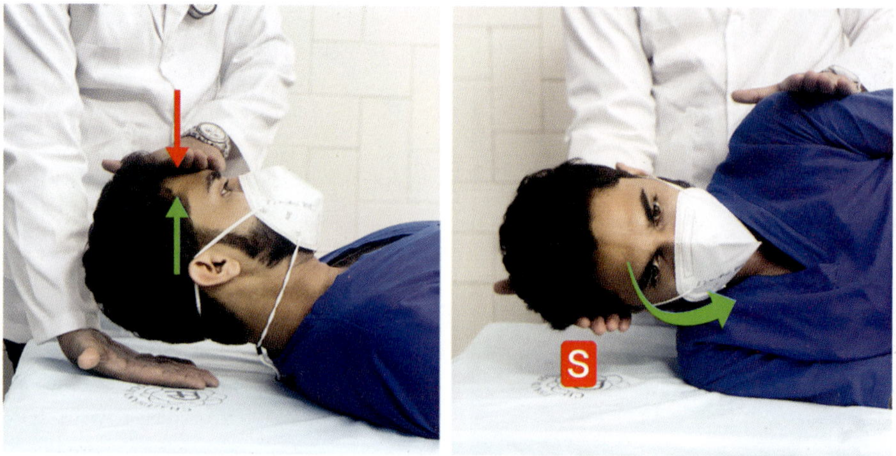

Fig. 2.5.2f: Testing the neck flexors against gravity (left) and with gravity eliminated (right)

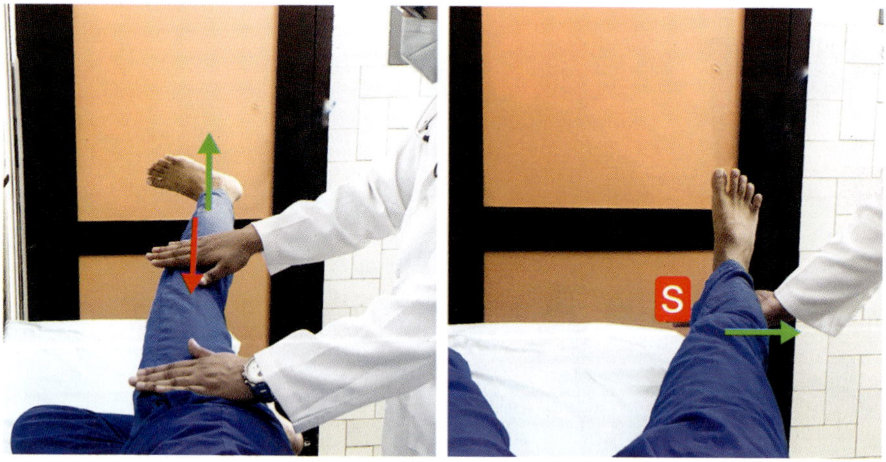

Fig. 2.5.2g: Testing the gluteus medius against gravity (left) and with gravity eliminated (right)

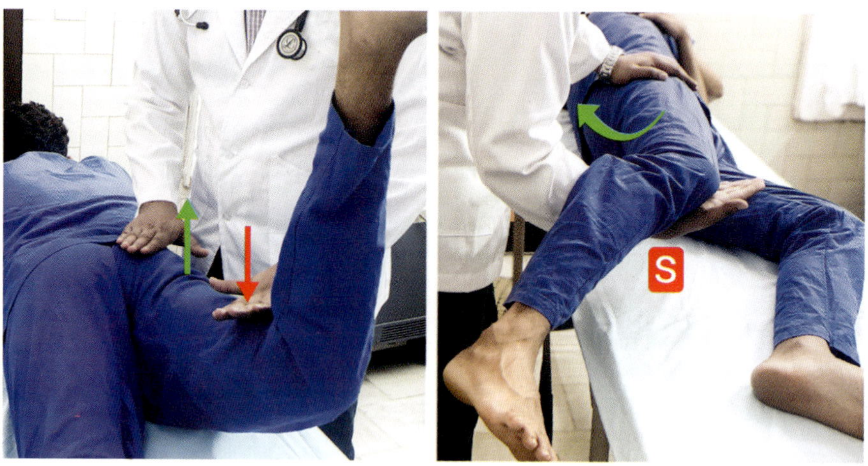

Fig. 2.5.2h: Testing the gluteus maximus against gravity (left) and with gravity eliminated (right)

Fig. 2.5.2a to h: Technique of muscle strength testing in MMT-8 (manual muscle testing-8). Green arrow—direction of force applied by the patient; Red arrow—direction of resistance applied by the examiner; S–support.

include MMT-8. CSM is easily performed, requires no equipment and, has adequate interrater and intrarater reliability and validity when performed by a trained examiner. The need for training the examiner is a major drawback of MMT-8. Poor sensitivity to change, a possible ceiling effect, the need for patient motivation and cooperation, and the effect of muscle atrophy are other problems encountered while performing MMT-8.

Short Physical Performance Battery (SPPB) for lower limb function and **IBM Weakness Composite Index** for muscle strength and endurance have been developed for the evaluation of IBM patients.

Patient-reported Outcome Measures (PROMs)

Several PROMs are available such as patient global assessment (PGA) and pain visual analog scale (pain VAS). Because of the various fallacies as well as intricacies of clinical examination, more objective ways of assessment are being investigated (using dynamometers and accelerometers, for example) and adequate training is important to minimize these biases. Pursuant to this, IMACS has designed a website and training module *(https://connect.niehs.nih.gov/imacs/module/training)*. Various PROMs used to measure physical function are detailed in Table 2.5.5.

Tests for Muscle Strength that can be Performed by the Individual at Home

Traditional methods of clinical examination remain the standard of care, however, in the remote setting, a number of patient maneuvers have been developed which are especially relevant in the present pandemic situation. The main advantage of all these tests is their ease of being performed by the patients themselves at their homes requiring minimal training and no specialized equipment (Fig. 2.5.3). These include:

Table 2.5.5: Various patient reported-outcome measures (PROMs) used to assess physical function in IIMs

PROM	*IIM subgroup*	*Comments*
HAQ-DI	DM, PM	8 ADL domains, Many language translations available
CHAQ	JDM	8 ADL domains, can be completed in 10 minutes
HAP	DM, PM	94 activities assessed
MAP	DM, PM	Takes 5 minutes to complete Correlates moderately to FI-2
MACTAR Semi-structured interview	DM, PM	Complicated scoring system
NSS	IBM	14 items scored from 0 to 3
IBMFRS	IBM	10 ADL domains
sIFA	IBM	Disease-specific PROM
CHQ-PF50	JDM	50 items assessed Complicated
NHP	DM, PM	38 items assessed including life areas
PedsQL	JDM	Fatigue scale has high responsiveness in JDM
INQoL	IBM	45 questions using Likert scale scoring

PROM: Patient-reported outcome measure; *IIM:* Idiopathic inflammatory myopathy; *HAQ-DI:* Health assessment questionnaire disability index; *DM:* Dermatomyositis; *PM:* Polymyositis; *ADL:* Activities of daily living; *CHAQ:* Child health assessment questionnaire; *JDM:* Juvenile dermatoymyositis; *HAP:* Human activity profile; *MAP:* Myositis activities profile; *FI-2:* Functional index-2; *MACTAR:* MacMaster Toronto arthritis patients preference questionnaire; *NSS:* Neuromuscular symptom and disability functional score; *IBM:* Inclusion body myositis; *IBMFRS:* IBM Functional Rating Scale; *sIFA:* sporadic inclusion body myositis physical functioning assessment; *CHQ-PF50:* Child health questionnaire-parent form 50; *NHP:* Nottingham health profile; *PedsQL:* Pediatric quality of life inventory; *INQoL:* Individual neuromuscular quality of life questionnaire.

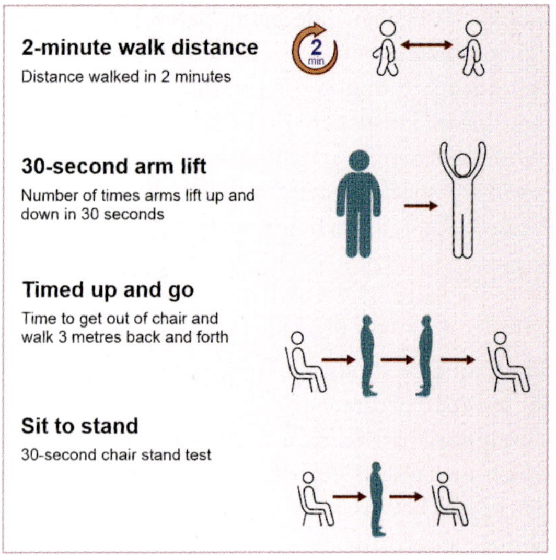

Fig. 2.5.3: Some commonly used remote tests of muscle strength useful in the present pandemic situation

- **2-minute walk distance:** It is the distance walked by the patient in two minutes. It requires no specialized equipment and can be done indoors. It does not take into account upper limb weakness and is more relevant in testing patients with IBM. The 6-minute walk distance may also be used but may be tiring to the patient.
- **30-second arm lift:** It is the number of times the arm can be lifted up and down in 30 seconds. It does not take into account lower limb weakness.
- **Ten times-arm lift test:** Record the time required for overhead abduction of the arms ten times at the fastest pace possible.
- **Timed up and go:** It is the time required to get up from a chair and walk 3 metres back and forth. The need to measure the distance of 3 meters and difficulty in getting up from a sitting position in moderate to severe weakness are its disadvantages. Usually, an arm-less chair is used but an arm-chair may also be used and this has to be documented.
- **Sit to stand test:** It is the number of times a patient can sit and stand from a chair alternately in 30 seconds. The disadvantage of needing enough muscle strength to get up from the chair applies to this test as well.
- **Leg-crossing capacity:** It is evaluated by asking the patient to cross legs without using hands.
- **Squatting capacity:** It is evaluated by asking the patient to bend his/her knees and hips at a 90° angle.
- **Endurance tests include:**
  - **Barré test:** Time in seconds during which patient can maintain his arms in flexion at a 90° angle with completely extended elbows
  - **Mingazzini test:** Time in seconds during which patient can maintain the supine position, with legs bent.

All these tests are more comprehensive if done together rather than individually. It is more important to see the results serially than considering a single test at a single point in time. With the almost ubiquitous presence of smartphones, it might soon enable the treating rheumatologist to observe the patient doing these tests on recorded video which can be shared through medical consultation apps or social media platforms, thus ensuring the test is reliable and reproducible.

Assessment of Muscle Function

Functional index: The IIMs are chronic and at times lead to muscle damage, in turn affecting functional performance. The functional index is a disease specific measure developed to quantify functional outcome (assessing muscle endurance) in myositis. Functional Index (FI) used in DM and PM patients consists of 14 tasks, which was reduced to 11 tasks in seven muscle groups in the Functional Index-2 (FI2) (Table 2.5.6). A Functional Index-3 (FI3), which is quicker and easier to perform, has recently been developed.

In IBM, due to its differing presentation from other IIMs, a new functional scoring system was developed that is called the Inclusion Body Myositis-Functional Rating Scale (IBM-FRS) which was adapted from the functional scale used in amyotrophic lateral sclerosis. A childhood myositis assessment scale (CMAS) has also been developed and validated. It uses 14 manoeuvres to assess muscle strength and endurance in children.

CONCLUSION

The primary objective of muscle examination is to identify true muscle weakness, and to rule out myositis mimics and muscle weakness due to other causes. Once true muscle weakness is established, the next important step is to objectively assess and record the muscle strength as well as maintain consistency in strength assessment over time.

Table 2.5.6: Components of Functional Index-2 (FI-2)

Muscle groups	*Description of task*
Shoulder flexion (right and left)	Sit on a back-less chair with a 1kg weight cuff around wrist and flex shoulder.
Shoulder abduction (right and left)	Sit on a back-less chair and abduct shoulder (no weight cuffs).
Head lift	Lie on a flat surface and lift the head up as much as possible.
Hip flexion (right and left)	Lie flat with a pillow under the head and do a straight leg raise with heel 40 cm from bench.
Step test (right and left)	Using a 25 cm high stool (40 cm from the wall) and balancing with one hand on the wall, climb using one leg and descend using the other.
Heel lift	Lift the heels at least 1 cm from floor, using the wall as a support.
Toe lift	With the heels 15 cm from the wall, the back and hips leaning on the wall, lift the toes up (MTP joints should not touch the floor)

LEARNING POINTS

- Examination of muscle strength is important for both the diagnosis and monitoring of disease activity of myositis.
- MMT-8 is specifically validated for this purpose and is an essential skill for the management of myositis patients.
- The limited scale of Medical Research Council grading for muscle strength may be suboptimal for monitoring disease activity.
- Integration of digital health services in the post COVID era may potentially pave the way for patient-reported outcome measures for objective assessment remotely.

FURTHER READING

1. Barohn RJ, Dimachkie MM, Jackson CE. A pattern recognition approach to patients with a suspected myopathy. Neurol Clin. 2014;32:569–93.
2. Gupta L, Chinoy H. Monitoring disease activity and damage in adult and juvenile idiopathic inflammatory myopathy. Curr Opin Rheumatol. 2020;32:553–61.
3. Oldroyd A, Little MA, Dixon W, et al. A review of accelerometer-derived physical activity in the idiopathic inflammatory myopathies. BMC Rheumatol. 2019;3:41.
4. Rider LG, Werth VP, Huber AM, et al. Measures of adult and juvenile dermatomyositis, polymyositis, and inclusion body myositis: Physician and Patient/Parent Global Activity, Manual Muscle Testing (MMT), Health Assessment Questionnaire (HAQ)/Childhood Health Assessment Questionnaire (C-HAQ), Childhood Myositis Assessment Scale (CMAS), Myositis Disease Activity Assessment Tool (MDAAT), Disease Activity Score (DAS), Short Form 36 (SF-36), Child Health Quevstionnaire (CHQ), physician global damage, Myositis Damage Index (MDI), Quantitative Muscle Testing (QMT), Myositis Functional Index-2 (FI-2), Myositis Activities Profile (MAP), Inclusion Body Myositis Functional Rating Scale (IBMFRS), Cutaneous Dermatomyositis Disease Area and Severity Index (CDASI), Cutaneous Assessment Tool (CAT), Dermatomyositis Skin Severity Index (DSSI), Skindex, and Dermatology Life Quality Index (DLQI). Arthritis Care Res (Hoboken). 2011; 63 Suppl 11(0 11):S118–57.
5. Rider LG, Aggarwal R, Machado PM, et al. Update on outcome assessment in myositis. Nat Rev Rheumatol. 2018;14:303–18.
6. Saygin D, Oddis CV, Moghadam-Kia S, et al. Hand-held dynamometry for assessment of muscle strength in patients with inflammatory myopathies. Rheumatology. 2021;60:2146–56.

Chapter 2.6

Skin Examination in Rheumatology

Logamoorthy Ramamoorthy, Laxmisha Chandrashekar

INTRODUCTION

Skin may be the initial site of involvement in many rheumatic diseases. Therefore, a properly done skin examination and early recognition of cutaneous signs help in the correct diagnosis of rheumatic disease. However, skin changes also occur in a patient with rheumatic disorders secondary to medications used to treat the rheumatic disorder. This chapter highlights principles of skin examination, and important cutaneous signs and symptoms of relevant rheumatic diseases.

SKIN EXAMINATION FOR THE RHEUMATOLOGIST

- First, principle of skin examination is to examine the patient in a well-lit room, with the patient appropriately disrobed. It is useful to have a pocket flashlight at hand in order to illuminate the area being examined.
- Secondly, do not forget to examine the nails, oral mucous membranes, hair, palms, and soles. Examine the patient overall from a seating distance, then focus on individual lesions.
- Thirdly, check whether the lesions are generalized or only in sun-exposed areas as is typically seen in lupus, or whether the lesions are distributed in a dermatomal pattern as seen in herpes zoster or whether the extensor surfaces of elbows and knees are involved as is seen in psoriasis. This is in contrast to atopic dermatitis where the lesions are present on the flexural surfaces. To determine whether the lesions are primary (namely macular or papular or vesicular, etc.) or secondary (fissure or crusts or ulcer, etc.) would often need the expertise of a dermatologist. Other things to look for are the size, shape, and color of the lesions.

CUTANEOUS FINDING IN RELEVANT CONNECTIVE TISSUE DISEASES

Systemic Lupus Erythematosus (SLE)

Cutaneous manifestation follows arthralgias as the most common clinical feature of SLE. About 1/4th patients have skin manifestations as the presenting feature. Classification of skin manifestations of SLE is challenging for a nondermatologist. Gilliam and Sontheimer developed the most widely accepted classification of cutaneous lupus erythematosus (Table 2.6.1). From among the lesions listed in Table 2.6.1, some are commonly encountered in day-to-day practice and some are rare.

A typical representation of malar rash, toxic epidermal necrolysis-like presentation of acute cutaneous lupus erythematosus, and classic discoid lupus erythematosus (DLE) are shown in Figures 2.6.1 to 2.6.3. Lupus hair shown in Figure 2.6.4 is considered a nonspecific LE skin lesion.

Dermatomyositis (DM)

Skin examination in dermatomyositis is important because characteristic cutaneous lesions are present that are diagnostic of dermatomyositis. In 60% of patients, there is simultaneous involvement of both skin and muscle, in 30% skin manifestations come before muscle disease and in 10% patients muscle weakness precedes the onset of skin lesions.

Table 2.6.1: Gilliam–Sontheimer classification of cutaneous lupus erythematosus (LE)

LE-specific skin lesions	*LE-nonspecific skin lesions*
1. Acute cutaneous lupus erythematosus (ACLE) • Malar rash (Fig. 6.2.1) • Maculopapular rash • Photosensitive lupus dermatitis • Toxic epidermolytic necrosis like ACLE (Fig. 6.2.2) 2. Subacute cutaneous lupus erythematosus (SCLE) • Papulosquamous SCLE • Annular SCLE 3. Chronic cutaneous lupus erythematosus • Classic Discoid lupus erythematosus (DLE) (Fig. 6.2.3) – Localized DLE (confined to head and neck) – Generalized DLE (involves head and neck and below the neck) • Hypertrophic/verrucous DLE • Mucosal DLE (conjunctival /oral DLE) • Lupus tumidus • Chilblain LE • LE/lichen planus overlap • Lupus profundus/lupus panniculitis	1. Cutaneous vascular disease • Vasculitis (leukocytoclastic vasculitis, urticarial vasculitis, polyarteritis nodosa like cutaneous lesions) • Vasculopathy (Degos' disease like lesions, livedoid vasculopathy) • Periungual telangiectasia • Livedo reticularis/racemose • Thrombophlebitis • Raynaud's phenomenon • Erythromelalgia 2. Nonscarring alopecia • Lupus hair (Fig. 2.6.4) • Telogen effluvium • Alopecia areata 3. Sclerodactyly 4. Rheumatoid nodules 5. Calcinosis cutis 6. LE-nonspecific bullous lesions 7. Urticaria 8. Papulonodular mucinosis 9. Cutis laxa/anetoderma 10. Acanthosis nigricans 11. Erythema multiforme 12. Leg ulcers 13. Lichen planus 14. Painless oral or nasopharyngeal ulcers

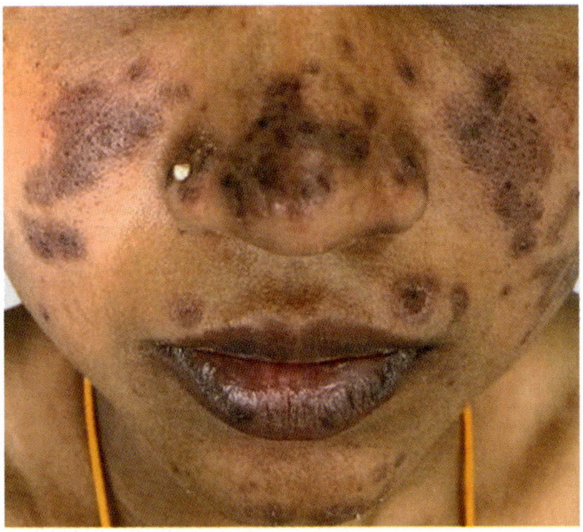

Fig. 2.6.1: Fixed erythema involving the bilateral malar area and dorsum of nose sparing the nasolabial fold (malar rash)

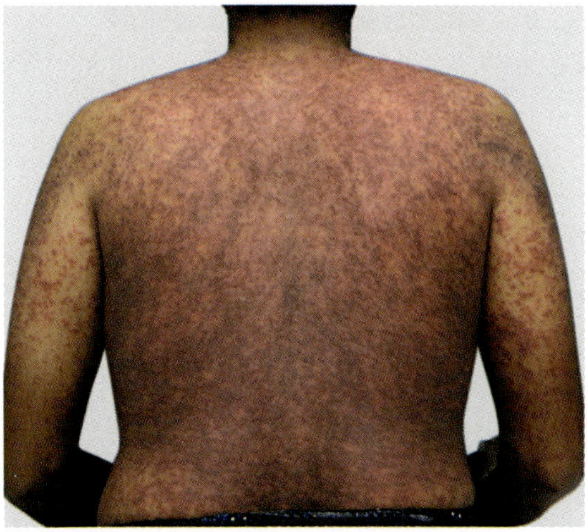

Fig. 2.6.2: Acute cutaneous lupus erythematosus: Toxic epidermal necrolysis presentation

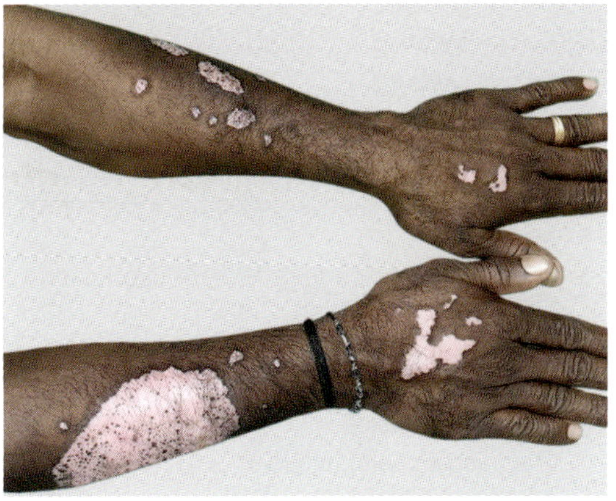

Fig. 2.6.3: Multiple well defined erythematous plaques symmetrically distributed over the bilateral forearm and arm with central depigmentation and atrophy with adherent scaling and peripheral hyperpigmentation (discoid lupus erythematosus)

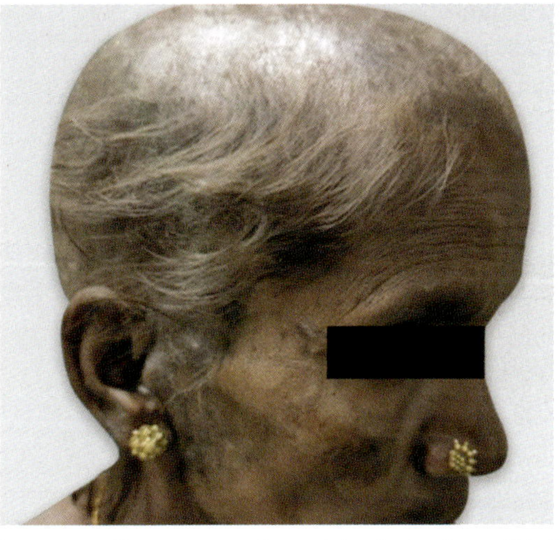

Fig. 2.6.4: Short coarse dry and fragile broken off hair predominantly over the frontal area (lupus hair)

Skin lesions that are characteristic of dermatomyositis are heliotrope rash (Fig. 2.6.5), Gottron's papules (Fig. 2.6.6), and Gottron's sign. Additionally, the presence of macular violaceous erythema over the malar eminence of the face, forehead, or chin (Fig. 2.6.7) can be mistaken for the malar rash of SLE. Macular violaceous erythema distributed over the neck and upper chest is called the V-neck sign (Fig. 2.6.7), the hip is called the holster sign (Fig. 2.6.8) and other areas of distribution are as detailed in Table 2.6.2. Calcinosis cutis (Figure 2.6.9) is also an important manifestation of dermatomyositis.

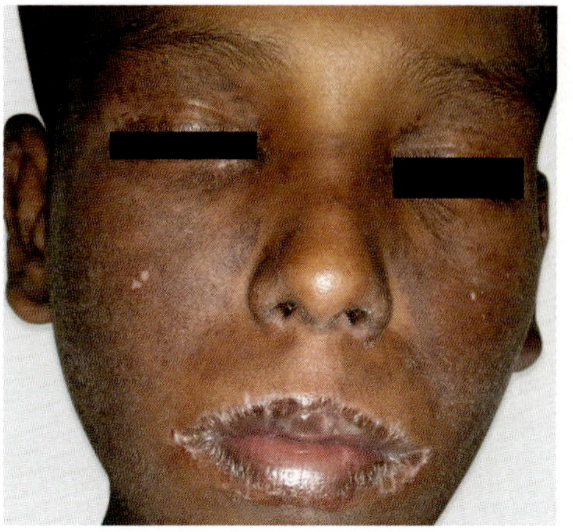

Fig. 2.6.5: Macular violaceous erythema over the periorbital area (heliotrope rash) and bilateral cheeks

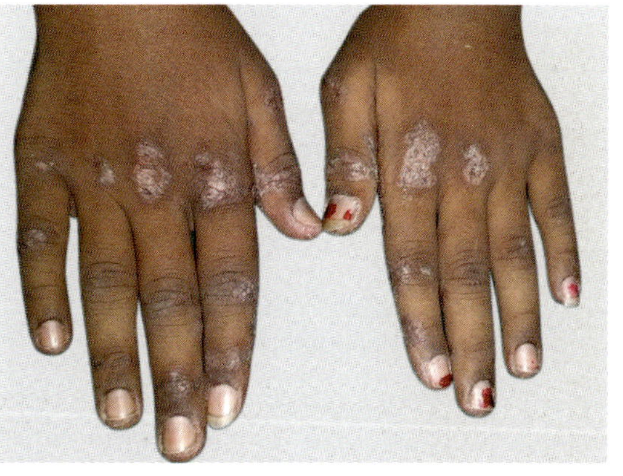

Fig. 2.6.6: : Gottron's papules are multiple erythematous scaly papules and plaques over the dorsal surface of the knuckles (metacarpophalangeal joints) and the interphalangeal joints of both hands

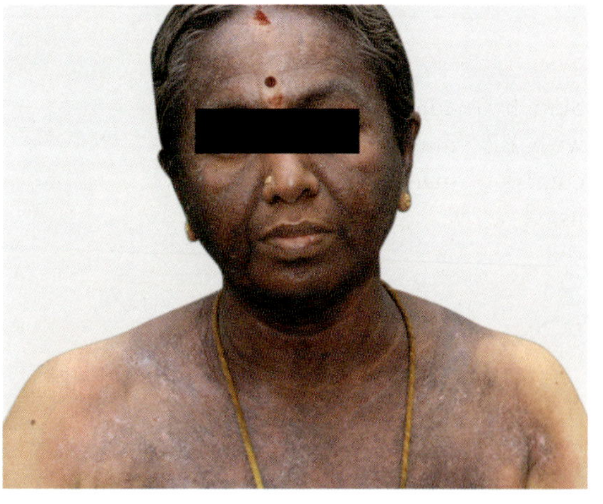

Fig. 2.6.7: Confluent macular violaceous erythema over the face and upper trunk (V-sign) in case of dermatomyositis

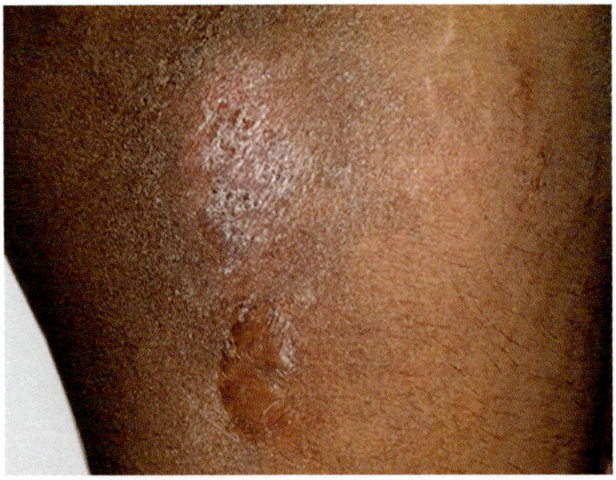

Fig. 2.6.8: Holster sign: A macular violaceous erythema with scaling over the lateral aspect of the right thigh is seen in this image

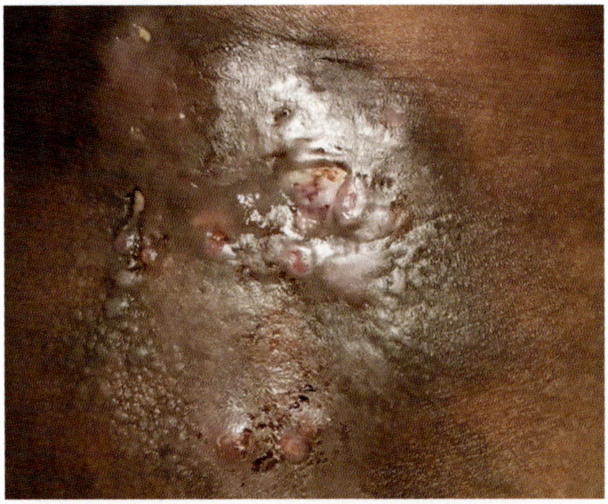

Fig. 2.6.9: Ill-defined hyperpigmented indurated plaque with chalky white discharging sinus over the right thigh (ulcerated calcinosis cutis)

Table 2.6.2: Sontheimer's criteria for cutaneous dermatomyositis

Major criteria

1. Heliotrope rash (Fig. 2.6.5)
2. Gottron papules (Fig. 2.6.6)
3. Gottron sign

Minor criteria

1. Macular violaceous erythema involving:
    - i. Scalp or the anterior hairline
    - ii. Malar eminences of face, forehead, or chin (Fig. 2.6.7)
    - iii. V-area of the neck or upper chest (V-neck sign) (Fig. 2.6.7)
    - iv. Posterior neck or posterior shoulders (shawl sign)
    - v. Extensor surfaces of arms or forearms
    - vi. Linear streaking overlying extensor tendons of dorsal hands
    - vii. Periungual skin
    - viii. Lateral thighs or hips (Holster sign) (Fig. 2.6.8)
    - xi. Medial malleoli
2. Nailfold capillary telangiectasia, hemorrhage-infarct
3. Flagellate erythema
4. Poikiloderma
5. Mechanic's hands
6. Cutaneous calcinosis (Fig. 2.6.9)
7. Cutaneous ulcers
8. Pruritus

Oral cavity

1. Palatal ovoid patch
2. Gingival telangiectasia
3. Lichen planus-like lesions

Sontheimer's criteria for cutaneous dermatomyositis is based on the presence of two major or one major and two minor criteria plus skin biopsy suggestive of cutaneous dermatomyositis.

Systemic sclerosis (SSc)

Skin involvement is a cardinal feature and manifests with Raynaud's and sclerodactyly. The various cutaneous manifestations of systemic sclerosis are listed below.

Cutaneous Manifestations of SSc

- Skin thickening in both limited and diffuse cutaneous systemic sclerosis.
- Typical scleroderma facies with hyperemia, microstomia with radial furrowing around the mouth, telangiectasia (mat-like), and beaked nose (Fig. 2.6.10)
- Inability to retract the lower eyelid is called Ingram's sign
- Tightening with ridging of the skin of the neck on extending the head with a visible and palpable tight band over platysma in the hyperextended neck is called Barnett's sign
- Salt and pepper pigmentation (Fig. 2.6.11)
- Sclerodactyly with dermatogenous contractures
- Raynaud's phenomenon
- Mechanics hands
- Digital ulcers with pitted scars (Fig. 2.6.12)

- The disappearance of the peaked contour on fingerpads and replacement with a hemisphere-like fingertip contour is called Mizutani's sign. This sign is especially marked on the ring finger.
- Calcinosis cutis

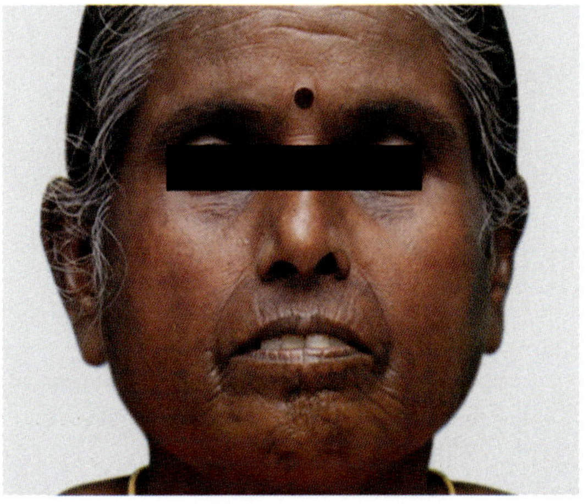

Fig. 2.6.10: Diffuse tightening of the skin over the face with perioral furrowing and beaked nose (systemic sclerosis)

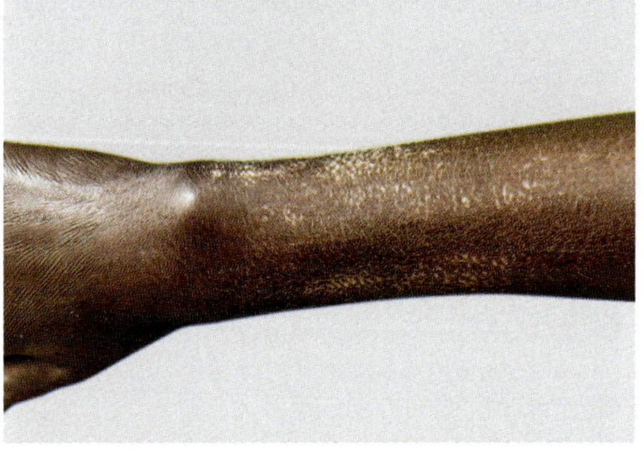

Fig. 2.6.11: Salt and pepper pigmentation with skin tightening in a case of systemic sclerosis

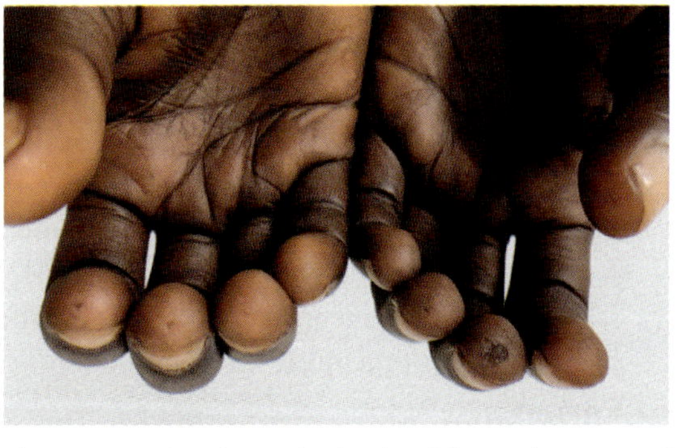

Fig. 2.6.12: Pitted scars in the tip of fingers in a case of systemic sclerosis

Rheumatoid Arthritis (RA)

RA is a systemic inflammatory autoimmune disease with debilitating chronic symmetric polyarthritis and extra-articular manifestations. Cutaneous manifestations occur in more aggressive forms of RA (Table 2.6.3). Of the cutaneous manifestations, pyoderma gangrenosum is particularly debilitating (Fig. 2.6.13).

Sjögren Syndrome

Cutaneous manifestations are common extra-glandular features and are classified as either vasculitis or non-vasculitic lesions.

Vasculitic Cutaneous Lesions Observed in Sjogren's Syndrome

- Hypergammaglobulinemic purpura
- Cutaneous vasculitis
  - Nonpalpable purpura
  - Palpable purpura (Fig. 2.6.14)
  - Urticarial vasculitis
  - Necrotizing vasculitis

Table 2.6.3: Cutaneous manifestations of rheumatoid arthritis (RA)

Specific cutaneous manifestations in RA

1. Palisading granuloma
   - Rheumatoid nodule
   - Granulomatous dermatosis (interstitial or palisading neutrophilic)
2. Neutrophilic dermatosis
   - Pyoderma gangrenosum (Fig. 2.6.13)
   - Sweet's syndrome
   - Rheumatoid neutrophilic panniculitis
3. Vascular cutaneous lesions
   - Bywaters lesion (small painful purpuric nodules over the pulp of digits)
   - Cutaneous small-vessel vasculitis
   - Capillaritis
   - Intravascular/intralymphocytic histiocytosis
4. Methotrexate triggered accelerated rheumatoid nodules

Nonspecific cutaneous manifestations

- Skin appears pale, atrophic and fragile, with easy bruising
- Palmar erythema
- Raynaud's phenomenon
- Brittle nails

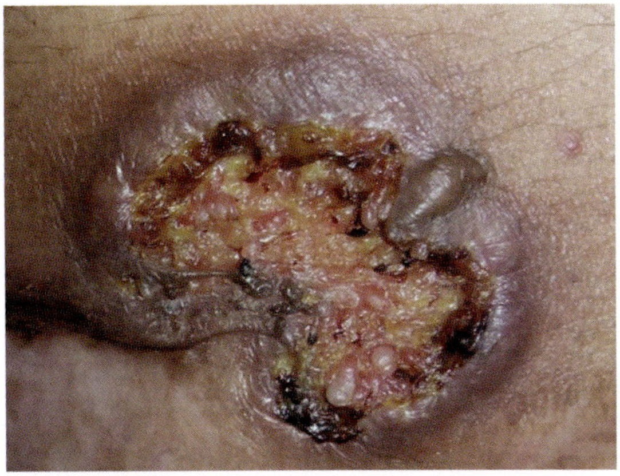

Fig. 2.6.13: Necrolytic ulcer with irregular violaceous undermined border (pyoderma gangrenosum)

- Annular erythema associated with Sjogren syndrome
- Erythema multiforme
- Erythema perstans
- Erythema nodosum

Nonvasculitic Cutaneous Lesions in Sjögren's Syndrome

- Oral cavity
  - Dry mucous membrane
  - Papillary atrophy of the tongue
  - Candidiasis
  - Angular cheilitis
- Eyelid dermatitis
- Alopecia
- Vitiligo

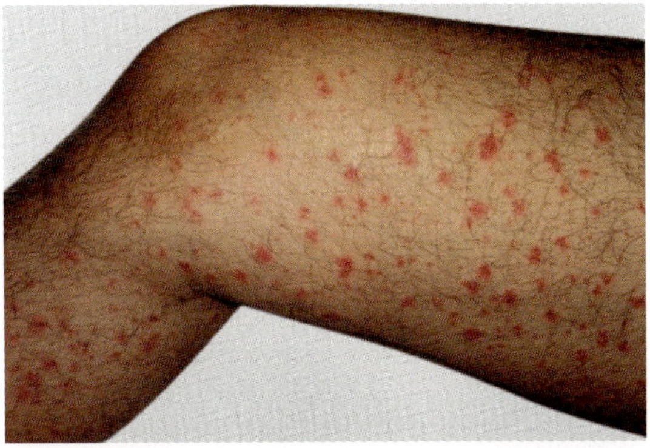

Fig. 2.6.14: Multiple palpable purpuric nonblanchable lesions over the right lower limb (small vessel vasculitis)

Still's Disease

Still's disease can be a severe debilitating systemic illness that is often difficult to diagnose. The majority of these patients have an exanthem, which is the most distinctive sign of this disorder.

Cutaneous Manifestations of Still's Disease

- Asymptomatic transient salmon-colored evanescent with linear macules, papules, and plaques at pressure or trauma sites.
- Periorbital edema
- Linear, persistent pruritic violaceous papules and nodules

LEARNING POINTS

- Examine the patient in a well-lit room, with the patient appropriately disrobed.
- Secondly, while doing a skin examination do not forget to examine the nails, oral mucous membranes, hair, palms, and soles. Also the natal cleft, behind the ears, and scalp where the lesions of psoriasis can hide.
- The majority of autoimmune rheumatic diseases will have a cutaneous manifestation at some point of time, some are specific and some are nonspecific.

FURTHER READING

1. Decker JL, Esdaile J, Hathaway DE, et al. American Rheumatism Association nomenclature and classification of arthritis and rheumatism (1983). Arthritis Rheum. 1983;2:1029–32.
2. Kittridge A, Routhouska SB, Korman NJ. Dermatologic manifestations of Sjögren syndrome. J Cutan Med Surg. 2011;15:8–14.
3. Lora V, Cerroni L, Cota C. Skin manifestations of rheumatoid arthritis. G Ital Dermatol Venereol. 2018; 153:243–55.
4. Pearson DR, Werth VP, Pappas-Taffer L. Systemic sclerosis: Current concepts of skin and systemic manifestations. Clin Dermatol. 2018;36:459–74.
5. Sontheimer RD. Skin manifestations of systemic autoimmune connective tissue disease: diagnostics and therapeutics. Best Pract Res Clin Rheumatol. 2004; 18:429–62.

Examination of Face and Oral Mucosa

Abhishek Zanwar

INTRODUCTION

Autoimmune rheumatic diseases have multisystem involvement. Orofacial manifestations in systemic autoimmune rheumatic diseases are like a window providing important clues for possible etiology. As an example, diseases such as systemic lupus erythematosus (SLE) and systemic sclerosis (SSc) characteristically involve the face, while the presence of a heliotrope rash is pathognomonic of dermatomyositis. This chapter gives an overview of manifestations of autoimmune rheumatic diseases over the face and oral mucosa.

FACE

Systemic Lupus Erythematosus

Of all the cutaneous manifestations of SLE, involvement of the face is most frequent in acute cutaneous lupus erythematosus (ACLE), followed by the presence of discoid lupus erythematosus (DLE) lesions in chronic cutaneous lupus, while lupus panniculitis can also be seen infrequently. Subacute cutaneous lupus usually spares the face.

- ACLE frequently manifests as malar rash, a characteristic confluent maculopapular rash that spares the nasolabial fold. ACLE can also manifest as diffuse erythematous lesions over the forehead, chin, and eyelid.
- Cold-induced tender, erythematous or violaceous papules or plaques over the nose and ears is a form of chronic cutaneous lupus known as chilblain lupus. Similar lesions are often present on acral areas.
- Lupus erythematosus tumidus is an exquisitely photosensitive edematous, erythematous plaques lesion with a smooth surface usually seen over the cheek.

Dermatomyositis

A characteristic feature of dermatomyositis is heliotrope rash (Fig. 2.7.1), a periorbital erythematous or violaceous rash usually accompanied by oedema. A malar rash is also seen in dermatomyositis but unlike the malar rash of SLE it involves nasolabial fold.

Sarcoidosis

Lupus pernio is a chronic raised, indurated and violaceous rash over the central part of the face, i.e. cheeks and nose. They are quite characteristic of sarcoidosis. Lupus pernio is a disfiguring lesion and can also occur over ears and lips, and other areas of the head and neck as a shiny nodule. Seen in approximately 25% of patients with sarcoidosis. Sometimes it can be the only manifestation and is a predictor of systemic disease.

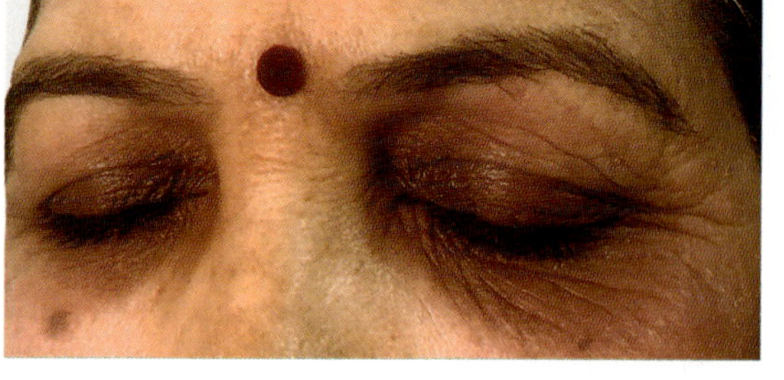

Fig. 2.7.1: A heliotrope rash over the upper eyelids in a patient with dermatomyositis

Systemic Sckrosis

Both limited and diffuse cutaneous SSc involves the face. Skin manifestations differ with the stages of the disease.

- Starting with nonpitting edematous swelling of the face in the "edematous phase" to less inflammatory thickened inflexible skin in the "fibrotic phase".
- Later stages of SSc are characterized by reduced mouth opening (oral aperture), the face appearing like "masked facies". Further, the reduced oral mouth aperture is accompanied by the furrowing of perioral skin and prominent front teeth. Pinched-up nasolabial folds are the other manifestations of SSc in the late stages.
- Salt pepper depigmentation can be evident over the face and scalp.
- Telangiectasis, one of the classifying features of SSc, is commonly distributed over the face (including the oral cavity), hands and upper extremities. They are markers of underlying pulmonary artery hypertension and gastric antral vascular ectasia.
- Localized scleroderma disorders can involve the face in various ways. One of them is "en coup de sabre" which is a linear dyspigmented scar over the forehead and scalp resembling the scar of a sabre sword wound (Fig. 2.7.2). Parry–Romberg syndrome is hemifacial atrophy of subcutaneous tissue, facial muscles and maxilla, and mandible bones.

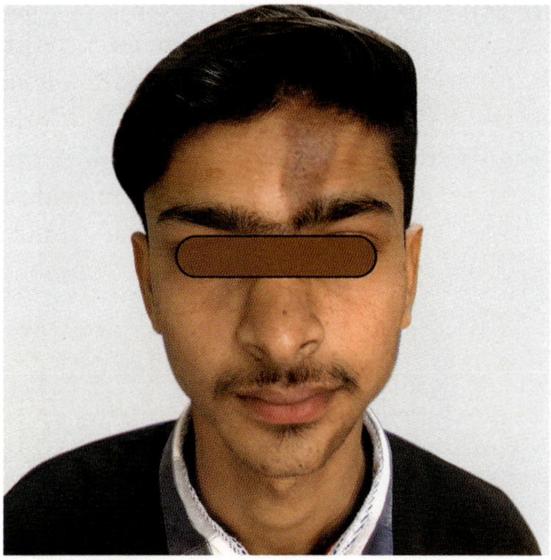

Fig. 2.7.2: A variant of linear morphea (a localized form of scleroderma) restricted to the forehead also called en coup de sabre from French for its resemblance to a scar from a sabre sword

Panniculitis

Lupus profundus is a form of panniculitis with an overlying discoid lesion usually seen in SLE. It can occur over the face and lead to lipodystrophy (Fig. 2.7.3) after the resolution of the nodular phase. Acquired lipodystrophy over the face can also be seen in dermatomyositis and other connective tissue disorders.

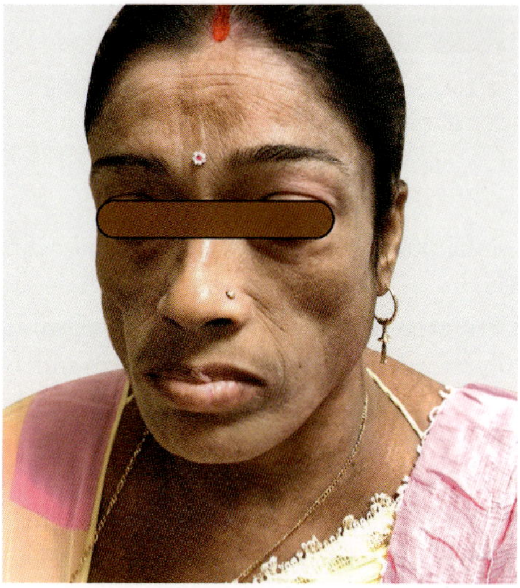

Fig. 2.7.3: Lipodystrophy in a case of SLE

Other Rheumatic Diseases

Nose: Saddle deformity of the nose occurs due to a variety of reasons including trauma, infections, inflammatory diseases, and malignancy. Relapsing polychondritis and granulomatosis with polyangiitis (GPA) (Fig. 2.7.4) are important inflammatory causes of saddle nose deformity.

Ears: Acute painful erythematous swelling of the upper two-thirds of the external ear is characteristic of relapsing polychondritis. Repeated episodes can result in deformed flaccid pinna. Tophi of gout can be deposited on the pinna of the ears (Fig. 2.7.5).

Parotid gland swelling: It can be due to various etiologies. Sarcoidosis, IgG4-related diseases, Sjögren's syndrome (SS), and GPA are usual rheumatic diseases that cause parotidomegaly.

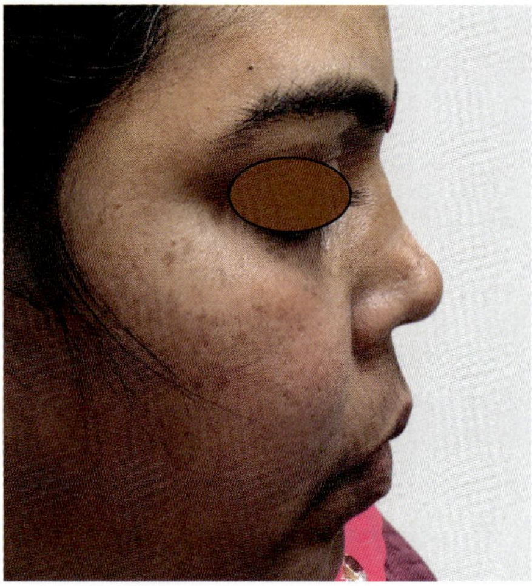

Fig. 2.7.4: Saddle nose deformity in a patient with granulomatosis with polyangiitis

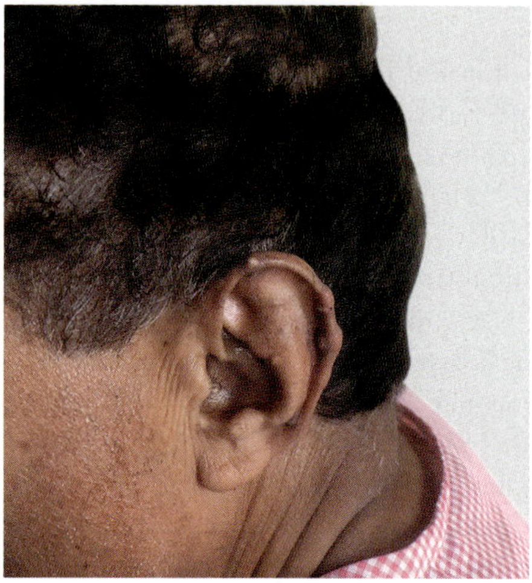

Fig. 2.7.5: Tophi over external ear pinna

Autoinflammatory Disorders

Autoinflammatory disorders can also cause a facial rash.

- Urticaria-like, nonpruritic, erythematous migratory skin rash over the face and body appear during infancy in most cases with the neonatal-onset multisystem inflammatory disorder (NOMID).
- Patients with chronic atypical neutrophilic dermatosis with lipodystrophy and elevated temperature (CANDLE) syndrome have annular-shaped erythematous edematous plaques with raised borders in all cases, usually seen over the trunk but can also occur over the face.
- Progressive lipodystrophy of the face and persistent purplish swelling of the eyelid is also common in CANDLE syndrome.

Other Manifestations in the Face

Temporomandibular joint (TMJ) synovitis is seen in juvenile idiopathic arthritis (JIA), rheumatoid arthritis, and sometimes Sjögren's syndrome. Up to 75% of children with JIA can have TMJ arthritis (2). Micrognathia is often observed in systemic and polyarticular subtypes of JIA.

ORAL MUCOSA

Systemic Lupus Erythematosis

The oral lesions of SLE can be acute, subacute or chronic.

- The most common site for oral lesions is the hard palate (Fig. 2.7.6), buccal mucosa, and the vermilion border though they can occur anywhere in the oral cavity. Acute lesions are usually painless, they range from palatal erythema, to erythematous macules to erosions and ulcerations.
- Subacute lesions in the form of round, well-demarcated red patches are rarely seen. A painful discoid red lesion with radiating hyperkeratotic white striae over buccal mucosa is a typical chronic oral lesion. They usually progress to honeycomb-like lesions.

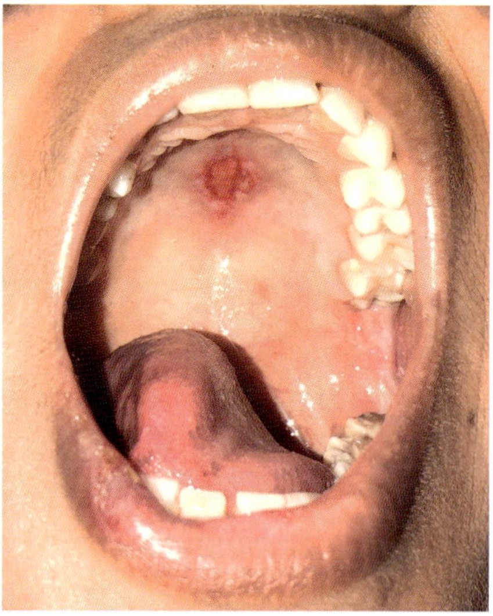

Fig. 2.7.6: Palatal ulcer in a patient with SLE

Sjögren's Syndrome

Oral mucosal dryness (xerostomia) is a hallmark feature of SS. It can present in different ways.

- A patient may present with difficulty in chewing and swallowing dry food or have difficulty in speaking for a prolonged period or present just with altered taste.
- Severe dysfunction might be evident with dry sticky erythematous oral mucosa.
- Another common complication of reduced salivary flow is recurrent and persistent dental caries, and loose and fragile teeth.

Vasculitis

- Painful oral ulcers accompanied by genital ulcers are presenting features of Behçet's disease. Other cutaneous manifestations of Behçet's disease over the face are erythema nodosum, pseudofolliculitis and acneiform nodules along the hairline.
- Reddish hyperplastic gingival swellings with petechial haemorrhages (strawberry gingivitis) are characteristic of GPA. In severe cases, it can cause palatal perforation.
- Extensive cutaneous necrosis over acral areas of the face like the tip of nose and ear lobule triggered by significant cold exposure can be features of cryofibrinogenemia.

To summarize the face and oral mucosa are quite common sites for manifestations of autoimmune rheumatic disease. One should not forget that leprosy can mimic most of the facial involvement of rheumatic diseases listed above.

LEARNING POINTS

- Many of the acute cutaneous manifestations of SLE manifest on the face and oral mucosa.
- Similarly, clues to the diagnosis of SSc and Sjögren's syndrome can be gathered by examining the face and oral cavity.
- Other lesions that have a predilection for the face are lupus pernio, heliotrope rash, lupus profundus.
- When examining the face, make it a point to carefully observe the bridge of the nose, the ear lobules, the pinna of the ear, parotid gland, temporomandibular joint, and the hairline as these structures can be involved characteristically in various autoimmune diseases.

FURTHER READING

1. Ghiasi M. Strawberry Gingivitis in Granulomatosis with Polyangiitis. N Engl J Med. 2017;377:2073.
2. Hamburger J. Orofacial manifestations in patients with inflammatory rheumatic diseases. Best Pract Res Clin Rheumatol. 2016;30:826–50.
3. Naji Rad S, Vashisht P. Malar Rash. [Updated 2021 Sep 13]. In: StatPearls [Internet]. Treasure Island (FL): StatPearls Publishing; 2022 Jan-. Available from: *https://www.ncbi.nlm.nih.gov/books/NBK555981.*

Eye Examination in Patients with Rheumatic Complaints

Ramesh Jois, Kalpana Babu

INTRODUCTION

Ocular involvement in patients with rheumatic diseases is not uncommon. Eye involvement can precede or follow the development of rheumatic diseases. Missed or delayed diagnosis of ocular disease can result in ocular morbidity and/or visual loss. An interdisciplinary approach between the rheumatologist and ophthalmologist is crucial for the effective management of inflammatory eye diseases. This chapter gives an overview of eye examination of relevance to the rheumatologist.

ANATOMY OF THE EYEBALL

Eyeball (Fig. 2.8.1) comprises an outer coat consisting of the transparent cornea and white sclera; the middle coat consists of the uveal tract, and the inner coat consists of the retina. The uveal tract consists of the iris (visible part of the uveal tract which gives color to the eye), the ciliary body (middle layer of the uveal tract which produces aqueous), and the choroid (posterior layer of the uvea rich in blood vessels). The conjunctiva and episclera are anterior to the sclera. Extraocular structures include the eyelids, extraocular muscles, lacrimal glands, nasolacrimal duct, and orbital tissue. All of these structures can be affected in various rheumatological diseases.

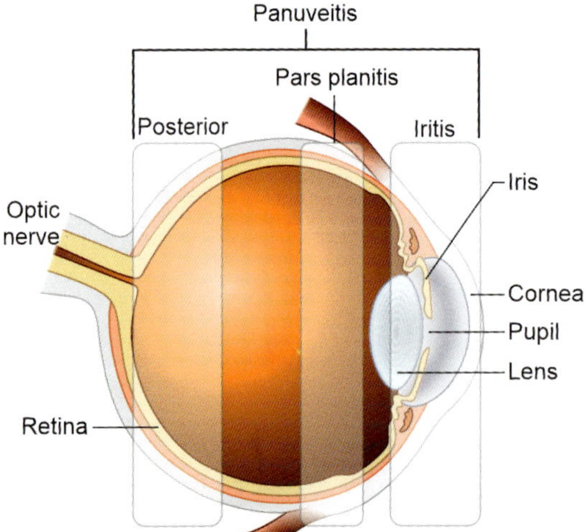

Fig. 2.8.1: Anatomy of the eyeball

EXAMINATION OF THE EYE

The purpose of eye examination in patients with rheumatic diseases or those presenting with rheumatological complaints is to help with anatomical localization, assessment of the severity of eye disease, and extent of ocular damage. All of these aid in diagnosis and can affect treatment decisions.

Essential Things a Rheumatologist must Know during Eye Examination

For a patient who complains of ocular symptoms, an initial torchlight examination is useful to assess whether it is conjunctivitis or scleritis or the presence of a hypopyon. However, the slit-lamp examination is the gold standard to document intraocular inflammation. Certain important terminologies (Table 2.8.1) are used to describe examination findings.

Table 2.8.1: A glossary of terms used by the ophthalmologist	
Anterior uveitis	Intraocular inflammation predominantly anterior to the lens of the eye
Band keratopathy	Deposition of calcium in the corneal epithelium. A sign of chronic inflammation and inadequate immunosuppression. A common finding in pediatric uveitis (associated with juvenile idiopathic arthritis, sarcoidosis)
Cells (in aqueous and vitreous)	Both the aqueous in the anterior chamber and the vitreous humor in the posterior chamber are technically not a part of the uveal tract. But leukocytes (cells) in either, usually indicate a uveitis
Cystoid macular edema (CME)	Common complication of uveitis that affects central vision and is often treated by a local corticosteroid injection
Central serous chorioretinopathy (CSR)	Collection of subretinal fluid in the macular area due to defective retinal pigment epithelial pump resulting in central vision loss. It occurs as a complication of systemic steroids. Treatment requires cessation of oral steroids. Refractory cases require laser photocoagulation to the area of leakage.
Episcleritis	Inflammation of the episclera
Flare	Due to the breakdown of the blood-aqueous barrier in uveitis, there is increased protein in the anterior chamber resulting in diffraction of the slit lamp beam (Tyndall effect). It guides monitoring of therapy.
Fluorescein angiography	Procedure to image the retinal vessels (detect vascular leakages and occlusions) using a special camera and a dye (fluorescein) injected intravenously. Also used to monitor therapy in uveitis.
Hypopyon	Pus or layering of WBCs in the anterior chamber. Indicates severity of inflammation. Seen in ankylosing spondylitis and Behçet's disease
Intermediate uveitis	Inflammation in the intermediate region predominantly in the vitreous humor
Keratic precipitates	Aggregations of cellular deposits adherent to the corneal endothelium seen on slit lamp examination. Fine cellular deposits are characteristic of non-granulomatous uveitis. Large aggregations of cellular deposits are seen in granulomatous uveitis seen in diseases like tuberculosis, sarcoidosis and viral uveitis
Keratitis	It indicates corneal involvement. Peripheral corneal involvement is seen in connective tissue disorders and systemic vasculitis and carry a grave prognosis. Central corneal thinning, perforation are seen in rheumatoid arthriti
Keratoconjunctivitis sicca	Severe dry eye (rheumatoid arthritis, Sjögrens syndrome, sarcoidosis)
OCT	Noninvasive imaging procedure to detect cystoid macular edema, retinal and choroidal inflammation. Commonly performed for monitoring therapy and HCQS toxicity
Panuveitis	Inflammation simultaneously in the anterior chamber, the vitreous humor and the retina and/or choroid
Posterior synechiae	Adherence of the iris to the lens. This is a nonspecific finding more common in acute forms of uveitis such as HLA B27 related anterior uveitis and or chronic uveitis like sarcoidosis and tuberculosis
Posterior uveitis	Inflammation involving the choroid and the adjacent retina and cells in the vitreous humor.
Retinal vasculitis	Inflammation resulting in abnormality of retinal vessels such as increased vascular permeability. A common feature in many forms of uveitis and does not correlate well with the occurrence of systemic vasculitis.
Scleritis	Inflammation of the sclera. It can be necrotising (rheumatoid arthritis, GPA) or non-necrotising scleritis.
SUN criteria	Standardization of uveitis nomenclature. An international consortium that has helped to define terms related to uveitis

The recommended screening tests are fundus examination, automated visual fields and spectral domain OCT.

OCULAR MANIFESTATIONS OF RHEUMATIC DISEASES

The ocular manifestations of rheumatic diseases are myriad, some are discussed below:

Uveitis

Symptoms of uveitis include redness, pain, photophobia, floaters, diminution of vision or it could be asymptomatic. Depending on the anatomic location of inflammation it could be anterior uveitis (iritis, iridocyclitis), intermediate uveitis, posterior uveitis (choroiditis, retinochoroiditis, chorioretinitis) or panuveitis (involving entire uveal tract) and the causes are different (Table 2.8.2). Figure 2.8.2 shows examples of anatomical subsets of uveitis.

Anterior uveitis is one of the most common reasons for ophthalmology consultation. Spondyloarthritis (SpA) associated uveitis is commonly unilateral and mild. Occasionally severe or fibrinous uveitis

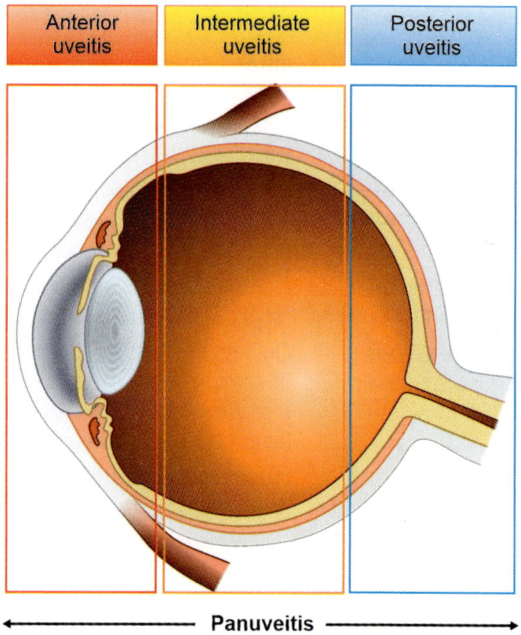

Fig. 2.8.2: Anatomical subsets of uveitis

Table 2.8.2: Symptoms, signs and rheumatic diseases associated with uveitis

Symptoms of uveitis	*Signs of uveitis*	*Rheumatic diseases associated with uveitis*
• Redness • Pain • Photophobia • Floaters • Diminution of vision • Asymptomatic	**Anterior uveitis** • Ciliary congestion • Hypopyon • Fibrin • Flare and cells • Posterior synechiae • Non-granulomatous • Granulomatous **Intermediate uveitis** • Vitritis • Cystoid macular edema **Posterior uveitis** • Retinitis • Choroiditis • Retinochoroiditis/chorioretinitis • Retinal vasculitis • Granulomas **Panuveitis** • Anterior chamber reaction and vitritis • Granulomatous • Optic disc edema • Occlussive retinal vasculitis and "fern-like pattern" of retinal vascular leakage on fluorescein angiography are characteristic findings in Behçet's disease	**Anterior uveitis (Nongranulomatous)** • Juvenile idiopathic arthritis (chronic cases can be granulomatous) • Ankylosing spondylitis • Psoariatic arthritis • Reiter's syndrome • Relapsing polychondritis • Rheumatoid arthritis • Tubulointerstitial nephritis and uveitis **Intermediate uveitis** • Sarcoid • Reiter's syndrome • Tuberculosis **Panuveitis** • Blau syndrome (granulomatous) • Sarcoid (granulomatous) • Tuberculosis (granulomatous) • Behçet's disease

is seen. Figure 2.8.3 illustrates the different forms of uveitis.

JIA is the most common cause of acute anterior uveitis in children. Oligoarthritis with a positive antinuclear antibody is strongly correlated with the development of uveitis in children. Regular eye screening is mandatory in JIA, because anterior uveitis in JIA is asymptomatic in up to 90% of cases, so children may present late with irreversible visual loss. Other causes of visual loss in children are cataracts, glaucoma, band keratopathy, and amblyopia.

Fundus Examination

It is important, especially in connective tissue diseases, systemic vasculitis, sarcoidosis, Blau syndrome, and Behçet's disease. Vitritis, retinitis, retinopathy (cotton wool spots, hemorrhages), vascular occlusions, retinal vasculitis, macular ischaemia, exudative retinal detachments, HCQ-related retinal toxicity, and optic nerve involvement including edema and atrophy can be detected on fundus examinations (Fig. 2.8.4).

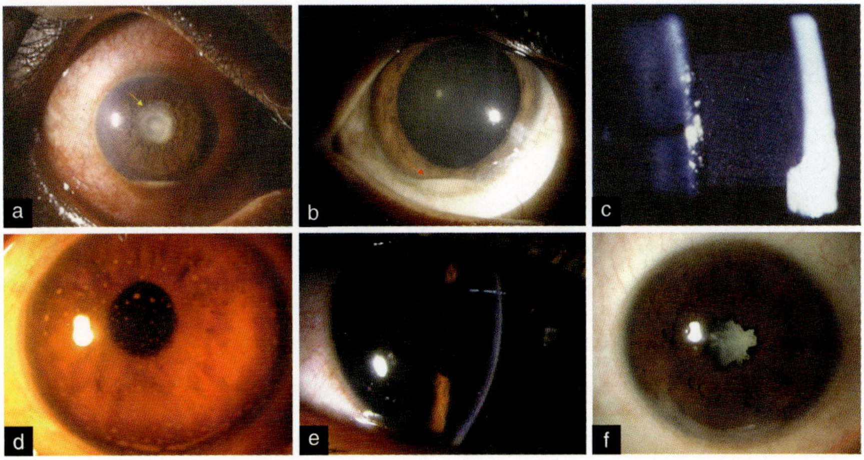

Fig. 2.8.3: (a) Composite slit lamp photographs showing uveitis with hypopyon and fibrin in pupillary area (yellow arrow) with a red eye in ankylosing spondylitis. (b) Hypopyon (red arrow) with a white eye in Behçet's disease. (c) Anterior chamber flare and cells—the Tyndall effect in uveitis on slit-lamp. (d) Mutton fat keratic precipitates in granulomatous uveitis. (e) Fine keratic precipitates in nongranulomatous uveitis. (f) Posterior synechiae with cataract

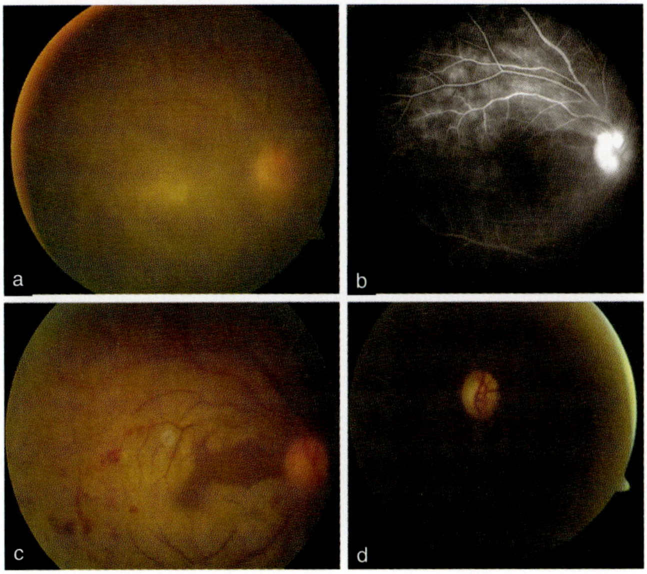

Fig. 2.8.4: Fundus photographs showing: (a) Vitritis with retinitis. (b) Characteristic fern-like pattern of vascular leakage in Behçet's disease. (c) Central retinal artery occlusion in giant cell arteritis. (d) Optic atrophy in Takayasu arteritis

Episcleritis and Scleritis

Association of scleritis and episcleritis (Table 2.8.3) with systemic diseases can occur in 80% of cases at some point in time. Scleritis can be anterior, posterior, or both. It can be nodular, diffuse, sectoral, or necrotizing (Fig. 2.8.5). Necrotizing scleritis and peripheral corneal involvement is associated with systemic vasculitis and collagen vascular diseases.

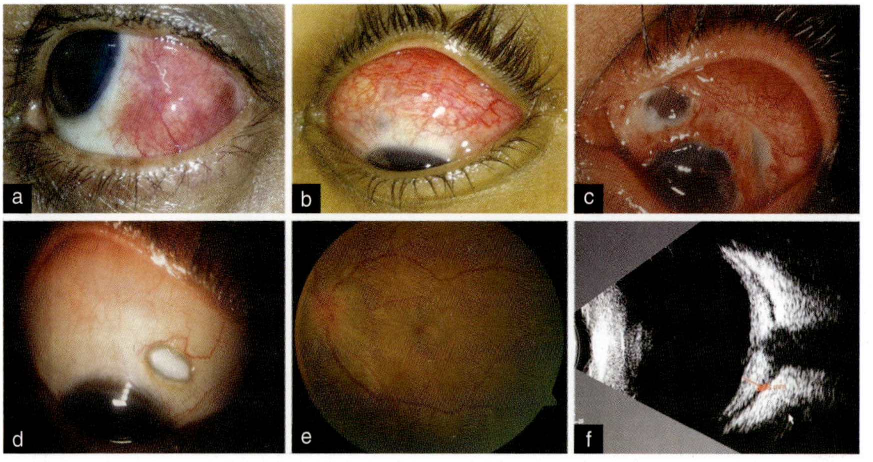

Fig. 2.8.5: Composite slit-lamp photographs showing: (a) Sectoral scleritis. (b) Diffuse scleritis. (c) Necrotizing scleritis with peripheral corneal involvement in ANCA associated vasculitis. (d) Early conjunctival and scleral melt in rheumatoid arthritis. (e) Disc edema with chorioretinal folds in posterior scleritis in SLE. (f) Ultrasonography (B-scan) showing T-sign in posterior scleritis in SLE

Table 2.8.3: Other ocular pathologies in rheumatologic diseases

Ocular symptoms	*Ocular signs*	*Rheumatologic diseases*
Dry eye (keratoconjunctivitis sicca) • Ocular burning • Ocular Itching • Foreign body sensation • Watering	• Decreased tear meniscus • Filaments on cornea • Corneal opacification / ulceration • Schirmer test <5 mm • Slit lamp examination decreased tear meniscus, increased tear debris	• Rheumatoid arthritis • Primary Sjögren's syndrome • Scleroderma • Systemic lupus erythematosus • Sarcoid
Conjunctivitis • Redness • Discharge • Irritation • Watering	• Conjunctival congestion • Discharge	• Reiter's syndrome
Episcleritis • Self limited • Mild pain/ discomfort	• Diffuse/segmental redness • May be nodular	• Rheumatoid arthritis • Vasculitis • Inflammatory bowel disease • Relapsing polychondritis
Scleritis • Redness • Unilateral pain • Headache • Diminution of vision (rarely)	**Non-necrotizing** • Diffuse • Nodular **Necrotizing** • With inflammation	• Rheumatoid arthritis • Granulomatosis with polyangiitis • Relapsing polychondritis **Rarely** • Dermatomyositis

(Contd.)

Table 2.8.3: Other ocular pathologies in rheumatologic diseases *(Contd.)*

Ocular symptoms	*Ocular signs*	*Rheumatologic diseases*
	• Without inflammation (scleromalacia perforans) **With or without Peripheral corneal involvement** • Infiltrates • Thinning • Peripheral ulcerative keratitis (PUK)	• Reiter's syndrome • Ankylosing spondylitis • Systemic lupus erythematosus. **Necrotizing** • Rheumatoid arthritis • GPA **With peripheral ulcerative keratitis (PUK)** • GPA
Corneal involvement • Redness • Pain • Watering • Photophobia	• Peripheral corneal infiltrates • Peripheral/central corneal thinning • Peripheral ulcerative keratitis • Corneal opacification/ulceration	• Sjögren's syndrome • Rheumatoid arthritis • Granulomatosis with angiitis • Eosinophilic granulomatosis with polyangiitis • Relapsing polychondritis • Systemic lupus erythematosis
Orbit involvement • Proptosis • Diplopia • Diminution of vision • Pain on movement of eyeball	• Pseudotumor/orbital mass • Superior oblique tendon sheath syndrome • Dacryoadenitis • Nasolacrimal duct obstruction • Periorbital edema and erythema	• Granulomatosis with polyangiitis • IgG4 disease • Systemic lupus erythematosus • Dermatomyositis
Retinal vasculitis • Diminution of vision • Amaurosis fugax • Transient ischemic attacks	• Cotton wool spots • Retinal hemorrhages • Perivasculitis with sheathing • Retinal vascular occlusions • Ocular ischemic syndrome	• Systemic lupus erythematosus • Large, medium and small vessel vasculitis • Behçet's disease • Sarcoidosis **Rarely,** • Relapsing polychondritis • Rheumatoid arthritis • Crohn's disease • HLA B27 related uveitis
Optic neuropathy • Vision loss (central or peripheral)	• Optic neuritis • Anterior ischaemic optic neruropathy	• Giant cell arteritis • Antiphospholipid syndrome • Systemic lupus erythematosus

Corneal Involvement

Dry eye is a common feature in most rheumatologic diseases (Table 2.8.3). Symptoms include redness, foreign body irritation, and diminution of vision. It is diagnosed on slit-lamp examination. Findings are decreased tear meniscus, increased tear debris, and Schirmer test <5 mm. In addition, corneal infiltrates, corneal scarring, corneal melts, peripheral ulcerative keratitis, subepithelial opacities (Blau syndrome) and band-shaped keratopathy are other findings seen (Fig. 2.8.6).

Orbital Involvement

The orbit can be involved in the form of an orbital mass, pseudotumors (Fig. 2.8.7), preseptal thickening or edema, lacrimal gland enlargements, periorbital edema, heliotrope rash, etc. in diseases like SLE, GPA, and dermatomyositis.

MANAGEMENT

1. **Anterior uveitis:** It is managed with topical steroids and cycloplegics while that for intermediate uveitis is local steroid injections and oral steroids.

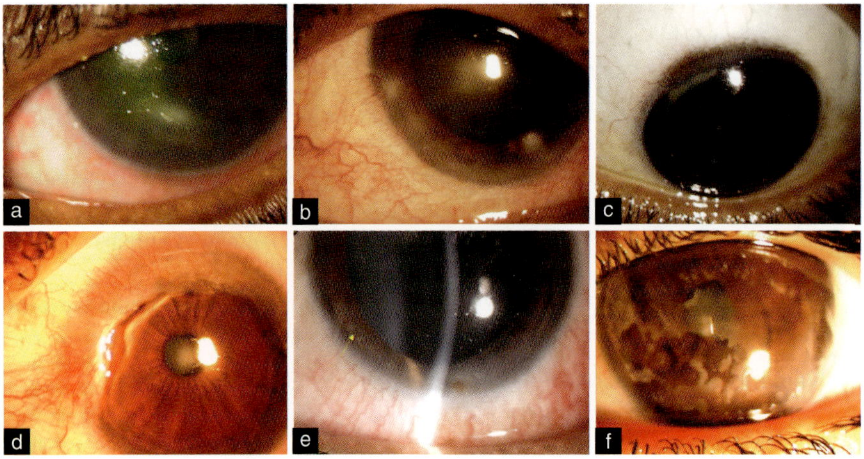

Fig. 2.8.6: Composite slit lamp photographs showing: (a) Keratoconjunctivitis sicca with corneal infiltrate in Sjögren's syndrome. (b) Multiple corneal infiltrates with dry eye in rheumatoid arthritis; (c) Peripheral corneal infiltrate with corneal thinning in SLE. (d) Advancing peripheral corneal melt and ulcerative keratitis in ANCA associated vasculitis; (e) Multiple peripheral round corneal infiltrates (yellow arrow) in SLE. (f) Band keratopathy in chronic uveitis in Juvenile idiopathic arthritis

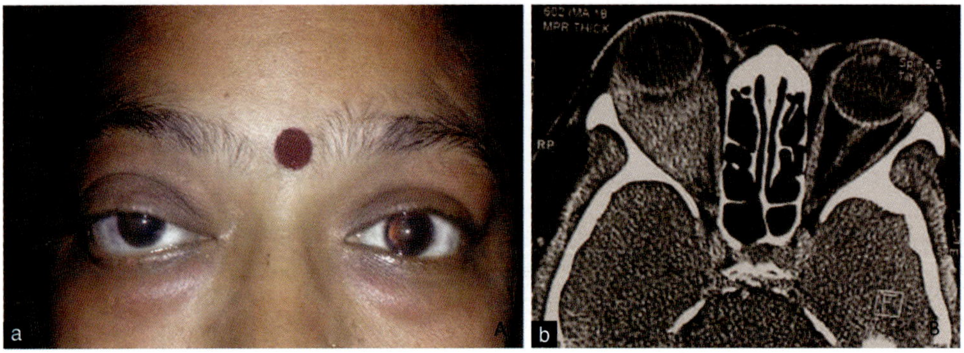

Fig. 2.8.7: (a) Proptosis of the right eye and (b) corresponding computed tomography showing orbital mass in GPA

Recurrent or chronic uveitis may require oral steroids and immunosuppressive drugs. The choice of second-line drugs depends on the underlying rheumatological disease, e.g. methotrexate, adalimumab for SpA and JIA associated uveitis. Methotrexate, mycophenolate or adalimumab in sarcoidosis. Azathioprine, cyclosporin, infliximab, adalimumab, interferon in Beçhet's disease.

2. **Posterior uveitis or retinal vasculitis:** It is preferably treated with oral steroids and second-line immunosuppressive drugs upfront. The choice of drugs is very similar to that used in anterior uveitis. However, retinal vasculitis in lupus would require cyclophosphamide in addition to steroids.
3. **Scleritis:** Nearly 60% of scleritis requires oral steroids and immunosuppression. Azathioprine or methotrexate are commonly used. Severe inflammation such as necrotising scleritis or refractory scleritis may require pulse doses of intravenous methylprednisolone and intravenous cyclophosphamide or rituximab especially when the underlying disease is vasculitis.
4. **Optic nerve and orbital involvement** generally is treated with pulse doses of intravenous methylprednisolone, intravenous cyclophosphamide or rituximab.
5. **Dry eye** or keratoconjunctivitis sicca is treated with topical lubricants, topical cyclosporine, sometimes punctal plugs and good lid hygiene.

Ocular Adverse Effects of Drugs

Ocular toxicity is known to occur with various drugs (Table 2.8.4) particularly HCQ and steroids.

Table 2.8.4 summarises the commonly used drugs used in rheumatology and their effect on the eye. Drug-induced ocular inflammation is reported with etanercept. Infections such as tuberculosis and CMV retinitis can occur when the patient is immunosuppressed. To prevent HCQ toxicity, recommendations are to do a baseline screening in the first year, and an annual screening after 5 years of use or sooner if major risk factors are present. The recommended screening tests are fundus examination, automated visual fields, and spectral domain OCT.

Table 2.8.4: Drugs and their impact on the eye

Medications	*Ocular involvement*	*Screening recommendations*
Hydroxychloroquine (HCQ) Chloroquine(CQ) **Risk of toxicity** • Up to 5 years: 1% • Up to 10 years: 2% • After 20 years: 20%	**Irreversible retinal damage:** Paracentral scotoma Bull's eye maculopathy Toxic maculopathy Toxic neuropathy Peripheral pigmentation In Asians, early damage is more peripheral pattern Corneal verticillata	**Screening frequency: Annual screening** • After 5 years of use • Sooner if major risk factors + **Major risk factors** • Daily dosage – HCQS: >5 mg/kg real weight – CQ: >2.3 mg/kg real weight • Duration of use: >5 years (with no other risk factors) • Renal disease with subnormal GFR • Tamoxifen use • Other macular diseases **Recommended screening tests** • Primary tests: Ideally do both – Automated visual fields – Spectral domain OCT • Other objective tests (as needed or available) – Multifocal electroretinogram – Fundus autofluorescence • Newer tests of possible value in future – Microperimetry – Adaptive optics • Not recommended for screening – Only fundus examination – Time-domain OCT – Fluorescein angiography – Full field ERG – Amsler grid – Color testing – EOG
Oral steroids	Cataract Glaucoma Central serous chorioretinopathy (CSR)	• Slit lamp, intraocular pressures and fundus examinations • Fluorescein angiography and OCT for diagnosis of CSR
Etanercept	Uveitis	• Slit lamp and fundus examinations
Intravenous biphosphonates	Uveitis	• Slit lamp and fundus examinations
Immunosuppression	Infections like tuberculosis, CMV retinitis	• Characteristic patterns on fundus examination confirmed by PCR from the ocular fluids

LEARNING POINTS

- A variety of ocular involvement can occur in rheumatological diseases and these may be asymptomatic or symptomatic.
- Medications used to treat rheumatological diseases may have adverse effects on the eye.
- There should be a low threshold for ophthalmic consultations when evaluating and treating rheumatological diseases.

FURTHER READING

1. Dick AD, Rosenbaum JT, Al-Dhibi HA, et al. Fundamentals of Care for Uveitis International Consensus Group. Guidance on Noncorticosteroid Systemic Immunomodulatory Therapy in Noninfectious Uveitis: Fundamentals of Care for UveitiS (FOCUS) Initiative. Ophthalmology. 2018;125:757–73.
2. Kim JS, Knickelbein JE, Nussenblatt RB, et al. Clinical trials in noninfectious uveitis. Int Ophthalmol Clin. 2015; 55:79–110.
3. Multicenter Uveitis Steroid Treatment Trial Research Group, Kempen JH, Altaweel MM, Holbrook JT, et al. The multicenter uveitis steroid treatment trial: rationale, design, and baseline characteristics. Am J Ophthalmol. 2010; 149:550–61.e10.
4. Rathinam SR, Babu M, Thundikandy R, et al. A randomized clinical trial comparing methotrexate and mycophenolate mofetil for noninfectious uveitis. Ophthalmology. 2014;121:1863–70.

Section

III

APPROACH TO THE PATIENT

Chapter 3.1

Approach to the Patient with Monoarthritis

SJ Gupta

INTRODUCTION

Inflammation of a joint that is confined to a single joint, is termed monoarthritis; Inflammation at more than one joint but less than 5, is termed oligoarthritis and when inflammation occurs at 5 or more joints, it is termed polyarthritis. Monoarthritis can occur in a previously normal joint or might occur in a joint that is abnormal due to a previous joint disease. Monoarthritis (MA) is termed: (a) Acute MA, when the inflammation is less than 6 weeks in duration or (b) Chronic MA, when inflammation has been present for 6 weeks and longer. The evaluation of a patient presenting with MA involves a systematic clinical approach, keeping in mind specific clinical features in the individual patient. Special mention needs to be made regarding the recent SARS CoV2-2019 disease (COVID-19) pandemic, as amongst its varied clinical manifestations, it may cause acute as well as chronic musculoskeletal complaints post-COVID infection. This chapter aims to provide an overview of the clinical approach to a patient with monoarthritis.

DIFFERENTIAL DIAGNOSIS

There can be many possible causes of MA and in order to determine the cause in an individual patient, it is obviously important to be aware of these. Specific conditions may present with and exhibit differing clinical features (Tables 3.1.1 and 3.1.2).

Though many causes are not immediately serious, evaluation of a patient with MA needs to be completed fairly soon, as the infection is one of the possible causes and if not recognized and treated adequately, can result in joint damage and considerable morbidity. It is also important to remember that occasionally, a polyarticular or systemic disease may present with an initial monoarticular involvement. Some patients may experience acute, reactive joint symptoms including MA following COVID-19 of whom about 10% will go on to experience chronic musculoskeletal complaints.

Acute Monoarthritis

Acute MA occurs fairly rapidly or suddenly. The patient will complain of pain, swelling, and stiffness at the affected joint over a matter of hours or at most, a few days, with the duration of symptoms being less than 6 weeks (Fig. 3.1.1). Acute MA constitutes a medical emergency. Prompt and rapid recognition of the cause in any given patient is important, to institute correct treatment. Septic arthritis is the most important cause of acute MA, because urgent treatment is essential in order to prevent

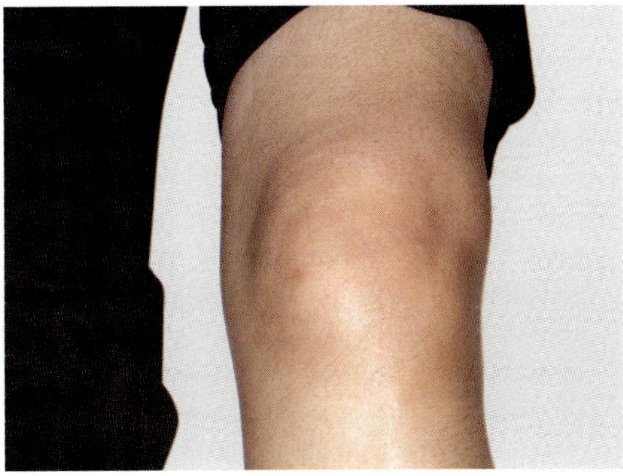

Fig. 3.1.1: Acute MA of the left knee (*Note* the obvious effusion at the joint)

Table 3.1.1: Possible causes of acute/chronic monoarthritis

Acute monoarthritis	*Chronic monoarthritis*
Infection Bacterial, mycobacterial, fungi, viral, lyme disease **Crystals** MSU (gout); CPPD (pseudogout); BCP (destructive arthropathy); calcium oxalate **Trauma** Fracture, internal derangement, hemarthrosis **Osteoarthritis** Presenting as MA-1st CMC joint, MTP joint, Hip or knee **Foreign body synovitis** **Ischemic/avascular necrosis** **Tumor** Metastasis, pigmented villonodular synovitis, osteoid osteoma **Systemic disease presenting as MA** SpA, Inflammatory bowel disease, PsA, ReA	**Infection** Plant thorn (foreign body) synovitis Sarcoidosis Enteropathic arthritis (Crohn's disease predominantly) Pigmented villonodular synovitis Synovial chondromatosis Synovial sarcoma **Monoarticular presentation of a** polyarticular disease (SpA, inflammatory bowel disease, PsA, ReA) **Other causes** Hemoglobinopathies, Loose bodies, Intermittent hydrarthrosis

MSU: Monosodium urate; *CPPD:* Calcium pyro-phosphate dihydrate; *BCP:* Basic calcium phosphate hydroxy-apatite; *SpA:* Spondyloarthritis; *PsA:* Psoriatic arthritis; *ReA:* Reactive arthritis.

Table 3.1.2: Causes of monoarthritis related to presence or absence of previous joint disease

Previously normal joint	*Abnormal joint (Previous joint disease or damage)*
Septic arthritis **Juvenile idiopathic arthritis** **Crystal synovitis** (gout or pseudogout) **Monoarticular presentation of oligo- or polyarthritis (initial)** Spondylorthritis (reactive/psoriatic); erythema nodosum; rheumatoid arthritis; Juvenile idiopathic arthritis **Trauma:** hemarthrosis **Foreign body reaction**	**Pseudogout** in association with osteoarthritis **Avascular necrosis** or subchondral collapse or fracture **Cartilage tear** **Hemarthrosis** **Septic arthritis**

joint damage and morbidity. Other common causes of acute MA are: crystal-induced synovitis; osteoarthritis (OA); trauma; and mono-articular presentation of a polyarticular or oligoarticular disease (Table 3.1.1).

1. **Septic arthritis:** Septic arthritis is caused by pathogenic bacteria, either by the hematogenous route or by direct inoculation of the joint such as following a trauma. This distinguishes septic arthritis from reactive arthritis (ReA) where the joint inflammation is due to an immunological reaction to the organism, which may be elsewhere in the body.

   A patient with joint infection will typically present with a painful, hot, and swollen joint, with restricted movements. The symptoms develop rapidly over a period of days and within about 2 weeks. Delayed treatment of septic arthritis can lead to irreversible joint damage and in addition, there is significant mortality, with an estimated case fatality rate of 11%. The presence of previous joint disease is one of the risk factors (Table 3.1.3) for septic arthritis. However, the diagnosis can be difficult and may be delayed, even in the hands of experienced clinicians. Usually, the presentation is at a large joint (knee or hip), but occasionally septic arthritis has oligo or polyarticular presentation.

   Once septic arthritis is suspected clinically, *prompt aspiration and analysis of synovial fluid from the affected joint is extremely important.* A Gram's

Table 3.1.3: Septic arthritis

Risk factors

1. The presence of existing joint disease such as rheumatoid arthritis (RA) or osteoarthritis (OA).
2. Acute inflammation in an artificial or prosthetic joint; Low socioeconomic status.
3. Intravenous drug abuse.
4. Chronic alcoholism.
5. Other associated medical conditions such as diabetes mellitus.
6. Previous intra-articular injections, particularly if appropriate asepsis is lacking or suspected.
7. Ulcers or frank infection of the skin overlying the affected joint.

Microbiological features

- *Staphylococcus* and *Streptococcus* are the most common organisms that cause septic arthritis and account for about 90% of cases.
- Gram-negative organisms are more common in immunocompromised or older patients and anaerobic bacteria may be responsible for septic arthritis following penetrating injuries.

stain and bacterial culture of the fluid enables confirmation of septic arthritis and examination for crystals under polarising light microscopy enables the diagnosis of crystal-induced arthritis. White blood cell (WBC) counts of >100,000/mm^3 are more likely to be due to joint infection and should be treated as septic arthritis unless proven otherwise; Counts of <50,000/mm^3 are less likely to be due to infection and more likely to be inflammatory in nature (Table 3.1.4).

Synovial fluid samples should be transported as rapidly as possible to the laboratory, and in order to improve the diagnostic yield from culture, it has been suggested that the synovial fluid should be inoculated into blood culture bottles in addition to direct culture on agar plates. Blood cultures may help isolate the causative organism in some cases and the serum WBC count, ESR and CRP levels may help monitor response to treatment.

Additional ways to improve rapid detection of infection that have been reported are:

(i) Assessing the synovial fluid glucose values by glucometer (low values around 1.4 nmol/L or 26 mg/dL) correlate well with infection.
(ii) Synovial fluid calprotectin-elevated calprotectin levels are found to correlate with infection.

There are no typical diagnostic imaging techniques to identify septic arthritis; however, isotope scanning may help distinguish osteoarthritis from sepsis (but will not necessarily distinguish sepsis from other inflammatory causes) and magnetic resonance imaging (MRI) may help identify appearances consistent with infection.

Table 3.1.4: Typical synovial fluid microscopy findings that aids in the diagnosis of acute monoarthritis

Microscopy/synovial fluid finding	Possible diagnosis
Presence of *crystals* under polarizing light microscopy	• Crystal arthritis
• Typical needle shaped negatively birefringent crystals	• Gout
• Larger rhomboidal shaped positively birefringent crystals	• Calcium pyrophosphate dihydrate deposition (CPPD)
Synovial fluid WBC count*	
• <2,000/mm^3 (2 × 10^9/ L)	• Non-inflammatory
• 2,000–100,000/ mm^3 (2–100 × 10^9/ L)	• Inflammatory arthritis
• > 100,000/ mm^3 (100 × 10^9/ L)	• Septic arthritis until proven otherwise
• Synovial fluid hemorrhagic or frankly bloody	• Trauma; internal derangement or tumor
• Large fat droplets visible	• Fracture

*occasionally, crystal synovitis, particularly acute gout can cause an intense inflammation with similar WBC counts.

2. **Crystal-induced synovitis**

Gout: Crystal-induced synovitis is an important cause of acute MA. A number of crystals can cause acute joint inflammation; the most common of these being monosodium urate (MSU) crystals that cause gout. Acute gout is eight times more common in men than women and the first attack commonly occurs between the third to sixth decades. It is extremely uncommon in women before the menopause. The most common joint to be affected is the first metatarsophalangeal (1st MTP) joint, also referred to as podagra. A typical attack is sudden in onset, develops rapidly with peak symptoms developing within 24 hours and even within 6–8 hours and may often awaken the patient from sleep. The joint becomes red, hot, and swollen, with shiny overlying skin, which may desquamate later. The joint is exquisitely painful and tender and the patient is usually unable to weight bear on it. The attack is not uncommonly misdiagnosed as local infection. During an acute attack there may be associated constitutional symptoms such as anorexia, nausea and fever. Leukocytosis and an elevated ESR may also be present. An elevated serum uric acid is usually (but not invariably) present. These clinical features will often allow a diagnosis of acute gout to be made with fair confidence. Occasionally, the initial attack may be polyarticular and the 1st MTP joint may be spared.

To establish the diagnosis of gout beyond doubt, synovial fluid should be aspirated from an affected joint whenever possible and examined under polarizing light microscopy to look for typical MSU crystals. These crystals will appear as needle shaped, negatively birefringent crystals (Fig. 3.1.2). Recurrent acute attacks may result in chronic tophaceous gout, with tophi being found typically in the periarticular tissues, cartilaginous helix of the ear, bursae and tendon sheaths. The tophi appear as periarticular swellings, filled with a soft, 'cheesy' or 'chalky' material (Fig. 3.1.3). The presence of tophi in a patient presenting with acute MA and a compatible history is a sure clinical sign confirming the diagnosis of gout and the tophaceous material will reveal numerous MSU crystals under polarizing light microscopy.

Pseudogout: Some calcium containing crystals may also cause acute episodes of synovitis. Calcium pyrophosphate dihydrate (CPPD) and basic calcium phosphate (BCP) are the common calcium crystals. CPPD crystals can cause an acute attack of synovitis, which may be indistinguishable from an attack of gout. This is termed pseudogout. The deposits can often be seen as a fine rim of calcification overlying the articular cartilage of the affected joint (chondrocalcinosis) (Fig. 3.1.4); and the crystals of CPPD can be identified on polarising light microscope, confirming the diagnosis.

BCP crystals include—hydroxyapatite, octacalcium phosphate and tricalcium phosphate. BCP crystals most often cause a periarthritis or calcific tendonitis, but may also cause a synovitis

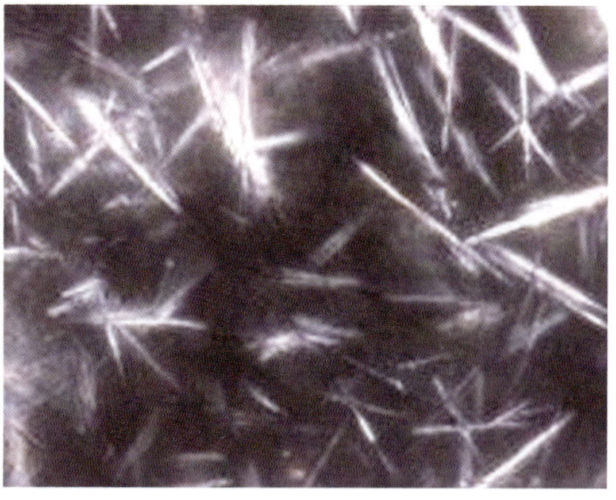

Fig. 3.1.2: Needle-shaped crystals of MSU (seen under polarizing light microscopy)

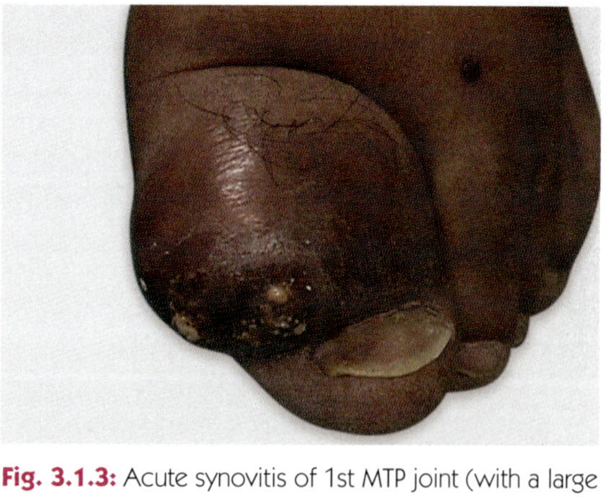

Fig. 3.1.3: Acute synovitis of 1st MTP joint (with a large overlying tophus and typical 'cheesy' material extruding from the tophus)

of a large joint such as the knee or shoulder (Milwaukee shoulder). Though this tends to be a more chronic synovitis, it may occasionally present as an acute MA and ought to be kept in mind in the evaluation of a patient with acute MA.

3. **Osteoarthritis:** Osteoarthritis (OA) is the most common joint disease and therefore, should always be borne in mind as a possible cause of joint symptoms including acute MA. Though usually a chronic, slowly progressive disease, OA can occasionally present with acute worsening of symptoms at a joint, with associated swelling. This is often seen at the knee joint, where mild trauma, overuse of the joint or chondrocalcinosis may cause an acute increase in symptoms with clinical signs of inflammation. However, these acute symptoms would be part of the overall clinical spectrum of OA, which commonly affects multiple joints (hands, feet, spine, and hips) and when associated with bony swelling at the DIP joints of the hands (Heberden's nodes) is referred to a primary generalized osteoarthritis (PGOA) or 'nodal' OA. Occasionally, OA may affect single large joints (knees or hips). The diagnosis of OA is not too difficult, keeping in mind the clinical picture and can be easily confirmed by radiology (Fig. 3.1.4).
4. **Trauma, hemarthrosis and foreign body reaction:** Trauma to a joint may cause acute pain due to internal derangement (particularly at the knee), hemarthrosis or fracture. This may be mistaken for acute synovitis. Milder episodes of trauma may cause a transient (reactive) synovitis at the joint and should be borne in mind in the evaluation of a patient with MA. Patients with coagulation or bleeding disorders (hemophilia or anticoagulant therapy) may present with bleeding into a joint, which clinically presents quite like an episode of acute MA. Joint aspiration will however confirm the diagnosis. Penetrating injuries from thorns (plant thorn synovitis), wood fragments and other foreign particles (foreign body synovitis) may cause an acute synovitis, due to a foreign body reaction, which may appear shortly after the injury or even a few weeks or months later. A careful history, eliciting possible trauma or even occupation of the patient (such as gardening) is therefore important, in reaching an accurate diagnosis.
5. **Monoarticular presentation of a polyarticular disease:** Many systemic or polyarticular diseases may initially present with an episode of acute MA. These conditions include: Rheumatoid arthritis, systemic lupus erythematosus, the arthritis of inflammatory bowel disease, psoriatic arthritis, Behçet's disease, Reiter's disease and other forms of reactive arthritis. Most of these conditions will however not persist as MA and in addition, the associated clinical features of the underlying disorder will enable an accurate diagnosis to be made.

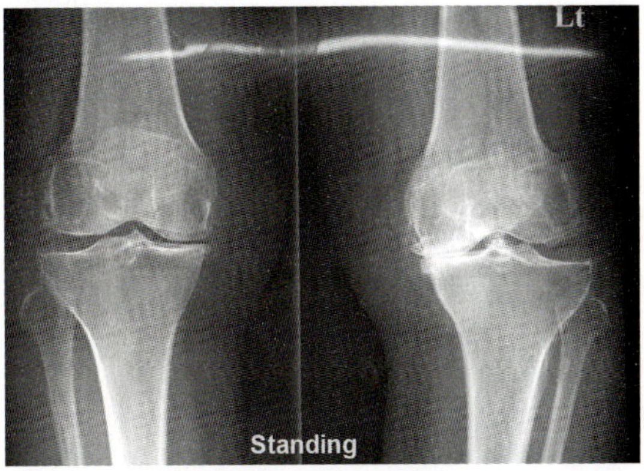

Fig. 3.1.4: Chondrocalcinosis, seen as a thin line of calcification over the articular cartilage of the right knee lateral compartment. (Also demonstrates OA changes at both knees, (left > right) with reduced joint space, osteophyte formation and varus deformities)

Chronic Monoarthritis

Inflammatory MA persisting beyond 6 weeks may have many causes (Table 3.1.1). As the duration of synovitis increases, infection (particularly chronic infection such as TB) becomes more likely and a synovial biopsy should be undertaken to confirm or exclude infection and also to exclude primary synovial conditions (such as villonodular synovitis). However, should there be associated radiological features suggesting the possibility of infection, such as periosteal reaction, osteopenia or bony erosion, the synovial biopsy should not be delayed. Some cases of chronic MA may eventually evolve to a polyarticular disease (OA or RA) but about 1/3rd may remain undiagnosed, particularly when the knee is involved.

APPROACH TO THE EVALUATION OF A PATIENT WITH MA

The process of evaluation of a patient presenting with joint symptoms, really commences even before the formal consultation, by careful observation of the patient as he/she enters the consulting room. The gait of the patient, how ill the patient appears, any visible extra-articular features (such as a rash) may all suggest possible diagnoses (Table 3.1.5).

History: The next and certainly the most important step in evaluation, is to take a detailed and full history.

Onset of symptoms is important in order to determine acute from chronic MA and often, patients may have some difficulty in recalling exactly when their symptoms began. Patients may not associate their present acute symptoms with pain at other joint(s) or even previous episodes of joint pain; however this would be important to elicit, even by specific questioning, as a history of previous similar episodes would suggest a noninfectious cause and the possibility of crystal arthritis. Likewise, a history of COVID-19 infection in the recent past must be sought specifically.

A history of fever, insect or tick bites, sexual contact, preexisting systemic disease, intravenous drug use, or travel, might all raise the possibility of infection. The presence of associated features, such as skin rash, ocular complaints, urethritis or genital ulcers and diarrhea, would suggest the possibility of Reiter's disease. History of trauma might suggest the possibility of traumatic synovitis or fracture.

A history of concurrent medical problems might be relevant such as the presence of psoriasis would make one consider psoriatic arthritis. History of drug therapy would also be important; the recent introduction of diuretics might suggest gout as a possibility.

Family history of gout, osteoarthritis or other inflammatory joint diseases should be sought and might often lead to a diagnosis.

Examination: The most crucial aspect of the physical examination would be to distinguish true synovitis (joint inflammation) from bursitis, cellulitis or tendonitis. The presence of joint effusion and synovial thickening, tenderness over the joint line and restricted active and passive movements at the joint, indicate joint inflammation. By and large, this is not difficult and one can recognize joint inflammation clinically, particularly at certain joints such as the knee joint. However, some clinical situations pose specific problems: olecranon bursitis may sometimes be difficult to differentiate from synovitis at the elbow; cellulitis around the ankle or knee may simulate synovitis; and deep seated joints such as the hip and sacroiliac joints can be difficult to evaluate.

Once the primary question is settled that one is dealing with a MA, one should attempt to look for specific clues that might suggest an underlying diagnosis on the further examination (Tables 3.1.6 and 3.1.7).

Investigations: The most important clinical investigation in the evaluation of a patient with MA is synovial fluid examination (particularly if an infection is suspected) and virtually every patient presenting with a MA should have the joint aspirated with this objective.

Table 3.1.5: Clues to a possible cause of arthritis: Based on initial clinical observation

Clinical observation	*Possible diagnosis*
1. Middle aged man with an acute, swollen, painful foot (MTP joint). *or* Elderly lady, single, swollen and painful joint, on diuretics.	Crystal synovitis/gout
2. Young male. Knee or ankle pain and enters with stiff neck and back	Spondarthritis/ankylosing spondylitis
3. Elderly, ill-looking individual with an acute, hot, swollen, painful joint.	Septic arthritis
4. Coagulopathy or anticoagulant use	Hemarthrosis
5. Erythema nodosum, hilar adenopathy	Sarcoid

Table 3.1.6: Diagnostic clues on examination of a patient with monoarthritis

Findings on examination	*Possible diagnosis/think of*
Significant lymphadenopathy	Infection (tubercular)
Oral ulcers	Behçet's disease; Reiter's syndrome; or systemic lupus erythematosus (SLE)
Cutaneous tophii	Gout
Nail pitting or onycholysis	Psoriatic arthritis
Specific skin rash • Erythematous facial rash • Psoriatic patches (natal cleft, behind ears or at umbilicus) • Erythema nodosum • Keratoderma blennorrhagicum • Pyoderma gangrenosum • Ulcers	 • SLE • Psoriatic arthritis • Sarcoidosis, inflammatory bowel disease, SLE • Reiter's disease • Inflammatory bowel disease • Infection
Sacroiliitis	Spondyloarthritis

Table 3.1.7: Possible systemic diseases presenting as acute monoarthritis

Clinical presentation	*Possible systemic disease(s)*
Acute monoarthritis	Psoriasis Reiter's disease Inflammatory bowel disease
Septic arthritis	Hypogammaglobulinemia Bacterial endocarditis Bacterial pneumonia HIV/AIDS
Pseudogout	Hemochromatosis Acromegaly Hypoparathyroidism

1. **Joint aspiration:** It is a simple, safe and easy bedside procedure with virtually no complications, providing a sterile no-touch technique with appropriate disposable equipment. The synovial fluid should be examined for:
   i. Gram's stain.
   ii. Bacterial culture
   iii. WBC count (total and differential); and
   iv. Crystals.
2. **Synovial biopsy:** Obtained by needle aspiration or arthroscopy, synovial biopsy might be indicated for the evaluation of chronic MA rather than in the acute situation. Often, the biopsy reveals "non-specific inflammatory" changes on histology, particularly so for the non-infective, inflammatory conditions. Synovial biopsy would be of specific help in identifying tuberculosis, amyloidosis, sarcoidosis, pigmented villo-nodular synovitis or other synovial tumours. Some recent advances in the processing of synovial biopsy specimens, by polymerase chain reaction (PCR) and immunoelectron microscopy, might help to identify tiny fragments of the aetiological agent and have been found to be useful for the diagnosis of Lyme disease, gonococci and chlamydiae.

Other investigations might be helpful depending upon the suspected clinical diagnosis. Leukocytosis might suggest infection and cultures of the blood and urine might also help in identifying the causative organism in some situations.

Radiology of the affected joint will seldom identify the cause of MA, but might help to identify fracture (suggesting trauma), chondrocalcinosis, sacroiliitis or changes of osteoarthritis. Magnetic resonance imaging is helpful in identifying possible infective changes at deep-seated joints (such as the sacro-iliac) and can also help to detect bone and soft-tissue involvement.

Finally, one should keep in mind that MA may occasionally be the first clinical sign of a systemic disease and therefore one may need to consider investigations depending upon the clinical features.

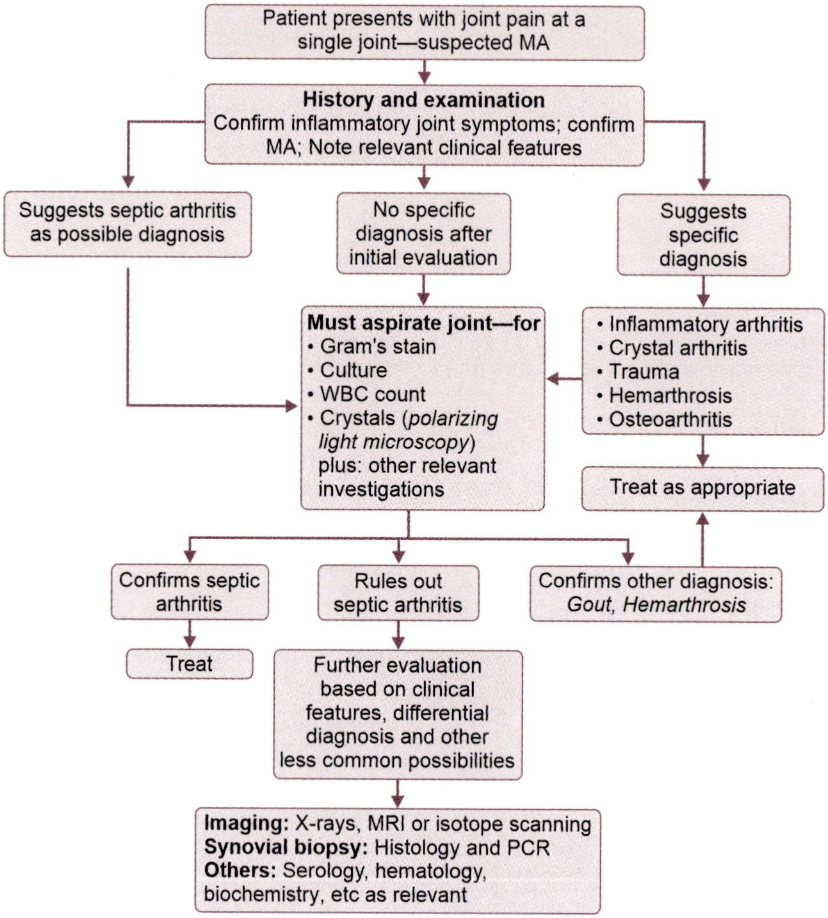

Fig. 3.1.5: Suggested algorithm for the evaluation of monoarthritis (MA)

An algorithmic approach to monoarthritis is presented in (Fig. 3.1.5).

LEARNING POINTS

- Acute monoarthritis is a medical emergency and the most significant cause to be excluded being septic arthritis.
- Trauma or non-inflammatory joint involvement needs to be excluded by a good history and physical examination.
- Crystal induced synovitis (gout) is another important cause of monoarthritis.
- Synovial fluid examination is crucial for the evaluation of acute monoarthritis and synovial biopsy for chronic monoarthritis.
- Gout is extremely uncommon in pre-menopausal women.
- Tuberculosis is an important differential diagnosis to consider in chronic monoarthritis.

FURTHER READING

1. Becker JA, Daily JP, Pohlgeers KM. Acute Monoarthritis: Diagnosis in Adults. Am Fam Physician. 2016; 94: 810–6.
2. Doherty M, Lanyon P, Ralston SH. Presenting Problems in Musculoskeletal Disease. In: Davidson's Principles and Practice of Medicine: 2006: Eds. Boon NA, Colledge NR, Walker BR, Hunter JAA. Churchill Livingstone Elsevier. 20th Edition; 1076–7.
3. Greenhalgh T, Knight M, A'Court C, et al. Management of post-acute covid-19 in primary care. BMJ. 2020; 370:m3026. doi: 10.1136/bmj.m3026.
4. Gupta SJ. Crystal induced arthritis: an Overview. J Indian Rheumatol Assoc 2002:10:5–13.
5. Gupta, SJ. Intra-articular steroid therapy. Journal Int Med Sci Aca 1998; 11:215–7.
6. Omar M et al. Rapid exclusion of septic arthritis using a glucometer. Clin Rheumatol: 2017;36:591–8.
7. Swan A, Amer H, Dieppe P. The value of synovial fluid assays in the diagnosis of joint disease: a literature survey. Ann Rheum Dis 2002;61:493–8.

Approach to the Patient with Polyarthritis

Anand N Malaviya

INTRODUCTION

Polyarthritis is the most common condition seen in the daily practice of rheumatology. Using history and physical examination, a skilled rheumatologist would quickly recognize patients with polyarthritis, make a short list of differential diagnoses, and then proceed to finalize the diagnosis with focused relevant laboratory and imaging investigations.

DEFINITION OF POLYARTHRITIS

Conventionally involvement of more than 4 joints is called polyarthritis, whereas less than 4 and more than 1 joint is oligoarthritis. Conditions that mimic polyarthritis are shown in Table 3.2.1. Usually, oligoarthritis is due to spondyloarthropathy (Table 3.2.2).

Table 3.2.1: Differential diagnosis of musculoskeletal pains that may mimic polyarthritis

- Multifocal osteonecrosis, periostitis, other primary bone diseases
- Muscle disorders
- Polymyalgia rheumatica
- Neuropathies
- Tendonitis, fibrositis, multifocal bursitis
- Functional, fibromyalgia and malingering

Table 3.2.2: Common conditions causing oligoarthritis

- Spondyloarthritis
- Psoriatic arthritis
- Löfgren's syndrome (a form of acute sarcoidosis)
- Poncet's disease
- A certain subset of juvenile idiopathic arthritis (JIA)

Note: Typically, inflammatory peripheral arthritis seen in the various forms of SpA is oligoarticular in nature with involvement of joints of the lower segment of the body with prominent asymmetry and associated enthesopathy.

POLYARTHRITIS: CLINICAL ANALYSIS FOR REACHING A DIAGNOSIS

The following points need to be ascertained:

1. Is it acute or chronic?
2. Is it inflammatory or noninflammatory?
3. The past, personal and family history
4. Review of systems and extra-articular manifestations
5. Pattern and topography of joint involvement

Acute or Chronic?

Involvement of less than 6-week duration is classified as acute polyarthritis. At one end of the spectrum could be self-limiting post-viral arthritis (e.g. chikungunya arthritis, others) that resolves completely within 6 weeks. At the other end of the spectrum could be a potentially life-threatening disease associated with high morbidity (acute presentation of systemic lupus erythematosus {SLE}).

In the majority of acute polyarthritis cases definitive diagnosis is usually not possible at the outset. The reason is that by-and-large clinical rheumatology is a science of recognizing patterns of joint involvement and its evolution and that remains central to making a rheumatological diagnosis. Therefore, in acute polyarthritis the symptoms may not have yet evolved into a recognizable pattern for a definitive diagnosis. An experienced rheumatologist realises the importance of patience; *evolution of pattern of symptoms over time* may give a clue to diagnosis.

However, recent good biomarkers provide diagnostic clues not only in the early stages of polyarthritis but even in preclinical phases. The best example is the presence of anti-citrullinated peptide antibodies (ACPA) in rheumatoid arthritis (RA). The presence of high titers of ACPA in a patient with acute polyarthritis is a strong clue that it would evolve into RA. In some of the patients presenting with polyarthritis (Table 3.2.3), a detailed history, review of systems, physical examination and diagnostic evaluation may give a clue to the diagnosis.

Is the Polyarthritis Inflammatory in Nature?

The next point is to evaluate whether it is *inflammatory* or *non-inflammatory* in nature. Inflammation namely redness (**rubor**), heat (**calor**), pain (**dolor**), swelling (**tumor**) and loss of function would be easily recognisable in joints for classifying polyarthritis as inflammatory. Unfortunately, joints may be tender, swollen and may not function normally even in some noninflammatory conditions, e.g. osteoarthritis (OA). On the other hand, redness and local heat may be difficult to perceive even in inflammatory joint disease especially in those with dark skin.

Table 3.2.3: Causes of acute polyarthritis

- RA, SLE, PsA, other CTDs, systemic vasculitides (May occasionally present as acute polyarthritis)
- Septic arthritis, Gonococcal arthritis, arthritis seen in infective endocarditis.
- Reiter's and other 'classical' reactive arthritides (Often HLA B27 positive, part of the SpA spectrum); 'non-classic' reactive arthritides (e.g. acute rheumatic fever, Poncet's, leprosy-related)
- Viral arthritis: Chikungunya, rubella, hepatitis-associated arthritis, parvovirus-B19, and others
- IBD-related arthritis
- Sarcoidosis (Lofgren's syndrome-type presentation)
- Erythema nodosum and other panniculitis-related arthritis
- Serum sickness
- Hematological causes: Sickle-cell anemia, leukemic arthritis, hemophilic arthritis
- Palindromic rheumatism

SLE: Systemic lupus erythematosus; *PsA:* Psoriatic arthritis; *SpA:* Spondyloarthritis; *CTDs:* Connective tissue diseases; *IBD:* Inflammatory bowel disease

However, in those with intense inflammatory arthritis as seen in the periankle-ankle involvement of acute sarcoidosis (Lofgren's syndrome) and acute gouty arthritis involving joints in the feet, the overlying skin would show indurated inflammatory edema with peeling off of the outer layer of skin as the inflammation subsides.

Certain clinical features (Table 3.2.4) distinguish inflammatory from non-inflammatory joint diseases with a high degree of sensitivity and specificity. However, in most of the common forms of inflammatory polyarthritides (RA, PsA) features of local inflammation may only be minimal or imperceptible.

Past, Personal and Family History

A transient episode of heel pain (Achilles' tendon enthesitis, plantar fasciitis) at the juvenile age or an episode of uveitis in the past may be due to ankylosing spondylitis/spondyloarthritis (AS-SpA) group. History in the recent past, of a febrile episode with or without exanthema, sexual contact or frank venereal disease, an episode of diarrhea, or acute conjunctivitis, may give a clue to the diagnosis of reactive arthritis, gonococcal arthritis, or peripheral spondyloarthritis.

Three most common diagnostic mistakes seen in day-to-day rheumatology practice involve tuberculosis, gout, and rheumatic fever. It is quite common that a juvenile was given treatment for tuberculosis or rheumatic fever (long-acting penicillin) in the past for a mono- or oligoarthritis

Table 3.2.4: Clinical features to distinguish inflammatory from noninflammatory joint disease

1. Early morning stiffness that takes at least 30 minutes for maximum improvement, more often it takes about 1 hour for maximum improvement.
2. Activity (gentle movement) improves the symptoms but inactivity does not (inactivity may actually increase the stiffness).
3. Spontaneous 'flares' with fluctuation in the severity of symptoms over time without any obvious extraneous cause.
4. Constitutional symptoms: Fatigue and tiredness, feverish feeling or actual fever, night sweats, loss of appetite, and weight.

Note: The presence of one, more or all of these manifestations would strongly suggest the inflammatory nature of the joint problem with increasing probability.

that evolved into rather typical enthesitis-related arthritis (ERA) over time. The other common mistake is to diagnose and treat the patient as 'gout' only based upon trivial increase in serum uric acid.

Cigarette smoking may be a trigger for most inflammatory arthritides, notably RA. Family history is equally important in making a diagnosis of polyarthritis. A so-called 'seronegative inflammatory polyarthritis' may be PsA if a blood relative is known to have psoriasis. The significance of family history is more obvious in frank hereditary conditions, e.g. AS and gout where invariably a positive history is elicited.

Review of Systems and Extra-articular Manifestations

a. History of *skin, mucosal* and *subcutaneous lesions* is highly relevant for making a diagnosis in many inflammatory polyarthritis. Thus, a psoriatic patch anywhere in the body points to a diagnosis of PsA. Facial 'butterfly' rash of systemic lupus erythematosus (SLE) along with mucosal ulcers, alopecia and vasculitic skin lesions is diagnostic of the disease. Gottron's papules, heliotrope-facial rash, 'mechanic's hands', 'shawl sign' along with periungual vasculitic infarcts are typical of dermatomyositis. Erythema nodosum and panniculitis are seen in association with several inflammatory arthritides. Subcutaneous nodules in association with polyarthritis are seen with several diseases including RA, SLE, OA (Heberden's and Bouchard's nodules), gout (gouty tophi), sarcoidosis, rheumatic fever, polyarteritis nodosa, dyslipidaemias, and others. Raynaud's phenomenon is associated with scleroderma skin changes.

   Mucosal ulcers in SLE (moderately painful), SpA (little pain), and Behçet's disease (severely painful) are helpful clinical features for diagnosis. Palpable as well as non-palpable purpuric lesions are seen in several polyarthritides including SLE, and Sjögren's syndrome (including hypergammaglobulinemia purpura of Waldenström). Leg ulcers (vasculitic or part of neutrophilic dermatosis, e.g. pyoderma gangrenosum) are seen in RA, SLE (subcutaneous inflammation that may ulcerate, e.g. lupus profundus), polyarteritis nodosa (including cutaneous polyarteritis), Behçet's disease and others.

b. The association of *eye* and *ear-nose-throat-mouth* with polyarthritis is equally important. Sicca symptoms are features of Sjögren's syndrome, but also occur secondary to RA, SLE, systemic sclerosis and others. Episcleritis-scleritis is common in RA. Iridocyclitis-uveitis is typically seen in association with SpA. Retinal lesions are seen in SLE, systemic vasculitides and others, retrobulbar lesions (causing proptosis) may be seen in granulomatosis with polyangiitis (GPA), and the involvement of rectus muscles may occur as part of inflammatory myositis.

   Inflammation of cartilage in the pinna and bridge of the nose is typically seen in relapsing polychondritis causing flail or deformed pinna giving the appearance of a 'boxer's ear' and 'saddle-nose' deformity. The latter is also seen in Wegener's granulomatosis which usually destroys the cartilage at the bridge of the nose. Involvement of the middle and inner ear is typically seen in GPA.

c. Inflammatory polyarthritis also has a close association with *genitourinary* and *gastrointestinal* systems. A urethritic form of 'reactive arthritis, and gonococcal infection with urethritis, cervicitis, and migratory inflammatory polyarthritis (and dorsum of the hands tenosynovitis) is a well-recognised association. IBD (Crohn's disease much more often than ulcerative colitis) also has a dual association with inflammatory polyarthritis. Behçet's disease is the other condition where IBD-type lesions may be seen. In fact, there are patients diagnosed with IBD who on detailed clinical evaluation may show features of milder forms of Behçet's disease including orogenital ulcers, erythema nodosum lesions, and eye inflammation.

d. *Renal disease* and inflammatory polyarthritis combination are among the most serious, often life-threatening forms of arthritic disorders. Urinary sediment abnormality indicative of glomerular inflammation (microscopic haematuria, a variety of casts and WBC), sub-nephrotic or nephrotic range proteinuria, frank nephrotic syndrome, renal arterial involvement with renal hypertension, rapidly progressive glomerulonephritis, and more recently podocytopathy is the manifestations of several diseases that may have associated inflammatory polyarthritis. This group mainly includes SLE, antiphospholipid syndrome, and anti-neutrophil cytoplasmic antibody (ANCA)-associated small vessel systemic vasculitides.

e. *Peripheral*, as well as *central nervous system* involvement and inflammatory polyarthritis, is another potentially serious, often life-threatening group of arthritides. These include SLE, antiphospholipid syndrome, systemic vasculitides of several types (mono neuritis multiplex is a common manifestation in some of them), and Behçet's disease.

f. Lung involvement is commonly seen with RA, connective tissue diseases, systemic vasculitides, sarcoidosis, relapsing polychondritis, and AS. There is an important clinical subset of pulmonary-renal syndrome where the kidney and lungs are affected in addition to inflammatory polyarthritis. SLE, systemic sclerosis and other connective tissue diseases, ANCA-associated vasculitides, Goodpasture's syndrome, pauci immune necrotising and crescentic glomerulonephritis (CGN), Henoch-Schönlein's purpura (HSP), and essential mixed cryoglobulinemia (EMC) are some of its causes.

g. Some hematological abnormalities may specifically point towards a certain diagnosis. Thus, low platelets may point towards the diagnostic possibility of SLE and antiphospholipid syndrome. The hypercoagulable state with widespread thrombo-embolic manifestations is rather typical of the antiphospholipid syndrome that is often associated with SLE.

What is the Pattern of Joint Involvement?

The next clinical feature to be analyzed toward making a diagnosis of the type of polyarthritis is the pattern of *evolution* of joint involvement. Basically, there are 3 patterns, namely *additive, intermittent,* and *migratory.*

In *additive* pattern joints are progressively recruited with many joints getting affected over time. RA is a typical example of such a pattern of involvement. In an *intermittent* pattern the joint involvement appears and then disappears till the next such episode with completely asymptomatic period in between these episodes. In its inflammatory form it is typically seen in palindromic rheumatism, acute gouty arthritis, relapsing polychondritis, and relapsing seronegative symmetrical synovitis with pitting edema (RS3PE). A condition called intermittent hydrarthrosis is an idiopathic noninflammatory intermittent arthritis.

In a *migratory* pattern, the joints become symptomatic then subside while different joints get involved. The tempo of migration may differ for example it could be only hours between one to the next joint involvement in rheumatic fever. On the other hand, the tempo of 'migration' may be much slower (days) in gonococcal arthritis.

The *topography* or distribution of joint involvement helps in narrowing down the diagnostic possibilities. For describing the *topography* of joint involvement, the following anatomical regions are taken into account: *peripheral joints* (in the extremities), *axial joints* (traditionally sacroiliac joints are considered part of axial joints), *root joints* (that overlap between peripheral and axial joints, namely shoulder and hip joints), and *upper segment* and *lower segment* of the body (above and below waist). In peripheral joints, *symmetry* or *asymmetry* is important to note. Table 3.2.5 lists some of the common causes of polyarthritis classified as inflammatory vs. non-inflammatory further categorised based on the *topographic pattern* of joint involvement. Figures 3.2.1 to 3.2.5 depict some of the typical topographic patterns of joint involvement in different forms of inflammatory and noninflammatory arthritides.

Examples

- Inflammatory synovitis of small as well as large joints in the extremities in a symmetrical distribution on both sides of the body, equally distributed in the upper and lower segments with predominant involvement of joints of the hands, wrists, and feet, with sparing of the distal interphalangeal (DIP) joints, is rather typical of RA (Fig. 3.2.1).
- Involvement of DIP joints without synovitis or inflammation is typically seen in primary nodular OA, but with synovitis, it is often seen in PsA, enteropathic arthritis.
- *Enthesitis* and lower extremity asymmetrical inflammatory arthritis, often associated with root joint involvement, is rather typical of the spondyloarthritis (SpA) group (Fig. 3.2.2).

Table 3.2.5: Common causes of polyarthritis classified as inflammatory vs. non-inflammatory further categorised on the topographic pattern of joint involvement (Modified from Ref. 3)

1. Inflammatory polyarthritis

a. *Peripheral polyarthritis, mostly symmetrical in distribution*
- i. RA
- ii. SLE and other connective tissue diseases
- iii. Wegener's granulomatosis and other systemic vasculitides
- iv. PsA

b. *Peripheral oligoarthritis* or *polyarthritis, often asymmetrical*
- i. PsA*
- ii. Peripheral involvement in SpA including Reiter's disease and other forms of 'classical' reactive arthritis.*
- iii. Enteropathic arthritis*
- iv. Behcet's disease
- v. Polyarticular gout and pseudogout
- vi. Infective endocarditis
- vii. Relapsing polychondritis
- ix. Sarcoidosis
- xi. Amyloid arthropathy

(Those marked by '*' may have axial disease as well)

Note: 1. PsA as well as sarcoid joint disease have several different patterns. Therefore, their names may appear in more than 1 list. 2. For labeling the condition as oligoarthritis (2–4 joints), the midfoot and wrist are taken as a single joint. 3. Several conditions mentioned above as 'oligoarthritis' may have a subset that presents mainly as oligoarthritis, in others it may only be a phase in the evolution of a polyarthritis).

2. Noninflammatory polyarthritis (generic term osteoarthritis)

a. Hereditary factors
- i. Primary nodular OA of the hands (distal and proximal interphalangeal joint involvement)
- ii. Generalized primary OA

b. Environmental factors and age-related osteoarthritis: lifestyle, occupational, trauma.
- i. First metatarsophalangeal joint (Bunion), the knee joints, the distal interphalangeal joints (including Heberden's nodes), proximal interphalangeal joints (including Bouchard's nodes), hip joints, lumbar and cervical spine–usually an obese elderly person.
- ii. OA following local injury (including surgery) in a joint.
- iii. OA in strenuous exercise-related cartilage damage (chondromalacia).

c. Metabolic conditions, some uncommon diseases
- i. Hypothyroidism
- ii. Acromegaly
- iii. Hemochromatosis
- iv. Ochronosis
- v. CPPD deposition disease

- Non-inflammatory involvement of the first carpometacarpal joint (floor of the 'snuff- box') is typically seen in primary OA (Fig. 3.2.3).
- Acute *dactylitis* is strongly suspicious of PsA (Fig. 3.2.4).
- In acute gout the first metatarsophalangeal joint involvement (Fig. 3.2.5) is often the first one to be affected with severe acute inflammatory response (podagra).
- Periankle-ankle inflammatory arthritis, usually associated with erythema nodosum is seen in acute sarcoid arthritis (Lofgren syndrome).
- Prominent involvement of metacarpophalangeal joints without synovitis is typically seen in haemochromatosis.

However, pattern recognition is only a rough guide to diagnosis since there is considerable overlap in the pattern of joint involvement among different types of polyarthritis.

Oligoarthritis

Involvement of 2–4 joints is called oligoarthritis (Table 3.2.2). It is to be noted that almost all forms of inflammatory arthritides may evolve through the

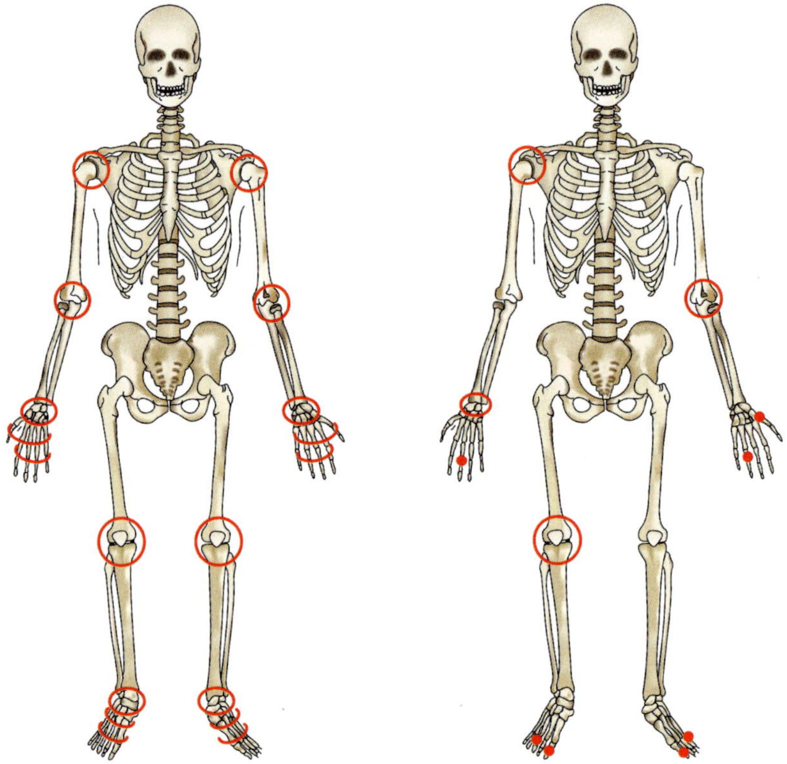

Fig. 3.2.1: Pattern of polyarthritis in rheumatoid arthritis (RA) versus psoriatic arthritis (PsA)

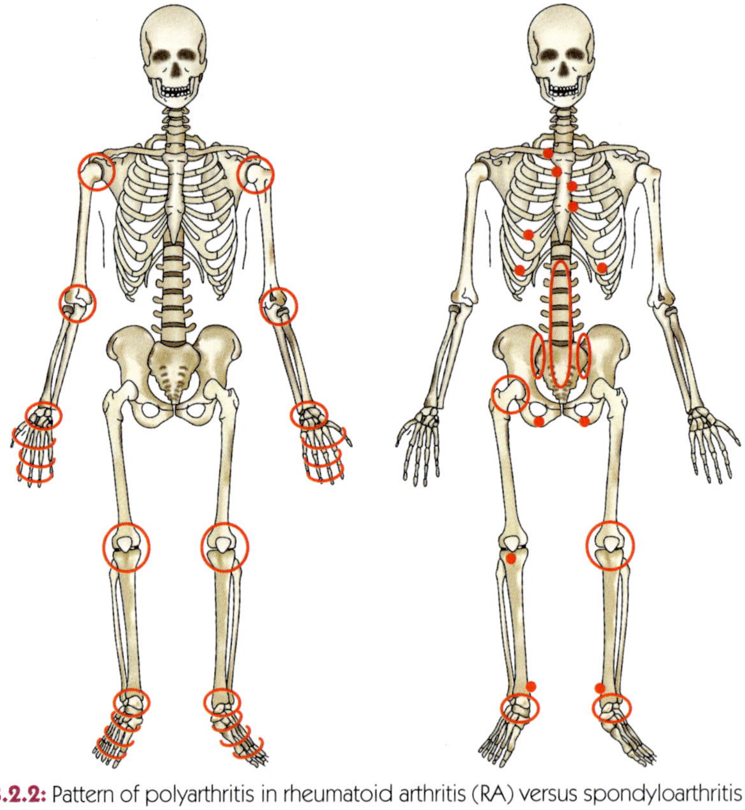

Fig. 3.2.2: Pattern of polyarthritis in rheumatoid arthritis (RA) versus spondyloarthritis (SpA)

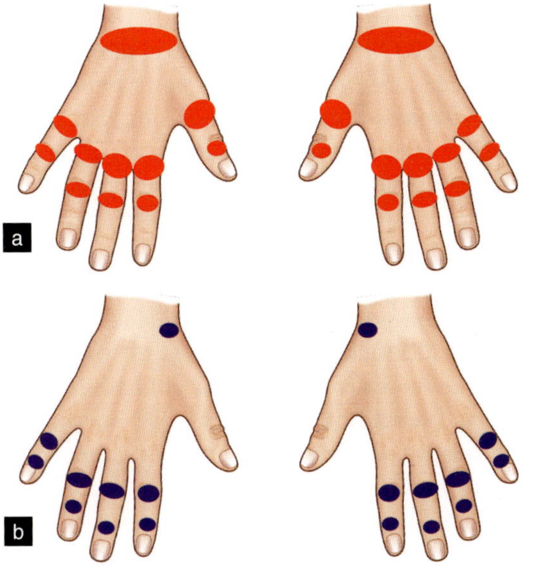

Fig. 3.2.3: Pattern of hand joints involvement in rheumatoid arthritis (RA) depicted as red circles (panel a); versus osteoarthritis (OA) (blue circles) (panel b). Both have symmetrical involvement of the PIPs, but the DIPS are spared in RA

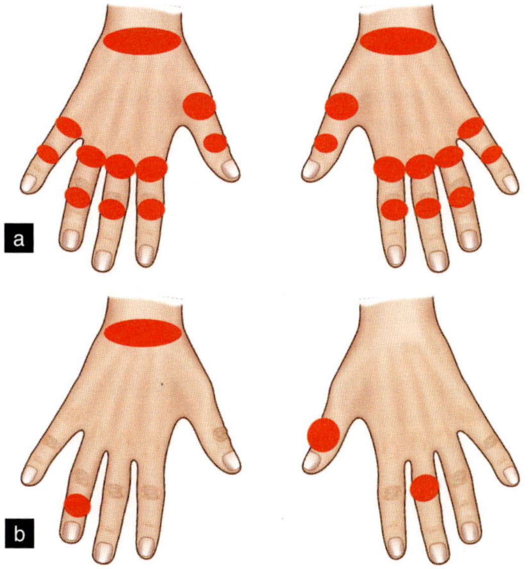

Fig. 3.2.4: Pattern of hand joints involvement in rheumatoid arthritis (RA) depicted as red circles (panel a); versus PsA (panel b). RA is symmetrical, but PsA is asymmetrical with DIP joint involvement

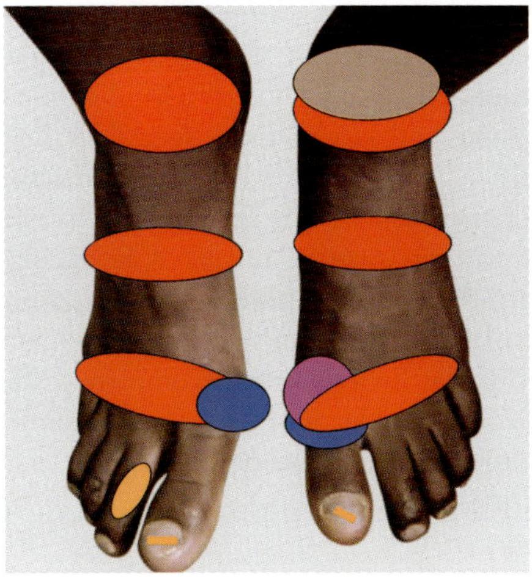

- **Rheumatoid**
  - Ankles, mid-tarsals, MTPs
- **Osteoarthritis**
  - 1st MTPs (noninflammatory)
- **SpA**
  - Ankles-asymmetrical
- **PsA**
  - Dactylitis (sausage digits), psoriatic nail involvement
- **Gout**
  - 1st MTP (podagra, inflammatory)

Fig. 3.2.5: Involvement of the feet in different forms of arthritis

oligoarticular stage but 'true' oligoarthritis would remain oligoarticular over time.

Joint Count

The simplest method of objective assessment of the disease activity is joint count, which must be carried out in every patient at the first and subsequent encounters. The original Disease Activity Score (DAS), its modification (DAS28), Clinical Disease Activity Index (CDAI) and Simplified Disease Activity Index (SDAI) are widely recommended for use in RA. Bath Ankylosing Spondylitis Disease Activity Index (BASDAI), Bath Ankylosing Spondylitis Functional Index (BASFI), etc. are available for objective assessment of SpA. The methodology is also available for objective assessment of noninflammatory diseases like the Western Ontario and McMaster (WOMAC) index for osteoarthritis.

INVESTIGATIONS

The inflammatory nature of polyarthritis can be confirmed by routine laboratory investigations (Table 3.2.6). Some exceptions, however, must be pointed out. In certain diseases ESR may not truly reflect the inflammatory state. This is often true of SLE, scleroderma and AS-SpA where ESR may be

Table 3.2.6: Commonly used nonspecific laboratory markers of inflammation (acute phase reactants)

1. Acute phase **reactants** that increase during inflammation:
   a. ESR
   b. Platelet count
   c. Total serum globulins with reversal of albumin/globulin ratio
   d. Leukocyte count (often but not always)
   e. C-reactive protein (CRP)
   f. Alkaline phosphatase
2. Acute phase reactants that **decrease** during inflammation:
   a. Hemoglobin (normocytic normochromic anemia of chronic disease)
   b. Serum albumin (with reversal of albumin/globulin ratio)

Note: The presence of one, more or all of these manifestations would strongly suggest the inflammatory nature of the joint problem with increasing probability.

disproportionately high or low. Similarly, platelet counts may be low in SLE as part of its clinical manifestation.

Examination of *synovial fluid* in polyarthritis only for confirming inflammatory nature of the joint disease is generally not recommended. However, on rare occasions with no definite clue in the history or examination and inconclusive results of acute phase reactants, joint fluid examination (if joints have effusion) for leukocyte count can help. A leukocyte count of >2000/mm^3 is a definite sign of inflammatory synovitis.

Imaging examination of the joints and other routine imaging investigations *do not distinguish* between inflammatory and noninflammatory conditions. They may, however, detect typical patterns of *radiographic abnormalities* associated with certain diseases (e.g. typical erosions of RA or characteristic juxta-articular new bone formation on plain radiograph of the hand or foot seen in PsA, etc.).

Magnetic resonance imaging (MRI) on the other hand can demonstrate bone marrow edema that has been demonstrated to be the earliest sign of inflammatory nature of the joint disease in recent studies.

In rare circumstances, a synovial biopsy may be necessary for making a diagnosis. Thus, it may be required in suspected polyarticular infection (mycobacterial infection, fungal), villonodular synovitis etc. On the other hand, skin or subcutaneous lesions may often yield useful diagnostic information (e.g. sarcoidosis, erythema nodosum, vasculitis). Specific tissue biopsy may be indicated in specific diseases, e.g. sural nerve biopsy in systemic vasculitis, muscle biopsy in inflammatory myositis.

Once a provisional diagnosis has been made, in the second step of diagnostic work-up, more specific investigations are usually required: example antibodies against anticitrullinated proteins (ACPA) for RA, and immunofluorescent antinuclear antibody test for SLE and related disorders. HLA B27 screening is particularly useful but only in a patient with a typical history of inflammatory back pain.

Nonspecific Arthralgias, Myalgias, Pain Amplification versus Polyarthritis

There are patients who present with vague pains in the joints, muscles, and other parts of the musculoskeletal system. Usually, the severity of the pain fluctuates and is often described as 'unbearable', and they have some features of fibromyalgia. In most cases the duration of symptoms is vague, e.g. 'since long'. They usually carry a handwritten list of complaints and another list of specialists they have already consulted, yet they have not been satisfied as no definite diagnosis has been made. Occasionally these patients may be mistaken as having true polyarthritis. Most require a limited workup, and some of them may require help from a counselor or a psychiatrist. However, a complete evaluation is called for in older age persons, and in those with constitutional symptoms or symptoms referable to other organ systems.

LEARNING POINTS

- As a rule, in musculoskeletal diseases, approximately 60–80% of the information towards making a diagnosis comes from clinical history.
- Polyarthritis and its diagnosis encompass almost the whole field of rheumatology. *Making a diagnosis of polyarthritis is really a test of the knowledge of general internal medicine.*
- It is necessary to follow a definite diagnostic algorithm for convenience and accuracy. Is it *polyarthritis*? → What is the *duration* (acute or chronic)? → What are the *circumstances of*

onset? → Is it *inflammatory* or *non-inflammatory*? What is the pattern of *evolution*? → What is the *topography* of involvement? → Is there a clue to diagnosis in the *past* clinical history, *family* history and review of *systems*? → Does physical *examination* give a diagnostic clue (e.g. a small psoriatic patch)?

- This approach narrows down the diagnostic possibilities and helps in requisitioning a limited number of *focused relevant investigations* to confirm the diagnosis.
- Acute inflammatory polyarthritis could be a self-limiting *benign* condition, the beginning of a *serious chronic* illness with significant morbidity that could even be life threatening or, a rheumatological *emergency* requiring urgent diagnosis and management.
- The distinction between benign, serious chronic illness and a rheumatological emergency requires deep knowledge of rheumatology as well as general internal medicine
- The addition of a few relevant investigations usually confirms the diagnosis that helps in initiating appropriate treatment.

FURTHER READING

1. Caines A, Samadi N, Ouimet G, et al. The sensitivity and specificity of pain diagrams in rheumatic disease referrals. Rheumatology (Oxford) 2012;51:1093–8.
2. Ellrodt AG, Cho M, Cush JJ, et al. An evidence-based medicine approach to the diagnosis and management of musculoskeletal complaints. Am J Med 1997;103:3S–6S.
3. Kush JJ, Dao KH. Polyarticular arthritis. In. Firestein GS, Budd RC, Gabriel SE, McInnes I, O'Dell, JR. (eds), Kelly's Textbook of Rheumatology (9th ed.), Elsevier-Saunders, Philadelphia, 2013, pp 587–98.
4. Lipsky PE. Algorithm for the diagnosis and management of musculoskeletal complaints. Introduction. Am J Med 1997;103:1S–2S.
5. Malaviya AN, Kumar A. Postgraduate Clinic: Polyarthritis. J Assoc Physicians India 1997;45:55–8.
6. Malaviya AN. A patient with musculoskeletal (MSK) pains-clinical approach. Bull Kuwait Inst Med Spec 2004; 3:72–81.
7. Malaviya AN. Clinical approach to patients with joint disease: importance of distinguishing inflammatory from non-inflammatory conditions. APLAR J Rheumatol 2006;9:11–7.
8. Peterson MC, Holbrook JH, Von Hales D, et al. Contributions of the history, physical examination, and laboratory investigation in making medical diagnoses. West J Med. 1992 Feb;156(2):163–5.
9. Pinals RS. Musculoskeletal signs and symptoms B. Polyarticular joint disease. In: Klippel JH (ed). Primer on the rheumatic diseases. Arthritis Foundation, Atlanta, Georgia, 2001:pp 160–5.
10. Robinson DB, El Gablawy HS, Evaluation of the patient – History and Physical Examination. In: 'Primer on the Rheumatic Diseases', (Eds) Klippel, J.H., Stone, J.H., Crofford, L.e.J., White, P.H. Pages 6–41;2008.

Chapter 3.3

Approach to Low Back Pain

N Subramanian

INTRODUCTION

Low backache or low back pain is one of the most common musculoskeletal symptoms in any general outpatient clinic. It affects both young and older people with an impact on social life, productivity, and quality of life. The prevalence of low back pain in any individual's lifetime is 65%. It is acute if the duration is within 6 weeks, subacute if the duration is 6–12 weeks, and chronic if back pain persists beyond 12 weeks.

CAUSES OF LOW BACKACHE

The causes of low back pain range from mild degenerative disease of the spine to referred pain and malignancy (Table 3.3.1). Degenerative diseases of the spine are fairly common causes of back in the older age groups. Tumors and metastases can affect any age however more common in the elderly. Ankylosing spondylitis will cause back pain in the age group 15–45 years. Often the etiology of low back ache is not identifiable, this group is called nonspecific low back ache.

APPROACH

From history we can gather whether the pain is mechanical or inflammatory. In clinical practice, almost 90% of low back pain is mechanical the most common etiology of which is degenerative spine disease. Degenerative changes of the spine

Table 3.3.1: Causes of low back pain

Cause	*Examples*
Mechanical back pain	Degenerative spine disease • Spondylolisthesis (protruded or herniated disc) with or without nerve compression (radiculopathy) • Spinal canal stenosis • Cauda equina syndrome • Spondylolysis Vertebral compression fractures
Infectious	Osteomyelitis, tuberculous spine, brucellosis, etc.
Inflammatory back pain	Sacroiliitis
Malignancy	Primary or metastasis Multiple myeloma
Referred pain	Renal stones Fibromyalgia Endometriosis
Miscellaneous	Osteitis condensans ilii Diffuse idiopathic skeletal hyperostosis (DISH)

can involve any component of the spine: the vertebral bodies, intervertebral discs, facet joints, and soft tissues surrounding it. The clinical feature of mechanical low back pain is a diffuse pain that occurs (and worsens) with activity and is often relieved with rest or inactivity. It is more common in people above the age of 30 years with slight female predominance.

Low back pain that radiates (shoots) down to the leg behind the thigh is indicative of associated radiculopathy and sciatica. History of low back pain and pain in the limbs on walking suggests spinal canal stenosis and neurogenic claudication.

Sudden onset of back pain, history of trauma, lower limb weakness, and urinary incontinence suggest a cauda equina syndrome.

Certain clinical features help identify inflammatory back pain (IBP) namely the presence of early morning stiffness, pain worse at rest, and relief with exercise (Table 3.3.2). IBP will wake the patient at night. Associated features include radiation to the buttocks, pain in the lateral part of the thigh due to trochanteric bursitis, and significant fatigue with some patients feeling pain in the neck. The presence of IBP is a pointer to spondyloarthritis (SpA), but not all IBP is SpA. Even infectious causes and degenerative conditions can cause an inflammatory type of back pain. A painful red eye, skin rash, hip arthritis, and peripheral arthritis, good response to NSAIDs will suggest SpA.

Systemic features like fever, weight loss, other system involvement point to infectious etiology. In contrast, back pain due to malignancy is present all the time and during sleep as well.

Red Flag Signs

In a patient with low back pain there are certain clinical manifestations that warrant urgent investigations. These are called red flags and mandate ruling out malignancy, vertebral compression fracture, tuberculosis, or cauda equina syndrome. Important red flags are: fever, weight loss, acute retention of urine, bladder or bowel incontinence (to rule out cauda equina syndrome), progressive neurological deterioration, history of cancer, thoracic pain, and anemia and bone pain (to rule out myeloma), and history of immunosuppressive medications.

Clinical Examination

General physical examination to look for anemia and lymphadenopathy in those with red flags. Clinical examination includes screening for gait, arms, legs, spine (GALS). If suspecting inflammatory rheumatic disease such as SpA the peripheral joint examination and spine examination is indicated. A simple test to assess L5 and S1 nerve root compression is the straight leg rising test.

Neurologic examination is essential if the pain shoots down the lower limb, and if there are sensory symptoms such as pins and needles or numbness. It is important to diagnose radiculopathies of L3, L4, L5, and S1 nerve roots, and cauda equina syndrome. In motor system examination look for motor power of the knee, ankle, and foot. Absent knee jerk indicates involvement of L4 nerve root, while absent ankle jerk indicates involvement of L5 and S1 nerve root. In the sensory system, look at whether there is any sensory loss. There may be a loss of sensations in the area of distribution of L2–L5, and sacral nerve roots indicating nerve root compression.

Table 3.3.2: Criteria for Inflammatory back pain (IBP)

Calin et al. (1977)	*Berlin criteria (2009)*	*ASAS criteria (2010)*
• Back pain in patients <40 years old • Early morning stiffness • Better with activity or exercise • Insidious onset • Duration >3 months	• Morning stiffness >30 min duration • Alternating buttock pain • Nocturnal awakening (second half of the night) • Improvement in back pain with exercise but not with rest	• Insidious onset • Age at onset <40 years • Pain at night (with improvement on getting up) • Improvement with exercise • No improvement with rest
*Requires the presence of four out of five to classify as IBP	The sensitivity is 70% and specificity 81% if two of the four criteria are fulfilled, for diagnosis of IBP	If at least four out of five parameters are present, sensitivity is 77.0% and specificity is 92% for the presence of IBP

ASAS: Assessment of SpondyloArthritis International Society.

Back Pain in Women

Osteoporotic vertebral fracture is a differential diagnosis of back pain in elderly women, the most common site being the mid thoracic and thoracolumbar junction (T12–L1). Osteoporosis is typically painless, and vertebral fractures occurring slowly over time are often incidentally detected on plain radiography, but sometimes vertebral compression fractures can occur acutely precipitated by a mild trauma or the patient can have sudden onset of low back pain after lifting a weight or bending forward.

Osteitis condensans ilii is an imaging diagnosis that is seen in women (predominantly) and can be confused with ankylosing spondylitis.

Imaging

Not all low back pain will need imaging. The American College of Radiology does not recommend imaging for uncomplicated low back pain (whether acute, subacute or chronic) except when pain persists beyond 6 weeks even with treatment. This is because degenerative changes in the MRI are common in the general population and do not correlate with back pain.

However those with red flags such as elderly, osteoporosis, chronic intake of glucocorticoids, or history of trauma where the vertebral fracture is most likely pathology it is reasonable to proceed with plain x-ray or CT or plain MRI. Similarly, imaging with CT or MRI is appropriate whenever there is suspicion that low back pain is of infectious or malignant cause. Young people with IBP (suspecting SpA) and positive inflammatory markers also merit imaging with plain X-ray followed by MRI.

Management

Management depends on the etiology. Discussion of management of degenerative spine diseases that includes intervertebral disc herniation, spondylosis, spondylolisthesis, spondylolysis, and cauda equina syndrome is beyond the scope of this chapter.

Chronic Nonspecific Low Back Pain

This is the major group of patients we encounter in general clinical practice, where no definite or major abnormality is present anatomically. There are various names ascribed to this group: lumbago, lumbar sprain, lumbar strain, etc. This group of patients may have severe pain and disability but surprisingly have no findings on imaging, indicating that there is a disconnect between clinical symptoms and imaging. Non-pharmacological treatment includes massage, heat therapy, and behavioral therapy should be the first line of treatment, followed by pharmacological therapy. Before assigning patients to this category, first, ensure there are no red flag signs.

CONCLUSION

History and clinical examination will enable us to narrow down the differential diagnosis. Patients with nonspecific low back pain require physical therapy, a structured exercise program, and cognitive behavioral therapy for a good outcome. Regular physical conditioning and exercises will help maintain good musculoskeletal health.

LEARNING POINTS

- More than 90% of low back pain is mechanical in nature.
- Inflammatory back pain is not specific to spondyloarthritis.
- A major chunk of low back pain seen in primary care is chronic nonspecific low back pain. Ensure red flag signs are absent before assigning the patient to this category.
- Imaging is indicated when there are red flag signs, or when the back pain is present beyond 6 weeks despite treatment.

FURTHER READING

1. Braun A, Saracbasi E, Grifka J, et al. Identifying patients with axial spondyloarthritis in primary care: how useful are items indicative of inflammatory back pain? Ann Rheum Dis. 2011;70:1782–7.
2. Chou R, Qaseem A, Owens DK, et al. Diagnostic imaging for low back pain: Advice for high-value health care from the American College of Physicians. Ann Intern Med. 2011;154:181–9.
3. Downie A, Williams CM, Henschke N, et al. Red flags to screen for malignancy and fracture in patients with low back pain: a systematic review. BMJ. 2013;347:f7095.
4. Markman JD, Czerniecka-Foxx K, Khalsa PS, et al. AAPT Diagnostic criteria for chronic low back pain. J Pain. 2020;21:1138–48.

Approach to Shoulder and Neck Pain

Keerthi Talari

SHOULDER PAIN

The shoulder girdle includes the clavicle, scapula, and humerus as the bony skeleton with four articulations—glenohumeral, acromioclavicular, sternoclavicular, and scapulothoracic. There are multiple bursae around the shoulder but the most important is the subacromial bursa that lies between the acromion and rotator cuff.

Approach to Shoulder Pain

There are four main causes of shoulder pain:

- Rotator cuff disorders (tendinopathy and tears) with bicipital tendinitis.
- Acromioclavicular disease.
- Glenohumeral joint disease (adhesive capsulitis).
- Pain that is referred from the neck and elsewhere.

The location of the pain can indicate the underlying cause (Fig. 3.4.1). A cervical spine

History

Location and type of pain

- Cervical spine involvement leads to suprascapular region pain with radiation or referral to upper limb, associated paresthesia
- Acromioclavicular or sternoclavicular joint: Localized pain and may radiate proximally into neck
- Rotator cuff: Upper part of arm (over deltoid)
- Adhesive capsulitis: Intense aching deep in shoulder
- Sharp night pain: Rotator cuff tendinopathy or acromioclavicular' joint pathology

↓

Examination

Inspection of the anterior, posterior and lateral aspects

- Assess how patient undress
- Look for erythema, bruising, swelling, deformity, muscle wasting
- Anterior bulge in upper arm indicates long head of biceps rupture
- Winging of scapula indicates serratus anterior weakness
- Dumping of scapula in abduction indicates trapezius weakness

↓

Examination

Palpation

- Range of motion (active and passive): Abduction, flexion, extension, internal and external rotation with arm by side and 90° abduction
- Acromioclavicular, sternoclavicular, and glenohumeral joints tenderness
- Tenderness at bicipital tendon in bicipital groove
- Tenderness at greater and lesser tuberosities for rotator cuff tendinitis
- Special tests

Fig. 3.4.1: Clinical approach to shoulder pain

pathology may manifest as pain over the *suprascapular region*, while acromioclavicular, and sternoclavicular joint disease produces local *pain over the respective joints* sometimes with swelling. Rotator cuff tendinopathy and tears lead to pain over the *upper part of the deltoid*. While adhesive capsulitis causes *deep aching pain in the shoulder*.

On examination, in rotator cuff disorders there is a painful **mid-range arc** of abduction (60–120°) with a painful catch while lowering the arm from full abduction. In adhesive capsulitis (glenohumeral disease) there is a **global restriction** of passive movement and joint line tenderness in the early stages. Disuse atrophy of the deltoid is detected on clinical examination in later phases.

In acromioclavicular joint disease, there is local tenderness and swelling sometimes. Special tests for the shoulder joint are summarized in (Table 3.4.1).

Other causes of shoulder pain are referred from the cervical spine, myocardial infarction (acute onset), and diaphragmatic pathology. In older individuals, bilateral shoulder pain should arouse a suspicion of polymyalgia rheumatica.

Table 3.4.1: Special tests in shoulder examination

Special Test	*Procedure*
Neer test	Passive flexion with pressure on shoulder Indicates supraspinatus and biceps brachialis pathology
Hawkin Kennedy test	Forced passive internal rotation Indicates supraspinatus pathology
Empty can sign	Abduct, flex and internal rotation Indicates supraspinatus pathology
Drop arm test	Drop from abduction and external rotation Indicates full thickness rotator cuff tears
Others	Resisted internal rotation for subscapularis Resisted external rotation for infraspinatus and teres minor
Speed test	Resists shoulder flexion with extended elbow Indicates biceps brachialis pathology
Yergason test	Resists supination with flexed elbow Indicates biceps brachialis pathology

Rotator Cuff Tendinopathy and Tears, and Bicipital Tendinitis

Risk factors of rotator cuff tendinopathy include trauma (fall on the shoulder), hyperabduction injury, and eccentric overload on the shoulder during throwing. Other risk factors are intrinsic, i.e. related to glenohumeral instability, acromion spur, and acromioclavicular joint degeneration. Subacromial bursitis can further worsen rotator cuff injury. Treatment is conservative with surgery reserved for pain persistent beyond a year. However acute tears, especially in young patients should be managed with immediate surgery.

Bicipital tendinitis is usually secondary to a rotator cuff pathology. Bicipital tendinitis ranges from painful tendinitis to a full tear with or without associated subacromial impingement. Primary bicipital tendinitis usually occurs after weight lifting, prolonged carrying of children, or rotation of shoulder during overhead abduction of arm.

Capsulitis

Capsulitis is characterized by a painful restriction of both passive and active shoulder movement in the absence of joint degeneration apparently of soft tissue origin. The predisposing factors are diabetes, thyroid disease, hyperlipidemia, and trauma. There are three phases of capsulitis– painful (3–8 months), adhesive (4–6 months), and resolution (1–3 years). True glenohumeral arthritis can occur. Diagnosis is clinical. MRI is primarily performed to exclude other causes.

NECK PAIN

Neck pain is quite common in primary care. It can either be acute or chronic depending on whether the duration is less than or more than 12 weeks.

Approach to Neck Pain

The causes of neck pain (Table 3.4.2) are varied. It is often difficult to pinpoint the exact cause in clinical practice. The most important prevalent cause would arguably be chronic musculoskeletal conditions namely cervical spondylosis which is highly prevalent in primary care and rheumatology clinics as well. Any of the cervical spine structures including disc, upper cervical synovial joints, lower cervical zygapophyseal synovial joints, muscles, or

Table 3.4.2: Causes of neck pain

Musculoskeletal conditions • Cervical spondylosis • Cervical disc protrusion and/or prolapse • Cervical strain • Whiplash injury • Facet joint arthritis • Myofascial pain • Diffuse idiopathic skeletal hyperostosis (DISH) • Referred pain from shoulder
Neurologic pain • Cervical nerve root compression (radiculopathy) • Cervical myelopathy • Atlantoaxial anomaly
Systemic causes of neck pain **(Most have red flags*)** • Myocardial ischemia • Infections: lymphadenitis due to tuberculosis, retropharyngeal neck abscess, Vincent's angina, meningitis. • Vertebral artery dissection • Thyroiditis • Takayasu arteritis (carotidynia) • Polymyalgia rheumatica • Rheumatoid arthritis • Malignancy and metastasis to cervical spine
***Red flags that indicates systemic cause of neck pain** • Acutely ill patients • Significant trauma • Fever • Elderly with shoulder girdle pain • Weight loss • Neurologic manifestations: paraesthesias, motor weakness, hyperactive deep tendon reflexes • Lhermitte's sign • Raised inflammatory markers

ligaments pathology can give rise to neck pain. They can be involved by degenerative mechanical and or inflammatory processes.

Secondly, cervical nerve root compression produces radicular pain and radiculopathy.

Thirdly systemic (non-cervical spine) causes have to be considered whenever "red flags" are present. These patients require imaging and investigations. An example is to consider polymyalgia rheumatica in older people with diffuse neck pain that cannot be localized. Acute onset neck pain with systemic symptoms such as fever indicates infections maybe meningitis or lymphadenitis or abscesses in the muscles. In a patient with rheumatoid arthritis, the presence of neck pain suggests underlying atlantoaxial joint subluxation or dislocation.

As illustrated in (Fig. 3.4.2), a good history of the location of pain and quality of pain helps narrow the differential diagnosis. The examination should cover general physical, neck palpation, and neurological examination for radiculopathy and myelopathy. A knowledge of nerve roots and their area of distribution is useful for localization (Table 3.4.3).

Cervical spondylosis: A condition of age-related degenerative changes in the cervical spine is one cause of neck pain. However degenerative changes in the spine do not always correlate with neck pain. Degenerative changes include osteophytes, which

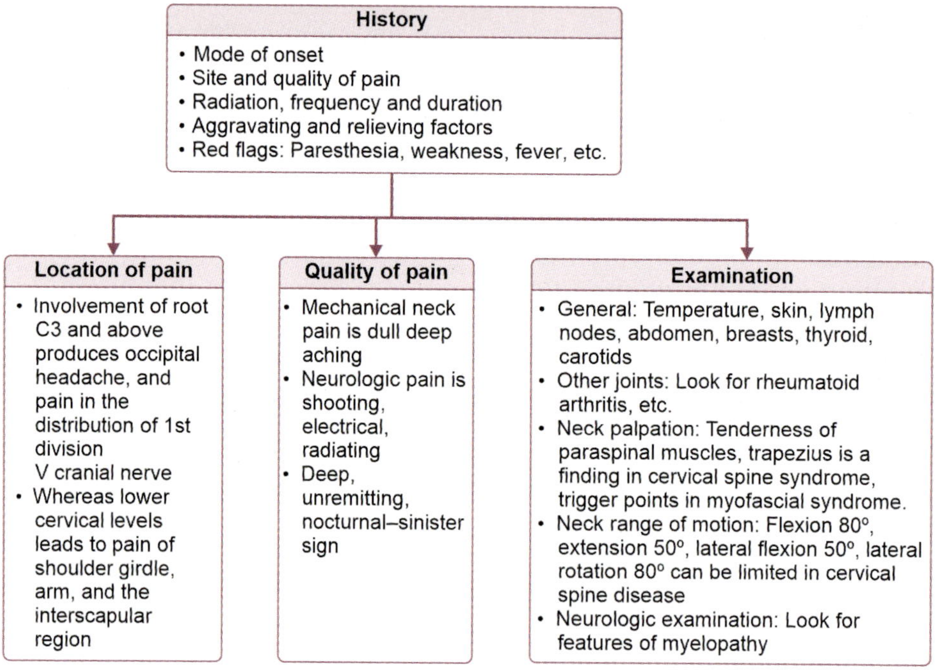

Fig. 3.4.2: Approach to a patient with neck pain

Table 3.4.3: Cervical spine nerve root value and their area of distribution

Root value	*Sensory distribution*	*Motor distribution*	*Deep tendon reflex*
C2	Above occipital protuberance	–	–
C3 C4	Posterior neck	Neck flexion/lateral flexion (along with spinal accessory)	Trapezius
C5	Lateral arm	Shoulder abduction, elbow flexion	Biceps
C6	Thumb	Wrist extension/pronation	Supinator
C7	Middle finger	Elbow extension	Triceps
C8	Little finger	Finger flexion/ extension	Finger flexion

can lead to intervertebral foraminal narrowing, and nerve root compression producing shooting pain down the arms with paraesthesias. Cervical radiculopathy is more commonly due to osteophytes and less commonly due to disc protrusion.

Specific tests for diagnosis of cervical nerve root compression include the **Spurling test**. The neck is placed in extension with rotation to the symptomatic side followed by tapping the head (axial pressure) from above to elicit symptoms. It has a good positive predictive value.

Disc degeneration: Disc degeneration with subsequent protrusion or herniation is another cause of neck pain, stiffness, and painful movements of the neck. Pain worsens during activities that involve holding the neck for prolonged periods and relief with rest. When the disc compresses on the spinal cord it leads to cervical myelopathy, manifesting with pain, weakness, and wasting of the upper limbs.

Whiplash injury: Hyperextension injury with axial compression of the cervical spine with double curvatures resulting in injury to the annulus fibrosus or anterior longitudinal ligament, articular pillar, articular surface, or end plate tears and fractures. Causes acute neck pain but can become chronic especially due to psychosocial factors. Facet (zygapophyseal) joint injury is also a common cause of neck pain. Reassurance, multimodal intervention, and resuming activities at the earliest are better than inactivity, cervical collars, and heat or ultrasound therapy.

Cervical strain: It is a common cause of neck pain/stiffness, particularly on neck movement. Patients often give a history of injury to the paraspinal muscles. Poor posture and sleeping habits are other predisposing factors. There may be tenderness on palpation of the neck and trapezius muscles. However, the Spurling test and other provocative tests for radiculopathy are negative.

Imaging

Those patients with red flags will need imaging on priority and other investigations

Management

Management consists of treating the primary cause—rheumatoid arthritis, infection or tumor, or other secondary causes. In case there are no red flags, management of musculoskeletal neck pain consists of analgesics, physical therapy, exercise (strengthening and proprioceptive training), posture correcting pillows, and correcting work ergonomics.

LEARNING POINTS

- Rotator cuff disorders, acromioclavicular joint disease, glenohumeral joint arthritis, adhesive capsulitis, and referred pain are the main causes of shoulder pain
- Impingement syndromes in the shoulder are secondary to rotator cuff injuries, mostly treated conservatively except when pain persists or in young individuals where surgery may be considered.
- Capsulitis causes loss of range of motion in all planes, unlike rotator cuff pathologies where the restriction is usually in abduction or any other plane.
- Whiplash injuries are better managed by returning to normal activities as early as possible rather than cervical collars and immobilization.

FURTHER READING

1. Burbank KM, Stevenson JH, Czarnecki GR, Dorfman J. Chronic shoulder pain: part I. Evaluation and diagnosis. Am Fam Physician. 2008;77:453–60.
2. Cohen SP, Hooten WM. Advances in the diagnosis and management of neck pain. BMJ. 2017;358:j3221.
3. Pattrick M, Doherty M. Clinical Examination in Rheumatology. London; Elsevier Health Sciences 1992.
4. Ramirez J. Adhesive Capsulitis: Diagnosis and Management. Am Fam Physician. 2019;99:297–300.

Approach to Regional Pain: Hand and Wrist

K Shanmuganandan, S Kartik

INTRODUCTION

Hand and wrist pain comprise a significant proportion of regional musculoskeletal disorders. The hands and wrists are involved in complex motor tasks. Repetitive use using hands and strain are integral parts of many professions such as computer operators, musicians, dentists, and artisans. Here we will give an overview on how to approach a patient with hand and/or wrist pain.

CAUSE OF HAND AND WRIST PAIN

The causes of hand and wrist pain (Table 3.5.1) can be local or general disorders. It could be benign causes such as due to repetitive use of the hand or could be the manifestation of systemic diseases such as rheumatoid arthritis (RA) or psoriatic arthritis (PsA). Some clues that help to ascertain the exact cause of hand and wrist pain are:

Table 3.5.1: Causes of hand and wrist pain

Local	*General*
Tenosynovitis	Fibromyalgia
deQuervain's disease	Cervical Spondylitis with radiation
Carpal tunnel syndrome	Cardiac angina
Cubital tunnel syndrome	Painful sensory neuropathy
Repetitive strain injury	Hypermobility
Fracture of carpal bones	
Cervical spondylosis	
Raynaud's phenomenon	
Peripheral vascular disease	
Osteoarthritis of the hand	
Rheumatoid arthritis	
Psoriatic arthritis	

1. **Age of the patient**
   a. **Young adults:** Causes of hand pain in young people could be trauma related, repetitive strain injury, smartphone overuse, or juvenile idiopathic arthritis (JIA).
   b. **Middle age:** Rhe causes to consider in this age group are inflammatory arthritis, Raynaud's phenomenon, ganglion, tenosynovitis, carpal tunnel syndrome, cubital tunnel syndrome etc.
   c. **Elderly:** Osteonecrosis, osteoporotic fracture, peripheral vascular disease, cervical spondylitis, crystal arthritis, nodal osteoarthritis, diabetic cheiroarthropathy, reflex sympathetic dystrophy.
2. **Gender**
   a. **Male:** Trauma, peripheral vascular disease, gout, pseudogout.
   b. **Female:** Carpal tunnel syndrome, inflammatory arthritis, Raynaud's phenomenon, osteoarthritis.
3. **Nature of pain**
   a. Neuropathic pain suggests carpal tunnel syndrome, radiculopathy, sensory neuropathy, reflex sympathetic dystrophy (complex regional pain syndrome).
   b. **Inflammatory joint pain:** RA, PsA.
   c. **Throbbing pain:** Acute gout, acute pseudogout.
   d. **Localized pain:** Carpal tunnel syndrome, osteonecrosis, ganglion.

SPECIFIC DISORDERS THAT PRODUCE HAND OR WRIST PAIN

deQuervain's disease: Is characterised by pain over the radial styloid, tender swelling of the first extensor compartment, and pain is reproduced by resisted thumb extension or positive Finkelstein's test.

Tenosynovitis of wrist: Pain on movement localised to tendon sheaths in the wrist and reproduction of pain by resisted active movement.

Carpal tunnel syndrome: Pain or paresthesia or sensory loss in median nerve distribution and any one of the following:

- Tinel's test positive
- Phalen's test positive
- Nocturnal exacerbation of symptoms with abductor pollicis brevis weakness
- Abnormal nerve conduction studies

DIAGNOSTIC MODALITIES

Clinical diagnosis: Fibromyalgia and hypermobility of the joints are diagnosed clinically.

Plain radiographs: Diagnosis of conditions such as RA, PsA, hand osteoarthritis, gout, and pseudogout are assisted by plain radiographic findings.

Musculoskeletal ultrasonography is increasingly being used to diagnose tendinitis, tenosynovitis, ganglion cyst.

Nerve conduction studies: Carpal tunnel syndrome, Cubital tunnel syndrome, peripheral neuropathy, radiculopathy are typically confirmed in nerve conduction studies.

Arterial doppler is useful to confirm peripheral vascular disease, Buerger's disease, Takayasu's arteritis.

Bone scintigraphy: Reflex sympathetic dystrophy (complex regional pain syndrome).

Magnetic resonance imaging: Tenosynovitis, Ganglion, Cervical radiculopathy.

Nail fold capillaroscopy: It is useful to evaluate Raynaud's phenomenon and look for patterns that may suggest systemic sclerosis or dermatomyositis or Raynauds disease.

Thermography: Raynaud's disease, Inflammatory arthritis, Peripheral vascular disease.

LEARNING POINTS

- Hand and wrist pain comprise a significant proportion of regional pain.
- The causes are manifold and may be local or systemic.
- Detailed clinical evaluation and appropriate investigations lead to early diagnosis.

FURTHER READING

1. Forman TA, Forman SK, Rose NE. A clinical approach to diagnosing wrist pain. Am Fam Physician. 2005;72:1753–8.
2. Shehab R, Mirabelli MH. Evaluation and diagnosis of wrist pain: a case-based approach. Am Fam Physician. 2013; 87:568–73. Erratum in: Am Fam Physician. 2013;88:427.

Chapter 3.6

Approach to a Child with Arthritis

Sujata Sawhney

INTRODUCTION

There are many differential diagnoses when confronted with a child with one or more swollen joints. This is because there are many triggers for a joint to swell up, these could range from infectious, inflammatory, neoplastic, to traumatic causes. Additionally, several metabolic and genetic conditions can cause joint deformities that can mimic arthritis. This chapter will outline the clinical approach to a child with arthritis and discuss briefly the appropriate investigations to arrive at a correct diagnosis.

Approach: Should address four questions:

1. Does the child have inflammatory, noninflammatory or sinister joint pains?
2. Is the clinical complaint acute or chronic?
3. Is the complaint limited to one joint or more?
4. Is it a standalone problem affecting only the joints or is it part of a multisystem disease process?

KEY FEATURES IN THE HISTORY AND CLINICAL EXAMINATION

As the differential diagnosis of arthritis in children is wide, a detailed history and careful top to toe clinical examination (Table 3.6.1) will give clues about the likely differential diagnosis. Armed with this information the clinician should order few relevant investigations and not order "rheumatological panels" which often cause more confusion rather than help. Let us address each of the four questions listed above.

1. Does the Child have Inflammatory, Noninflammatory or Sinister Joint Pains?

It is important to distinguish these 3 major categories of arthritis (Table 3.6.2). The most common cause of joint pains in children is *non-inflammatory pains* of which benign joint hypermobility syndrome is the most frequent. In the true sense, there is no frank joint swelling and therefore these patients do not have arthritis. They may have small transient joint effusions but predominantly have arthralgia. Amongst *inflammatory joints* juvenile idiopathic arthritis (JIA) is the most frequent. This is seen in 1:1000 children, as frequent as insulin dependent diabetes. Finally, young infants may have neuroblastoma as a cause of arthritis and the older child with acute leukaemia may have arthritis as the presenting feature-the *sinister joint pain* category. Screening joint examination and further regional assessment is detailed online: *(http://www.arthritisresearchuk.org).*

2. Is the Clinical Complaint Acute or Chronic?

Acute arthritis: It is defined as arthritis of less than 6 weeks duration. The most common cause in children is viral arthritis. The most important differential diagnosis that needs urgent exclusion here is the child that presents with septic arthritis where a diagnostic tap of the synovial fluid is critical. The fluid should be sent for cell count and culture. A cell count of more than 50,000/dL with predominant neutrophils is usually highly suggestive of a septic process. This is supported by a positive gram stain and culture. Table 3.6.3 gives descriptors and causes of several important reasons for children

TABLE 3.6.1: General points to be covered in history and clinical examination	
Clinical characteristics	*Example*
Age at presentation and sex of the child	**Neonate:** most common joint involvement is because of septic arthritis **Preschool female child:** likely oligoarticular juvenile arthritis **Adolescent male:** inflammatory joint disease likely to be enthesitis related arthritis, non-inflammatory disease likely to be sports related such as Osgood Schlatter disease or developmental disorders such as slipped capital femoral epiphysis or Perthes disease. Kawasaki Disease presents most often in children < 5 years. Lupus, other CTDs and primary vasculitides are unusual in young infants, seen over 8–10 years.
Joint pain Location, onset, progress, severity, night disturbance, pattern (additive vs migratory), triggers, etc.	Severe pain is seen in infection, trauma, bleed and with a neoplastic process. Night awakening if focal and accompanied by constitutional features is characteristic of neoplastic lesions. Migratory arthritis is classically seen in acute rheumatic fever.
Joint swelling Onset, location, and pattern of joint involvement.	The pattern of joint involvement can be identified by seeing involvement of upper versus lower limbs, symmetric versus asymmetric involvement, large joint versus small joint, involvement of the axial skeleton.
Is the joint disease pattern additive or migratory? In additive pattern the patient has involvement of several joints either acutely or indolently. In migratory pattern there is involvement of the joints one after the other with resolution of the previous joint as the next one gets involved.	**Additive arthritis** is seen in most inflammatory rheumatic diseases such as juvenile arthritis, lupus or juvenile dermatomyositis. **Migratory arthritis** is classically described in the child with acute rheumatic fever. It can also be seen in patients with acute leukaemia, Henoch–Schonlein purpura or Lyme disease.
Fever Duration, pattern and associated complaints	Only systemic onset JIA has classical quotidian fever with evanescent rashes, organomegaly and associated serositis and lymphadenopathy. Other subcategories of JIA have no fever. Reactive arthritis, CTDs, vasculitis, infections and malignancies have presentation with fever.
Constitutional features	Profound weight loss and loss of appetite point to a malignancy. Myalgias and joint pains can be seen in many rheumatological diseases such as lupus and primary systemic vasculitis.
Systems review	To define if the joints alone are involved or this is part of a systemic disease, detailed in Table 3.6.5.
Clinical examination Head to toe clinical examination and detailed MSK examination, measurement of blood pressure in all four limbs	Define organs involved: Skin, mucosa, organomegaly, lymphadenopathy Blood pressure Joint pattern and assessment of all systems. Can define if the broad category is JIA, CTD, vasculitis, infection, malignancy or a mimic

CTD: Connective tissue disease

Table 3.6.2: Nature of joint disease

Clinical feature	*Inflammatory*	*Noninflammatory**	*Sinister ***
Early morning stiffness	Present	Absent	Absent
Joint swelling	Present	Absent /transient	+/–
Improves with gentle mobility	Yes	No	No
Night awakening because of pain	No	Yes, bilateral lower limb pain	Yes, with focal pain and constitutional features, bony tenderness, hepatosplenomegaly.
Example	Juvenile idiopathic arthritis	Benign joint hypermobility	Acute lymphoblastic leukemia
Investigations	Complete blood count, ESR, CRP, rheumatoid factor, antinuclear antibody and HLA B27 as appropriate	Clinical examination adequate, no laboratory investigations required	Initial basic investigations should include complete blood count, peripheral smear, uric acid, LDH, chest X-ray, screening ultrasound abdomen. Proceed as per specific malignancy detected.

*Non-inflammatory pains such as that occurs with hypermobility usually do not have frankly swollen joints and patients have more joint pain than frank arthritis, the effusion seen (if at all) is minor and transient.

*It is important to distinguish joint contractures from arthritis. Mimics of juvenile idiopathic arthritis (JIA) that present with joint *contractures* but no frank arthritis include a wide range of metabolic arthropathies. Amongst these are mucopolysaccharidoses especially the mild variant such as Scheie syndrome and Morquio syndrome.

**The classic presentation of acute lymphoblastic leukemia to the rheumatologist is that of acute migratory monoarthritis. These children have significant pain and clinically can have both arthritis and periarthritis. This can be associated with anaemia, bony tenderness, hepatosplenomegaly, and lymphadenopathy.

Table 3.6.3: Acute arthritis: Etiology and descriptors

Etiology	*Causes*	*Descriptor*
Infections	Bacterial *Staphylococcus aureus* *Streptococcus pneumonia* Leptospirosis Viral Fungal Lyme disease Tuberculosis (unusual)	Septic arthritis is a rare but potentially serious disorder. The presentation is usually with acute monoarthritis where the joint is red hot and swollen. Some viral infections may present with symmetric polyarthritis.
Inflammatory	JIA: Spondyloarthropathy or ERA Plant thorn synovitis Reactive Acute rheumatic fever Other reactive arthritis	Patients with JIA usually have an indolent onset, but sometimes ERA and SJIA present acutely. Reactive arthritis can have an acute onset and often presents in older children with a triad of red eyes, urethritis/ diarrhea, and swollen lower limb joints.
Vasculitis	Henoch–Schonlein purpura (HSP) Kawasaki disease (KD)	HSP may present with large lower limb joint swelling. Arthritis is described in the 2nd to 3rd week of illness in children with KD.
Bone/cartilage	Tumor Osteonecrosis	Can present with severe bone pain and clinical examination can reveal periarthritis.

(*Contd.*)

Table 3.6.3: Acute arthritis: Etiology and descriptors *(Contd.)*

Etiology	*Causes*	*Descriptor*
Trauma	Fracture Internal derangement of the knee (IDK)	History of significant trauma followed by abrupt onset swelling of the joint within 12–24 hours, the child is unable to bear weight after trauma.
Hematological	Hemarthrosis Infarctive crisis of sickle cell disease Malignancies (acute leukemia)	Hemophilia can present with an abrupt swelling of the joint in young male infants who have just begun weight bearing. Infarction crisis in sickle cell disease presents severe symmetric pain in the small joints of the hand and feet.

JIA: Juvenile idiopathic arthritis; *ERA:* Enthesitis-related arthritis

to develop acute arthritis. Figure 3.6.1 outlines the clinical approach when evaluating a child with acute monoarthritis.

Chronic arthritis: It is defined as one that persists for more than 6 weeks. One of the most common causes of chronic arthritis is JIA, defined as arthritis that begins in a child less than 16 years, which lasts for more than 6 weeks whereas all other known causes have been excluded. Therefore, a history of connective tissue disease, vasculitis and malignancy must be taken when any patient presents with arthritis of any duration.

3. Is it One Joint or More?

Figure 3.6.2 details the differentials for chronic monoarthritis and Table 3.6.4 outlines diseases

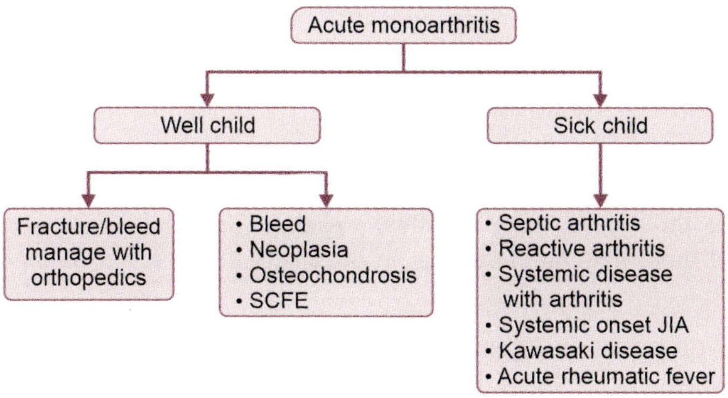

Fig. 3.6.1: Approach to a child with acute monoarthritis

SCFE: Slipped capital femoral epiphysis; *JIA:* Juvenile idiopathic arthritis

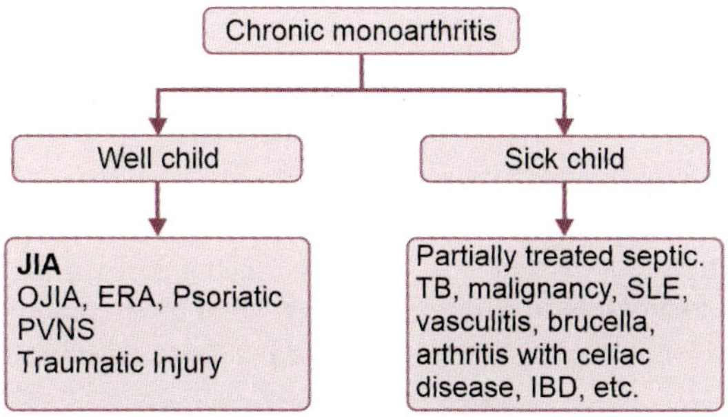

Fig. 3.6.2: Differential diagnosis of chronic monoarthritis

OJIA: Oligoarticular juvenile idiopathic arthritis; *ERA:* Enthesitis related arthritis; *PVNS:* pigmented villonodular synovitis; *TB:* Tuberculosis; *SLE:* Systemic lupus erythematosus; *IBD:* inflammatory bowel disease

Table 3.6.4: Polyarthritis (Acute and Chronic)

Acute Polyarthritis	*Disease*
Not sick child	**Post viral arthritis** HSP, Kawasaki disease Reactive arthritis
Sick child	Acute onset of PJIA, ERA, SJIA Acute rheumatic fever cSLE Other CTDs: JDM, scleroderma Malignancy Miscellaneous: arthritis with infective endocarditis (IE), Inflammatory bowel disease, immunodeficiency
Chronic polyarthritis	**Disease** All categories of JIA CTDs: cSLE, JDM, SSc, overlap and MCTD Systemic vasculitides **Miscellaneous** Chronic infections Malignancies Mimics

PJIA: Polyarticular juvenile idiopathic arthritis; *ERA:* Enthesitis-related arthritis; *SJIA:* Systemic juvenile idiopathic arthritis; *HSP:* Henoch-Schonlein purpura; *CTD:* Connective tissue disease; *cSLE:* Childhood systemic lupus erythematosus; *JDM:* Juvenile dermatomyositis; *SSc:* Systemic sclerosis; *MCTD:* Mixed connective tissue disease

that present with more than one joint involvement. It is very important to examine the child and precede that with a comprehensive history. The child or parent may point to the joint causing the most difficulty but several more may be picked up on examination.

4. Is it only Joint Involvement or is this Part of a Multi-system Disease?

This is the final question that the clinician should address. It is often the extra-articular features that lead one to the correct diagnosis.

In addition to giving attention to the age and sex of the child, the onset, duration and the pattern of joint involvement, further history taking and clinical examination should focus on a careful systems review which is detailed in Table 3.6.5.

INVESTIGATIONS TO BE ORDERED

There is no battery or panel of rheumatological investigations that should be ordered for every child. There should be only a few relevant investigations per the clinical context (Table 3.6.6).

Table 3.6.5: Extra-articular features (systems review) mandatory during examination

Organ	*Feature*	*Associated disease*
Eye	To look for acute or chronic anterior uveitis, scleritis, and a careful retinal examination.	• Silent chronic anterior uveitis is a common feature in oligo-JIA especially the young preschool female child. • Scleritis may be a presenting manifestation of systemic vasculitis such as granulomatosis with polyangiitis. • Choroidal tubercles or intermediate uveitis may be associated with patients with tuberculosis. • Retinal vasculitis can also be seen in childhood lupus and other connective tissue diseases.

(Contd.)

Table 3.6.5: Extra-articular features (systems review) mandatory during examination (*Contd.*)

Organ	*Feature*	*Associated disease*
Skin	Psoriasiform rashes, photosensitivity, clinical hallmarks of juvenile dermatomyositis or systemic sclerosis, palpable purpura, nodules or skin ulcers.	• Malar rash with nasolabial sparing seen in childhood lupus. • Gottron's papules, heliotrope rash, extensor surface erythematous rash-juvenile dermatomyositis. • Sclerodactyly and Raynaud's phenomena suggestive of limited or diffuse-systemic sclerosis. • Lower limb palpable purpura with arthritis-Henoch Schonlein purpura.
Reticuloendothelial system	Lymphadenopathy, Hepatosplenomegaly.	• Exclude infections especially tuberculosis in the correct clinical context. • Review for childhood lupus, malignancy, sarcoidosis, etc.
Serositis	Identify pleural or pericardial effusion or ascites.	• Consider infections such as tuberculosis. • Look for connective tissue diseases such as childhood lupus. • Systemic JIA juvenile idiopathic and some autoinflammatory diseases can also have polyserositis.
Neurology	History of seizures, mononeuritis multiplex, focal neurological deficit, severe headache.	• All of these point to systemic diseases that could either be connective tissue disease or primary systemic vasculitis, and occasionally antiphospholipid syndrome.
Heart and lungs	Heart murmurs, pericardial friction rub, pulmonary parenchymal disease.	• Acute rheumatic fever present with pancarditis. • Childhood lupus can have small pericardial and pleural effusions, rarely tamponade. • Parenchymal lung disease warrants exclusion of infection. • Cavitating lung lesions may be the presentation of a child with granulomatosis with polyangiitis.
Pulses	Renal bruit, peripheral pulses Unequal BP.	• Childhood Takayasu

Table 3.6.6: Investigative approach for evaluation of arthritis in children

Investigation	*Utility*
CBC, ESR, CRP	Can help distinguish between inflammatory and non-inflammatory pains. These are only a guide and not absolute. Thus the child with one swollen joint in the context of juvenile arthritis can have all acute phase response is normal.
Chest X-ray, abdomen ultrasound, liver and renal function tests	Helps define any underlying organ involvement.
Infection screen	Tuberculosis, brucellosis, Lyme disease, acute rheumatic fever depending upon the clinical context.
ANA by IIF, HLA-B27, RF, ACPA	These tests are ordered in the context of JIA. No test can rule in or rule out JIA which remains a clinical diagnosis to date.
ANCA IIF, antimyeloperoxidase, antiproteinase 3	Should only be done in the relevant clinical context when ANCA associated vasculitis such as granulomatosis with polyangiitis (GPA), eosinophilic granulomatosis with polyangiitis or microscopic polyangiitis are suspected.

(*Contd.*)

Table 3.6.6: Investigative approach for evaluation of arthritis in children *(Contd.)*

Investigation	*Utility*
Angiographic study	In those who are suspected to have polyarteritis nodosa or aortoarteritis.
CT chest	When lung involvement is suspected.
Ultrasound examination	This is especially useful in monoarticular disease, when the diagnosis is in doubt, and for evaluation of the sacroiliac joint which is difficult to define clinically.
MRI of the involved joint	

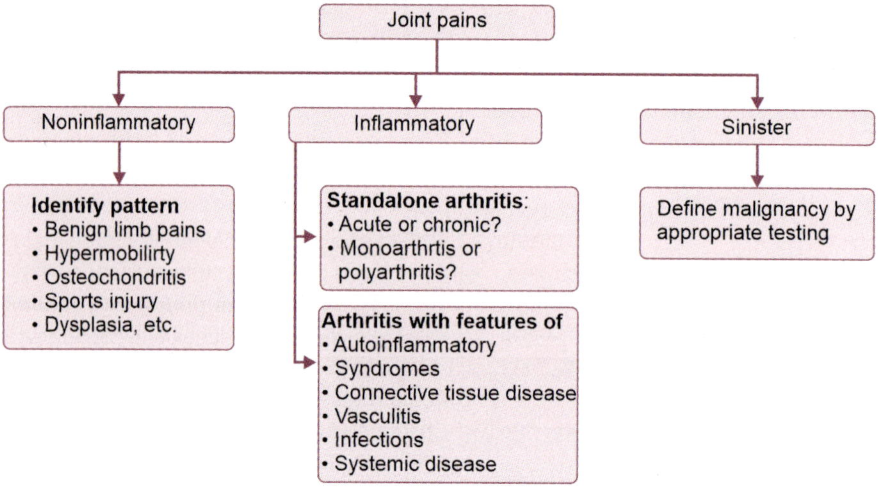

Fig. 3.6.3: Summary of approach to a child with arthritis

SUMMARY

The differential diagnosis of arthritis in children is wide. It ranges from infections, to inflammatory and sinister causes. There can be several mimics where children present with joint contractures and not frank arthritis. Thus, a careful history, clinical examination and few relevant investigations will help clinch the final diagnosis for the child (Fig. 3.6.3).

LEARNING POINTS

- There is a wide differential diagnosis for the child that presents with arthritis.
- Detailed history and clinical examination with few relevant investigations will point one in the correct direction.
- Basic classification into acute/chronic, additive/migratory arthritis, with/without systemic symptoms (fever) can help narrow down possibilities.
- Order only a few relevant investigations in the correct clinical context there is no role for ordering "Rheumatology panels".
- Distinguish between arthritis and joint contractures, the latter can mimic childhood arthritis.

FURTHER READING

1. Haines KA. The Approach to the Child with Joint Complaints. Pediatr Clin North Am. 2018;65:623–38.
2. Quartier P, Prieur AM. Immunodeficiency and genetic conditions that cause arthritis in childhood. Curr Rheumatol Rep. 2002;4:483–93.
3. Rezaei E, Hogan D, Trost B, et al. BBOP Study Group. Associations of clinical and inflammatory biomarker clusters with juvenile idiopathic arthritis categories. Rheumatology (Oxford). 2020;59:1066–75.
4. Rumsey DG, Laxer RM. The Challenges and Opportunities of Classifying Childhood Arthritis. Curr Rheumatol Rep. 2020;22:4.
5. Weiser P. Approach to the patient with noninflammatory musculoskeletal pain. Pediatr Clin North Am. 2012; 59:471–92.

Chapter 3.7

Approach to Fever in Rheumatic Diseases

Bidyut Das, Saumya Ranjan Tripathy

INTRODUCTION

Fever can be the presenting manifestation of SLE, vasculitis, and adult-onset Still's disease among others. Thus while working up patients with fever of unknown origin a systemic autoimmune/ inflammatory disease may have to be ruled out. Secondly, in a known case of an inflammatory rheumatic disease the presence of fever may be due to infection that has to be differentiated from active disease. In children, the presence of intermittent periodic fevers can be due to monogenic autoinflammatory disorders.

PATTERN OF FEVER

The fever is intermittent in adult onset Still's disease (AOSD) and acute rheumatic fever. Other conditions such as vasculitis can also occur with intermittent fever. Periodic fever syndromes are diseases of children except for familial mediterranean fever which can also present in adolescent age group (Table 3.7.1). Among those conditions that give rise to continuous fever (Table 3.7.2), macrophage activation syndrome, SLE, myositis, septic arthritis are important.

FEVER AND ARTHRITIS

The combination of 'fever and arthritis' in rheumatology has a wide differential diagnosis (Table 3.7.3). Rheumatological differential diagnosis for fever and monoarthritis includes septic arthritis, acute gout, and pseudogout. The important rheumatology causes of 'polyarthritis and fever' are acute rheumatic fever, and AOSD where fever is almost always part of the presenting manifestation.

Table 3.7.1: Intermittent fever

Rheumatic Conditions	*Non-rheumatic conditions*
Adult-onset Still's disease	**Infections:** Malaria, urinary tract infections, infective endocarditis, osteomyelitis, spondylitis
Rheumatic fever	
Crystal arthritis	
Vasculitides	Neoplasms
Sarcoidosis	Pulmonary embolism
Behcet's disease	Drug-induced fever
Relapsing polychondritis	
Familial periodic fever syndromes	

Table 3.7.2: Continuous fever

Rheumatic conditions	*Non-rheumatic conditions*
SLE	Acute osteomyelitis
Antisynthetase syndrome	Chronic osteomyelitis
Macrophage activation syndrome	Brodie's abscess
Septic arthritis	Bacterial spondylodiscitis
Viral arthritis	
Prosthetic joint infections	
Septic bursitis	

Table 3.7.3: Fever and arthritis

Type of arthritis	*Differential diagnosis*	*Fever prevalence*	*Diagnostic clues*
Monoarthritis	Gout	9–18%	Episodic attacks that are self-resolving within 2 weeks, tophi and erosions on the radiograph, negatively birefringent needle shaped crystals in synovial fluid.
	Calcium pyrophosphate deposition disease	Up to 50%	Affects elderly, radiographs show chondrocalcinosis, positively birefringent rhomboid crystals in synovial fluid.
	Septic arthritis	>90%	Red, hot, tender and swollen joints. Synovial fluid >50,000 cells/mm³.
	Reactive arthritis	Fever is uncommon	History of preceding urinary tract infection or diarrhea.
Polyarthritis	Acute rheumatic fever	Fever is a hallmark	1st episode between 3 and 15 years of age, arthritis is migratory. Other features are subcutaneous nodules, pancarditis, erythema marginatum, chorea
	AOSD	High-spiking intermittent fever, diurnal, peak >39°C	Evanescent salmon-pink rash, arthritis, lymphadenopathy, hepatosplenomegaly, serositis and neutrophilic leukocytosis
	SLE	Up to 41% at some point of time in the course of illness	Other clinical features of SLE
	Sarcoidosis	66% of cases.	Heerfordt syndrome: fever, parotidomegaly, arthritis, uveitis, facial nerve palsy. Lofgren syndrome: Erythema nodosum, bilateral hilar lymphadenopathy, arthritis.
	IBD associated arthritis	Fever is a sign of severe IBD	Bloody diarrhea, oral ulcers, oligoarthritis or polyarthritis in 5–20%
	Rheumatoid arthritis	<5%	Low-grade fever may occur during a flare

Fever is less common in rheumatoid arthritis if it does we have to rule out infection, vasculitis, or a flare, or drug fever. Sarcoidosis, one of whose manifestations is arthritis, may present as pyrexia of unknown origin. In case of inflammatory bowel disease, fever indicates severe disease.

There is another situation where fever occurs along with musculoskeletal manifestations such as myalgia, arthralgia, back pain, tenosynovitis, bursitis, neck pain, where the etiology is infectious (Table 3.7.4). These conditions are Chikungunya arthritis, dengue, HIV, acute lepra reaction, musculoskeletal tuberculosis, and brucellosis. Most often than not all these conditions are acute to subacute in onset.

Fever in Vasculitis

Almost all forms of systemic vasculitis have fever as a manifestation. Giant cell arteritis (GCA) occurs in people older >50 typically presenting with temporal headache, jaw claudication, loss of vision (15–20%). Almost half of GCA patients can have low grade fever. Similarly polymyalgia rheumatica (PMR) can have low grade fever (40%) at presentation. Thus

Table 3.7.4: Infectious diseases that have fever and musculoskeletal manifestations

Infection	*Musculoskeletal manifestation*
Chikungunya	Acute chikungunya presents with high-grade fever and arthritis/arthralgia
Dengue	Dengue fever causes fever, myalgia, arthralgia, arthritis (12–20%)
HIV	HIV can present with fever. Other clinical features are polyarthralgia, increased severity of psoriasis, HIV associated myopathy, vasculitis
Leprosy (Hansen's disease)	Acute lepra reaction presents with fever and cutaneous lesions, there can be symmetric polyarthritis resembling RA, tenosynovitis, swollen hand and feet syndrome
Tuberculosis (TB)	TB arthritis of the hip, knee, and Pott's spine all manifest with fever albeit variably
	Reactive arthritis (Poncet's disease) in response to active extra-articular tuberculosis (e.g. pulmonary TB or lymphadenitis)
Brucellosis	Brucellosis is a rare zoonotic infection manifesting with fever and back pain and polyarthalgia. Important musculoskeletal manifestations are sacroiliitis (usually asymmetric), spondylodiskitis, bursitis and osteomyelitis

low grade fever in older people with fatigue, girdle pain, and raised ESR should prompt one to consider large vessel vasculitis ie GCA and PMR.

Similarly Takayasu arteritis is known to present as fever of unknown origin. Thus it is important to consider Takayasu in young people (especially women) with fever of unknown origin. Examination of all peripheral pulses is often rewarding.

Polyarteritis nodosa (PAN), a systemic necrotizing medium vessel vasculitis often present with marked constitutional symptoms, and fever can be present in about 60%. Diagnostic clues to PAN are hypertension, proteinuria, abdominal pain, high inflammatory markers, thrombocytosis.

Kawasaki disease is an important cause of persistent fever in children. It is often accompanied by other hallmark clinical manifestations such as cervical lymphadenopathy, oral and pharyngeal mucosal erythema, etc.

The small vessel vasculitides: eosinophilic granulomatosis with polyangiitis (EGPA), granulomatosis with polyangiitis (GPA), microscopic polyangiitis (MPA) all are known to have fever as an accompanying manifestation. The challenge of fever in these cases (just like in SLE) lies in differentiating active vasculitis from infection, especially those are on immunosuppressants.

Fever in Connective Tissue Disorders (CTDs)

Antisynthetase syndrome is characterized by fever, arthritis, Raynaud's phenomenon, mechanic's hands, interstitial lung disease, myositis and the presence of antisynthetase antibodies.

Fever in Children with Arthritis

Systemic onset JIA has fever as a dominant manifestation, which can further be complicated by macrophage activation syndrome (MAS) (Table 3.7.5). Also the infections should be ruled out in a child with JIA who has fever. Additionally, fever and arthritis in a child can be hematological malignancy. Autoinflammatory syndromes (discussed in Chapter 12.5) is characterized by periodic fever amongst other manifestations.

Differentiating Active Disease from Infection in SLE or Vasculitis Patients

Though fever can be a manifestation of SLE indicating active disease, ruling out infections is challenging. The predictors of infections in SLE are very high CRP (usually >11 mg/L), presence of comorbidities, patients who have received immunosuppressive agents such as cyclophosphamide, moderate doses of glucocorticoids, damage accrual, a higher baseline disease activity, and those who have experienced an infection before. The most common sites of infections in SLE are pneumonia, urinary tract infections, and skin and soft tissue infections. Tuberculosis should be considered in the differential diagnosis of a SLE patient with fever.

Table 3.7.5: Fever in children with joint symptoms

Type of arthritis	*Pattern of fever*
Systemic onset juvenile idiopathic arthritis (SoJIA)	Temperature >40°C (104°F), quotidian with 1–2 spikes/ day, wide diurnal fluctuation, child is normal between fever episodes
Macrophage activation syndrome (MAS)	In SoJIA, a change in the pattern of fever from intermittent to continuous fever, transaminitis, cytopenias is a harbinger of MAS. Other features are increased triglyceride, CRP, ferritin, low albumin, ESR, and fibrinogen. Bone marrow aspirate/biopsy may reveal hemophagocytosis
Toxic (transient) synovitis	Characterized by mild fever. It is the most common cause of acute hip pain in children (2–12 years), following an episode of viral infection. Synovial fluid aspiration is essential to rule out septic arthritis. High-grade fever favors septic arthritis over toxic synovitis
Juvenile dermatomyositis	Fever is more common than in adult dermatomyositis. The most common pattern of myositis in children. Calcinosis is more common

Increased CD64 expression on neutrophils measured by flow cytometry is a good marker to diagnose infection and sepsis. High serum procalcitonin is a sensitive (70%) and specific (90%) marker for the presence of sepsis and bacterial infections, especially in the acute episodes of fever. Whereas active lupus patients will have low complements, high titers anti-dsDNA, active urinary sediment, and high SLEDAI or new BILAG scores. More often than not SLE patients with fever have both active disease and infection.

There are new promising biomarkers for infections that have been tested in small cohorts of SLE. One of these, the triggering receptor expressed on myeloid cells type 1 (TREM-1) is identified on the surface of mature neutrophils and monocytes responding to bacterial and fungal infections. Soluble TREM-1 (sTREM1) are elevated in SLE patients with infections, it is also higher in flares without infection when compared to SLE without flare.

OAS, i.e. 2'5'-Oligoadenylate synthetase, is an enzyme involved in the degradation of RNA and protection from viral infections. It is induced by type I IFN. Increased expression of OAS1 are and low OAS-L expression are suggestive of infections in SLE. Also an increased CD27 expression on plasma cells has been found to be a good and promising biomarker for disease activity of SLE.

Other differential diagnoses of fever in SLE are drug related fevers, macrophage activation syndrome, and rarely malignancies.

To summarize in patients with a known autoimmune disease such as lupus or vasculitis and are on immunosuppressants, we have to differentiate infections from disease activity. While for the patient who presents for the first time with fever and musculoskeletal manifestations apart from a rheumatology diagnosis one has to rule out infectious diseases. This is possible with good history, and judicious investigations (Fig. 3.7.1).

LEARNING POINTS

- Rheumatic disorders in children that present with fever include acute rheumatic fever, Kawasaki disease, SoJIA, MAS, autoinflammatory syndromes. Hematological malignancies must be ruled out.
- In adult patients, rheumatic disorders that have fever as a dominant manifestation include AOSD, MAS, FMF, sarcoidosis, antisynthetase syndrome, septic arthritis.
- Certain infectious diseases have fever and musculoskeletal manifestations as dominant manifestations.
- Malignancies must also be ruled out before considering rheumatologic diseases.
- In those patients with systemic autoimmune rheumatic disease who are on immunosuppressants and have fever the challenge lies in differentiating active disease from infection.

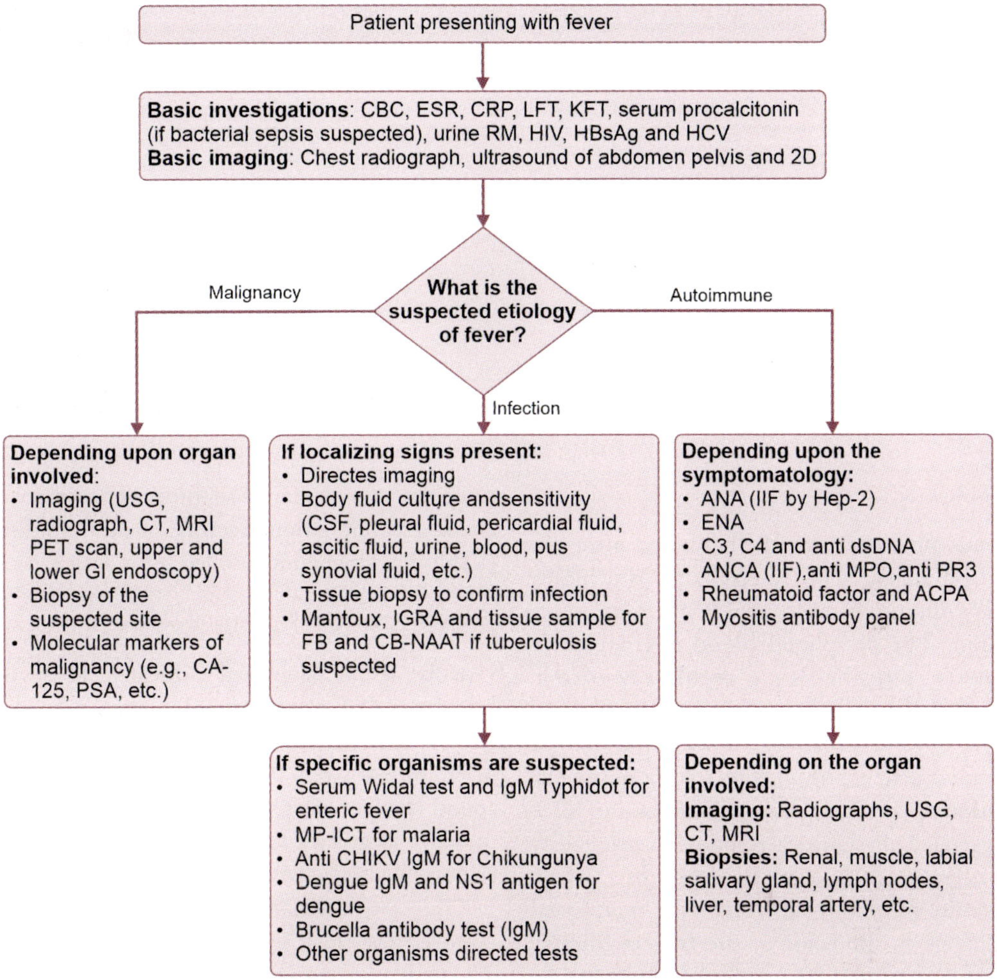

Fig. 3.7.1: Investigations for a patient presenting with fever to a rheumatologist.

FURTHER READING

1. Galloway J, Cope AP. The yin and yang of fever in rheumatic disease. Clinical Medicine. 2015;15: 288–91.
2. Ospina FE, Echeverri A, Zambrano D, et al. Distinguishing infections vs flares in patients with systemic lupus erythematosus. Rheumatology (Oxford). 2017;56:i46–i54.
3. Toth E, Speer G. Febrile conditions in Rheumatology. Clin Rheumatol. 2012;31:1649–56.

Chapter 3.8

Approach to Raynaud's Phenomenon

Vivek Vasdev, Ramakant

INTRODUCTION

Raynauds phenomenon (RP), named after the French physician Maurice Raynaud, is a highly variable symptom complex due to aberrant digital perfusion. The peripheral blood circulation in humans is controlled by a regulatory system involving neurons and mediators released from the local environment. The normal physiologic response on cold exposure is to reduce peripheral circulation to preserve the core temperature. RP is an exaggerated physiological response manifested by vasospasm of microvasculature on exposure to cold temperature or emotional stress. It is manifested by a change in the color of the fingers (digits); however, other sites and vascular beds can be affected, e.g. toes, ears, lips, nipples and nose. RP can occur as a primary phenomenon (primary RP) and as a manifestation of several medical conditions (Table 3.8.1) when it is called secondary RP.

ESTABLISHING THE DIAGNOSIS OF RP

Usually, RP is diagnosed clinically. The typical history is of a triphasic color change in digits (pallor, cyanosis and redness) on exposure to cold or emotional stress (Fig. 3.8.1). However, not all colour changes are necessary for the diagnosis. The presence of at least two colour changes ('biphasic' response) is sufficient to diagnose RP.

Objective measures of blood flow are rarely required for the confirmation of the diagnosis. The Cold challenge test is one of the widely used methods for this purpose. Recently, a 3-step

Table 3.8.1: Causes of Raynaud's phenomenon (RP)

Underlying cause	*Examples*
AIRDs	SSc, MCTD, SS, SLE, RA, IIM, PBC
Occupation	HAVS, polyvinyl chloride exposure, cold injury
Drugs	Antimigraine, beta blockers, bromocriptine, cytotoxic drugs, cocaine, sulfasalazine, minocycline
Infections	Hepatitis B, hepatitis C, CMV, parvovirus B-19
Miscellaneous	CRPS-I, carcinoids, hypothyroidism
RP mimics	
Vascular occlusions	Atherosclerosis, arteritis, thromboangiitis obliterans, microembolism, diabetic microangiopathy
Hyperviscosity	Paraproteinemia, polycythemia, cryoglobulinemia, cryofibrinogenemia

AIRDs: Autoimmune rheumatic diseases; *SSc:* Systemic sclerosis; *MCTD:* Mixed connective tissue disease; *SS:* Sjogren's syndrome; *SLE:* Systemic lupus erythematosus; *RA:* Rheumatoid arthritis; *IIM:* Idiopathic inflammatory myositis; *PBC:* Primary biliary cholangitis; *HAVS:* Hand arm vibration syndrome; *CMV:* Cytomegalovirus; CRPS: Complex regional pain syndrome.

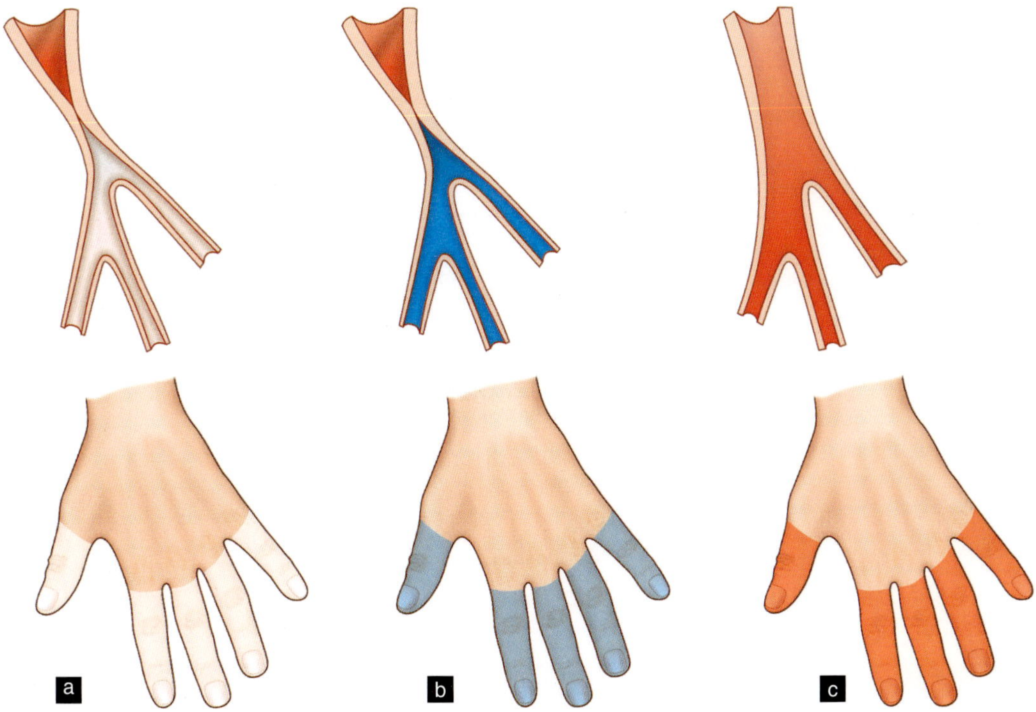

Fig. 3.8.1: Triphasic response in Raynaud's phenomenon: (a) White digits due to intense vasoconstriction, (b) Hypoxemic venous stasis causing blue digits and (c) hyperemic reperfusion leading to redness

approach to the diagnosis of RP has been proposed. It is based on the presence of unusual sensitivity in fingers and biphasic color changes during vasospastic episodes along with the presence of three or more of the following features:

- Episodes triggered by things other than cold
- Associated numbness or paresthesias
- Bilateral hand involvement (even if asynchronous or asymmetric)
- Clear cut demarcation between affected and unaffected skin
- Involvement of other body sites like nose, ear, feet, areola, and others
- Triphasic response
- Photographs highly suggestive of RP

Primary or Secondary RP: Why and How to Differentiate?

RP is called primary when there's no identifiable underlying aetiology whereas secondary RP has an underlying disorder. Primary RP is considered purely vasospastic. Secondary RP is associated with a variety of clinical conditions like autoimmune rheumatic diseases (AIRD), drugs and occupational exposures. Besides, there are various conditions that mimic RP (Fig. 3.8.2).

Classifying RP as primary or secondary has therapeutic and prognostic implications. The absence of nail fold capillary abnormalities, autoantibodies and clinical features of AIRDs suggest primary RP. RP with underlying AIRDs tends to be severe and may precede the diagnosis of underlying pathology by up to two decades, especially in scleroderma spectrum disorders (SSD). The occurrence of certain clinical features may suggest a greater likelihood of disease progression to overt AIRD. These include older age at onset (>35 years), male sex, recurrence of chilblains as adult, vasospasm all year round, asymmetric attacks, sclerodactyly or any other sign of AIRDs, digital ulceration and pitting scars involving the finger pulp. The combination of positive ANA and abnormal nail fold capillaries confers a high risk of progression to full-blown AIRDs, especially SSD.

Assessment of Patients with RP

Detailed history to ascertain the presence of RP, and clinical features suggestive of underlying

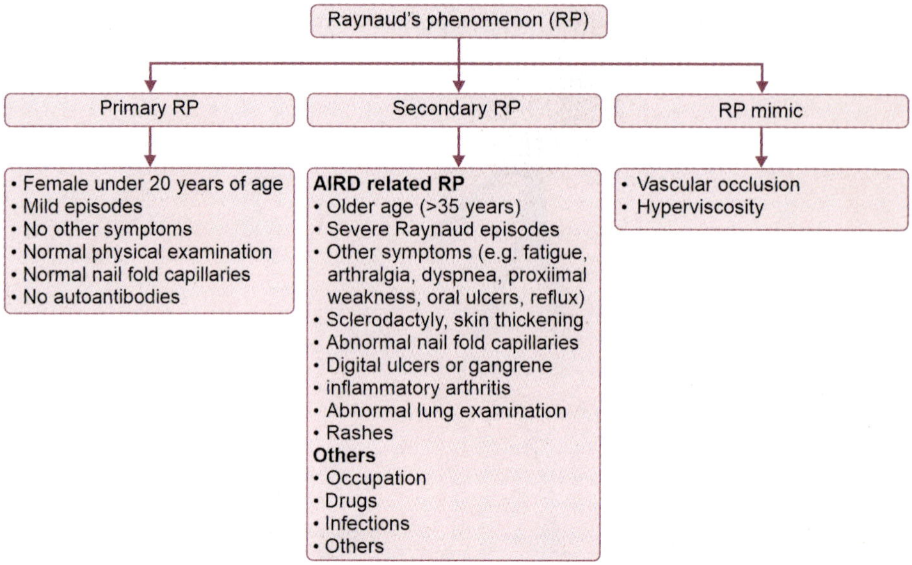

Fig. 3.8.2: Diagnostic approach to Raynaud's Phenomenon

Table 3.8.2: Assessment of patients with Raynaud's Phenomenon (RP)

History	Triphasic or biphasic colour change in digits. capturing of RP attacks by patients on their mobile phones, photosensitivity, mouth ulcers, tightening of the skin, and dryness of eyes or mouth.
Physical examination	Sclerodactyly, puffy hands, digital tip pitting, digital ulcers, telangiectasias
Serological investigations	Full blood count, biochemistry, ANA (ENA if ANA is positive)
Nail fold capillaroscopy (NFC)	Capillary density, distribution, morphology, dilatation and hemorrhages

ANA: Antinuclear antibodies, *ENA:* Extractable nuclear antigen

disease are important clues to differentiate primary from secondary RP. The diagnosis can be further substantiated by nail fold capillaroscopy and serological tests for autoantibodies (Table 3.8.2).

Nail fold capillaroscopy (NFC): NFC should be carried out in all cases of RP to differentiate between primary from secondary RP. Autoantibodies and NFC findings used in combination are an important diagnostic tool to predict (evolving) AIRD. The NFC changes (Fig. 3.8.3) predates other clinical signs and symptoms by several years, especially in SSD. The major morphological parameters that are assessed during NFC are capillary density, distribution, morphology, dilatation, giant capillaries, avascular areas and microhemorrhages.

Infrared thermography (IRT): IRT records the surface temperature of the human body and is an indirect measure of blood flow (Fig. 3.8.4). This modality for the diagnosis of RP requires validation studies before finding a suitable place in clinical practice.

CONCLUSION

There are clinical and serological pointers towards the presence of an underlying disorder (secondary RP) that is usually severe and invariably requires pharmacological treatment. The management depends on the severity of symptoms and includes non pharmacological measures (first) and pharmacological treatment of which calcium channel blockers are first line treatment. NFC is used even in the absence of such pointers to predict the progression of RP to frank CTD, especially SSD. Thermography is a simple technique which is emerging as a modality to define an underlying vascular abnormality to RP.

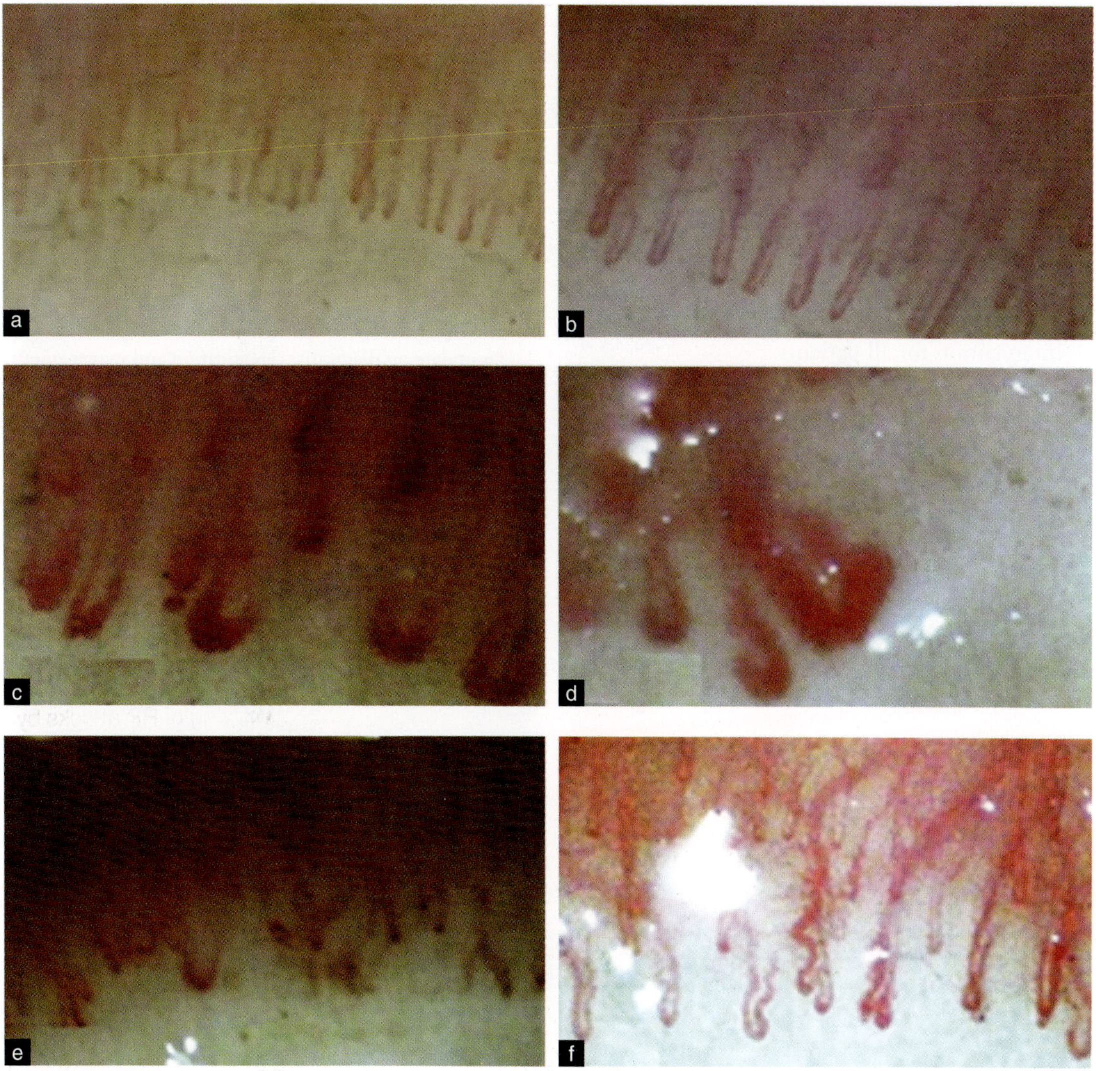

Fig. 3.8.3: Nail fold capillaroscopy (NFC) patterns: (a and b) Normal, (c) Early systemic sclerosis (SSc), (d) Active SSc, (e) Late SSc, (f) Nonspecific changes

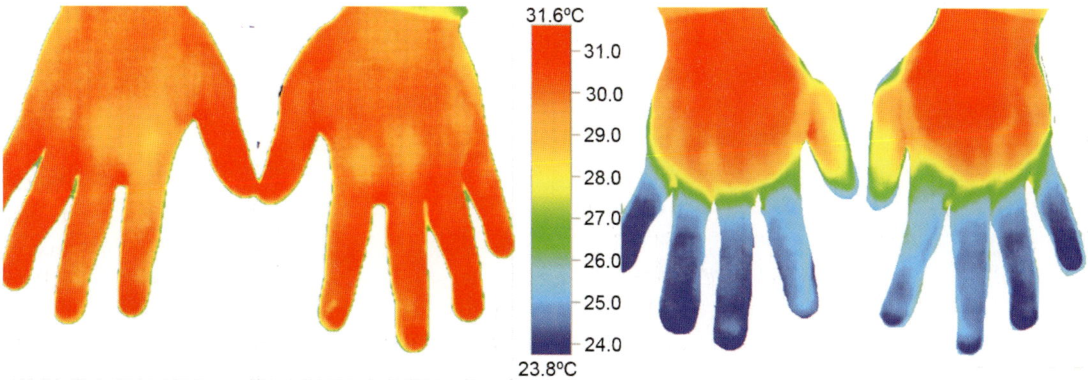

Fig. 3.8.4: Thermal imaging in a case during the intervening (asymptomatic) period and during Raynaud's episode

LEARNING POINTS

- The primary objective for evaluation of RP is to differentiate between primary and secondary RP.
- NFC is an important tool for differentiating between Primary and secondary RP
- Young patients with mild RP with normal NFC do not require detailed work up or serology and can be followed up.
- Nonpharmacologic measures remain the first line intervention for all patients.
- Calcium channel blockers are the first-line drugs and should be titrated to the maximum tolerated dose before adding or switching to other agents.

FURTHER READING

1. Cutolo M, Sulli A, Smith V. How to perform and interpret capillaroscopy. Best Practice and Research Clinical Rheumatology. 2013;27:237–48.
2. Herrick AL, Wigley FM. Raynaud's phenomenon. Best Pract Res Clin Rheumatol. 2020;34:101474.
3. Maverakis E, Patel F, Kronenberg DG, et al. International consensus criteria for the diagnosis of Raynaud's phenomenon. J Autoimmun. 2014; 48–49:60-5.
4. Pauling JD, Hughes M, Pope JE. Raynaud's phenomenon-an update on diagnosis, classification and management. Clin Rheumatol. 2019;38:3317–30.
5. Shapiro SC, Wigley FM. Treating Raynaud phenomenon: Beyond staying warm. Cleve Clin J Med. 2017; 84:797–804.

Approach to Digital Gangrene in Rheumatology Practice

Hima Shreekumar, Vishad Viswanath

INTRODUCTION

Gangrene denotes the death of body tissue due to a lack of adequate blood supply. The risk of amputation is inevitable unless a proper evaluation brings out the underlying cause and a multipronged treatment is initiated in a timely manner.

PATHOPHYSIOLOGY

Digital gangrene is usually a marker of underlying systemic disease and hence the mechanism of peripheral extremity ischemia leading to gangrene is varied. These can be broadly grouped as five mechanisms as follows:

1. Thrombotic occlusion
2. Embolic occlusion
3. Vasospasm
4. Vasculopathy
5. Extrinsic compression of the vascular lumen.

ETIOLOGY

There are numerous conditions that present with features of peripheral extremity ischemia and digital gangrene. Infections are one of the common causes of digital gangrene. However, atherosclerosis and autoimmune diseases remain the two major causes described so far. For ease of patient assessment, the causes of peripheral extremity ischemia can be broadly classified into five categories viz ischemic, rheumatologic diseases, infective, malignancy, and others (Table 3.9.1).

Digital gangrene can be the presenting or late feature of autoimmune rheumatic disease. An

Table 3.9.1: Causes of peripheral extremity ischemia and digital gangrene

Cause	*Examples*
Ischemic	**Intrinsic occlusion:** Atherosclerosis, embolism, cholesterol embolism. **Extrinsic occlusion:** Cervical rib, compartment syndrome, vascular dissection. **Hypovolemia:** Vascular access steal syndrome, congestive heart failure, dehydration, sepsis.
Rheumatologic diseases	**Autoimmune:** SLE, scleroderma, APS, Sjogren's syndrome, MCTD, RA. **Vasculitis:** Beurger's disease, temporal arteritis, takayasu arteritis, cryoglobulinemia, polyarteritis nodosa, ANCA-associated vasculitis, hypersensitivity angiitis, hypereosinophilic syndrome.
Malignancy	Paraproteinemia, lymphoma, leukemia, carcinoma lung
Thrombophilia	Factor V Leiden mutation Hyperhomocystinemia Protein C, protein S deficiency Anti-thrombin III deficiency
Infective	Infective endocarditis, septic emboli, syphilis, Chlamydia, filariasis, COVID-19
Others	**Drugs:** Ergot abuse **Trauma:** Accidental intra-arterial injection Disseminated intravascular coagulation Symmetrical peripheral gangrene

example is rheumatoid vasculitis which is a late presentation of rheumatoid arthritis (Fig. 3.9.1). The mechanism of ischemia in these settings could be due to vasospasm, thrombosis, or vasculitis.

Systemic sclerosis: It is one of the major autoimmune causes of digital ischemia. In systemic sclerosis patients, around 95% have manifest secondary Raynaud, often being the first presentation. Almost 20% of patients present with active digital ulcers, whereas nearly 40–50% of patients report a history of digital ulcers at some point in the disease. Thus in systemic sclerosis, secondary Raynaud's is the most common cause of digital gangrene; rarely vasculitis and thrombotic occlusions have been described as a cause of digital gangrene. Patients with anti-centromere antibodies have higher susceptibility to develop digital gangrene. Apart from this, antibodies to β2 glycoprotein 1 (β2GP1) is also associated with a higher risk for digital ischemia in systemic sclerosis.

Other connective tissue diseases: Mixed connective tissue disease, SLE, Sjogren's syndrome can present with secondary Raynaud's phenomenon, or thrombotic occlusions leading to digital gangrene. Other than Raynaud's phenomenon, the digital gangrene in these diseases could be due to underlying vasculitis or secondary antiphospholipid syndrome.

Antiphospholipid syndrome (APS) is another cause of digital ischemia. APS patients usually have persistently elevated levels of antibodies against membrane anionic phospholipids

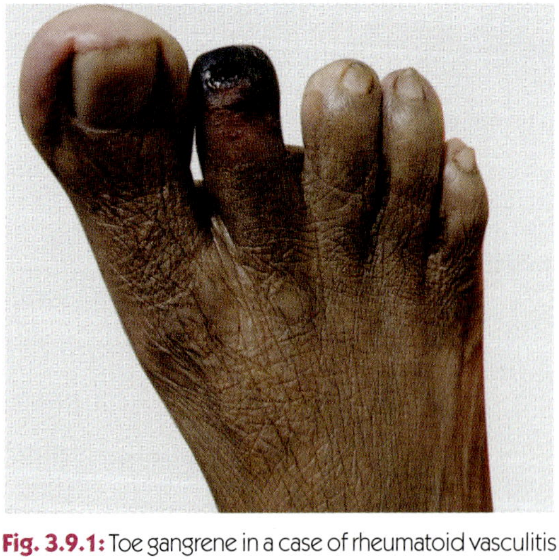

Fig. 3.9.1: Toe gangrene in a case of rheumatoid vasculitis

(i.e. anticardiolipin antibody) or their associated plasma protein (predominantly β2GP1). Thrombosis is especially common in those with triple-positive antiphospholipid antibodies, referring to elevated titers of anti-cardiolipin, anti-β2GP1 antibodies and positive lupus anticoagulant.

Systemic vasculitis: These disorders especially those that involve medium-sized vessels can present with digital gangrene. The classical example of such a presentation is polyarteritis nodosa. Often the gangrene in this condition is associated with other manifestations of medium vessel vasculitis as livedo reticularis or vasculitis neuropathy. Granulomatous polyangiitis, microscopic polyangiitis, and eosinophilic polyangiitis can involve medium vessel vasculitis along with small vessels and present with digital gangrene. Large vessel vasculitis such as Takayasu arteritis is an improbable cause of digital gangrene and if gangrene occurs in their background alternate pathology needs to be excluded.

Hypereosinophilic syndrome (HES): It is a rare heterogeneous condition with different subtypes. It comprises a group of disorders with persistent blood hypereosinophilia (>1500/mm^3) for more than 6 months with obvious signs of organ involvement. Cutaneous necrotizing eosinophilic vasculitis along with Raynaud's phenomenon and digital gangrene may occur as cutaneous manifestations of HES.

Symmetrical peripheral gangrene (SPG): It is yet another rare clinical syndrome, characterized by symmetrical digital ischemia leading to gangrene of two or more sites, in the absence of large vessel vasculitis or obstruction. Usually, the arterial pulse is intact in SPG as large vessels are spared. Few rheumatological diseases such as APS are noted to have an association with SPG. Data suggests a strong correlation between SPG and DIC as well.

Cryoglobulinemic vasculitis: It is a small vessel vasculitis associated with chronic infections such as hepatitis C, autoimmune disorders, and B cell lymphoproliferative diseases. It involves skin, joints, peripheral nervous system, and kidneys. Skin is the most commonly involved target organ, mainly as palpable purpura but chronic cutaneous ulcers are not uncommon. Raynaud's phenomenon and acrocyanosis can lead to digital ulceration and gangrene. One in three noninfectious cases of cryoglobulinemia can be due to Sjogren's syndrome.

CLINICAL FEATURES

Historically, the classical presentation of peripheral vascular disease is the 6 P's: Pain, Pallor, Poikilothermia, Pulselessness, Paresthesia, and Paralysis.

The clinical spectrum of peripheral extremity ischemia is a continuum of 5 stages:

1. Asymptomatic stage
2. Intermittent claudication
3. Rest pain
4. Ischemic ulceration
5. Critical ischemia

CLINICAL HISTORY

In a patient with digital gangrene, the evolution of the disease is very important and a thorough history is the only tool to access this information. Certain key points in history might be considered insignificant by the patient and hence care should be taken not to miss such points which may help to clinch the diagnosis (Table 3.9.2).

CLINICAL SIGNS

The affected extremities are usually pale with mild hypothermia and a mottled cyanotic appearance. There may be dependent erythema in the early stages of the disease whereas a woody limb with rigidity usually suggests an unsalvageable limb. Usually palpation of the peripheral pulse is a starting point to narrow the differential diagnosis (Fig. 3.9.2).

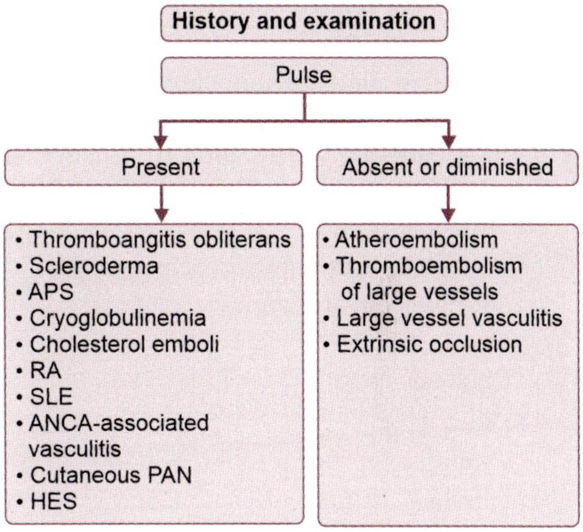

Fig. 3.9.2: Approach to a patient who presents with gangrene

Table 3.9.2: Clues to the etiology of gangrene from symptomatology

Symptom	*Significance*
Intermittent claudication and claudication distance	Atherosclerosis
Rest pain	Advanced disease
Worsening on exposure to cold	Raynaud phenomenon, cryoglobulinemia, frostbite
Skin color changes: White→Blue→Red	Raynaud's phenomenon
Cardiac symptoms—palpitation	May suggest embolic pathology
Personal history—smoking/drug abuse	Accelerated atherosclerosis
Fever	Infective/autoimmune pathology
History of recurrent abortions, unprovoked DVT	Antiphospholipid syndrome
Loss of weight and loss of appetite	Malignancy/autoimmune pathology
Prior thrombotic episodes	Hypercoagulable states
Prior trauma/burns	Compartment syndrome
Rash, photosensitivity, hair loss, oral ulcers	SLE, systemic vasculitis
Epistaxis, asthma, skin lesions, hematuria, allergy, polyps, nasal ulceration	ANCA-associated vasculitis
PUO, skin lesions	Infective endocarditis/autoimmune pathology
Kidney disease/prior dialysis	Vascular access steal syndrome, SLE, systemic vasculitis

Other relevant physical examination findings are listed below:

- General examination—look for pallor, pedal edema, and lymph node enlargement.
- Capillary refill time—a capillary refill time greater than 5 seconds has a likelihood ratio of 1.9 for moderate to severe peripheral arterial disease.
- Thorough neurological examination with special attention to the affected limbs.
- Auscultate for bruits
- The pattern of involvement: Digital gangrene involving all digits of four limbs is a sign of systemic diseases, such as infections like syphilis, leprosy, endocarditis, hepatitis B, hepatitis C, human immunodeficiency virus, fungal and parasitic infection.
- Signs of chronic extremity ischemia namely:
  - Subcutaneous atrophy
  - Hair loss
  - Coolness
  - Pallor
  - Cyanosis, dependent rubor, or both
  - Petechiae, fissures, ulceration, and gangrene with critical limb ischemia.
- Bedside tests:
  - **Ankle brachial pressure index (ABPI):** This is useful, especially for the lower extremities. ABPI <0.9 implies definite evidence of arterial disease with 95% sensitivity and 100% sensitivity.
  - **Allen's test:** This is useful to assess arterial patency of the hand.
- In addition, look for features of systemic diseases such as:
  - Petechiae, splinter hemorrhages, changing murmur—infective endocarditis.
  - Sclerodactyly, telangiectasias, hypopigmentation, digital pitting, loss of digital pulp, calcinosis cutis—scleroderma.
  - Livedo reticularis is seen in both antiphospholipid syndrome and cutaneous PAN.
  - Features of other connective tissue disorders like purpuric rashes, painless oral ulcers, malar erythema, alopecia, etc.
  - Purpura fulminans (purpuric patches leading to skin necrosis)—seen in SPG.
  - Features of kidney failure, purple toes, livedo reticularis, sudden blindness, altered mental state, stroke, etc. could indicate cholesterol embolism.

INVESTIGATIONS AND MANAGEMENT

From the wide array of investigations available, specific investigations should be chosen based on the clinical scenario. Along with the preliminary clinical assessment, a Duplex ultrasonography helps to categorize the patient according to the Rutherford classes adapted from the Society of Vascular surgery (Table 3.9.3). This shall aid to prevent the

Table 3.9.3: Categorization of patients with gangrene according to the Rutherford classification (adapted from the Society of Vascular Surgery)

Class	*Category*	*Sensory loss*	*Muscle weakness*	*Arterial Doppler signal*	*Venous Doppler signal*	*Prognosis*
I	Viable	None	None	Audible	Audible	No immediate threat
IIA	Threatened: Marginal	Minimal in the toes–none	None	Often inaudible	Audible	Treat promptly
IIB	Threatened: Immediate	Involves forefoot ± rest pain	Mild to moderate	Usually inaudible	Audible	Treat immediately
III	Irreversible	Anaesthetic	Paralytic/rigor	Inaudible	Inaudible	Permanent damage/ Amputation

Class I and IIA patients can be worked up for the underlying cause and treated accordingly, whereas Class IIB and III patients require urgent angiography and revascularization procedures to salvage the extremity and prevent further damage.

amputation of a salvageable extremity. Class I and IIA patients can be worked up for an underlying cause and treated accordingly, whereas Class IIB and III patients require urgent angiography and revascularization procedures to salvage the extremity and prevent further damage.

Investigations are Ordered Based on the Clinical Scenario

- Complete blood count
- Lipid profile
- Renal function test
- Urinalysis: Urinary eosinophils may be seen in cholesterol embolism
- Hepatitis B and C
- Rheumatologic workup
  - ANA (immunofluorescence)
  - ENA
    - Anti-Scl-70 antibodies, anticentromere antibody specific for scleroderma.
    - Anti dsDNA and anti-Smith antibody in SLE.
  - Antiphospholipid antibodies
    - Anti-β2 glycoprotein antibody—IgG and IgM.
    - Anticardiolipin antibody—IgG and IgM.
    - Lupus anticoagulant.
  - ANCA ELISA—anti-MPO and anti-PR3.
  - Rheumatoid factor and anticitrullinated peptide antibodies.
  - Serum cryoglobulins and cold agglutinins.
- Thrombophilia profile: Protein C, protein S, factor V Leiden mutation, homocysteine.
- Disseminated intravascular coagulopathy (DIC) evaluation.
  - Fibrin degradation product, D-dimer, Fibrinogen levels
- Work up for hypereosinophilic syndrome (HES)
  - IgE levels
  - Stool routine including parasites
  - Presence of the FIP1L1-PDGRFA-mutation when strongly considering HES
  - BCR ABL mutation
  - Bone marrow examination to rule out myeloproliferative diseases.
- Serum protein electrophoresis to assess paraproteinemias.
- Chest X-ray to rule out cervical rib.
- Echocardiography—transthoracic and transesophageal to diagnose infective endocarditis.
- Nail fold capillaroscopy—dilated or enlarged loops with areas of capillary loss are seen in scleroderma.

IMAGING

Doppler ultrasound: Useful as an initial evaluation to demonstrate the size of the vessel and is cost-effective. Luminal narrowing and decreased digital pulsations can be demonstrated.

Laser Doppler imaging: A newer modality that can assess more than one area at the same time; it can also differentiate between primary and secondary Raynaud's phenomenon.

Catheter-based arteriography: As mentioned above, patients with Class IIB and III occlusions need immediate catheter-based angiography. Arteriography can usually distinguish between thrombosis and embolism. In the case of upper limb ischemia, complete arteriography of both upper extremities is necessary to establish the diagnosis and institute effective treatment. Arteries of the upper extremities must be clearly visualized starting from the arch of the aorta up to the digits. In peripheral arterial disease, atheroma may be visible, however, in connective tissue disease, angiography does not show atheromatous obstruction; instead, features of vasculitis may be seen (Table 3.9.4). In scleroderma, the radial artery is usually spared and the ulnar artery is more commonly involved.

CT angiography: Patients with viable or marginally threatened limbs are usually candidates for either CT angiography or catheter-based angiography to evaluate arterial anatomy and potentially initiate thrombolytic therapy. CT angiography is limited by the artifact from possible heavy calcification of vessel walls.

MR angiography: Is faster, noninvasive, and gives high-quality images. Since it does not use vasodilators unlike conventional angiography, the exact degree of vasospasm can be appreciated.

Table 3.9.4: Findings that suggest vasculitis in catheter-based angiography
1. Tapering of ulnar, radial, and digital arteries
2. Superimposed vasospasm
3. Areas of narrowing between normal areas

LEARNING POINTS

- There are five major mechanisms of digital gangrene: Thrombotic occlusion, embolic occlusion, vasospasm, vasculopathy, and extrinsic compression of the vascular lumen.
- There are five major categories of causes of digital gangrene: ischemic, rheumatologic diseases, infective, malignancy, and others (example drugs).
- A proper history and clinical examination of the peripheral pulses can significantly narrow down the differential diagnosis.
- Doppler ultrasound is a useful initial diagnostic modality.
- Catheter-based arteriography is immediately indicated in those with limb-threatening ischemia. It helps in determining the etiology. In peripheral arterial disease, atheroma may be visible, however, in connective tissue disease features of vasculitis may be seen.

FURTHER READING

1. Abdel-Gadir A, Patel K, Dubrey SW. Cryoglobulinaemia induced digital gangrene in a case of hepatitis C. BMJ Case Rep. 2010 Dec 20; 2010:bcr1020103439. doi: 10.1136/bcr.10.2010.3439.
2. Al-Rudaini HEA, Han P, Liang H. Comparison Between Computed Tomography Angiography and Digital Subtraction Angiography in Critical Lower Limb Ischemia. Curr Med Imaging Rev. 2019;15:496–503.
3. Archer KA, Lembo T Jr, Haber JA. Protein S deficiency and lower-extremity arterial thrombosis: complicating a common presentation. J Am Podiatr Med Assoc. 2007;97:151–5.
4. Nihtyanova SI, Brough GM, Black CM, Denton CP. Clinical burden of digital vasculopathy in limited and diffuse cutaneous systemic sclerosis. Ann Rheum Dis. 2008;67:120–3.
5. Ravindran V, Rajendran S. Digital gangrene in a patient with primary Raynaud's phenomenon. J R Coll Physicians Edinb. 2012;42:24–6.

Approach to Muscle Weakness

Sajal Ajmani

INTRODUCTION

Finding out the cause of muscle weakness depends on good history, neurological, and muscular examination. The causes of muscle weakness are widely varied ranging from central neurological up to the local muscle cause. The neurological origin of weakness could be either due to upper motor neuron (UMN) or lower motor neuron (LMN) lesions. Localizing the site of deficit in the neural axis either UMN or the LMN will help to narrow down the differential diagnosis (Table 3.10.1). So, probably the first step is to determine whether it is true muscle weakness (myopathy) or a neurological cause.

Table 3.10.1: Causes of muscle weakness comprises neurologic diseases and intrinsic muscle disease
Upper motor neuron lesions
Cerebral ischemia, hemorrhage, or mass lesions (tumor or abscess)
Degenerative: amyotrophic lateral sclerosis
Demyelinating diseases: Multiple sclerosis, transverse myelitis, neuromyelitis optica
Extrinsic compression of the spinal cord (compressive myelopathy)
Subacute combined degeneration: Vitamin B_{12} deficiency
Lower motor neuron lesions
Anterior horn disease
Amyotrophic lateral sclerosis
Spinal root
Compressive (degenerative disc disease)
Guillain–Barre syndrome
Peripheral nerve
Metabolic (diabetes), toxic (ethanol, heavy metals, drugs), nutritional (vitamin B_{12} deficiency), autoimmune (e.g. vasculitis, lupus), entrapment of nerve
Neuromuscular junction
Myasthenia gravis, Lambert–Eaton syndrome
Muscle (intrinsic muscle weakness)
Infectious: HIV, other viruses, bacterial (Lyme disease), syphilis, etc.
Rheumatological: Idiopathic inflammatory myositis
Genetic: Muscular dystrophies
Toxic and medication induced myopathy: glucocorticoids, ethanol, statins
Endocrine myopathy: Thyroid disease, Cushing's syndrome

Modified from Harrison's manual of medicine 20th edition

Table 3.10.2: Common causes of muscle weakness in rheumatology practice

- A patient with lupus or Sjogren's syndrome might present with weakness due to transverse myelitis as a result of neuromyelitis optica
- A patient on high dose steroids might present with myopathy as part of Cushing's syndrome
- A lupus patient may present with stroke due to antiphospholipid syndrome
- Weakness in a patient with Sjogren's syndrome may due to hypokalemia and distal renal tubular acidosis
- Vitamin B_{12} deficiency due to pernicious anemia or nutritional deficiency
- Vitamin D deficiency and resultant osteomalacia is one cause of weakness
- A patient with muscular dystrophy might be referred to rule out inflammatory myositis

One might assume that peripheral nerve disease and inflammatory myositis might be the only muscle weakness-causing diseases that one would see in a rheumatological clinic. However, in rheumatology practice, the causes of muscle weakness are varied (Table 3.10.2).

HISTORY

The onset, duration, progression of symptoms, and distribution of weakness are important.

Acute onset of weakness (hours to days) of lower limbs indicates metabolic cause namely hypokalemia, or a Guillain–Barré syndrome, or acute transverse myelitis. Other causes of acute weakness are neurotoxic snakebite, and if fever is present with the acute weakness it could be infectious etiology such as a subdural abscess causing compressive myelopathy.

If the weakness is subacute (days to weeks), we need to consider inflammatory myositis or neuropathies. Whereas a gradually progressive weakness suggests genetic, metabolic, or inclusion body myositis.

The pattern of weakness should be ascertained from the history (whether the weakness is proximal or distal): Common causes of proximal muscle weakness are inflammatory myositis, muscular dystrophies, and osteomalacia. Distal muscle weakness can be caused by an early stage of inclusion body myositis, hereditary motor neuropathy, and toxins like organophosphates.

Asymmetric weakness or those involving only side or with specific nerve distribution is usually caused by central nervous lesions or peripheral nerve inflammation, or compressive lesion. The presence of sensory loss along with muscle weakness would suggest a neuropathic disorder.

Some specific history might point to a diagnosis; for example, dysphagia or dysarthria would suggest pharyngeal muscle weakness a clue to myositis, vision loss could be optic neuritis as part of multiple sclerosis or neuromyelitis optica, and diplopia with variable weakness and fatigability would suggest myasthenia gravis.

In addition, a history of fever, arthralgia, skin rash, and Raynaud's phenomenon would suggest a rheumatologic disease. A detailed family history in case of chronic weakness, and medicine review are essential as there are many drugs that are associated with muscle weakness such as antithyroid drugs (carbimazole), statins, fibrates, glucocorticoids, and anti-retroviral agents scuch as zidovudine.

EXAMINATION

The aim of examination is to differentiate muscle weakness that is an outcome of neurological deficit from an inherent muscle weakness. See whether the patient UMN or LMN signs (Tables 3.10.3 and 3.10.4). Cranial nerve examination to check for ptosis and diplopia should not be forgotten. Amyotrophic lateral sclerosis would have both UMN and LMN signs. Additionally, there will be fasciculations. A patient with transverse myelitis will have motor weakness, brisk deep tendon relexes, sensory loss with a distinct sensory level, and extensor plantars. However, if the weakness is muscle in origin the muscle tone would be normal or decreased, weakness is proximal, atrophy is mild, deep tendon reflexes would be normal, or reduced in severe weakness, and plantar response vis flexor.

The findings from history should be confirmed during the examination, especially the distribution of weakness. Muscle power should be graded

Table 3.10.3: Clinical examination features: UMN vs LMN vs myopathic

Sign	*Upper motor neuron (UMN)*	*Lower motor neuron (LMN)*	*Myopathic*
Muscle tone	Increased (spastic)	Decreased	Normal or decreased
Distribution of weakness	Pyramidal*/regional	Distal/segmental	Proximal
Atrophy	None	Severe	Mild
Fasciculation	None	Common	None
Deep tendon reflexes	Brisk response	Hypoactive or absent	Normal to hypoactive
Plantar reflex	Extensor response	Flexor response	Flexor response

*Pyramidal—sparing of antigravity muscles.

Table 3.10.4: Clinical signs depending on the area of the motor unit involved

Motor neuron	Diffuse weakness may involve speech and swallowing, muscle fasciculations, atrophy, and no sensory loss
Spinal root	Dermatomal sensory loss, radicular pain
Polyneuropathy	Distal weakness, feet>>hands, usually symmetric, distal sensory loss
Mononeuropathy	Weakness and sensory loss in the distribution of single nerve
Neuromuscular junction	Fatigable weakness, ocular involvement. No sensory loss, no reflex change
Muscle	Proximal weakness, no sensory loss, muscle tenderness may be present

according to the Medical Research Council (MRC) and Manual Muscle Testing (MMT) Scale. Extramuscular findings such as heliotrope rash, Gottron's rash and cushingoid appearance should be looked for.

INVESTIGATIONS

Based on the history and examination, the clinician should order a focused list of investigations. Though a raised creatine kinase is nonspecific but can confirm myositis and help in monitoring disease. Since metabolic abnormalities can cause muscle weakness, calcium, potassium, phosphate, and magnesium levels should be checked. Thyroid function tests and cortisol levels should be checked if indicated. Antiacetylcholine receptor antibodies should be checked if myasthenia gravis is suspected. Autoantibodies in myositis, such as anti-Mi 2 and anti-Jo1 help in diagnosis and predicting prognosis.

Electrophysiology and Imaging

A nerve conduction study is indicated to look for demyelination or axonal pathology. Electromyography helps in confirming myopathic patterns. However, it is usually not pathognomonic for a particular condition. MRI brain and spine will help rule out central lesions and spinal cord disease. MRI of muscle aids in the diagnosis of inflammatory myositis and decides the site for muscle biopsy.

Muscle Biopsy

The indications and use of muscle biopsy for diagnosis have decreased in recent years. It is used in suspected inflammatory myositis patients without any skin changes to confirm the diagnosis. Doing a biopsy from a severely weak muscle should be avoided since it usually shows fibrosis and fatty infiltration at that stage. To summarize evaluation of muscle weakness requires a good knowledge of neuroanatomy and muscle and their examination. A simplified approach is illustrated in Figure 3.10.1.

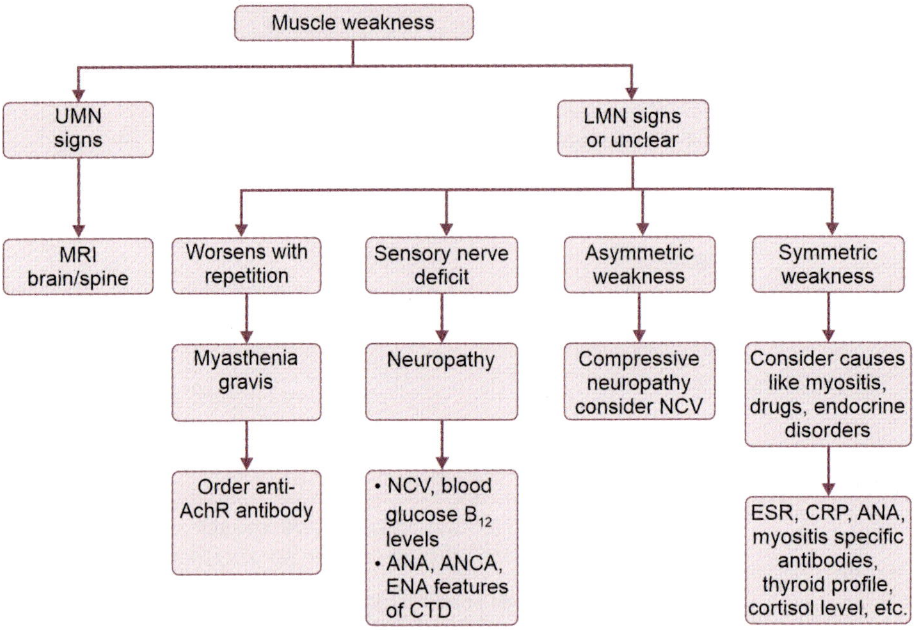

Fig. 3.10.1: A simplified approach to the patient with muscle weakness. A good neurological examination will be able to differentiate UMN from LMN weakness, from which we can further localize to either a neuropathy or neuromuscular junction disease or muscle disease.

Anti-AchR: Anti-acetylecholine receptor; *VNC:* Nerve conduction velocity; *ANA:* Antinuclear antibodies; *ANCA:* Anti-neutrophilic cytoplasmic antibodies; *ENA:* Extractable nuclear antigens; *CTD:* Connective tissue disease.

LEARNING POINTS

- There are easily treatable causes of acute weakness such as hypokalemia that should not be missed.
- The approach to muscle weakness requires good neurological examination, to distinguish whether the weakness is UMN or LMN or both signs are present, so as to ascertain whether the weakness is neurological disease or a myopathy.
- Myopathies are caused by infectious agents, medications or toxins, endocrine disorders, genetic causes, or inflammatory myositis to name a few. The presentation is usually symmetric, while asymmetric weakness and sensory loss is often due to neuropathy or compression.

FURTHER READING

1. Jackson CE. A clinical approach to muscle diseases. Semin Neurol. 2008; 28:228–40.
2. Larson ST, Wilbur J. Muscle Weakness in Adults: Evaluation and Differential Diagnosis. Am Fam Physician. 2020; 101:95–108.

Approach to Uveitis

Bhavya Chintala, Lalit Duggal

INTRODUCTION

A patient with uveitis would naturally seek help from an ophthalmologist. The role of a rheumatologist is in investigation and management of noninfectious causes of this condition. In this chapter, we shall discuss the approach in such a patient after briefly enumerating various causes of uveitis.

PRESENTATION

Uveitis can be acute with a sudden onset and brief duration as seen in spondyloarthritis, recurrent uveitis (sudden brief repeated attacks) and chronic uveitis with insidious onset and prolonged duration as seen in juvenile idiopathic arthritis (JIA). Patients with acute anterior uveitis present with painful red eye and vision abnormalities. Inflammatory infiltrate can be seen in the anterior chamber on slit lamp examination and at times it gets deposited on posterior corneal endothelium which is referred as keratic precipitates. In some cases it can be so intense which appears as a layering in the anterior chamber referred as hypopyon (Fig. 3.11.1). Flare is the protein exudation in the anterior chamber and in chronic conditions it can form synechiae.

CLASSIFICATION AND CAUSES

Depending upon the site of involvement uveitis is classified as anterior (anterior chamber involved–also known as iritis or iridocyclitis), intermediate uveitis (involving vitreous) and posterior uveitis (retina and choroid are involved).The diffuse involvement of all three chambers is termed as panuveitis. The causes of uveitis ranges from infections (toxoplasma, herpes simplex, herpes zoster, syphilis, cytomegalovirus), to immune-mediated disorders, and even malignancies like leukemia and lymphoma (Fig. 3.11.2). About 40% of the patients with uveitis will have some systemic illness. Rheumatologists are generally consulted to identify a systemic immunological disease associated with uveitis.

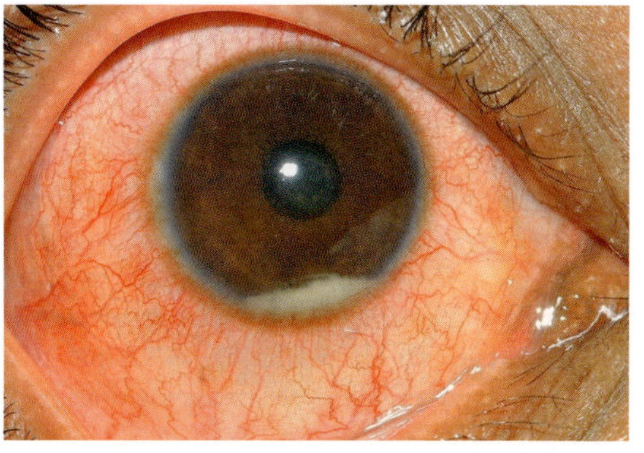

Fig. 3.11.1: Anterior uveitis with hypopyon

NONINFECTIOUS CAUSES

HLA B27 Association

The prevalence of HLA B27 positivity in acute anterior uveitis is about 50%. The HLA B27 associated uveitis is acute, unilateral and recurrent. Bilateral and chronic presentation is rare. Nearly 80% of patients with HLA B27 uveitis will have spondyloarthritis. Acute anterior uveitis can be seen in 25–30% of ankylosing spondylitis. In reactive arthritis, it is seen in about 10–20% of cases and chronic uveitis is not rare. Uveitis is common in inflammatory bowel disease (IBD) associated

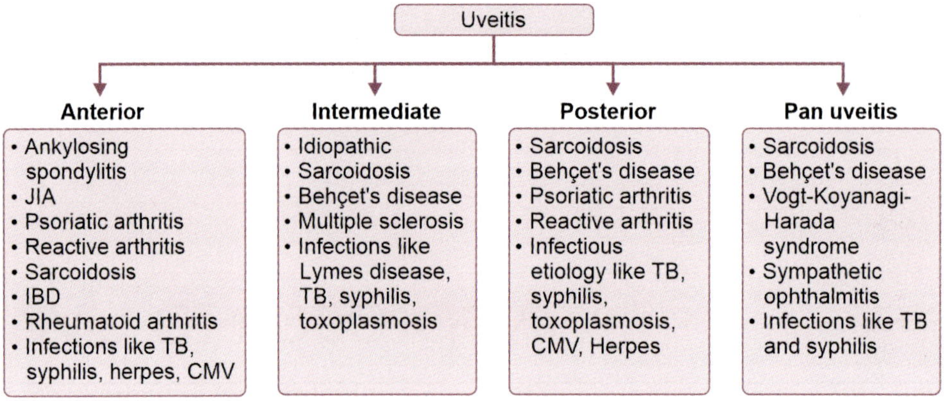

Fig. 3.11.2: Causes of uveitis based on anatomical sites

spondylitis than in isolated IBD. In psoriatic arthritis, the incidence of uveitis is 7–10%.

Rheumatological disease most commonly associated with chronic anterior uveitis is JIA. The prevalence is around 10–15% in children and it rises to around 30% with ANA positive particularly in oligoarticular JIA. Its course is insidious in onset with mild symptoms (also referred as white eye uveitis), hence children who are ANA positive should undergo periodic eye examination preferably every 3 months.

Sarcoidosis

In sarcoidosis any structure of the eye can be involved ranging from orbit, lacrimal gland, uvea, retina and optic nerve. Even in some cases the initial presentation of disease can be with eye manifestation. Sarcoid is one of the few causes of panuveitis, with posterior uveitis more common than anterior uveitis. Uveitis is granulomatous in nature with big mutton fat keratic precipitates. Retinal vasculitis is also one of the common manifestations of sarcoidosis.

BEHÇET'S AND OTHER VASCULITIDES

Behçet's disease is another rheumatological disorder associated with uveitis. The classical feature in Behçet's disease is recurrent bilateral uveitis with incomplete resolution between the attacks. The spectrum of uveitis ranges from isolated posterior uveitis and retinal vasculitis to panuveitis. The therapy for uveitis is always systemic in Behçet's disease. Other vasculitis syndromes associated with uveitis are Cogan's syndrome and Kawasaki disease. Cogans is classically associated with sensorineural hearing loss and interstitial keratitis. The eye manifestations can range from keratitis to uveitis and retinal vasculitis. In other vasculitis syndromes like Kawasaki disease and granulomatosis with polyangitis, scleral and conjunctival involvement is more common than uveal involvement.

Others

Certain auto inflammatory conditions like Blau syndrome and neonatal onset multisystem inflammatory disease (NOMID) are associated with uveitis. Blau syndrome is characterized by arthritis, uveitis and dermatitis. Single nucleotide polymorphism (SNP) in NOD2 gene is associated with Blau syndrome and histologically it is a non caseating granulomatous inflammation similar to sarcoidosis. NOMID is a multisystem inflammatory disease with variable presentation. Papillodema and uveitis are most common eye manifestations in NOMID.

Treatment

Treatment of uveitis depends on the etiology, severity, duration, recurrence rate. In case of isolated anterior uveitis, treatment usually starts with topical steroids (Fig. 3.11.3). Intraocular steroid injection particularly with triamcinolone is used when the inflammation is posterior to lens. Long-term intraocular therapy will cause a raise in intraocular pressure leading to glaucoma. Systemic steroid therapy is preferred to active, bilateral, noninfectious inflammation affecting the quality of

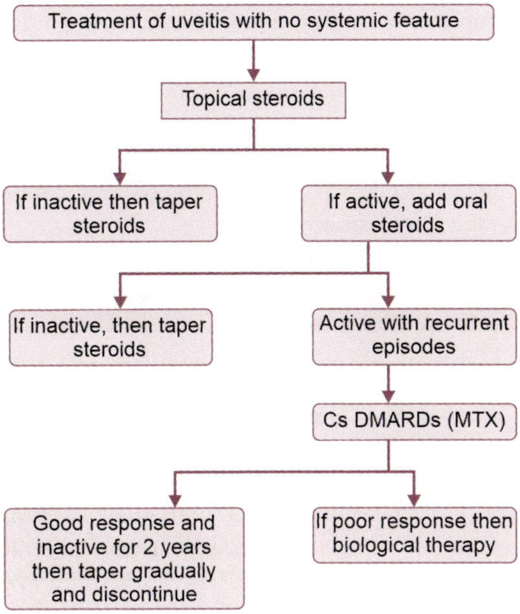

Fig. 3.11.3: Approach to management of uveitis with no systemic features

life. Figure 3.11.4 shows approach to management of noninfectious uveitis with systemic features. Conventional synthetic disease modifying anti rheumatic drugs (csDMARDS) can be considered in below mentioned settings.

1. Uveitis not responding to steroids
2. >/= 2 flares per year with disease flares on tapering of steroids and unable to taper the steroid dose to less than or equivalent to 7.5 mg per day.
3. Side effects and contraindications to steroids.

Few studies have described methotrexate as a better tolerated immunomodulatory and steroid sparing agents compared to others. Other drugs in this category are azathioprine, sulfasalazine, mycophenolate mofetil, leflunomide, calcineurine inhibitors (cyclosporine) and alkylating agents (cyclophosphamide).

Biologicals are considered especially in conditions with significant extraocular involvement like musculoskeletal, skin, gut, etc. Biological agents in

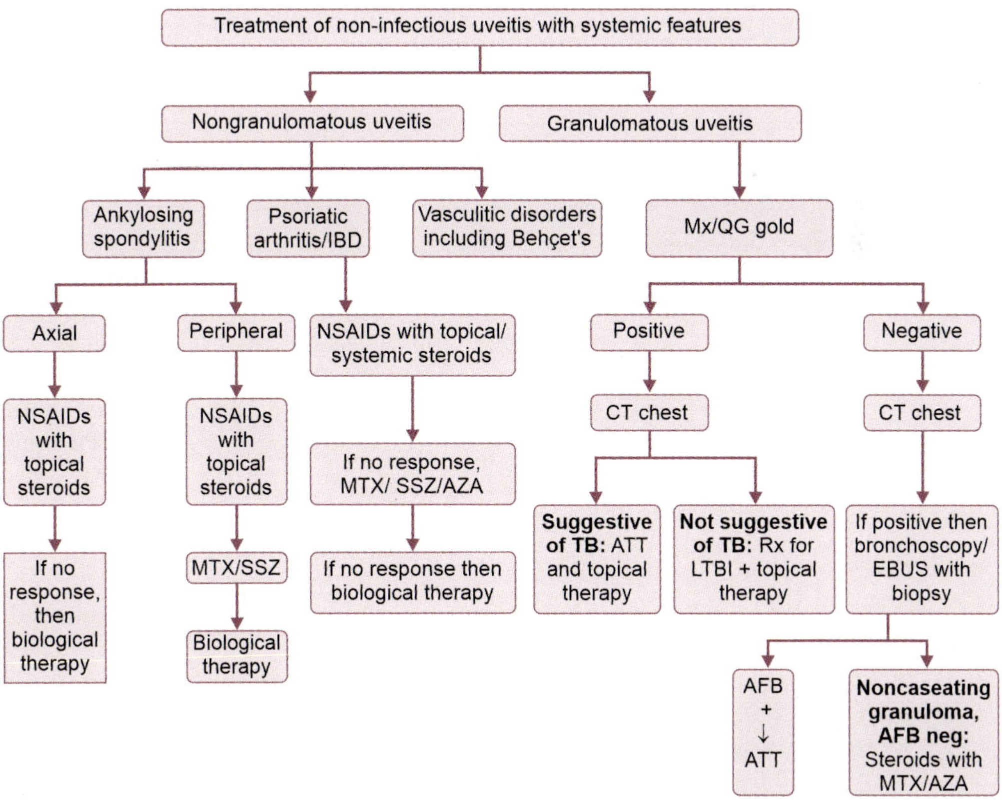

Fig. 3.11.4: Approach to management of noninfectious uveitis with systemic features.

NSAIDs: Nonsteroidal anti-inflammatory drugs; *MTX:* Methotrexate; *SSZ:* Sulfasalazine; *AZA:* Azathioprine; *Mx:* Mantoux test; *QG gold:* QuantiFERON-TB gold; *TB:* Tuberculosis; *ATT:* Anti tubercular therapy; *LTBI:* Latent TB infection; *AFB:* Acid-fast bacilli; *Cs DMARDs:* Conventional synthetic disease-modifying antirheumatic drugs; *IBD:* Inflammatory bowel disease.

use are TNFi (Infliximab, adalimumab), IL17/23 inhibitors and anti-CD20 monoclonal antibodies (Rituximab). In 2017 FDA approved adalimumab as the first biological agent in management of intermediate, posterior and panuveitis based on results of VISUAL 1 and 2 clinical trials. Infliximab is specifically indicated in Behçet's disease. The upcoming newer therapeutics are the small molecules (JAK inhibitors) being studies for various rheumatological indications. Tofacitinib has been approved for psoriatic arthritis and further trials are to be needed for its use in isolated uveitis.

LEARNING POINTS

- A patient with uveitis is referred to rheumatology to rule out inflammatory immune-mediated causes of uveitis.
- HLA B27 associated uveitis is acute, unilateral and recurrent.
- The most common cause of HLA B27 associated uveitis is spondyloarthritis.
- Acute anterior uveitis can be seen in 25–30% patients with ankylosing spondylitis.
- Sarcoidosis causes posterior uvietis > anterior uveitis. It is one of the few causes of panuveitis.
- The uveitis in JIA is often chronic anterior uveitis. It is insidious onset, mild symptoms, hence children with JIA especially ANA positive and oligoarticular JIA has undergo eye examination every three months.

FURTHER READING

1. Constantin T, Foeldvari I, Anton J, Boer J de, et al. Consensus-based Recommendations for the Management of Uveitis Associated With Juvenile Idiopathic Arthritis: The SHARE Initiative. Ann Rheum Dis 2018; 77(8):1107–17.
2. Dick DA, Rosenbaum JT, Al-Dhibi HA, et al. Guidance on Noncorticosteroid Systemic Immunomodulatory Therapy in Noninfectious Uveitis: Fundamentals of Care for UveitiS (FOCUS) Initiative. Ophthalmology 2018; 125:757–73.
3. Rosenbaum JT. The eye in spondyloarthritis. Semin Arthritis Rheum. 2019;49:S29–S31.
4. Rosenbaum JT. Uveitis: Etiology, clinical manifestations and diagnosis. UpTo date 2021.

Approach to a Patient with Multisystem Disease

Ashok Kumar

INTRODUCTION

Human body comprises various organ systems. Exponential growth of medical science over the years necessitated the development of various specialties and superspecialties. Thus a patient with leukemia is best managed by a medical oncologist, a patient with abnormal movements is best managed by a neurologist, and so on. A multisystem disease poses unique challenges with regard to the cost-effective utilization of health resources in modern practice. One needs to link all the manifestations in order to reach a working diagnosis which can explain most of the clinical features. Internists, rheumatologists, and endocrinologists frequently see multisystem disorders in clinical practice.

The diagnostic process in such cases involves a comprehensive clinical approach followed by an appropriate laboratory/imaging work-up. Numerous 'panels' are available like cardiac panel for chest pain and arthritis/autoimmune panel for joint pain, etc. Major drawback of this approach is the frequent occurrence of false-positive results, thus adding to the confusion instead of clearing it. Only a thorough history and examination can help in narrowing down the differential diagnosis. The relevant differential diagnoses can then be ruled in/out with tests, to reach a final diagnosis. Multisystem involvement is commonly seen in infectious, rheumatological, endocrinological, and neoplastic disorders (Table 3.12.1). Let us consider an instructive clinical vignette:

An 18-year-old boy presents with fever, cough, polyarthritis, and reduced appetite for 1 month. He is wheel-chair bound due to severe joint pains. Examination reveals scattered crepitations in the chest, and tenderness and effusion in the knees, elbows, and ankles. As the patient is suffering from a multisystem disease, a thorough examination of all the systems is performed (summarized in Table 3.12.2). Given the fact that infections are more common than primary rheumatic diseases in our country, important differential diagnoses pertinent to this case include infective endocarditis, tuberculosis with Poncet's arthritis, and sarcoidosis.

He undergoes routine laboratory investigations (Table 3.12.3), namely complete blood count (CBC), erythrocyte sedimentation rate (ESR), C-reactive protein (CRP), liver and kidney function tests, chest radiograph, ultrasound of the abdomen, blood cultures, and urine examination. Salient findings include leukocytosis, anemia, thrombocytosis, reversal of A/G ratio, raised inflammatory markers, and bilateral infiltrates on chest X-ray (Fig. 3.12.1). These point towards an infection but the same abnormalities can also be seen in sterile inflammation typical of systemic rheumatic diseases.

Next level of work-up (Table 3.12.4) probes these results in a greater detail. Contrast-enhanced computed tomography (CT) of the chest, Mantoux test, interferon-gamma release assay, echocardiogram, and sputum examination are requested. While awaiting the test results, the patient is started on broad-spectrum antibiotics and non-steroidal anti-inflammatory drugs.

CT of the chest shows multiple cavitating nodules in both lungs with bilateral pleural effusion (Fig. 3.12.2). Tests for histoplasmosis, aspergillosis,

Table 3.12.1: Causes of multisystem diseases

Infections	**Tuberculosis** Meningococcemia, staphylococcal septicemia Parvovirus B19, EB virus, CMV, COVID-19 HIV, HBV, HCV Histoplasmosis, cryptococcosis, angioinvasive aspergillosis
Rheumatological conditions	**Arthritides** RA, SpA, PsA, SAPHO syndrome, JIA, gout
	Connective tissue diseases SLE, scleroderma, inflammatory myopathy, Sjögren's syndrome Antiphospholipid syndrome **Vasculitides** HS purpura, cryoglobulinemic vasculitis, Urticarial vasculitis GPA, EGPA, MPA Takayasu arteritis, giant cell arteritis Kawasaki disease Polyarteritis nodosa Behçet's disease
Endocrinological conditions	Diabetes mellitus, hypothyroidism, thyrotoxicosis, Addison's disease, Cushing's syndrome Autoimmune hypophysiitis Obesity and metabolic syndrome
Malignancies	Multiple myeloma, lymphoma, leukemia Paraneoplastic syndromes

EB: Epstein-Barr; *CMV:* Cytomegalovirus; *COVID-19:* Coronoavirus disease-2019; *HIV:* Human immunodeficiency virus; *HBV:* Hepatitis B virus; *HCV:* Hepatitis C virus; *RA:* Rheumatoid arthritis, *SpA:* Spondyloarthritis; *PsA:* Psoriatic arthritis; *SAPHO:* Synovitis acne pustulosis hyperostosis osteitis; *JIA:* Juvenile idiopathic arthritis; *SLE:* Systemic lupus erythematosus; *HS:* Henoch–Schönlein; *GPA:* Granulomatosis with polyangiitis; *EGPA:* Eosinophilic granulomatosis with polyangiitis; *MPA:* Microscopic polyangiitis.

and HIV infections are reported as negative. A discussion between clinician and radiologist acknowledges the rare but well known possibility of granulomatosis with polyangiitis (GPA) as the cause of cavitating nodules in the lungs.

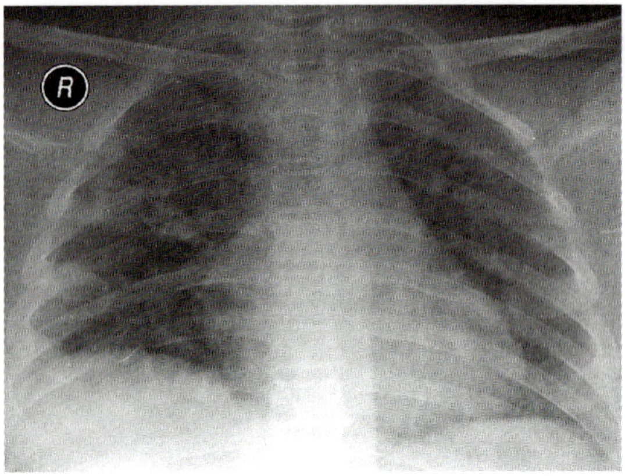

Fig. 3.12.1: Chest X-ray posteroanterior projection of the patient, showing bilateral infiltrates with cavities

The young boy has sterile blood culture. ANCA is negative by immunofluorescence assay (IFA) and enzyme linked immunosorbent assay (ELISA). His fever and joint effusions do not improve. Synovial fluid from knee joint reveals polymorphonuclear leucocytosis; culture is sterile. A repeat blood culture is sent for melioidosis in view of exposure to pooled water during rain (this history is revealed later) and probable internal abscesses in lungs and joints. Result is found negative for melioidosis but delayed growth of *Staphylococcus aureus* is found in the sample sent earlier. It is also grown from brochoalveolar lavage. He is started on intravenous antibiotics according to sensitivity results. In spite of that, the patient's symptoms are not relieved.

Considering that 10% cases of GPA can be ANCA negative, this possibility is revisited and a surgical lung biopsy from one of the nodules is obtained. Histopathology of the lung shows granulomatous vasculitis typical of of GPA and that clinches the diagnosis.

APPROACH TO RHEUMATIC MULTISYSTEM PRESENTATION

As emphasised earlier, when a systemic rheumatic disease is suspected, the work-up should not start with an 'autoimmune panel'. This approach amounts to sheer waste of resources. Therefore, the provisional diagnosis should first be categorized into arthritides, connective tissue disease (CTD), vasculitides, and so on, before proceeding with the relevant investigations.

Table 3.12.2: Systemic examination in a patient with multisystem disease

Organ system	*Findings*	*Clinical relevance*
General physical examinatin	Fever Peripheral pulse discrepancy Regional lymph nodes Thickened peripheral nerves Major salivary glands	Infections, SARD, malignancy Vasculitis Infection, SLE, malignancy Leprosy Sialadenitis, Sjögren's syndrome, T2DM, sarcoidosis, GPA
Skin (the largest organ system!)	Xerosis Erythema nodosum Papules, macules, purpurae, nodules Echymoses and gangrene in the extremities Cutaneous bleeding, hemorrhagic bullae Abnormal nail-fold capillaroscopy	Hypothyroidism, Sjögren's syndrome Tuberculosis, reactive arthritis and sarcoidosis Vasculitis Meningococcal septicemia Large differential diagnosis
Nails	Platynychia and koilonychias Pits, transverse ridges, 'oil-drop' pigmentation, onycolysis, subungual keratosis Nicotine stain Clubbing	Chronic and severe anemia Psoriasis Chronic smoking, e.g. in COPD Various cardiac, respiratory and hepatic diseases
Respiratory system	Bronchial breath sounds Reduced breath sounds Fine crepitations Expiratory wheeze	Lung consolidation, cavity Pleural effusion, collapse, fibrosis ILD Obstructive airway diseases
Cardiovascular system	Jugular venous pressure Muffled heart sounds Valvular murmurs	Cardiac and respiratory diseases Pericardial effusion due to tuberculosis, SLE Infective or lupus endocarditis
Gastrointestinal system	Organomegaly Ascites Renal or abdominal aortic bruit Features of peritonitis	Chronic infections like tuberculosis, SLE, infiltrative diseases and malignancies Large differential diagnosis Large vessel vasculitis or syphilis Mesenteric vasculitis due to lupus or abdominal angina of IgA-associated vasculitis besides other surgical causes
Musculoskeletal system	Joint examination Tenderness in muscle planes Spine abnormalities Periarticular abnormalities	Synovitis and range-of-motion Myositis or fibromyalgia Mobility restriction in SpA, DISH, etc. deformities like gibbus in TB Rheumatoid nodules, tophi, calcinosis, etc.
Oral cavity	Stomatitis, mucositis and gingivitis. Strawberry tongue Absent salivary pool under the tongue Dental carries and oral thrush	Large differential diagnosis including SLE, Sjögren's syndrome, Behçet's disease, etc. Kawasaki disease Sjögren's syndrome Sjögren's syndrome

(Contd.)

Table 3.12.2: Systemic examination in a patient with multisystem disease (Contd.)

Organ system	*Findings*	*Clinical relevance*
Ear and nose	Crusting of nasal mucosa 'Saddle-nose' deformity Nasal polyps Inflammed cartilage of the ear	GPA GPA, Hansen's, syphilis, cocaine EGPA, atopy Relapsing polychondritis
Ocular system	Redness Fundus: Haemorrhages, retinitis, Roth's spots, papilloedema, etc. Pupillary abnormalities Xerophthalmia	Tiredness or excessive visual strain, uveitis, scleritis T2DM, vasculitis, infective endocarditis, raised intracranial tension Anisocoria in ICSOL, intracranial hemorrhage, orbital inflammatory disease. Sjögren's syndrome
Nervous system	Headache Encephalopathy and myelitis Focal neurological deficit Peripheral neuropathy	Very nonspecific symptom and may occur due to stress, uncorrected refractory error, ICSOL, APS, CVA, etc. Metabolic causes—dyelectrolytemia, uremia, etc. infection or autoimmune causes like SLE CVA due to cardiovascular causes, antiphospholipid syndrome or septic embolisation in infective endocarditis. Large differential diagnosis including T2DM, leprosy, SLE, vasculitis, sarcoidosis, etc.
Renal system	Prerenal failure Proteinuria Nephritis	Compromised renal blood flow due to various possible causes Nephrotic syndrome, T2DM, SLE Vasculitis
Drugs	Cutaneous ulcers which mimic vasculitis Drug-induced lupus	Pentazocine Isoniazid, propylthiouracil, hydralazine, TNF-inhibitors, etc.

GPE: General physical examination; *SARD:* Systemic autoimmune rheumatic disease; *SLE:* Systemic lupus erythematosus; *T2DM:* Type 2 diabetes mellitus; *GPA:* Granulomatosis with polyangiitis; *COPD:* Chronic obstructive pulmonary disease; *ILD:* Interstitial lung disease; *SpA:* Spondyloarthritis; *ECG:* Electrocardiogram; *IgA:* Immunoglobulin A; *DISH:* Diffuse idiopathic skeletal hyperostosis; *TB:* Tuberculosis; *EGPA:* Eosinophilic granulomatosis with polyangiitis; *ICSOL:* Intracranial space-occupying lesion; *APS:* Antiphospholipid syndrome; *CVA:* Cerebrovascular accident; *TNF:* Tumor necrosis factor.

Table 3.12.3: Baseline screening investigations which should be obtained in patients with multisystem diseases

Investigation	*Findings*	*Clinical relevance*
Hemogram, liver and kidney function tests	Wide range of abnormalities.	Deranged in infections, vasculitis, organ dysfunction.
Peripheral blood smear examination	Toxic granules, schistocytes, immature cells.	Bacterial septicemia, hemolysis, etc.
Urine examination	24 hour protein, RBCs (including dysmorphic) and casts of various types.	Diabetic nephropathy, nephrotic and nephritis syndrome, ATN, interstitial nephritis, APS related nephropathy.
Chest X-ray and ultrasound examination of the abdomen	Essential part of initial work-up of a multisystem disease which may reveal vital information	

RBC: Red blood cell; *ATN:* Acute tubular necrosis; *APS:* Antiphospholipid syndrome.

Table 3.12.4: Special investigations

Investigation	*Utility*
CECT of chest and abdomen, PET scan	Better characterization of findings observed on plain radiography and ultrasound; useful for obtaining tissue sample for histopathological examination
Histopathology	Skin and minor salivary gland biopsies are least invasive Skeletal muscle, kidney, liver, lymph nodes, nasal mucosa, synovium and pleura are the other common sites Superficial temporal artery for giant cell arteritis Immunofluorescence examination for deposition of autoantibodies and complement
Serum protein electrophoresis	Plasma cell dyscrasias
Investigations for nervous system	Imaging including CT, MRI, PET and spectroscopy Lumbar puncture for meningitis, neuropsychiatric lupus and CNS vasculitis Nerve conduction studies for evaluation of peripheral nervous system Venous or arterial angiogram may be obtained to assess CNS vasculitis or venous thromboembolism Rarely, sural nerve biopsy or brain biopsy for suspected vasculitis
Investigations for cardiovascular system	ECG may reveal features suggestive of myocarditis or pericarditis CK-MB and troponin are elevated in myocarditis, coronary artery disease and congestive heart failure Echocardiogram for chamber dimensions, pressures across various cardiac chambers, contractility of myocardium and fluid in the pericardium Transoesophageal echocardiogram for infective or lupus endocarditis Cardiac MRI for diagnosing cardiac sarcoidosis; guiding myocardial biopsy
Endocrinological investigations	Blood glucose levels, glycated haemoglobin, serum insulin and C-peptide levels to assess diabetes TSH, FT3 and FT4 for thyroid disorders, which give rise to systemic features Anti-thyroglobulin and anti-TPO antibodies for autoimmune thyroiditis Cushing's syndrome and Addison's disease have multi-organ features which are assessed by respective hormonal assays including various stimulatory and suppression tests Autoimmune hypophysiitis is a rare cause of panhypopituitarism which can be diagnosed with reduced levels of all the pituitary hormones
ANA	Screening by IFA–pattern of immunofluorescence and end-titres Positive ANA should be investigated further by assessing anti-ENA profile
ANCA	Screening by IFA–pattern of immunofluorescence (cytoplasmic [cANCA] or perinuclear [p-ANCA]) and end-titers Positive test should be further tested by ELISA for characterising the exact antibody (anti-PR3 or anti-MPO)
Serum complement levels	Levels are reduced in lupus nephritis, cryoglobulinaemic vasculitis, urticarial vasculitis, etc. where there is consumption of complement components
Muscle enzymes like CPK, LDH, Aldolase	Elevated in myositis (inflammatory or infective) or muscular dystrophies

CECT: Contrast-enhanced computed tomography; *PET:* Positron emission tomography; *CT:* Computed tomography; *MRI:* Magnetic resonance imaging; *ECG:* Electrocardiogram; *CK-MB:* Creatine kinase-muscle brain; *TSH:* Thyroid stimulating hormone; *T3:* Tri-iodothyronine; *T4:* Tetra-iodothyronine; *TPO:* Thyroid peroxidase; *ANA:* Antinuclear antibody; *IFA:* Immunofluorescence assay; *ENA:* Extractable nuclear antigen; *ELISA:* Enzyme linked immunosorbent assay; *ANCA:* Antineutrophil cytoplasmic antibody; *PR3:* Proteinase-3; *MPO:* Myeloperoxidase; *CPK:* Creatine phosphokinase, *LDH:* Lactate dehydrogenase.

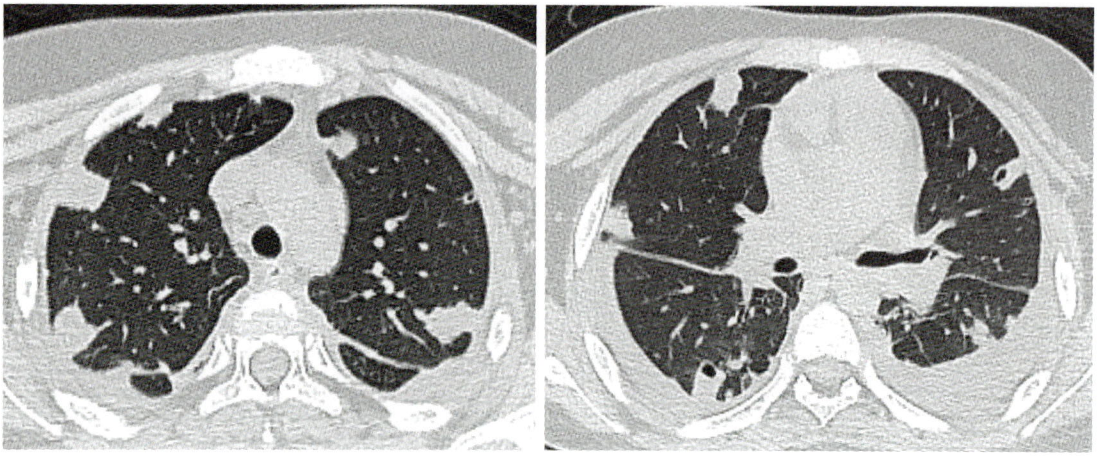

Fig. 3.12.2: CT scan of the chest of the patient, showing cavitating nodules with bilateral pleural effusion. CT computed tomography.

Identifying the pattern of arthritis is important. Thus, a long-standing case of rheumatoid arthritis (RA) with classical deformities does not require serological markers for diagnosis. In such a patient, obtaining antinuclear antibody (ANA), antineutrophil cytoplasmic antibody (ANCA), etc. as part of an autoimmune 'panel' is irrelevant. In contrast, the recent onset of polyarthritis involving small joints of hands in a symmetrical pattern points towards RA and rarely, SLE or Sjögren syndrome.

Predominantly lower limb oligoarticular arthritis favors the peripheral form of spondyloarthritis. Dactylitis raises the possibility of psoriatic arthritis. Monoarticular flares occur in gout and reactive arthritis. Predominant involvement of ankle joints and their peri-articular tissues is typically seen in sarcoidosis. ANA must be obtained when a CTD or vasculitis is suspected. On the other hand, ANCA, serum cryoglobulins and cryofibrins are essential for evaluating vasculitis.

Lymphoma and leukemia often mimic rheumatological conditions in presentation. Solid organ malignancies can have multisystem paraneoplastic syndromes. Histopathological examination is required in almost all cases of malignancies.

There is no diagnostic marker for polyarteritis nodosa (PAN). Compatible clinical features on the presence of negative results for all the autoimmune markers is an indirect pointer towards PAN. Classical beaded appearance of mesenteric and renal arteries on CT angiography supports the diagnosis.

The possibility of a test being falsely-positive must be remembered. Further, treating the derangements in investigations alone is not appropriate, unless they have a clinical correlation. Elevated leucocyte count, ESR and CRP may be seen in infections as well as vasculitis. Positive blood cultures and significantly raised procalcitonin favor infection. Some patients may have constitutionally raised ESR without any clinical abnormality. In addition, obesity contributes to elevated inflammatory markers. Treating such patients with antibiotics or immunosupressants empirically is inappropriate.

LEARNING POINTS

- There is no replacement of a thorough history and diligent physical examination while evaluating a patient with multisystem disease.
- Use of 'panels' of laboratory investigations should be avoided.
- Colleagues from other subspecialties should be involved when required.
- The patient's clinical profile should be assessed through a 'panoramic' rather than 'tubular' view.
- Relevance of a positive test should always be interpreted in view of the clinical features.

FURTHER READING

1. Crouser ED, Maier LA, Wilson KC, et al. Diagnosis and detection of sarcoidosis. An Official American Thoracic Society Clinical Practice Guideline. Am J Respir Crit Care Med 2020;201:e26–51.

2. National Institute for Health and Care Excellence (NICE) 2015. Procalcitonin testing for diagnosing and monitoring sepsis (ADVIA Centaur BRAHMS PCT assay, BRAHMS PCT Sensitive Kryptor assay, Elecsys BRAHMS PCT assay, LIAISON BRAHMS PCT assay and VIDAS BRAHMS PCT assay). ISBN: 978–14731–1463–0. [accessed May 2021].
3. Pujalte GGA, Albano-Aluquin SA. Differential diagnosis of polyarticular arthritis. Am Fam Physician 2015; 92:35–41.
4. Sharma A, Kumar A, Jha A, et al. The impact of obesity on inflammatory markers used in the assessment of disease activity in rheumatoid arthritis-a cross-sectional study. Reumatologia 2020;58:9–14.

Section

IV

DRUGS

Nonsteroidal Anti-inflammatory Drugs

Annil Mahajan, Vishal R Tandon, Akhil Mahajan

INTRODUCTION

Nonsteroidal anti-inflammatory drugs (NSAIDs) are among the most widely prescribed medications in many inflammatory rheumatic diseases. Because they are easily available over-the-counter they are also consumed on a nonprescription basis as well.

MECHANISM OF ACTION

NSAIDs blocks the cyclooxygenase (COX) enzyme involved in the conversion of arachidonic acid to prostaglandins (PGs) (Fig. 4.1.1). There are two types of COX enzyme namely COX-1 and COX-2. The COX-1 enzyme is constitutively present in most tissues and it generates good PGs that are essential for housekeeping functions, namely maintenance of gastric mucosal integrity, platelet homeostasis and renal blood flow. COX-2 production is induced by macrophages, it is involved in producing PGs that are responsible for inflammatory reactions. Thus inhibition of COX-2 is responsible for anti-inflammatory actions of NSAIDs, whereas inhibition of COX-1 isoenzyme causes the unwanted side effects of conventional NSAIDs such as gastrotoxicity. However both COX-1 and COX-2 inhibition causes renal toxicity, and additionally selective inhibition of COX-2 causes cardiovascular toxicity. Inhibition of COX-3 might be the mechanism by which paracetamol and other NSAIDs decrease fever.

Table 4.1.1 shows the classification of NSAIDs, while a pictorial representation of various NSAIDs is shown in Figures 4.1.2 and 4.1.3. There are many other mechanisms (Table 4.1.2) by which NSAIDs produce their clinical effects (Table 4.1.3).

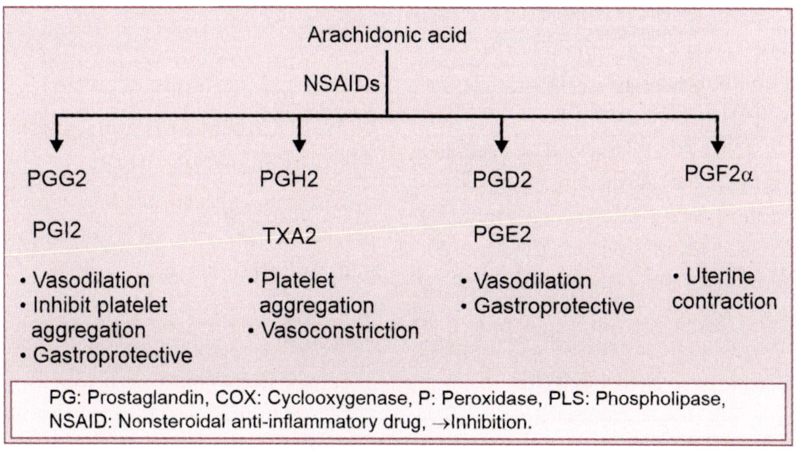

Fig. 4.1.1: COX dependent mechanism of action

Table 4.1.1: Classification of NSAIDs on the basis of COX Selectivity

Nonselective NSAIDs	
Aspirin	600–900 mg 4–6 hourly
Diclofenac	50 mg 8 hourly
Aceclofenac	100 mg 12 hourly
Indomethacin	50 mg 8 hourly
Ketorolac	10 mg 6 hourly
Sulindac	50–200 mg twice daily
Ibuprofen	600–800 mg 8 hourly
Flurbiprofen	100 mg 8 hourly
Naproxen	500 mg 12 hourly
Mefenamic acid	500 mg 8 hourly
Piroxicam	20 mg once daily
Tenoxicam	20 mg once daily
Preferential COX-2 (Show preferential COX-2 inhibition over COX-1)	
Nimesulide	100 mg 12 hourly
Nabumetone	1000 mg once daily
Etodolac	200 mg twice daily
Meloxicam	7.5 mg once daily
Selective COX-2 Inhibitors	
Celecoxib (FDA alert)	100 mg 12 hourly
Etoricoxib	60–120 mg once daily
Lumiracoxib	400 mg once daily
Parecoxib	10 mg/kg daily dose (Injectable)
Rofecoxib (withdrawn from market)	
Valdecoxib (withdrawn from market)	

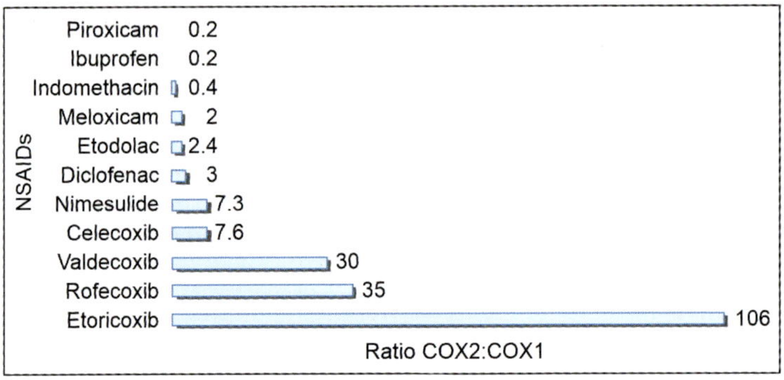

Fig. 4.1.2: COX-2:COX-1 selectivity of NSAIDs

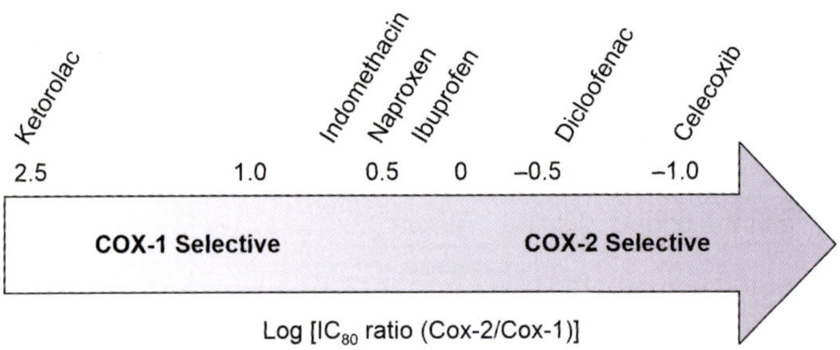

Fig. 4.1.3: Relative COX-1 and COX-2 selectivity for commonly used non-aspirin NSAIDs

Table 4.1.2: COX independent mechanisms of action of NSAIDs

• Inhibitor effects on lipooxgenase products (sulindac, diclofenac)
• Inhibition of superoxide formation (indomethacin, piroxicam)
• Inhibition of neutrophil aggregation, adhesion and enzyme release (salicylates, indomethacin, aceclofenac)
• Depression of lymphocyte transformation (salicylates)
• Inhibition of rheumatoid factor production (piroxicam)
• Inhibition of cytokine production by inhibiting factor kappa B (salicylates)
• Suppression of proteoglycan production in cartilage (salicylates, piroxicam, ibuprofen, fenoprofen)
• Stimulation of adenosine receptors (salicylates)
• Peroxisome proliferators activated receptor (PPAR) Activation
• COX independent apoptosis and angiogenesis (COX-2 inhibitors)
• Inhibition of IL-beta and TNF in inflammatory cells and stimulation of synthesis of the extracellular matrix of human articular cartilage (Aceclofenac)

Table 4.1.3: Beneficial effects of NSAIDs

• **Anti-inflammatory action:** Utilizes various mechanism but main is PGs inhibition
• **Analgesic effects:** Most effective against inflammation associated pain
• **Antipyretic effect:** By inhibiting synthesis of PGE_2 in hypothalamus
• **Anti-platelet effect:** Low dose aspirin selectively inhibits thromboxane A_2(TXA_2)
• **Closure of ductus arteriosus:** Indomethacin causes closure of ductus arteriosus by inhibiting PGE_2 and I_2
• **Cancer chemoprevention:** For familial adenomatous polyposis, colorectal cancer/adenoma)
• **Alzheimer's disease:** Ibuprofen reduces the risk of Alzheimer's disease by an unknown mechanism

TOXICITY

Various toxicities are associated with NSAIDs; the major ones are gastrointestinal (GI), cardiovascular, and renal (Tables 4.1.4 to 4.1.6). The mechanisms by which NSAIDs produce GI, cardiovascular, and renal toxicity are depicted in Figures 4.1.4 to 4.1.6.

Table 4.1.4: Toxicity profile of NSAIDs

1.	Gastrointestinal (GI) toxicity	Older age, history of ulcer, *H. pylori* infection, smoking, alcohol are risk factors for GI toxicity. Other are concomitant use of steroid, higher dosess of NSAIDs, use of multiple NSAIDs, and anticoagulants
2.	Renal toxicity	This is manifestated by acute tubular necrosis, acute tubulointerstitial nephritis, glomerulonephritis, renal papillary necrosis, salt and water retention, and progression of CKD.
3.	Cardiovascular toxicity	Thrombotic events namely myocardial infarction, unstable angina, ischemic stroke, transient ischemic attacks, resuscitated cardiac arrest, sudden or unexplained death have been linked to rofecoxib, celecoxib, valdecoxib. The risk of myocardial ischemia is present even with dicofenac and ibuprofen; however, naproxen is considered safe.
4.	Hepatic toxicity	Transient rise in liver enzymes. Reye's syndrome has been reported with aspirin, whereas cholestasis is seen with sulindac and diclofenac therapy. Fulminant hepatitis, with the use of nimesulide in children has been reported
5.	Bone	NSAIDs also interfere with and suppress bone repair and remodeling. The drugs can decrease sleep
6.	Endocrinological effects	Aspirin and ibuprofen augment insulin secretion
7.	Psychiatric	There are reports of depressive disorders and suicidal tendencies with NSAIDs

(*Contd.*)

Table 4.1.4: Toxicity profile of NSAIDs (*Contd.*)		
8.	CNS	Aseptic meningitis, drowsiness, headaches are reported
9.	Hematologic	Phenylbutazone or oxyphenbutazone can cause aplastic anemia and thrombocytopenia. However, COX-2 specific inhibitors do not affect platelet functions
10.	Dermatologic and respiratory	Urticaria, macular rashes, pseudoporphyria, and erythema multiforme are reported

Table 4.1.5: Mechanism of gastrointestinal (GI) toxicity
• GI toxicity is mediated through COX-1 inhibition with a subsequent decrease in gastroprotective prostaglandins, leading to superficial damage such as mucosal hemorrhages and erosions, endoscopically documented silent ulcers and symptomatic ulcers that can bleed
• To minimize the risk of GI complications, avoid using >1 NSAID at a time, concomitant use of oral corticosteroids and/or anticoagulants
• Misoprostol is an efficacious protective agent
• Other potential protective agents are histamine2 (H_2) receptor antagonists, sucralfate, and proton pump inhibitors
• In patients with at least one GI risk factor use NSAID with a protective agent or choose a COX-2 inhibitor

Table 4.1.6: Mechanisms of cardiovascular toxicity
• COX-2 enzyme is cardioprotective, has anti-proliferative effects toward vascular smooth muscle cells in conjunction with nitric oxide (NO)
• COX-2 inhibition lead to decrease vasodilatory prostacyclin (PGI 2), cause an imbalance between prothrombotic and antithrombotic eicosanoids
• COX-2 inhibitors may destabilize plaques.
• Inhibition of COX-2 may cause increase of arachidonate through lipoxygenase (LO) pathways, leading to LDL oxidation and worsens inflammatory atheromatous plaque
• COX-2 inhibitors increases blood pressure, by medaiting in the renin angiotensin pathway, renal sodium and water retention, inhibition of vasodilating PGs and production of vasoconstrictors (endothelin)

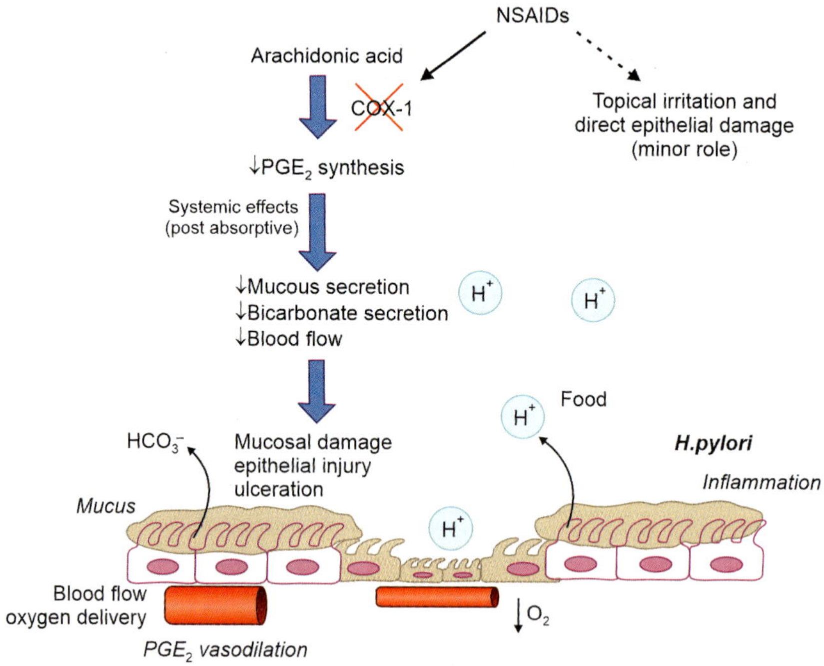

Fig. 4.1.4: Pathogenesis of gastric damage by NSAIDs

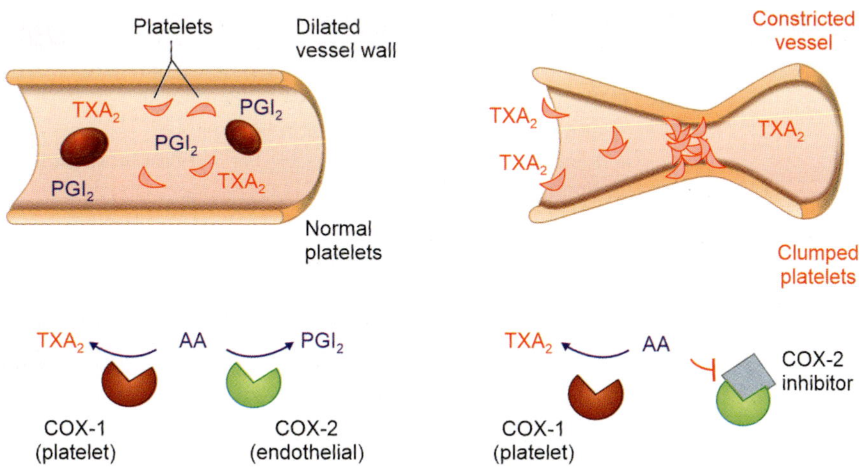

Fig. 4.1.5: COX-2 inhibitors and cardiovascular risk: Thromboxane/prostacyclin imbalance hypothesis

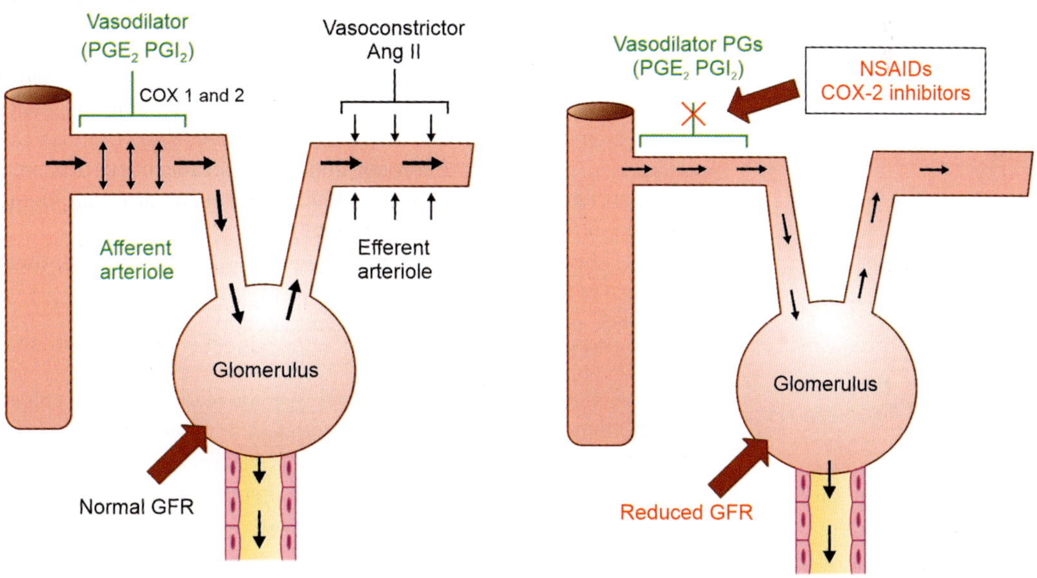

Fig. 4.1.6: Prostaglandin in renal blood flow regulation and effect of NSAIDs: Prostaglandins normally maintain renal perfusion by causing enhanced pre-glomerular vasodilation (left panel). NSAIDs and COX-2 inhibitors adversely affect renal function by blocking the production of autoregulatory prostaglandins, resulting in a decline in GFR that can ultimately result in acute kidney injury (right panel).

INDICATIONS

NSAIDs are used in many inflammatory rheumatic diseases (Table 4.1.7). A guide on how to choose an NSAID and the FDA recommendations are summarized in Tables 4.1.8 and 4.1.9. Osteoarthritis (OA) and gout are two diseases where NSAID is strongly recommended. Topical NSAIDs are recommended by the ACR for patients with knee OA and conditionally recommendation for patients with hand OA. Oral NSAIDs remain the mainstay of treatment in OA. Acetaminophen is conditionally recommended for patients with knee, hip, and/or hand OA.

Regarding gout, the ACR 2020 guideline strongly recommends concomitant anti-inflammatory prophylaxis in the form of either colchicine, NSAIDs, or prednisolone when initiating urate lowering therapy.

Table 4.1.7: Indications for NSAIDs in rheumatic diseases

Disease	Indications
Rheumatoid arthritis (RA)	• NSAIDs provide both analgesic and anti-inflammatory benefits • They do not modify the course of the disease and joint damage may continue despite symptomatic relief • Long acting NSAIDs may be added at night for those patients who have significant morning stiffness
Gout	• Indomethacin is the traditional choice • NSAIDs are indicated in patients with acute gout (uncomplicated) • Other agents include ibuprofen, naproxen, ketoprofen, sulindac, piroxicam, etc.
Osteoarthritis (OA)	• NSAIDS are symptom modifiers, they have no disease modifying effect • Paracetamol is recommended as initial therapy, others like ibuprofen, naproxen, diclofenac, etc. are considered when there is no pain relief with paracetamol • COX-2 inhibitors provide a better GI safety profile • Opioids (codeine) and paracetamol in combination provide better analgesia than paracetamol alone
Low back pain	• NSAIDs are indicated for acute low back pain
Juvenile idiopathic arthritis (JIA)	• NSAIDs form an important part of the initial management of children with oligoarticular, polyarticular, spondyloarthritis, enthesitis related, and systemic onset JIA • Naproxen, meloxicam, ibuprofen, and celecoxib are all approved in JIA • A word of caution: There are reports that naproxen can induce pseudoporphyria in children with JIA • Aspirin should be avoided when there is a suspicion of viral illness because of fear of development of Reye's syndrome • Analgesic nephropathy is also known to occur
Ankylosing spondylitis (AS)	• NSAIDs are firstline treatment in AS • No one NSAIDs have clear superiority over the other in terms of efficacy • Most clinicians choose either indomethacin or naproxen • It is not well known whether continuous treatment with NSAIDs has a long-term advantage over intermittent therapy in terms of functional ability and prevention of structural damage
Undifferentiated Spondyloarthritis and reactive arthritis	• First-line treatment for all these patients is still NSAIDs • NSAIDs provide maximum suppression of pain and inflammation within 2 weeks
Psoriatic arthritis	• NSAIDs are used in the initial treatment for joint disease for symptomatic relief
Systemic lupus erythematosus (SLE)	• NSAIDs are employed in SLE for relief of arthritis, arthralgia and myalgia • Certain agents (ibuprofen, sulindac, rofecoxib) can cause aseptic meningitis • NSAIDs in patients with SLE through salt and water retention can lead to hypertension and pedal edema • There is a higher chance of hepatotoxicity, thus patients should be monitored for renal, and hepatic side effects
Acute rheumatic fever	• NSAIDs (salicylates) are used in management of arthritis in acute rheumatic fever
Soft tissue rheumatism	• Indicated also in acute and chronic bursitis, tendinitis, radiation synovitis and sport injuries

Table 4.1.8: Factors to be considered while prescribing NSAIDs

	Factors	*Choice of NASIDs*
1.	Efficacy	Nonspecific NSAIDs or COX-2 specific NSAIDs show comparable efficacy in different rheumatological conditions
2.	Safety	Greater the potency more is the chance ADRs Nonselective NSAIDs lead to more chances of GI toxicity The COX -2 inhibitors have increased risk of cardiovascular related events and deaths. Nimesulide is safe in asthmatics. Sulindac has incidence of renal side effects Increased risk of acute myocardial infarction with selective COX-2 inhibitors and treatment with diclofenac and ibuprofen Naproxen is the safest NSAID for those with CVD
3.	Pharmacokinetics	Compliance is better with once daily or twice daily dosing Higher dose has a faster onset and a longer duration of action Start with a high dose of a short-life drug (e.g. ibuprofen) and when analgesic effect is achieved the dose is reduced For management of chronic pain, it is better to give NSAIDs having long half-lives such as naproxen and COX-2 inhibitors
4.	Dosage/formulation	Entero-coating-better tolerated by GI tract, rapid onset and prolonged duration of analgesic activity
5.	Concomitant treatment	Avoid using when patient is on steroids, warfarin to minise GI toxicity Antineoplastic drugs can cause thrombocytopenia and can increase risk of bleeding. NSAIDs can decrease efficacy of antihypertensives such as beta-blockers, calcium channel blockers, and angiotensin converting enzyme inhibitors
6.	Disease	Indomethacin is the traditional choice in gout. Ankylosing spondylitis (AS) is better treated with indomethacin or naproxen. RA is better treated with drug having a long half life such as piroxicam and naproxen
7.	Target symptom	Morning stiffness may be better controlled with long half-life drugs such as piroxicam or a night time dose of indomethacin
8.	Concomitant disease	GI dysfunction, renal disease, cardiovascular dysfunction, diabetes mellitus and hypertension influence the choice in between COX selective Vs nonselective Vs preferential COX inhibitors
9.	Old age	Chances of drug interaction and serious adverse effects are more
10.	Pregnancy	Paracetamol may be considered as safe analgesic
11.	Lactation	Most NSAIDs are safe during breastfeeding

Table 4.1.9: FDA Expert Advisory Committee Recommendations

- NSAIDs have to display black box warnings for risk of cardiovascular and GI adverse effects
- COX-2 inhibitors and NSAIDs should be prescribed at lowest effective dose and for minimum duration of time
- Avoid in patients with high risk for GI and CVD toxicity
- Any patient with a previous GI toxicity, concurrently receiving aspirin, warfarin or steroids or warfarin should also receive PPI with NSAID or instead use a COX-2 inhibitor

NSAIDs IN COVID-19

NSAIDs are useful to provide pain relief of arthritis in patients with rheumatic diseases having concomitant novel SARS CoV2 disease (COVID-19). At the start of the pandemic there were concerns that ibuprofen exacerbated COVID-19 symptoms, theoretically by increasing the expression of angiotensin converting enzyme inhibitor (ACE-I) receptors. Thus there was a general reluctance among physicians not to use NSAIDs in COVID-19. More recently, analysis of a large database from the UK comprising more than 70,000 individuals with COVID-19 found that there was no association of NSAIDs exposure and severe outcomes.

NITRIC OXIDE NSAIDs

NSAIDs having a nitric oxide (NO) moiety linked to a conventional NSAID is called a nitric oxide NSAID. They donate NO to the gastric mucosa to counterbalance the harmful effects of prostaglandin deficiency. Licofelone, a 5-lipoxygenase (5-LOX) and COX inhibitor was tried in OA (mixed results) but never submitted for regulatory approval. NO releasing aspirin (acetylsalicylic acid) has potentially more antithrombotic action than aspirin. The released NO at the vascular level theoretically has anti-atherogenic effects (similar to endogenous NO). In animal models, NO-flurbiprofen was demonstrated to be devoid of nephrotoxicity and improve renal function. Therefore, hybrid NSAIDs have a potential to be effective with reduced GI and cardiovascular side effects.

LEARNING POINTS

1. NSAIDs are effective in reducing pain and inflammation in various rheumatological disorders.
2. The therapeutic approach is to use low dose NSAID for a shorter duration, to avoid adverse events. During this initial stage paracetamol/acetaminophen is used to supplement analgesic activity.
3. The choice of an NSAID for a particular patient is based upon efficacy, toxicity, concomitant drug use, patient's age, renal function, cost, etc.
4. Different NSAIDs exhibit different anti-inflammatory activity between NSAIDs.
5. It is important to give each NSAID an appropriate therapeutic trial before switching to another.

FURTHER READING

1. Abdellatif KR, Abdelall EK, Bakr RB. Nitric Oxide-NASIDS Donor prodrugs as hybrid safe anti-inflammatory agents. Curr Top Med Chem. 2017; 17(8):941–55.
2. FitzGerald JD, Dalbeth N, Mikuls T et al. 2020 American College of Rheumatology Guideline for the Management of Gout [published correction appears in Arthritis Rheumatol. 2021;73(3):413]. Arthritis Rheumatol. 2020;72:879–95.
3. O'Dell JR. Treatment of rheumatoid arthritis. In: Firestein GS, Budd RC, Gabriel SE, Kortezky GA, McInnes IB, O'Dell JR, editors. Firestein and Kelley's Textbook of Rheumatology. Vol-I, 11th edition. Philadelphia: Elsevier; 2020. p.1258–83.
4. Polston GR, Wallace M. Analgesic agents in Rheumatic disease. In: Firestein GS, Budd RC, Gabriel SE, Kortezky GA, McInnes IB, O'Dell JR, editors. Firestein and Kelley's Textbook of Rheumatology. Vol-I, 11th edition. Philadelphia: Elsevier; 2020. p. 1135–55.
5. Robert LJ, Morrow D. Analgesic-antipyretic and anti-inflammatory agents and drugs employed in the treatment of gout. In: Hardman JG, Limbird LE, Gilman AG, editors. Goodman and Gilman's The Pharmacological basis of Therapeutics. 13 edition. New York: McGraw-Hill; 2018. p. 687–731.

Methotrexate

Arup Kumar Kundu, Arghya Chattopadhya

INTRODUCTION

Methotrexate (MTX) is a structural analog of folic acid that interferes the binding of folic acid to various enzymes where it (folic acid) acts as a cofactor for the synthesis of purines and pyrimidines, and thus interrupting DNA replication and consequently cellular proliferation. It was Food and Drug Administration (FDA) approved for use in rheumatoid arthritis (RA) in 1988, and since then it is the most commonly employed conventional synthetic disease-modifying antirheumatic drugs (cs-DMARDs).

Formerly known as amethopterin, MTX was discovered by a Harvard-based Indian biochemist Dr. Yellapragada Subbarow in 1947. Initially it was used in high dose for the treatment of childhood leukemias. In 1951, Gubner et al. first published the utility of MTX for the management of RA and psoriatic arthritis (PsA), and for the first time demonstrated the steroid-sparing effect of this anti-proliferative medicine. Later the use of MTX got suppressed due to both difficulty in manufacturing, and more and more use of corticosteroid by the clinicians. During the 1960s–70s use of low-dose MTX gained popularity in RA and PsA, which subsequently got FDA approval in 1988 for the management of RA. Due to the limited oral bioavailability, two different preparations of MTX for subcutaneous use got FDA approval in 2013 and 2014.

Mechanism of Action

Low-dose (LD) MTX is practically different from high-dose (HD) MTX in terms of mechanism of action, pharmacokinetics and pharmacodynamics. The anti-inflammatory effect of MTX is through increasing intracellular and extracellular adenosine level by inhibiting aminoimidazole carboxamide ribonucleotide (AICAR) transformylase (ATIC), and anti-proliferative action by inhibiting TYMS (thymidylate synthetase) and DHFR (dihydrofolate reductase) resulting in decreased pyrimidine synthesis and inhibition of transmethylation reactions essential for cell function respectively (Table 4.2.1).

INDICATIONS

Unless contraindicated, low-dose MTX is the first-line csDMARD for most rheumatological disorders. It is the sheet anchor drug for RA, Felty's syndrome, PsA, juvenile idiopathic arthritis. It is also used for management of arthritis and skin manifestations in systemic lupus erythematosus, in psoriasis, as a steroid-sparing maintenance agent in polymyositis-dermatomyositis, MCTD, scleroderma, vasculitis, sarcoidosis, and rarely, in multicentric reticulohistiocytosis.

Amongst non-rheumatological disorders, MTX is useful in the management of childhood leukemia, meningeal carcinomatosis, chorio-carcinoma, breast/ovary/bladder/head-neck cancer, osteosarcoma, cranial lymphoma, and along with misoprostol for medical termination of pregnancy.

Table 4.2.1: Pharmacology of methotrexate

Features	*Oral*	*Parenteral (SC or IM)*
Absorption	Rapid, peak at 1–2 hours.	Rapid, peak at 0.1–1 hours
Bioavailability	• Plateau after single oral dose of 15 mg • No relation with food, except milk which hampers absorption • Reduced absorption in patients with malabsorption syndrome	• Linear increase with the dose • NA • NA
Half-life	~ 6 hours	
Distribution	50–60% plasma protein bound. Can accumulate in third space	
Elimination	Excreted in urine in the first 12 hours except MTX-PG. Median half-life for elimination of MTX-PG is 3.1 weeks	
Pharmacogenomics	• 80G>A variant of the reduced folate carrier gene 1(RFC1) linked with MTX efficacy • Solute carrier family 19-member 1(SLC19A1) associated with MTX treatment response • AITC 347 C>G single nucleotide polymorphism rs2372536 linked with MTX toxicity; although not replicated consistently	

NA: Not applicable; *MTX-PG:* Methotrexate polyglutamates

DOSING AND ADMINISTRATION

The therapeutic dose of MTX in inflammatory rheumatic diseases ranges from 7.5 mg to 25 mg/week. The starting dose could be 7.5 mg/week to 15 mg/week, which depends on the severity of the disease process and other special situations (Table 4.2.2). The dose may be escalated by 2.5–5 mg increments at an interval of 4 weeks with careful surveillance on disease activity and drug toxicity. On a single day, the dose is given in a gap of 12 hours to improve tolerability.

MTX is available in oral (2.5 mg, 5 mg, 7.5 mg, 10 mg, 15 mg, 20 mg and 25 mg tablets) and parenteral (7.5 mg/mL, 15 mg/mL, 20 mg/mL and 25 mg/mL solution for subcutaneous (SC) or intramuscular (IM) injections) forms. Many a time, parenteral regimen is preferred when the dose requirement is 15–25 mg/week. MTX can be used as monotherapy or along with other cs-DMARDS.

SIDE EFFECTS AND TOXICITY

The side effects of MTX are broad as shown in Table 4.2.3. MTX toxicity may be dose-dependent, e.g. bone marrow depression and oral mucosal ulcerations (Fig. 4.2.1), idiosyncratic (e.g. pneumonitis) or multifactorial (e.g. cirrhosis of liver). Concomitant use of folic acid (5–10 mg/week, other than on the day of MTX) decreases the toxicity of MTX, especially mucositis and nausea, without hampering the efficacy of MTX. Acute MTX toxicity is mostly due to accidental overdose or daily dosing (Table 4.2.4).

Nodulosis/MTX induced accelerated nodulosis (MIAN) was first described by Kremer et al. in 1986. It presents as an acute onset, multiple, small, painless or painful nodules over fingers (Fig. 4.2.2), pulp spaces. Other areas of nodulosis are ear helix, sole of feet, penis, meninges, scalp, chest, heart, lung, surgical incision site. The genetic risk factor is HLA DRB1* 0401 in Caucasians. Time to develop MTX nodulosis is a few months to several years. Histopathologically they are similar to RA nodules, the suggested pathogenesis are increased levels of adenosine. The points that favor MIAN over rheumatoid nodules are: acute onset multiple nodules, in atypical site, quiescent arthritis, absence of other extra-articular symptoms, and rheumatoid factor negativity.

Once a patient is started on MTX the blood counts and liver functions need to be monitored periodically (Table 4.2.5).

Table 4.2.2: Use of methotrexate in special situations

Situations	*Comments*
Geriatric	• Start lower dose 5–7.5 mg/week • Maximum dose not more than 20 mg/week • Dose depends on CrCl
Pediatric	Weight-based dose: • Dose range 0.3–1 mg/kg/dose once weekly • Starting dose 0.3 mg/kg/dose once weekly
Pregnancy	• Contraindicated, FDA category X drug (teratogenic) • Women (men too) should discontinue the drug for at least 3 months before conception
Lactation	• Contraindicated
Fertility	• No effect on female fertility • Reversible sterility in males
Renal impairment	Dose adjustment required based on CrCl: • 61–80 mL/min: reduced by 25% • 51–60 mL/min: reduced by 30% • 10–50 mL/min: reduced by 50–80% • <10 mL/min: avoid use
Hepatic impairment	• MTX-induced nausea, dyspepsia or severe anorexia may be overcomed by addition of folic acid or parenteral administration
Drug interaction	• Caution while using with concomitant hepatotoxic drugs • Concomitant administration with trimethoprim-sulfamethoxazole daily dose can cause cytopenia
Vaccination	• MTX>0.4 mg/kg/week is considered as immunosuppressive as per CDC definition. Temporary discontinuation of MTX, 2 weeks prior and 2 weeks post-vaccination, has shown to improve immunogenicity for seasonal influenza vaccine; although not recommended for the same • For COVID-19 vaccine, discontinuation 1 week post-vaccination after each dose of vaccine has been suggested by the ACR
Combination with other drugs	• Can be used with other cs-DMARDs and biologic DMARDs (i.e. adalimumab, tofacitinib, etc.) • Strongly advised to use in combination with infliximab as it prevents development of Human Anti-Chimeric Antibodies (HACA)
Non-rheumatological use	• Malignancy • Abortifacient
Contraindications	• Ongoing infection • Severe renal, pulmonary and hepatic impairment • TLC <3,000/mm^3, platelet <50,000/mm^3 • HBV or HIV infection • Pregnancy and lactation • Alcoholic liver disease; LFT>2 × ULN • Recent lymphoproliferative malignancy/myelodysplasia

CrCl: Creatinine clearance; *CDC:* Centers for Disease Control and Prevention; *ACR:* American College of Rheumatology; *TLC:* Total leucocyte count; *LFT:* Liver function tests; *ULN:* Upper limit of normal

Table 4.2.3: Side effects and toxicity of methotrexate (MTX)

Systems involved	*Types of involvement*	*Comments*
Gastrointestinal (GI) and hepatic	• Nausea, anorexia ~20–70% cases; diarrhea • Hepatic toxicity–1/1000 after 5 years use; elevated transaminases, hepatic fibrosis, cirrhosis	Risk factors for hepatotoxicity—alcohol abuse, obesity, diabetes, concomitant hepatotoxic drug use, chronic HBV and chronic HCV infection, α1-antitrypsin deficiency
Hematology	• Dose-dependent bone marrow toxicity–cytopenia (leukopenia > anemia > thrombocytopenia) ~1–2%	Risk factors–renal impairment, hypo-albuminemia, dosing errors (taking daily instead of weekly), concomitant use of probenecid or trimethoprim sulfamethoxazole
Pulmonary	• Hypersensitivity pneumonitis • Pleurisy • Pleural effusion • Pulmonary nodules	ILD in RA has been linked with the use of MTX, however, recent trials have shown there is no such conclusive evidence to prove the fact. Rather uncontrolled disease could be a risk factor
Mucocutaneous	• Mostly minor oral ulceration (Fig. 4.2.1), dose-dependent • Severe ulcers involving mouth, GI tract and vagina are reported with toxicity • Alopecia	Folate replacement indicated
Malignancy	• Lymphoma: Conflicting evidence, disease itself is a confounding factor	Potential benefits > small risks
Flu-like syndrome	• Soon after taking the weekly dose; with nausea, mild fever, myalgia and chills	Helped by–dose reduction, folic acid supplementation, changing from oral to parenteral route, or change of timing to bed time dose
Vasculitis	Leukocytoclastic vasculitis reported	Rare

HBV: Hepatitis B virus; *HVC:* Hepatitis C virus; *ILD:* Interstitial lung disease; *TMP-SMX:* Trimethoprim-sulfamethoxazole; *LCV:* Leukocytoclastic vasculitis

Table 4.2.4: Treatment of acute methotrexate toxicity

Treatment of acute MTX toxicity can be divided into three major components:

Folinic acid rescue	*Elimination of MTX from body*	*Organ specific care*
• Folinic acid (leucovorin) is the antidote of choice, the dose is 15 mg/m^2 every 6 hourly • Ideally serum MTX level should be measured every 24 hours until level fall <0.2 µmol/L	Hydration: • >90% cleared by kidneys • Urine output target 2 L/m^2/day until MTX level falls <0.2 µmol/L Urine alkalization: • 40–50 mEq of sodium bicarbonate/L of IV fluid reduces the risk of intratubular crystal formation Management of delayed MTX excretion: • Glucarpidase—approved by US FDA for treatment of plasma MTX >1 µmol/L in patients with delayed MTX clearance due to renal impairment. It has no effect on intracellular MTX, hence folinic acid should be continued	MTX-induced myelosuppression: • Reverse barrier nursing • Fever: treatment as per febrile neutropenia protocol • G-CSF (granulocyte colony-stimulating factor) therapy Oral care: • Small frequent meals. Straws may be used to sip water and liquid food. Food should be at room temperature • Hot food/drinks, acidic foods/fruits to be avoided • Oral saline rinse. Folinic acid mouth wash 15 mg QDS (15 mg/2 mL injection diluted to 10 mL with water) • Syrup viscous lignocaine 2 tea spoon full taken 10 minutes before meal

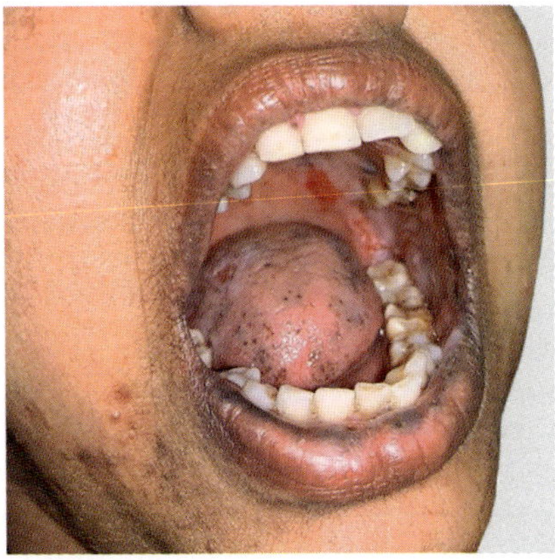

Fig. 4.2.1: Painful oral ulceration (mucositis) following methotrexate therapy (*Courtesy:* Dr Prasanta Padhan, Professor of Clinical Immunology and Rheumatology, KIMS, Bhubaneswar)

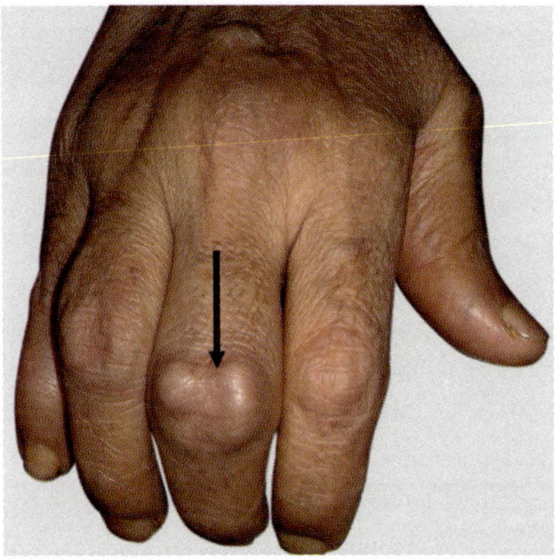

Fig. 4.2.2: Methotrexate-induced nodules formation (arrow) over dorsal aspect of right middle finger

Table 4.2.5: Monitoring plan of a patient on low dose methotrexate (MTX)

Time after initiation of MTX	*Baseline evaluation— CBC, LFT (transaminases, albumin), renal function, HBV, HCV, HIV screening, chest X-ray*
At <3 months of treat-ment on stable dose	Monitor with CBC, LFT, creatinine every 4 weeks
At 3–6 months of treat-ment on stable dose	Monitor with CBC, LFT, creatinine every 8–12 weeks
At >6 months of treat-ment on stable dose	Monitor with CBC, LFT, creatinine every 12 weeks
Drug discontinuation	In persistence of LFT abnormality

CBC: Complete blood counts; *LFT:* Liver function test; *HBV:* Hepatitis B virus; *HCV:* Hepatitis C virus; *HIV:* Human immunodeficiency virus

LEARNING POINTS

1. MTX is the cornerstone of combination DMARD therapy in most of the autoimmune rheumatic disorders.
2. MTX is a safe and time-tested drug, if administered judiciously by a rheumatologist/physician who is surveillant about drug toxicity.
3. MTX toxicity is not uncommon and is mostly due to accidental overdose from patients' part. Detailed communication regarding the dose and side effects can help in reducing the incidence of toxicity.
4. The physician should be cautious when MTX is used in an alcoholic, renal failure or cytopenic patient, or along with other hepatotoxic drugs.
5. MTX is a category X drug for pregnancy. Both men and women should hold MTX for 3 months before conception.
6. MTX has shown no deleterious effect on RA-ILD, and stoppage of MTX is not required in those patients.

FURTHER READING

1. Chan ES, Cronstein BN. Methotrexate–how does it really work? Nat Rev Rheumatol. 2010;6:175-8.
2. Cronstein BN, Aune TM. Methotrexate and its mechanisms of action in inflammatory arthritis. Nat Rev Rheumatol. 2020;16:145–54.
3. Malaviya AN. Landmark papers on the discovery of methotrexate for the treatment of rheumatoid arthritis and other systemic inflammatory rheumatic diseases: a fascinating story. Int J Rheum Dis. 2016;19:844–51.
4. Weinblatt ME. Methotrexate in rheumatoid arthritis: a quarter century of development. Trans Am Clin Climatol Assoc. 2013;124:16–25.

Leflunomide

Pradip Kumar Sarma

INTRODUCTION

Leflunomide is an oral conventional synthetic disease-modifying antirheumatic drug (csDMARD) with anti-inflammatory and immunomodulatory properties. It originated in the 1980s from an anti-inflammatory drug development program at Hoechst Marion Roussel (Aventis). In the initial animal studies, it was shown to prevent proliferation of mitogen-stimulated lymphocytes in autoimmune diseases and prolonged graft survival.

MECHANISM OF ACTION

Pyrimidine requirement is increased in activated lymphocytes in autoimmune diseases in order to progress from G1 through the S phase of the cell cycle. Leflunomide inhibits the mitochondrial enzyme dihydroorotate dehydrogenase (DHODH), which is required for *de novo* synthesis of the pyrimidine ribonucleotide uridine monophosphate. So when DHODH is inhibited, activated lymphocytes get arrested in the G1 phase. As a result, proliferation of autoimmune T cells and production of autoantibodies by B-cells are inhibited.

Nonlymphoid cells have a salvage pathway for pyrimidine synthesis and therefore are not much affected by leflunomide. Other mechanisms of action are inhibition of tyrosine kinases, NFκB pathways, etc. (Table 4.3.1).

Table 4.3.1: Pharmacology of leflunomide
• It is a pro-drug with molecular a weight of 270 Da
• Absorption is almost 100% from the intestinal mucosa and it undergoes rapid nonenzymatic conversion predominantly in the intestine and plasma to its active form, a malononitrilamide named A77–1726 or teriflunomide
• There is no interaction with food
• Plasma level of A 77–1726 is not affected by body size, age, or sex at steady state
• Conversion by the liver during "first-pass" metabolism may also occur
• Over 99.5% of A77–1726 is protein bound, predominantly to albumin
• The t1/2 of A77–1726 is approximately 15 days (5–40 days)
• Though it can be excreted in bile, it is efficiently reabsorbed by enterohepatic recirculation
• About 60–70% of the drug is ultimately excreted in the urine as trifluoromethylaniline oxanilic acid
• Leflunomide has no drug interaction with oral anticoagulants, oral contraceptives, cyclosporine, prednisolone or oral hypoglycemic agents. It may weakly displace certain NSAIDs and thus lead to increased blood levels of these drugs. Rifampicin may increase the blood level of A77–1276. No pharmacokinetic interaction was seen with methotrexate in rheumatoid arthritis patients.

INDICATIONS

Rheumatoid arthritis (RA): Leflunomide improves disease activity, and the retardation of radiological progression is similar to methotrexate or sulfasalazine. It is indicated when patients fail or are intolerant to first line methotrexate therapy. It is used as monotherapy or as combination therapy with other csDMARD or biological DMARD.

Psoriatic arthritis: Effective for arthritis; although not very effective for skin manifestations.

Juvenile idiopathic arthritis (JIA): There are few studies of leflunomide specially in polyarticular JIA. The usual indication of leflunomide in children is when there is failure or intolerance to methotrexate or sulfasalazine. However, it is still not officially recommended because of lack of long-term data and lack of studies in younger children <3 years.

Systemic lupus erythematosus: It is useful for arthritis, and difficult cases of proliferative lupus nephritis where standard treatment has failed.

Vasculitis: For nonsevere refractory or relapsing ANCA associated vasculitis or large-vessel vasculitis.

Sarcoidosis: Alternative agent for pulmonary and extrapulmonary sarcoidosis.

Others: It has also been evaluated for other conditions like Sjögren's syndrome, Crohn's disease, bullous pemphigoid, prevention of rejection of organ transplantation, etc. Cancer is another field as it inhibits DHODH, important for cell proliferations.

DOSING

In children the dose is 10–20 mg/1.73 m^2/day. In adults the dose is 20 mg daily. If 20 mg/day is not well tolerated, the dose may be decreased to 10 mg/day. The previous practice of loading dose (100 mg/day for initial 3 days) is nowadays not used by most rheumatologists because of toxicity concerns.

In patients with increased risk for toxicity, for example, in the elderly, those with concomitant methotrexate therapy, it is better to start with 10 mg daily for 2 months, and increase to 20 mg/day in case of inadequate response. The patient should be monitored for development of transaminitis and cytopenias (Table 4.3.2).

SIDE EFFECTS AND TOXICITY

Leflunomide, though generally well-tolerated, is associated with several adverse effects (Table 4.3.3). An important toxicity is hepatotoxicity, so should not be used in those with liver disease. Though data from clinical trials show that only <5% of patients develop liver function abnormalities, rates that are similar to methotrexate and sulfasalazine. It carries a black box warning for severe liver damage including fatal liver failure, and should not be used in patients with preexisting liver disease or who have transaminitis.

Other contraindications are given in Table 4.3.4. It is also best to avoid leflunomide in patients with preexisting interstitial lung disease (ILD), and previous methotrexate pneumonitis.

CHOLESTYRAMINE WASHOUT

Leflunomide is contraindicated during pregnancy and lactation. Women who are planning pregnancy are advised to undergo a drug washout with cholestyramine to bring down the active metabolite levels to below 0.02 mg/L in 2 separate tests at least 14 days apart before pregnancy is contemplated. Without cholestyramine washout it may take up to 2 years for metabolites to come down to this level. Cholestyramine washout is also required in case of inadvertent pregnancy. The procedure consists of oral cholestyramine 8 g every eight hours for 11 days,

Table 4.3.2: Monitoring plan for a patient who is on leflunomide

Baseline, every month for 6 months, then 6–8 weeks thereafter	CBC, LFT, and measurement of blood pressure
When to discontinue Leflunomide*	Leflunomide should be stopped if AST, ALT is >3 times ULN, total leukocyte count is <4,000/mm³, Hb is <7 g/dL or platelet count is <100,000/mm³.

CBC: Complete blood count; *LFT:* Liver function tests; *ULN:* Upper limit of normal.

*Caution is necessary when leflunomide is used with other hepatotoxic drugs. It can be combined with methotrexate; however, the incidence of elevated liver enzymes is higher and careful monitoring is required.

Table 4.3.3: Side effects and toxicities associated with leflunomide

System involved	*Side effects*
Hepatotoxicity	It carries a black box warning for severe liver damage including fatal liver failure. But, in clinical trials only <5% of patients develop liver function abnormalities, similar to sulfasalazine or methotrexate
Gastrointestinal	The most common adverse events are gastrointestinal, namely diarrhea, nausea, oral ulcer and abdominal pain. These are generally mild to moderate and resolve in a week. However, the most common reasons for discontinuation of leflunomide are diarrhea, nausea, vomiting and abnormal liver tests
Cutaneous	Alopecia, rash, infection is also reported Hypersensitivity reactions are reported
Constitutional	Some patients lose weight without any other adverse effects
Cardiovascular	Leflunomide can aggravate preexisting hypertension or cause hypertension in a small number of patients
Nervous system	Peripheral neuropathy, which is reversible if the drug is discontinued, is also reported in a small number of patients.
Hematological, pulmonary	Less common adverse effects are hematological like cytopenias Pulmonary toxicity include development of hypersensitivity pneumonitis, especially with preexisting abnormalities interstitial lung disease

Table 4.3.4: Contraindications to treatment with leflunomide

1. Pregnancy
2. Lactation
3. Liver disease
4. Hypersensitivity
5. Previous or current skin reactions to leflunomide
6. Impaired bone marrow function
7. Current infections

followed by measurement of drug levels. It can be repeated if plasma level is >0.02 mg/L.

Other indications for washout with cholestyramine is acute toxicity in the liver, lung or bone marrow toxicity.

LEARNING POINTS

1. Leflunomide a pyrimidine synthesis inhibitor, is effective in the management of RA, PsA, and has been tried in refractory lupus nephritis.
2. It can be given in combination with methotrexate in RA, but the liver functions need to be closely monitored.
3. The major adverse event associated with leflunomide is hepatotoxicity. It is also associated with development of hypertension, and peripheral neuropathy that is reversible once the drug is stopped.
4. It is contraindicated in pregnancy and lactation.

FURTHER READING

1. Cannon GW, Kremer JM. Leflunomide. Rheum Dis Clin N Am. 2004:295–309.
2. Fox RI, Herrmann M L, Frangou CG, et al. Mechanism of action for leflunomide in rheumatoid arthritis. Clin Immunol. 1999;93:198–208.
3. Zhang M, Qi C, Zha Y, et al. Leflunomide versus cyclophosphamide in the induction treatment of proliferative lupus nephritis in Chinese patients: a randomized trial. Clin Rheumatol. 2019;38:859–67.

Hydroxychloroquine

Ankit Jain, Sundeep Grover

INTRODUCTION

The antimalarial drugs chloroquine and hydroxychloroquine (HCQ) are derivatives of aminoquinoline. Both are well established, safe and well tolerated oral disease modifying anti-rheumatic drugs (DMARDs). The various beneficial effects of HCQ makes it one of the most widely used pharmacotherapeutic agents in rheumatology.

MECHANISM OF ACTION

HCQ is an important immunomodulating drug in systemic autoimmune diseases. It accumulates in the lysosome and inhibits lysosomal activity and autophagy, thus preventing MHC class II mediated antigen presentation. It also accumulates in the endosome and inhibits toll-like receptor (TLR) activity, preventing TLRs from binding to its ligands (DNA and RNA), and thus preventing TLR signaling and proinflammatory cytokine production, especially type I interferons. HCQ acts at various levels of the adaptive and innate immune system.

It also has antilipidemic effects, and hypoglycemic action due to which occurrence of incident diabetes is reduced. It has anti-angiogenic, antiplatelet, antithrombotic effects, and is also a good antioxidant. Moreover, it also has photoprotective properties.

INDICATIONS IN SYSTEMIC AUTOIMMUNE INFLAMMATORY DISEASES

1. **RA:** HCQ improves joint pain and swelling in RA patients. However, it does not prevent erosions. It is best suited for use in mild RA, early disease, palindromic rheumatism, as an agent in combination DMARD therapy, and management of RA during pregnancy.
2. **SLE:** Because of its multiple mechanisms of actions like anti-inflammatory, antithrombotic effects and photoprotection it is the standard of care in all patients with SLE. HCQ prevents flares, there are studies showing that HCQ withdrawal in patients with SLE led to flares. Other benefits in SLE include: reduction of risk of thrombosis and infection, delays progression to SLE in prelupus, reduces damage accrual, protection from avascular necrosis, reduced SLE related hospitalization and also has survival benefit.
3. **Antiphospholipid antibody syndrome (APS):** HCQ has been shown to reduce the risk of thrombosis in patients with antiphospholipid antibodies. In animal models, it reduces thrombus size, and retards platelet activation. Despite the lack of randomized trials evaluating use of HCQ in APS, experts recommend its use in patients with refractory APS, in whom optimum anticoagulation is difficult, and in patients with secondary APS. It also has a role in obstetric APS due to its beneficial effect in preeclampsia.
4. **Cutaneous LE:** Most patients with discoid lupus erythematosus (DLE) respond to HCQ.
5. **Sjögren's syndrome:** HCQ improves ocular and oral symptoms, arthralgia and myalgia in Sjogren's syndrome besides the other immunomodulatory and anti-inflammatory actions.
6. **Prevention of congenital heart block:** HCQ has been found useful for prevention of autoimmune congenital heart block in the fetus of patients with SSA/SSB/Ro52 antibodies.

DOSING

Adults: 5 mg/kg/day according to actual body weight. Maximum dose: 400 mg/day.
Children: 5 mg/kg/day according to actual body weight. Maximum dose: 400 mg/day.
Geriatric population: No dose adjustment.
Chronic kidney disease (CKD) stage III: 75% of dose, CKD stage IV: 50% of dose, CKD stage V: 25% of dose.

TOXICITY

Ocular Toxicity

Damage to retinal pigment epithelium is the most important toxic effect of HCQ. Retinopathy is irreversible, and may progress despite withdrawing the drug. It is manifested by the appearance of Bull's eye maculopathy in the later stages. Hence early detection of retinopathy is a must. Among the risk factors for ocular toxicity (Table 4.4.1) one of them is continuous usage for >20 years. Thus the risk of ocular toxicity is <2% for 10 years use, 20% for 20-year use.

Prevention

Baseline ophthalmology evaluation should be done within the first few months of starting HCQ. It is needed to detect underlying retinal pathology that may in itself cause retinopathy or create difficulty in recognition of drug related retinopathy, e.g. advanced macular degeneration, severe diabetic retinopathy, or hereditary retinopathies.

Annual ophthalmologic screening should begin after 5 years of starting therapy, if there are no special risk factors (such as a high daily dose, kidney disease, or concurrent tamoxifen usage). In presence of these risk factors, annual screening should begin from the first year of therapy. Screening tools are Optical Coherence Tomography (OCT), and automated visual fields.

Table 4.4.1: Risk factors of ocular toxicity of hydroxychloroquine (HCQ)

1. A daily dose ≥5 mg/kg/actual body weight or ≥6.5 mg/kg/ideal body weight
2. Prolonged HCQ use (minimal risk <5 years, increases after 10–25 years of use)
3. High cumulative dose ie > 600–1000 g
4. Chronic kidney disease (CKD) when eGFR <60 mL/min/m^2
5. Concomitant use of Tamoxifen for >6 months

Cardiac Toxicity

HCQ seems to be generally well tolerated by patients with rheumatic diseases, cardiac toxicity is a rare adverse effect. A predominantly restrictive or diastolic cardiomyopathy presenting as heart failure, although rare, has been reported following long-term use (more common with chloroquine). Risk factors associated with cardiotoxicity are listed in Table 4.4.2. Additionally, conduction abnormalities, e.g. AV block, sick sinus syndrome, bundle branch block and pulmonary hypertension have been reported. Cardiomyopathy can be asymptomatic. It may or may not reverse on discontinuation. It happens over a long duration of therapy and the exact mechanism is unknown. It is probably related to the drug binding to phospholipids within the myocyte leading to accumulation of toxic metabolic end products. A population-based study from Olmsted Minnesota found that there was no association between HCQ use and heart failure in patients with RA.

Prolonged QT Interval

Long-term use or high doses of antimalarials especially chloroquine have been associated with prolonged QT interval on ECG (Table 4.4.2) and subsequent ventricular arrhythmias including torsades de pointes, syncope, and sudden cardiac death. Exact mechanism is unknown but probably related to the drug affecting ionic currents leading to electrophysiological abnormalities. In recent times where HCQ was increasingly used in patients having disease due to the novel severe acute respiratory syndrome coronavirus 2 (SARS CoV2) or coronavirus disease-2019 (COVID-19), meta-analysis data showed that CQ/HCQ is associated with prolonged QT in 10% patients and the prevalence was more in those who concomitantly received azithromycin.

However, recent data demonstrate that HCQ in lupus patients without cardiovascular disease is not associated with QTc prolongation. Because of the variability and non-specificity of HCQ-associated cardiac toxicity, accurate diagnosis is difficult, especially in patients with RA and SLE, who often have cardiovascular comorbidities.

Table 4.4.2: Risk factors for cardiac toxicity, and prolonged QT interval due to hydroxychloroquine

Risk factors for cardiotoxicity
1. Longer duration of therapy
2. Higher cumulative doses
3. Older age
4. Women
5. Preexisting cardiac disease
6. Renal impairment
Risk factors for prolonged QT interval*
1. Women
2. Structural heart disease (e.g. history of myocardial infarction or heart failure)
3. Genetic defects of cardiac ion channels
4. Congenital long QT syndrome
5. Baseline QTc interval prolongation
6. Electrolyte disturbances (e.g. hypokalemia or hypomagnesemia)
7. Bradycardia
8. Hepatic impairment
9. Renal impairment
10. Coadministration of multiple drug which can prolong the QT interval or drug interactions that increase serum concentration of QT-prolonging medications

*risk factors for prolonged QT interval listed here are as noted in the general population and not specifically to autoimmune diseases.

Dermatologic Toxicity

Cutaneous adverse effects of HCQ in the form of photosensitivity, skin hyperpigmentation, psoriasiform dermatitis, stomatitis, and alopecia are rare. Hyperpigmentation of the skin is commonly described as slate gray pigmentation, is not considered to be very rare, it appears to be unrelated to cumulative dose. More common is a maculopapular and erythematous rash that occurs within 4 weeks of initiation and disappears once the drug is discontinued.

Neuromuscular Toxicity

Headaches, tinnitus, insomnia, and irritability are common. Neuromyotoxicity has been reported. Skeletal muscle myopathy or neuropathy leading to proximal myopathy, depressed tendon reflexes, and abnormal nerve conduction can happen. Creatine kinase (CK) may be normal or mildly elevated. Muscle biopsy reveals vacuolar degeneration with preferential involvement of type I fibers. The underlying primary rheumatic disease can mask these symptoms rendering the diagnosis of drug induced myopathy difficult.

Gastrointestinal Toxicity

Symptoms such as anorexia, nausea, vomiting, diarrhea, abdominal pain are quite common.

Metabolic Toxicity

HCQ has a favorable effect on blood glucose and lipids. Administration of HCQ leads to a lower risk of diabetes among RA and SLE patients.

DRUG INTERACTIONS

The most significant drug interactions are increases in retinal toxicity when coadministered with tamoxifen. Coadministration with albuterol, amiodarone, amitriptyline, artemether, azithromycin, digoxin is contraindicated or need close monitoring as they can prolong the QT interval.

CONCLUSION

The antimalarial HCQ is an anchor drug in the management of SLE. It is also a particularly useful agent in the management of APS and Sjogrens syndrome. A sound knowledge of its adverse effects will help the clinician detect them early.

LEARNING POINTS

1. Hydroxychloroquine is an antimalarial drug.
2. It is an immunomodulatory agent by virtue of its action at various levels of the innate and adaptive immune system.
3. Important first-line DMARD in treatment of mild and moderately severe RA.
4. HCQ prevents disease flares in SLE, and decreases the risk of infections in SLE.
5. However, long-term use may be associated with ocular toxicity: need to monitor for it.
6. Dose of HCQ needs to be adjusted in CKD.
7. Can cause QT prolongation, therefore avoid co-prescription with other drugs causing QT prolongation.

FURTHER READING

1. Dima A, Jurcut C, Chasset F, et al. Hydroxychloroquine in systemic lupus erythematosus: overview of current knowledge. Ther Adv Musculoskeletal Dis. 2022; 14:1759720X211073001.
2. Nishiyama T, Kondo Y, Tsuboi H, et al. QTc interval prolongation in patients with systemic lupus erythematosus treated with hydroxychloroquine. Mod Rheumatol. 2021;31:1107–12.
3. Schrezenmeier E, Dörner T. Mechanisms of action of hydroxychloroquine and chloroquine: implications for rheumatology. Nat Rev Rheumatol. 2020;16:55–66.
4. Sorour AA, Kurmann RD, Shahin YE, et al. Use of Hydroxy-chloroquine and Risk of Heart Failure in Patients With Rheumatoid Arthritis. J Rheumatol. 2021; 48:1508–11.
5. Tselios K, Gladman DD, Harvey P, et al. Hydroxy-chloroquine-Induced Cardiomyopathy in Systemic Lupus Erythematosus. J Clin Rheumatol. 2016; 22:287–8.
6. Tleyjeh IM, Kashour Z, AlDosary O, et al. Cardiac Toxicity of Chloroquine or Hydroxychloroquine in Patients With COVID-19: A Systematic Review and Meta-regression Analysis. Mayo Clin Proc Innov Qual Outcomes. 2021;5:137–50.

Chapter 4.5

Sulfasalazine

Darshan Singh Bhakuni, Anuj Singhal

INTRODUCTION

Sulfasalazine (SSZ) is an important disease-modifying anti-rheumatic drug (DMARD) in the management of inflammatory rheumatic diseases. It is composed of the antibiotic sulfapyridine that is linked via an azo bond to 5 amino-salicylic acids (5-ASA), an anti-inflammatory agent. It was developed by Professor Svartz at the Karolinska Institutet Sweden in 1938–1939. However, it was not widely used in rheumatology due to the simultaneous development of glucocorticoids. Subsequently, interest in SSZ was rekindled when the anti-inflammatory properties of a closely related drug dapsone were found.

MECHANISM OF ACTION

After an oral dose, >90% of SSZ reaches the large intestine, where bacterial enzymatic action splits the molecule into sulphapyridine and 5-ASA. Sulfapyridine is almost completely absorbed, and is responsible for its immunomodulatory effect in rheumatic diseases, whereas nearly all of the 5-ASA is excreted fecally and is responsible for its anti-inflammatory effect in inflammatory bowel disease (IBD).

The exact mechanism by which SSZ acts as an immunomodulatory agent is not known. Proposed mechanisms are inhibition of the Nuclear Factor Kappa B (NF-κB) pathway, inhibiting TNF alpha by causing caspase 8 induced apoptosis of macrophages, inhibition of osteoclastogenesis, and stimulating the anti-inflammatory activity of adenosine.

The onset of action is slow and it takes more than three months to achieve any significant clinical benefit.

INDICATIONS IN RHEUMATOLOGY

RA: SSZ is an important conventional synthetic DMARD (csDMARD) in the management of RA. Its efficacy is modest and it is used for the treatment of early, mild and most commonly as adjunctive therapy with methotrexate (MTX). The combination of SSZ, MTX and hydroxychloroquine is popularly known as triple therapy. There is good quality evidence that has shown triple therapy is comparable to biological agents in RA.

The advantages of SSZ as a DMARD are that it is affordable and has good long-term tolerance, safe, and has serious side effects that are encountered infrequently. But the disadvantages are its frequent dosing schedule, which may cause patients to miss their dose.

The American College of Rheumatology (ACR) and European Alliance for Rheumatology (EULAR) recommend

- SSZ as an add-on therapy if MTX monotherapy fails to achieve the treatment target of low disease activity after 3–6 months of therapy.
- As a first-line in treatment of RA in DMARD naïve patients where there are contraindications to MTX.

Spondyloarthritis (SpA): It is useful in the management of peripheral arthritis in axial SpA, psoriatic arthritis (PsA), and reactive arthritis (ReA). Other uses include inflammatory bowel disease (IBD) ulcerative colitis and Crohn's disease.

Table 4.5.1: Pharmacology of sulfasalazine

Sulfasalazine	*Pharmacological properties*
Route of administration and absorption	SSZ is orally administered More than 90% reaches the large intestine, wherein the colon bacterial enzymatic action splits the molecule into sulfapyridine and 5-ASA. Sulfapyridine is almost completely absorbed, whereas nearly all of the5-ASA is excreted faecally
Metabolism	Sulfapyridine is primarily metabolized by the liver by N-acetylation with a half-life of 5.5 hours in fast acetylators and 15.3 hours in slow acetylators. However, the difference is not clinically significant and there are no major drug interactions with SSZ
Excretion	Absorbed, intact SSZ is mainly excreted unchanged in the urine with an elimination of 6–11 hours

Juvenile idiopathic arthritis (JIA): SSZ is also indicated in enthesitis-related JIA and in polyarticular JIA. SSZ is not used in children younger than two years of age.

DOSE

The effective dose is 2–3 g/day in divided doses, taken after meals to reduce gastrointestinal (GI) side effects. It is started as 0.5–1 g/day and then titrated to the maximum tolerated dose with an average of 0.5–1 g/day increase every 5–7 days. Even higher doses are used in IBD.

SSZ is also available in enteric-coated tablets to reduce the GI side effects and improve tolerance.

ADVERSE EFFECTS

The common adverse reactions to SSZ are GI-related, namely anorexia, nausea, and headache. Other rare adverse events are anaphylaxis, cyanosis, nephrolithiasis, folate deficiency, agranulocytosis, and hepatic toxicity. Peripheral neuropathy has been reported as a rare adverse drug reaction to SSZ.

It can cause a skin rash. Like other sulfonamides, SSZ can cause a characteristic idiosyncratic liver injury that has features of drug allergy or hypersensitivity. The typical onset is the sudden development of fever and rash followed by jaundice within a few days or weeks of starting the medication, leading to a syndrome of drug rash, eosinophilia and systemic symptoms (DRESS).

It can cause severe hemolytic anemia in those who are deficient in glucose-6-phosphate dehydrogenase (G6PD). There is a very rare but possibly fatal risk of agranulocytosis. SSZ inhibits dihydropteroate synthase and can cause folate deficiency and megaloblastic anemia.

SSZ decreases sperm counts, and sperm motility causing functional azoospermia. The sperm effects are reversible by discontinuing the drug. So male patients must be informed about the risk of oligospermia and temporary infertility.

Pregnancy and lactation: SSZ is safe to use during pregnancy and lactation.

CONTRAINDICATIONS

1. Known history of hypersensitivity to sulfa drugs or salicylates
2. SSZ can trigger acute attacks in porphyria
3. It can induce nephrolithiasis by causing crystalluria; hence, it is avoided in nephrolithiasis, and in obstructive uropathy
4. G6PD deficiency
5. Blood dyscrasias

LEARNING POINTS

1. SSZ has modest efficacy in the treatment of RA. It is often used in combination with HCQ and MTX as triple therapy in the treatment of RA.
2. It is also effective for peripheral arthritis in SpA.
3. It can cause hemolytic anemia in people with G6PD deficiency.
4. It causes oligospermia and infertility that is reversible on discontinuation of the drug.
5. It is safe in pregnancy and lactation, thus it is useful to manage female patients who are planning on pregnancy.

FURTHER READING

1. Donovan S, Hawley S, McCarthy J, et al. Tolerability Of enteric-coated sulfasalazine in rheumatoid arthritis; results of a cooperating clinics study. Br J Rheumatol. 1990;29:201–4.
2. Farr M, Tunn EJ, Symmons DP, et al. Sulphasalazine in rheumatoid arthritis: haematological problems and changes in haematological indices associated with therapy. Br J Rheumatol. 1989;28:134–8.
3. Pullar T, Hunter JA, Capell HA. Sulphasalazine and hepatic transaminases. Ann Rheum Dis. 1987;46:421.
4. Smolen JS, Landewé RBM, Bijlsma JWJ, et al. EULAR recommendations for the management of rheumatoid arthritis with synthetic and biological disease-modifying antirheumatic drugs: 2019 update. Ann Rheum Dis. 2020;79:685–99.
5. Tett SE. Clinical pharmacokinetics of slow-acting antirheumatic drugs. Clin Pharmacokinet 1993; 25:392–407.

Glucocorticoids

Vinod Ravindran

INTRODUCTION

Glucocorticoids (GCs) are being used in the management of not only rheumatoid arthritis but also in many more autoimmune rheumatic diseases for the past several decades. However, therapeutic advances in the management of these conditions and concerns regarding the safety of GCs have led to continuous reappraisal of their relevance. At the same time, effective strategies to deal with the adverse effects of GCs have been developed. Newer GCs molecules hold promise for optimum use of GCs in future.

MECHANISMS OF ACTION

GCs produce their anti-inflammatory effects by their action on the glucocorticoid receptor (GCR) and block various inflammatory signaling. They inhibit inflammation by three mechanisms: direct genomic, indirect genomic, and non-genomic mechanisms. These mechanisms are activated depending on the dose of GC employed (Table 4.6.1). Genomic action is via action on the cytosolic GCR that translocates to the nucleus, binding with transcription factors that lead to induction or repression of transcription of genes involved in inflammation. This is called transactivation and transrepression, respectively. Most of the anti-inflammatory beneficial effects of GCs is due to transrepression, while transactivation is generally responsible for the unwanted (particularly metabolic) adverse effects.

DEFINITION OF DOSES

Based on the recognition of different mechanisms of action and resulting clinically recognisable differences, the dose of GCs can be classified as 'low', 'medium' and 'high' doses of GC (Table 4.6.2).

Doses <7.5 mg of prednisone-equivalent are low dose; between 7.5 and 30 mg prednisone-equivalent are medium dose; >30 mg and up to 100 mg prednisone-equivalent per day are high dose; very high doses >100 mg prednisone-equivalent per day. When the dose is >250 mg of prednisone-equivalent per day, usually for no more than 5 days, it is called as pulse therapy (Table 4.6.2). Pulse therapy is typically used when a rapid onset of action is desired such as induction therapy in lupus nephritis or severe vasculitis which may be offset by accompanying adverse events (Tables 4.6.1 and 4.6.2).

Table 4.6.1: Key differences between genomic and nongenomic actions of glucocorticoids

Characteristics	*Mechanism*	
	Genomic	*Nongenomic*
Glucocorticoid dose	Low	High
Onset of action	Hours to days	Minutes
Efficacy	Moderate	High
Adverse effects	Low	High

Table 4.6.2: Glucocorticoid utilization in rheumatic diseases	
Routes	*Strategies*
Oral	Short-term, high dose Medium-term, low to moderate dose Long-term, low dose
Intramuscular	At initiation and for flares
Intravenous	Pulse therapy
Intra-articular	Single or more affected joints, refractory joint
Intra-lesional	Epicondylitis, bursitis, tendinosis etc.

A GC dose of ≤7.5 mg prednisolone equivalent is considered a low dose GC because this dose occupies less than 50% of the GC receptors. Low-dose GC is the most commonly employed dose for the maintenance therapy of many immuno-inflammatory rheumatic diseases. Relatively fewer adverse effects are expected with low-dose GCs. In chronic inflammatory conditions such as rheumatoid arthritis a relative hypocortisolism is often present, thus low-dose GC treatment is considered a means of replacement therapy for reduced adrenal production. Therefore most authors now regard ≤7.5 mg prednisolone/day to be near the physiologic range.

TYPES AND POTENCY

There are various types of GCs preparations (Table 4.6.3), that differ from one another in terms of relative mineralocorticoid and glucocorticoid potency. While selecting a GC preparation based on the clinical indication, it is usual to refer to their mineralocorticoid and glucocorticoid potency. So equivalent GC doses are usually calculated using prednisone as the comparator (Table 4.6.3).

Table 4.6.3: Potency comparison of selected therapeutic glucocorticoids		
Agent	*GC Potency*	*MC Potency*
Hydrocortisone	1	0.002
Deflazacort	4	No data
Prednisolone	4	0.002
Methylprednisolone	5	0.0013
Betamethasone	25	0
Dexamethaosne	25	0

GC: Glucocorticoid; *MC:* mineralocorticoid

GLUCOCORTICOID USE IN RHEUMATOLOGICAL CONDITIONS

In rheumatology GCs are utilized in several different ways and by various routes (Table 4.6.2).

Rheumatoid arthritis (RA): Scenarios of GC use in RA presented in Box 4.6.1 is representative of its wide scope. Its use as a "bridge" therapy (typical starting dose 10 mg/day with planned tapering) not only allows rapid reduction in the inflammatory burden but also gives the conventional synthetic disease modifying antirheumatic drugs (csDMARDs) such as methotrexate the time (typically takes 6–10 weeks) to be effective.

Systemic lupus erythematosus (SLE): GCs are indicated in the treatment of SLE both for induction and maintenance of remission. Concomitant use of antimalarials and another immunosuppressive agents is vital to maintain remission. The goal is to keep daily doses of prednisone <7.5 mg/day, or even to withdraw it in some patients. In patients with severe lupus disease activity a higher dose of GC (prednisolone 1 mg/kg/day) is being used, though recent evidence suggests that significantly lower doses (prednisolone 0.5 mg/kg/day) might be equally effective and have less adverse effects. With regard to pulse methylprednisolone, recent evidence underscores similar efficacy of 500 mg/

Box 4.6.1: Indications for the possible use of glucocorticoids in rheumatoid arthritis (RA)

- Bridge therapy for patients who have experienced a severe functional decline with limitations interfering with necessary daily living or vocational activities
- Patients who have moderate-to-severe disease activity when NSAID is contraindicated and DMARDS are taking time to act
- Rheumatoid vasculitis or other serious life-threatening or organ damaging conditions
- Men or women not at reduced risk of bone loss, for whom GCs may be reasonable in combination therapy regimens with a single daily dose of less than 7.5 mg/day
- Pregnant or lactating women with active RA

day during three consecutive days vs. 1000 mg/day for three to five consecutive days in treating severe lupus flares including nephritis. Upfront usage of biologic DMARDs potentially could reduce GC accrued damage in many rheumatologic diseases including SLE.

ADVERSE EFFECTS

Table 4.6.4 lists some of the important adverse effects of GCs. A special mention has to be made of GC-induced osteoporosis (GIOP). Long-term GC use even in moderate doses is associated with reduced bone mineral density, particularly loss of trabecular bone, and increased fracture risk at the hip and spine. The main mechanism of GIOP is osteocyte and osteoblast apoptosis, which occurs very early as soon as GCs are initiated. The risk of fracture risk increases soon after GCs are commenced; the good news is that fracture risk returns to baseline risk when GCs treatment is stopped and this is independent of effects on bone mineral density. Other contributing factors are disturbed calcium homeostasis and osteoclast dysfunction.

GENERAL PRINCIPLES OF USE IN RHEUMATIC DISEASES

The patient must be informed of the adverse effects of GC therapy that should be discussed at the start of therapy. Relevant information such as weight gain, hyperglycemia, hypertension, risk for infections, fracture risk, etc. can be discussed. A recommendation by the EULAR on the management of systemic GC therapy in rheumatic diseases is presented in Box 4.6.2.

Use in Special Situations (Perioperative Period, Pregnancy, and Children)

In the perioperative period those patients on long-term low dose GC therapy need to continue their usual dose. For minor surgery, those on medium-dose GC can receive intravenous (IV) hydrocortisone 25–100 mg on the day of surgery; for major surgery 100 mg eight hourly on the day of surgery, and the dose can be tapered off to the usual GC dose on the next day. In situations where a patient is on high dose GC, IV hydrocortisone 100 eight hourly can continue till the usual oral dose can be resumed.

Table 4.6.4: Toxicity of glucocorticoids

Organ system	*Dose*		
	Probably with high dose only	*High or low dose*	
		Probably	*Definitely*
General	Infections		Weight gain Redistribution of body fat Facial edema Withdrawal symptoms
Musculoskeletal	Osteonecrosis	Osteoporosis	
Gastrointestinal	Pancreatitis Bowel rupture	Peptic ulcer	
Cardiovascular	Hypertension Dyslipidemia Atherosclerosis		
Reproductive	Fetal wastage		
Neurological	Psychosis		
Cutaneous	Delayed wound healing		Purpura Skin atrophy Acne Easy bruising
Eye			Glaucoma Cataract
Endocrine		HPA dysfunction	Diabetes

Box 4.6.2: General principles on the use of glucocorticoid (GC) in rheumatic diseases as per EULAR recommendations

- Initial dose, dose reduction and long-term dosing depend on the underlying rheumatic disease, disease activity, risk factors and individual responsiveness of the patient.
- When it is decided to start GC treatment, comorbidities and risk factors for adverse effects should be evaluated and treated where indicated; these include hypertension, diabetes, peptic ulcer, recent fractures, presence of cataract or glaucoma, presence of (chronic) infections, dyslipidemia and comedication with non-steroidal anti-inflammatory drugs (NSAIDs).
- For prolonged treatment, the GC dosage should be kept to a minimum, and a GC taper should be attempted in case of remission or low disease activity; the reasons to continue GC therapy should be regularly checked.
- During treatment, patients should be monitored for body weight, blood pressure, peripheral edema, cardiac insufficiency, serum lipids, blood and/or urine glucose and ocular pressure depending on the individual patient's risk, GC dose and duration.
- If a patient is started on prednisone >7.5 mg daily and continues on prednisone for more than 3 months, calcium and vitamin D supplementation should be prescribed.
- Antiresorptive therapy with bisphosphonates to reduce the risk of GC-induced osteoporosis (GIOP) should be based on risk factors, including bone-mineral density measurement.
- Patients treated with GCs and concomitant NSAIDs should be given appropriate gastro-protective medication, such as proton pump inhibitors or misoprostol, or alternatively could switch to a cyclo-oxygenase-2 selective inhibitor.

For those patients who have recently been on GC and are scheduled to undergo surgery, it is presumed that some amount of suppression of the hypothalamic–pituitary axis, so adequate stress dose GC replacement in the perioperative management is needed to avoid potential adrenal insufficiency.

GCs are safe during pregnancy both for mother and child. Children receiving GCs are prone to linear growth impairment, so height should be checked regularly and considered for growth-hormone replacement if necessary.

CONCLUSION

GCs remain an important treatment option in many conditions in rheumatology, and a new understanding of disease-specific and dose-specific effects has resulted in a renewed efforts to make full use of their potential.

LEARNING POINTS

1. Glucocorticoids (GCs) are important therapeutic options in several rheumatic diseases.
2. Although no dose of GC is without adverse effects, low dose and high dose GC have different mechanisms of action, therapeutic effects and adverse effects.
3. A better understanding of GC mechanism of actions (genomic and nongenomic) helps in understanding issues with GC adverse effects observed at a particular dose.
4. A disease-modifying effect of GC therapy in RA has become established.
5. Several newer GCs molecules have the potential to enhance the current role of GCs by selective augmentation of the beneficial effects.
6. Adherence to relevant guidelines such as for GC induced osteoporosis is mandatory in minimizing the GC adverse effects.

FURTHER READING

1. Dua A, Das P, Ravindran V. Glucocorticoids: A review of its adverse effects including bone loss. Indian J Rheumatol 2019;14:S90–8.
2. Hoes JN, Jacobs JWG, Boers M, et al. EULAR evidence-based recommendations on the management of systemic glucocorticoid therapy in rheumatic diseases. Ann Rheum Dis. 2007;66:1560–7.
3. Mithun MC, Gonzalez-Perez O, Ramos-Remus C, Ravindran V. Deflazacort in rheumatology: Where does it stand? Indian J Rheumatol. 2014;9;161–2.
4. Pandey A, Ravindran V. Glucocorticoids in rheumatology. 1st Edition. Mumbai: National Book Depot; 2022.
5. Ravindran V. Glucocorticoid therapy in rheumatic diseases: What's latest? In: Narsimulu G, editor. Progress in Medicine. Indian College of Physicians; 2019. pp 401–3.
6. Ravindran V. Newer glucocorticoids: Overcoming mechanistic hurdles. Indian J Rheumatol. 2012;7:221–5.

Chapter 4.7

Azathioprine and Cyclophosphamide

Abhilasha Manwatkar, John Mathew

AZATHIOPRINE

Introduction

The effect of 6-mercaptopurine (6-MP) on the primary and secondary immune response was identified by Robert Schwartz in 1958. Azathioprine (AZA), a prodrug of 6-MP was found to be better tolerated than 6-MP and since then it has been used in various autoimmune disorders.

Mechanism of Action

AZA's main mechanism of action is inhibition of leukocyte proliferation by affecting the purine synthesis pathway. In the body it is first converted to 6-MP, then by enzymatic action of thiopurine methyltransferase (TPMT) it is converted to its primary active metabolite 6-thioguanine, which inhibits purine metabolism (adenine and guanine) by inhibiting inosine monophosphate. Inhibition of purine synthesis leads to decreased DNA, RNA, and protein synthesis. This reduces B lymphocytes, T lymphocytes (mainly CD8 +T cells), IgM, IgG, and interleukin-2 syntheses.

Pharmacokinetics

AZA is well absorbed from the gastrointestinal tract, in the plasma it is 30% protein bound. It is metabolised to 6-MP, which is further metabolized either into 6-thiouric acid by xanthine oxidase or to 6-methyl mercaptopurine (6-MMP) by TPMT. It gets converted into active form 6 thioguanosine monophosphate by multiple steps. The site of metabolism is liver and kidney. The main route of excretion is the kidney (20–50%). Its serum t½ is 0.2–0.5 hours and biologic t½ of 24 hours.

Indications in Autoimmune Rheumatic Diseases

- **Systemic lupus erythematosus (SLE):** AZA is used in cutaneous manifestations, arthritis, and as maintenance treatment for major organ involvement including lupus nephritis, neuropsychiatric lupus, pneumonitis, myocarditis, and vasculitis. For maintenance therapy for lupus nephritis AZA is as effective as mycophenolate mofetil.
- **ANCA-associated vasculitis:** It is as effective as oral cyclophosphamide for maintenance therapy and to prevent relapse. It is equivalent to methotrexate in terms of effectiveness and adverse effects.
- **Idiopathic inflammatory myositis**, for long-term management of myositis.
- **Systemic sclerosis:** It is an option for long-term management of interstitial lung disease, skin disease and myositis
- Autoimmune hemolytic anemia
- Immune-mediated thrombocytopenia
- Autoimmune hepatitis
- Behçet's syndrome and its various manifestations.
- Sarcoidosis with joint, lung, myocardium, or other major organ involvement
- Rheumatoid arthritis: It is less effective than methotrexate. It is one of the treatment options for RA in pregnancy
- Psoriatic arthritis

Adverse Effects

The most common side effects are gastrointestinal intolerance (21%) such as nausea, vomiting, diarrhea and cholestasis. Rarely it causes pancreatitis and stomatitis. Infection increases in a setting of leukopenia caused by AZA, including herpes zoster. It can cause dose-related bone marrow suppression. Thus the blood counts must be monitored especially while escalating the dose (Table 4.7.1). Cytopenia can be due to genotype and phenotype variants of TMPT and nucleoside diphosphate-linked moiety X-linked motif (NUDT15). Routine testing of TPMT before starting AZA is not required.

Important drug interactions: Allopurinol inhibits xanthine oxidase and can increase AZA toxicity. Therefore when coprescribing with allopurinol it is advisable to decrease the dose of AZA. AZA reduces warfarin action.

Pregnancy and lactation: AZA is safe during pregnancy. It is compatible with breastfeeding since excretion in breast milk is very low.

CYCLOPHOSPHAMIDE

Introduction

Cyclophosphamide (CYC) is an immunosuppressive agent used in different types of solid cancers, hematological malignancies, renal transplantation and various autoimmune diseases. It was first made from nitrogen mustard such that after a structural change it affects only cancer cells (target cell).

Mechanism of Action

It is an alkylating agent. It inhibits DNA replication by incorporating itself in DNA strands and causes crosslinking of DNA. CYC inhibits both active and resting lymphocytes.

Table 4.7.1: Dosing of azathioprine and monitoring

Azathioprine dosing	*Monitoring*
Usual dose: 1–2 mg/kg/day	Complete blood counts: 2 weekly during escalation, 6 weekly when on stable dose
Maximum dose: 3 mg/kg/day	
Starting dose: 25–50 mg/day	
Weekly/fortnightly dose escalation	

Pharmacokinetics

Oral CYC is well-absorbed and the leading site of metabolism is the liver by cytochrome 450 system. Serum elimination half-life is 2–8 hours. It is eliminated mainly by the kidneys. In autoimmune rheumatic diseases it is used as daily oral dose of 2–3 mg/kg/day, as pulse (intermittent high dose) intravenous dose 10–15 mg/kg, and less commonly as oral pulse 10–15 mg/kg.

Indications in Autoimmune Rheumatic Diseases

- In SLE it is used in proliferative and membranous lupus nephritis (Table 4.7.2). The Euro–Lupus Nephritis Protocol showed less toxicity by way of less cumulative dose and the same relapse rate as NIH protocol. It is also used in neuropsychiatric lupus, lupus with secondary vasculitis, lupus pneumonitis, myocarditis, and enteropathy.
- ANCA-associated vasculitis (AAV): It is an important agent for induction of remission of AAV. Pulse CYC is particularly useful in generalised AAV, and severe organ threatening diseases such as renal involvement with high serum creatinine, diffuse alveolar hemorrhage, and myocarditis, etc.

  [The readers are referred to Chapter 9.6 for a description of the EUVAS protocol of IV CYC in AAV (granulomatosis with polyangitis)].
- Polyarteritis nodosa
- Beçhet syndrome
- Secondary vasculitis due to RA or other connective tissue diseases
- Cryoglobulinemic vasculitis
- Interstitial lung disease related to connective tissue disease viz scleroderma, idiopathic inflammatory myositis, rheumatoid arthritis, mixed connective tissue disease and Sjören's syndrome.

Adverse Effects

Bone marrow suppression is the most common adverse effect, which mainly starts with neutropenia. Irrespective of the dose used, rapid recovery occurs in 2–3 weeks. Nausea and vomiting are more common after CYC infusion which can be decreased using 5-hydroxytryptamine receptor antagonist (ondansetron) or dexamethasone. It can also cause reversible transient alopecia. Rare adverse effects include hyponatremia due to the syndrome of inappropriate antidiuretic hormone

Table 4.7.2: Cyclophosphamide (CYC) dosing in SLE and monitoring

Oral cyclophosphamide	*National Institutes of Health (NIH) Protocol*	*Euro–Lupus Nephritis Trial Protocol*
1–2.5 mg/kg/day (Needs reduction in renal dysfunction)	Seven monthly infusions of 500–750 mg/m^2 of body surface area followed by 18 months of quarterly infusions	Six fortnightly IV CYC pulses at a fixed dose of 500 mg
CBC fortnightly and later monthly when on stable dose Creatinine, electrolytes, LFT monthly	CBC, LFT and creatinine before each infusion	CBC, LFT and creatinine before each infusion

CBC: Complete blood counts; *LFT:* Liver function tests; *IV:* Intravenous

secretion (SIADH), central pontine myelinolysis, cardiotoxicity and hemorrhagic cystitis.

Some centers use Mesna (2-mercaptoethane sodium sulfonate) to prevent cystitis when intermittent dosing is used. Since the CYC dose is lower compared to use in malignancy, many centers do not use it.

Baseline investigations before the start of CYC therapy are complete blood count (CBC), liver function tests (LFT), serum creatinine, urinalysis, serologic testing for hepatitis B and C virus infection and chest radiograph.

Gonadal failure is one of the biggest concerns with the use of CYC. Patient age and cumulative dose are significant determinants. Amenorrhea is more common in women older than 30 years (50%) than younger women (12%). The risk of ovarian failure is less in short course CYC even when used in higher doses. It can cause azoospermia in males. Cryopreservation of ejaculated semen in men and embryos or oocytes in women can be offered prior to treatment when possible. In women gonadotropin-releasing hormone (GnRH) analog, leuprolide can be given 2 weeks prior to CYC infusion to suppress the ovaries in order to preserve fertility.

Pregnancy and lactation: CYC is teratogenic and is contraindicated in pregnancy and lactation.

LEARNING POINTS

1. Azathioprine and cyclophosphamide have made a major contribution in improving the morbidity and mortality of various autoimmune rheumatic diseases over the past 40 years.
2. They are medications with a narrow therapeutic window and needs precise dosing and monitoring for toxicity.
3. We need medications with better toxicity profile and better response, also medications for specific situations like during pregnancy and lactation.
4. Azathioprine can be used during pregnancy and lactation.
5. Lower dose of cyclophosphamide use, as in Euro–Lupus Nephritis Trial Protocol can achieve the same response rates than higher dose with fewer side effects.

FURTHER READING

1. Austin HA 3rd, Klippel JH, Balow JE, et al. Therapy of lupus nephritis. Controlled trial of prednisone and cytotoxic drugs. N Engl J Med. 1986;314:614–9.
2. Chung SA, Langford CA, Maz M, et al. American College of Rheumatology/Vasculitis Foundation Guideline for the Management of Antineutrophil Cytoplasmic Antibody-Associated Vasculitis. Arthritis Rheumatol. 2021;73:1366–83.
3. de Groot K, Harper L, Jayne DR, et al. EUVAS (European Vasculitis Study Group). Pulse versus daily oral cyclophosphamide for induction of remission in antineutrophil cytoplasmic antibody-associated vasculitis: a randomized trial. Ann Intern Med. 2009;150:670–80.
4. Elion GB. The purine path to chemotherapy. Science. 1989;244:41–7.
5. Fanouriakis A, Kostopoulou M, Cheema K, et al. 2019 Update of the Joint European League Against Rheumatism and European Renal Association-European Dialysis and Transplant Association (EULAR/ERA-EDTA) recommendations for the management of lupus nephritis. Ann Rheum Dis. 2020;79:713–23.
6. Houssiau FA, Vasconcelos C, D'Cruz D, et al. The 10-year follow-up data of the Euro-Lupus Nephritis Trial comparing low-dose and high-dose intravenous cyclophosphamide. Ann Rheum Dis. 2010;69:61–4.

Mycophenolate Mofetil

Molly Mary Thabah, Abhishek Rai, Paul T Antony

INTRODUCTION

Mycophenolic acid was isolated from the mold *Penicillium brevicompactum* in the late 19th century and used as an antibiotic. Later in 1986, its immunosuppressive properties were discovered. Mycophenolic acid (MPA) is available in two forms as mycophenolic sodium salt and as mycophenolate mofetil (MMF) a morpholinoethyl ester of MPA (Table 4.8.1).

MECHANISM OF ACTION

The mechanism of immunosuppressive action of MPA and MMF is by a potent non-competitive and reversible inhibition of inosine monophosphate dehydrogenase isoform 2, an enzyme critical in *de novo* purine synthesis. Lymphocytes mainly depend on the *de novo* guanosine nucleotide synthesis for DNA synthesis and cell division while the salvage pathway is primarily used by other cell types. Thus, MPA has selective inhibitory action on activated T and B lymphocytes without causing major myelosuppression.

MPA decreases the synthesis of guanine nucleotides, hinders DNA synthesis and consequently reduces lymphocyte proliferation, antibody production and even microRNA (miR) expression. The effect of MPA on miR expression is attributed to histone modifications in CD4+ T cells. In CD4+ T cells from patients with SLE, this effect can result in a downregulation of CD40 ligand (CD40L). CD40L-mediated co-stimulation of antigen-presenting cells has a crucial role in various rheumatic diseases.

INDICATIONS IN RHEUMATIC DISEASES

The clinical indications of MMF cover a wide range of autoimmune and inflammatory rheumatic diseases (Table 4.8.2). The efficacy of MMF in systemic lupus erythematosus (SLE), scleroderma, anti-neutrophil cytoplasmic antibodies (ANCA) associated vasculitis is established.

Table 4.8.1: Pharmacokinetics properties of mycophenolic acid and mycophenolate mofetil

Absorption and bioavailability	MMF is available in both oral and intravenous formulation. It has good oral bioavailability, though absorption is delayed with food intake. As a result, MMF is best administered on an empty stomach, one hour before meals or two hours post meals
Plasma levels and protein binding	It undergoes extensive presystemic de-esterification in the liver to MPA, the active moiety which reaches its maximum plasma concentration within one hour. MPA is 98% protein bound. MPA undergoes enterohepatic circulation, resulting in a secondary peak in its plasma concentration at 6–12 hours after intravenous or oral dosing
Half-life and elimination	The mean half-life of MPA in the systemic circulation is ~17 hours, and is metabolized mainly in the liver to inactive glucuronide metabolites. More than 95% of an administered MMF dose is eliminated through the kidney

Table 4.8.2: Clinical indications of mycophenolate mofetil (MMF) in adults with autoimmune inflammatory rheumatic diseases
Systemic lupus erythematosus Class III, class IV, and class V lupus nephritis Neuropsychiatric lupus Refractory cutaneous lupus such as lupus panniculitis or discoid lupus
Vasculitis ANCA-associated vasculitis Takayasu arteritis Giant cell arteritis IgA vasculitis
Systemic sclerosis-related interstitial lung disease **Systemic sclerosis** with rapidly progressive diffuse skin involvement
Inflammatory myositis Dermatomyositis, polymyositis, antisynthetase syndrome, clinically amyopathic dermatomyositis, MDA-5 associated dermatomyositis.
Others: In patients with gout who receive pegloticase, coadministration of MMF results in reduced pegloticase immunogenicity

Systemic Lupus Erythematosus

Lupus nephritis: MMF is an established agent useful for induction and maintenance of remission in proliferative and membranous lupus nephritis. In a landmark study by Contreras et al. (Table 4.8.3) patients with proliferative lupus nephritis received induction with intravenous (IV) cyclophosphamide (CYC), then randomized to one of three arms: quarterly IV CYC, MMF, and azathioprine (AZA). Patients on MMF had a better 72-months event-free survival, lower renal relapse, marked reduction of adverse effects, hospitalization days, amenorrhea, and infections.

The Aspreva Lupus Management Study (ALMS) evaluated the role of MMF vs IV CYC as both induction and maintenance of remission in lupus nephritis. There was no difference between IV CYC and MMF in the urine protein/creatinine ratio and stabilization/improvement in creatinine at 24 weeks. Patients who had achieved remission after induction were randomized to either MMF or AZA. MMF was non-inferior to AZA in maintaining renal response and preventing relapse. However, in the

Table 4.8.3: Important clinical trial of mycophenolate mofetil in systemic lupus erythematosus

Trial	*Study population*	*Intervention*	*Primary endpoint*	*Results*
Contreras et al. (2004)	WHO Class III and IV lupus nephritis ($n = 59$) predominantly Black and Hispanic females	Induction with monthly boluses of IV CYC (0.5–1 g/m^2) for 7 months and glucocorticoid. Maintenance either IV CYC (0.5–1.0 g/m^2 every 3 months) or oral AZA (1–3 mg/kg daily) or oral MMF (500– 3000 mg daily), all with oral prednisone (up to 0.5 mg/kg/day)	Patient and renal survival	Higher survival in AZA vs IV CYC, similar survival in the MMF vs IV CYC Better composite endpoint of death or chronic renal failure in both the AZA and MMF groups vs IV CYC group at 72 months
The Aspreva Lupus Management Study (ALMS), 2009	ISN/RPS Class III -V lupus nephritis ($n = 370$) predominantly non-Caucasian patients	Induction with MMF (target dosage 3 g/d) vs IV CYC (0.5–1.0 g/m^2 in monthly pulses) for 6 months. Tapering dose of prednisone Maintenance MMF vs AZA	Renal response at 6 months (24 weeks)	No difference in urine PCR and serum creatinine at 24 weeks. Complete renal remission, systemic disease activity and damage, and safety was also similar suggesting equivalency of MMF to IVC In maintenance MMF was not inferior to AZA

(Contd.)

Table 4.8.3: Important clinical trial of mycophenolate mofetil in systemic lupus erythematosus (*Contd.*)

Trial	*Study population*	*Intervention*	*Primary endpoint*	*Results*
MAINTAIN nephritis trial, 2011	Lupus nephritis WHO class III, IV, Vc, or Vd	Induction with IV CYC + methyl-prednisolone Maintenance with AZA (target dose 2 mg/kg/day) or MMF (target dose 2 g/day). Mean follow-up 48 months	Time to treatment failure (death, end stage renal disease, doubling of creatinine, renal flare)	AZA was superior to MMF in maintaining remission and in preventing flares

IV CYC: Intravenous cyclophosphamide; *AZA:* Azathioprine; *MMF:* Mycophenolate mofetil; *ISN/RPS:* International Society of Nephrology/Renal Pathological Society

MAINTAIN trial, AZA was superior to MMF for maintenance.

Thus the clinical uses of MMF in SLE are:

- As a remission induction agent in proliferative and membranous lupus nephritis. The decision to choose MMF over IV CYC induction depends on affordability, ovarian preservation, and severity of disease, etc. However, in more severe cases of lupus nephritis for example presence of high serum creatinine, crescents in the renal biopsy, poor GFR, IV CYC is the preferred induction agent.
- Either AZA or MMF for maintenance of remission the latter is preferred if MMF is used for induction.
- It is also used in patients with severe discoid cutaneous lupus, and panniculitis.

Systemic Sclerosis (SSc)

The role of MMF for the stabilization of lung functions in SSc-related interstitial lung disease (ILD) has been proven by the scleroderma-related interstitial lung disease (SLS II) study (Table 4.8.4). MMF for two years led to comparable improvements in the % forced vital capacity and dyspnea compared to one year of oral CYC, with a better safety profile. Thus, MMF is a good agent for the management of SSc-related progressive ILD.

Idiopathic Inflammatory Myositis

Data showing the clinical efficacy of MMF is only from case series.

- One case series reported on the effectiveness of MMF for cutaneous lesions of dermatomyositis that were recalcitrant to other therapies.
- There are also large case series documenting that MMF is as effective as AZA in myositis-related interstitial lung disease (ILD).
- There are also case reports of the usage of a combination of MMF with other therapies in rapidly progressive ILD of myositis.
- In clinical practice MMF is employed as a second-line agent in the treatment of dermatomyositis, polymyositis, anti-synthetase syndrome, and MDA-5 associated myositis specifically for those patients who are refractory to methotrexate, AZA, and CYC.

ANCA-Associated Vasculitis (AAV): Role of MMF

MMF has been tried for induction and maintenance of remission of AAV.

Induction of remission: A study by Han et al. compared oral MMF versus IV CYC combined with corticosteroids for remission induction of microscopic polyangiitis in Chinese patients. It was found that MMF is effective for inducing remission in microscopic polyangiitis and may represent an alternative therapy to monthly IV pulses of IVC. The MYCYC (2019) trial found that MMF was non-inferior to CYC for remission induction in nonlife-threatening AAV, but there were more relapses in the MMF group when compared to those receiving maintenance with IV CYC, especially in the PR3 positive patients (Table 4.8.4).

Maintenance of remission: To maintain remission AZA is a better agent as compared to MMF. The International Mycophenolate Mofetil Protocol to Reduce Outbreaks of Vasculitides (IMPROVE) trial showed that after induction

Table 4.8.4: Important clinical trials that studied mycophenolate mofetil (MMF) in systemic sclerosis and ANCA-associated vasculitis

Trial	Study population	Intervention	Primary endpoint	Study outcome
Systemic sclerosis-related interstitial lung disease (SSc-ILD)				
Scleroderma Lung Study (SLS II) 2016	SSc-ILD patients (n = 126) meeting defined dyspnea, pulmonary function and HRCT criteria	MMF (dose 1.5 g BD) for 24 months vs oral CYC (dose 2 mg/kg/day) for 12 months then placebo for 12 months	Improvement in adjusted FVC % (baseline to at 24 months)	Both MMF and CYC-treated patients achieved some improvements in FVC, but was not significantly different in MMF compared to CYC
ANCA-associated vasculitis (AAV)				
IMPROVE trial (2010)	Newly diagnosed granulomatosus with polyangiitis (GPA), microscopic polyangiitis (MPA) (n = 156)	Induction with CYC PO/IV and glucocorticoid ± plasma exchange. Maintenance MMF 2 g/day, reduced to 1.5 g/day after 12 months, 1 g/day after 18 months, and discontinued after 42 months vs AZA 2 mg/kg/day, reduced to 1.5 mg/kg after 12 months, 1 mg/kg after 18 months, and discontinued after 42 months. Prednisolone until month 24 in both arms.	Relapse–free survival	Relapses were more common in the MMF group compared to AZA group Thus, MMF was less effective than AZA for maintaining remission in AAV
MYCYC trial (2019)	Newly diagnosed non-life threatening AAV (n = 140)	Induction with MMF 2–3 g/day vs IV CYC 15 mg/kg, given 2 weeks apart, followed by pulses at 3-week intervals until remission, and then every 3 months. Prednisone 1 mg/kg/day tapered to 5 mg by 6 months in both the groups	Remission by 6 months	MMF was not inferior to IV CYC in remission induction but relapses were higher in MMF. Relapses were particularly higher in patients who were PR3 positive

IV CYC: Intravenous cyclophosphamide; *AZA:* Azathioprine; *MMF:* Mycophenolate mofetil

with glucocorticoids and IV CYC, maintenance therapy with MMF led to more frequent relapses when compared to AZA.

Therefore,

- MMF is an alternative induction and maintenance agent in AAV in cases of intolerance to IV CYC, or cases with high cumulative dose of CYC, in cases with insufficient response to standard agents including rituximab
- The 2016 EULAR recommendations for the management of AAV state that MMF could be used as remission induction of non-organ threatening vasculitis and as an agent to maintain remission.

Other Indications

MMF is useful in the management of Takayasu's arteritis, giant cell arteritis, and IgA vasculitis. It might be useful in gout. It has been shown to prevent formation of anti-polyethylene glycol (PEG) antibodies which hinder treatment with pegylated uricase in gout.

DOSAGE, CONTRAINDICATIONS AND ADVERSE EFFECTS

Clinicians need to be aware of the adverse events related to MMF, the most common of which is gastrointestinal symptoms (Table 4.8.5).

Table 4.8.5: Dosage of mycophenolate, adverse effects, and contraindications

Dosage, duration of treatment	*Adverse effects*	*Contraindications*
In lupus nephritis **Induction of remission** The dose of MMF is based on the ALMS trial. The starting dose is 500 mg twice a day for one week, followed by 1 g twice daily in the second week, to a target dosage of 1.5 g twice daily in the third week. The maximum induction dose is 2–3 g per day **For maintenance of remission** the dose is 1 to 2 g per day **Timing with food** Best taken one hour before food or two hours after a meal Absorption also decreases with co administration of antacids and cholestyramine. In ANCA-associated vasculitis, SSc-related ILD, inflammatory myositis the duration of treatment is typically 2 years or more. Dose is typically similar as in lupus nephritis	Most patients do not tolerate 3 g per day because of gastrointestinal (GI) adverse effects. Most will tolerate only 2–2.5 g in a day. The common GI adverse events are nausea, abdominal pain, and diarrhea. Persistent diarrhea is one reason that patients discontinue MMF or take lower doses. Increasing the frequency of dosing often helps reduce the GI symptoms. Substituting MMF with enteric-coated formulation also helps. Cytopenia can also occur; therefore, blood counts should be monitored every 6–8 weeks	*Pregnancy* is a contraindication to MMF therapy. Caution should be exercised when prescribing to women as it is teratogenic. MMF must be discontinued a minimum of 6 weeks before planning pregnancy *Lactation* is a contraindication *Active infections* are a contraindication
Dosing in special situations		
Dose modification is rarely required in hepatic and mild renal disease however with creatinine clearance of <30 ml/min, concentration of glucuronide metabolite may contribute to gastrointestinal (GI) side effects.		
Renal insufficiency	Avoid >1 g twice daily if GFR <25 mL/min.	
Liver function abnormalities	No recommendations available. In general, no dose adjustment required	
Pancytopenia	If the absolute neutrophil count <1300/mm^3 the dose should be interrupted or dose reduction is advised.	

LEARNING POINTS

1. MMF is a drug with good oral bioavailability, with gastrointestinal symptoms being the most common reason why full dose cannot be given in most patients.
2. Caution must be exercised when prescribing in women of reproductive age group as its safety in pregnancy is not yet known, so women must be advised to discontinue the drug at least six weeks before planning a pregnancy.
3. Its clinical efficacy is established in lupus nephritis both for induction and maintenance of remission.
4. It stabilizes lung function in SSc-ILD.
5. In AAV it can be used as an induction regimen in non-life-threatening disease. For maintenance of remission AZA is a better agent to prevent relapse as compared to MMF.
6. Randomized clinical trials are needed to study its efficacy in inflammatory myositis, myositis related ILD, and large vessel vasculitis.

FURTHER READING

1. Bullingham RE, Nicholls AJ, Kamm BR. Clinical pharmacokinetics of mycophenolate mofetil. Clin Pharmacokinet. 1998;34:429–55.
2. Contreras G, Pardo V, Leclercq B, et al. Sequential therapies for proliferative lupus nephritis. N Engl J Med. 2004;350:971–80.
3. Hiemstra TF, Walsh M, Mahr A, et al.; European Vasculitis Study Group (EUVAS). Mycophenolate mofetil vs azathioprine for remission maintenance in antineutrophil cytoplasmic antibody-associated vasculitis: a randomized controlled trial. JAMA. 2010;304:2381–8.
4. Jones RB, Hiemstra TF, Ballarin J, et al.; European Vasculitis Study Group (EUVAS). Mycophenolate mofetil versus cyclophosphamide for remission induction in ANCA-associated vasculitis: a randomised, non-inferiority trial. Ann Rheum Dis. 2019;78:399–405.
5. Tamirou F, D'Cruz D, Sangle S, et al.; MAINTAIN Nephritis Trial Group. Long-term follow-up of the MAINTAIN Nephritis Trial, comparing azathioprine and mycophenolate mofetil as maintenance therapy of lupus nephritis. Ann Rheum Dis. 2016;75: 526–31.
6. Tashkin DP, Roth MD, Clements PJ, et al. Sclerodema Lung Study II Investigators. Mycophenolate mofetil versus oral cyclophosphamide in scleroderma-related interstitial lung disease (SLS II): a randomised controlled, double-blind, parallel group trial. Lancet Respir Med. 2016;4:708–19.

Apremilast and Iguratimod

Phani Kumar Devarasetti, Challa Madhuri

INTRODUCTION

Apremilast and iguratimod are new oral small molecules for the treatment of inflammatory rheumatic diseases. Apremilast has proven efficacy in psoriatic arthritis, whereas Iguratimod has a role in rheumatoid arthritis.

APREMILAST

Apremilast is an oral phosphodiesterase-4 (PDE4) inhibitor. It is approved for treatment of psoriasis and psoriatic arthritis (PsA) by the US FDA in 2014 and Drug Controller General of India in 2017.

Mechanism of Action

PDE4 degrades cyclic adenosine 3',5'-monophosphate (cAMP), an essential intracellular second messenger that regulates inflammatory response. Apremilast inhibits the enzyme PDE4 thus increasing cAMP in turn resulting in decreased production of pro-inflammatory cytokines, namely interferon-ϒ, tumor necrosis factor-α, interleukin-12 (IL-12), IL-17, IL-23 and an increase in expression of anti-inflammatory cytokine particularly IL-10.

Pharmacokinetics

Apremilast is metabolized extensively by CYP-mediated oxidative mechanisms (mainly by CYP3A4) followed by glucuronidation. It is metabolized by non-CYP mediated hydrolysis as well.

Indications

In rheumatology its main clinical use is in PsA typically in patients with mild disease who have not responded to conventional synthetic DMARDs and are not candidates for JAK inhibitors or a biologic DMARD (bDMARD). The guidelines issued by various professional bodies regarding its usage in PsA is summarized in Table 4.9.1.

Its efficacy in PsA over placebo has been shown (Table 4.9.2). The American College of Rheumatology 20 (ACR 20) response defined as the improvement of 20% in the number of tender and number of swollen joints, and a 20% improvement in three of the following five criteria: patient global assessment, physician global assessment, functional ability, visual analog pain scale, and erythrocyte sedimentation rate or C-reactive protein (CRP).

Table 4.9.1: Guidelines on use of apremilast in psoriatic arthritis

GRAPPA 2022	*ACR/NPF 2018*	*EULAR 2019*
• Indicated in peripheral arthritis DMARD naïve, DMARD intolerant, enthesitis, dactylitis, and nail disease • Conditionally recommended against in axial disease	• Recommendation for apremilast not clearly defined • Considered along with other oral small molecules in DMARD naïve or DMARD intolerant patients.	• For mild arthritis with previous inadequate response to at least one csDMARD, and when neither a bDMARD nor a JAK inhibitor is appropriate

Table 4.9.2: Summary of clinical trials that has shown the efficacy of apremilast (APR) in psoriatic arthritis (PsA)

Author/year of study	*Study design*	*Population*	*Intervention*	*ACR 20 response*
PALACE 1 and PALACE 2	Double blind RCT 52 weeks	Active PsA despite prior conventional synthetic or biologic DMARDs	APR-20 mg BD (n = 168) APR-30 mg BD (n = 168) Placebo (n = 168)	37% vs 32% vs 19%
PALACE 3	Double blind RCT 52 weeks	Active PsA despite DMARDs along with active skin	APR-20 mg BD (n = 169) APR-30 mg BD (n = 167) Placebo (n = 169)	28% vs 41% vs 18%
PALACE 4	Double blind RCT 52 weeks	DMARD-naive	APR-20 mg BD (n = 175) APR-30 mg BD (n = 176) Placebo (n = 176)	28% vs 31% vs 16%
Kavanaugh et al.	Open-label extension 52–260 weeks	Participants pooled from PALACE 1–3 trials	APR-20 mg BD APR-30 mg BD	67% at 260 weeks

In these clinical trials of apremilast in PsA listed in table 2, ACR 20 response was observed in about 30 to 40% individuals at 52 weeks.

Apremilast also is effective in extra-articular domains of PsA. In the PALACE 1, PALACE 2, and PALACE 3 trials it was shown that in patients with a baseline ≥ 3% body surface area involvement of psoriasis approximately 43% achieved ≥75% reduction from the baseline Psoriasis Area and Severity Index (PASI) scores. In patients with baseline enthesitis and dactylitis about 62% achieved a Maastricht Ankylosing Spondylitis Enthesitis Score of 0, and 81% achieved a dactylitis count of 0 respectively compared to placebo. Apart from PsA it has been tested in rheumatoid arthritis, ankylosing spondylitis and Behcet's disease (Table 4.9.3).

Dosing and Administration

The dose in psoriasis and PsA is 30 mg twice daily by mouth. Treatment starts with a 10 mg once a

Table 4.9.3: Summary of evidence for apremilast (APR) in rheumatoid arthritis, ankylosing spondylitis and Behçet's disease

Author/year of study	*Study design*	*Population*	*Intervention*	*Primary oucome*
Genovese et al., 2015	Double blind RCT 52 weeks	**Rheumatoid arthritis** who are methotrexate intolerant	APR-20 mg BD (n = 82) APR-30 mg BD (n = 76) Placebo (n = 79)	ACR 20 at 16 weeks was similar 28% vs 34% vs 35%
Taylor et al., 2021 POSTURE 3	Double blind RCT 24 weeks	**Ankylosing spondylitis** BASDAI ≥4 with or without stable doses of DMARDs/NSAIDs or low dose steroids	APR-20 mg BD (n = 163) APR-30 mg BD (n = 163) Placebo (n = 164)	ASAS20 response at week 16 was similar 35% vs 33% vs 39%
Hatemi et al., 2019	Double blind RCT 12 weeks followed by a 52 week extension	**Behçet's disease** At least two oral ulcers, refractory to topical or systemic therapy (biologics excluded) and no significant organ involvement	APR-30 mg BD (n = 104) Placebo (n = 103)	Number of oral ulcers was significantly lower with apremilast

day with a daily increment of 10 mg until a dose of 30 mg twice a day is reached. No dose change is required in mild to moderate renal dysfunction or moderate to severe hepatic dysfunction. However, dose reduction is advised in patients with severe renal dysfunction.

Adverse Effects

The most common adverse effects are nausea, headache, diarrhea, nasopharyngitis, and upper respiratory tract infections. These are more during the initial stages of therapy and most resolve over time. Less common adverse events (noted in clinical trials) are depression, suicidal tendency, and weight loss. But long-term safety analysis has not shown any increase in the incidence of depression. Weight loss can occur especially the first year of treatment in those with higher baseline body mass index.

IGURATIMOD

Introduction

Iguratimod is a small-molecule antirheumatic drug developed and used for rheumatoid arthritis (RA) in Japan since 2012. It is also approved in a few Southeast Asian countries.

Mechanism of Action

Its immunomodulatory role in RA is by inhibiting cytokines and immunoglobulin production without altering B cell proliferation. It inhibits inflammatory T cell mainly Th17 by suppressing the mRNA expression of IL-17-related genes and reducing the phosphorylation of mitogen-activated protein kinases (MAPKs). The principal mode of action is through nuclear factor-κB (NF-κB) activity inhibition. It has favorable effects on bone metabolism by osteoblast differentiation and inhibiting osteoclastogenesis.

Efficacy of Iguratimod in RA

The 2015 Asia Pacific League against Rheumatism (APLAR) guidelines on the treatment of RA recommend iguratimod as one of the options for the management of treatment-naïve RA patients who do not tolerate methotrexate (MTX). Iguratimod in combination with MTX has good efficacy as compared to MTX alone (Table 4.9.4).

Table 4.9.4: Summary of clinical trials of Iguratimod (IGU) in rheumatoid arthritis

Author/year	*RCT duration*	*Intervention*	*Primary outcome*
Hara et al., 2007	28 weeks	IGU* vs SSZ 500 mg BID vs Placebo (PB)	ACR 20 response at 24 weeks: IGU superior to placebo, not inferior to SSZ.
Lü et al., 2008	24 weeks	Group 1 IGU:25 mg QD vs Group 2 IGU: 25 mg BID vs Placebo (PB)	ACR 20 and ACR 50 response better in IGU
Lü et al., 2009	24 weeks	Group 1 IGU* vs Group 2 IGU: 25 mg BID vs MTX group: 15 mg/week	ACR 20 response at 24 weeks IGU vs MTX was similar
Hara et al., 2014	52 weeks	IGU+MTX x 52 weeks vs PB/IGU+MTX [PB x 28 weeks, IGU 25 mg QD from 28–32 weeks, then 25 mg BID from 32–52 weeks + MTX 6 or 8 mg/week]	ACR20 response was similar at 24 weeks. The switch to IGU treatment improved ACR responses at 52 weeks.

(Contd.)

Table 4.9.4: Summary of clinical trials of Iguratimod (IGU) in rheumatoid arthritis *(Contd.)*

Author/year	*RCT duration*	*Intervention*	*Primary outcome*
Ishiguro et al., 2013	24 weeks	IGU* and MTX 6 or 8 mg /week vs Placebo + MTX 6 or 8 mg /week	ACR20 response at 24 weeks better in IGU compared to placebo Significant improvements in ACR50 and ACR70.
Duan et al., 2015	24 weeks	MTX + IGU vs MTX 12.5/week *25 mg QD x 4 wks, then 25 mg BID	ACR50 response at 24 weeks better in MTX + IGU group

This is based on the results of randomised controlled trials conducted in Japan, China, and other observational studies. It is noninferior to methotrexate monotherapy. Its efficacy as an add-on therapy in those with inadequate response to biologics such as tocilizumab or TNF inhibitors has been reported. But overall the evidence is limited.

Future clinical trials in diverse populations in RA are required, for example comparing iguratimod as monotherapy or combination therapy with DMARDs (other than MTX). Clinical trials of iguratimod in Sjogren's syndrome, IgG4 disease, ankylosing spondylitis and lupus nephritis are ongoing.

Dosing and Administration

It is given orally 25 mg twice a day, either when administered with food or after fasting, as food does not affect its absorption, and is extensively metabolized by the liver.

Adverse Effects

Similar to MTX the most common adverse effects are gastrointestinal symptoms. Elevation in AST and ALT is also common. In combination with MTX given for 24 weeks, about 5.5% and 9.8% of patients have an increase in ALT and AST, while at 52 weeks AST and ALT were reported in 16 and 14%, respectively. So, a close watch on transaminases is advised.

Serious adverse events reported are bacterial pneumonia, interstitial lung disease, and *Pneumocystis jiroveci* pneumonia. Risk factors for severe infections are concomitant glucocorticoid use and the presence of comorbidities. Firtunately meta-analysis and real-world data of >2600 RA patients who have received iguratimod have not shown any significant difference in adverse effects (including transaminitis) as compared to standard agent MTX. A higher risk of bleeding has been reported, therefore it is to be cautiously administered to those who are concomitantly receiving warfarin.

CONCLUSION

In summary, apremilast and iguratimod are two new immunomodulatory agents in the management of autoimmune inflammatory diseases, with good safety profiles.

LEARNING POINTS

Apremilast

- Apremilast a phosphodiesterase-4 inhibitor exerts anti-inflammatory role by increasing cellular cyclic adenosine 3', 5'-monophosphate (cAMP)
- Apremilast is indicated in DMARD naïve or DMARD intolerant peripheral arthritis domain of PsA, enthesitis, dactylitis, and nail disease
- It is not yet recommended in axial disease
- Gastrointestinal side effects and headaches are common with apremilast.

Iguratimod

- Iguratimod as monotherapy in RA is noninferior to MTX.
- Iguratimod+MTX combination therapy in RA has better efficacy than MTX monotherapy.
- Liver enzyme elevation and gastrointestinal side effects are common but not more than MTX.

FURTHER READING

1. Coates LC, Soriano ER, Corp N, et al.; GRAPPA Treatment Recommendations domain subcommittees. Group for Research and Assessment of Psoriasis and Psoriatic Arthritis (GRAPPA): updated treatment

recommendations for psoriatic arthritis 2021. Nat Rev Rheumatol. 2022;18:465–79.

2. Jiang H, Gao H, Wang Q, et al. Molecular mechanisms and clinical application of Iguratimod: A review. Biomed Pharmacother. 2020;122:109704.
3. Keating GM. Apremilast: A Review in Psoriasis and Psoriatic Arthritis. Drugs. 2017;77:459–72.
4. Li J, Bao J, Zeng J, et al. Iguratimod: a valuable remedy from the Asia Pacific region for ameliorating autoimmune diseases and protecting bone physiology. Bone Res. 2019;7:27.
5. Nozaki Y. Iguratimod: Novel Molecular Insights and a New csDMARD for Rheumatoid Arthritis, from Japan to the World. Life (Basel). 2021;11:457.

Cyclosporine and Tacrolimus

Joe Thomas

INTRODUCTION

The calcineurin inhibitors (CNIs) cyclosporine and tacrolimus are key immunosuppressives used in organ transplantation and certain autoimmune rheumatic diseases. They exert their immunosuppressive effect by inhibiting calcineurin which is a calcium and calmodulin dependent phosphatase which is a regulator of nuclear translocator and subsequent activation of NFAT transcription factors.

MECHANISM OF ACTION

Both cyclosporine and tacrolimus are isolated from fungi. Cyclosporine (also spelt ciclosporin or cyclosporin) is a lipophilic cyclic peptide of 11 amino acids, while tacrolimus is a macrolide antibiotic. Cyclosporine binds to cyclophilin, while tacrolimus (which is 10–100 times more potent than cyclosporine) binds to FK-binding proteins. The drug-protein complexes competitively bind calcineurin and inhibits the translocation of transcription factors NFAT leading to reduced transcription of IL-2 and other cytokines, and ultimately reduced T cell proliferation and activity.

Voclosporin is a new CNI structurally similar to cyclosporine except for modification of a functional group on the amino acid 1 residue. Voclosporine has improved metabolic profile and is more potent when compared to cyclosporine.

Another mechanism of action of cyclosporine is by blocking JNK (c-Jun N-terminal kinase) and the p38 signalling pathway leading to specific reduction and inhibition of T cell activity.

PHARMACOKINETIC PROPERTIES

The oral bioavailability of CNIs is only 20% due to low solubility, extensive hepatic first-pass metabolism. After absorption, approximately 99% of CNIs binds to erythrocytes and remaining 1% enters the lymphatic system and exerts its main therapeutic effects. Since they are lipophilic they are distributed extensively in the body. CNIs metabolites are predominantly excreted through the bile.

INDICATIONS OF CNIs IN RHEUMATOLOGY

Systemic lupus erythematosus (SLE): Tacrolimus in combination with mycophenolate mofetil (MMF) is used for remission induction of lupus nephritis that is not responding adequately to initial standard therapy. The combination tacrolimus + MMF + low dose steroid is called the multi-targeted therapy approach, mostly employed to treat refractory lupus nephritis. Though in the past few years there is also data showing that multitarget approach is superior to cyclophosphamide and steroid for remission induction of (non-refractory) lupus nephritis. Further it is also shown that voclosporin added to low dose steroid and MMF produces a superior complete renal response as compared to standard care alone (AURORA 1 study).

Topical tacrolimus 1% is effective in the treatment of cutaneous lupus erythematosus.

Idiopathic inflammatory myositis (IIM): CNIs are second-line agents for treatment of IIM refractory to a standard regimen of prednisone plus methotrexate (MTX) or azathioprine (AZA).

Behçets disease: Cyclosporine is a valuable agent in the management of uveitis and thrombophlebitis of Behcets disease.

Autoimmune disorder and concomitant chronic HCV infection: Cyclosporine suppresses the replication of hepatitis C virus (HCV); therefore, it is useful in the management of autoimmune rheumatic diseases when HCV infection is a co-morbidity.

Connective tissue disease-related interstitial lung disease (CTD-ILD): In CTD-ILD as well as interstitial pneumonia with autoimmune features (IPAF) CNIs have been widely used as induction and maintenance.

Psoriatic arthritis: Cyclosporine is recommended in the management of moderate or severe peripheral arthritis, moderate to severe skin, and nail disease.

Rheumatoid arthritis (RA): Tacrolimus currently approved in management of RA in Canada, Japan, Korea. It is used mainly as add-on to other DMARDs in patients who do not achieve an adequate response.

Macrophage activation syndrome: Cyclosporine in combination with steroids is used in treatment of macrophage activation syndrome (MAS) associated with Adult-onset Still's Disease or SLE.

Sjögren's syndrome: Topical cyclosporine appears to be a useful agent in the management of dry eye in Sjogren's syndrome.

Juvenile dermatomyositis (JDM) and systemic onset juvenile idiopathic arthritis (SoJIA): In JDM patients unresponsive to immunosuppressive drugs, cyclosporine treatment have shown good response. ACR guidelines recommends cyclosporine as third-line treatment for SoJIA children with active systemic features.

Adverse Effects

The most commonly encountered adverse effects of CNIs are neurotoxicity, hypertension, and nephrotoxocity (Table 4.10.1). Voclosporin is better tolerated, safer, and has an improved metabolic profile when compared to cyclosporine. Though inferior to cyclosporine in psoriasis, it is efficacious in lupus nephritis. Nevertheless monitoring (Table 4.10.2) is important especially in the initial few months, and the greatest challenge is nephrotoxicity, because once chronic nephrotoxicity develops it is irreversible.

Pregnancy and lactation: Tacrolimus is compatible with pregnancy and lactation. Cyclosporine can also be used during pregnancy and lactation but blood

Table 4.10.1: Adverse effects associated with calcineurin inhibitors (CNIs)

Adverse effect	*Comment*
Nephrotoxicity	Nephrotoxicity of CNIs is both acute and chronic. Most commonly it manifests as an increase in creatinine, that is reversible on reducing the dose. Tubulopathy and thrombotic microangiopathy with cyclosporine are also reported.
Hypertension	Hypertension is caused by sodium retention and vasoconstriction, generally occurs within first few weeks of therapy, and needs anti-hypertensive therapy in most patients.
Neurotoxicity	Mild tremors occur commonly in both cyclosporine and tacrolimus. However, akinetic mutism, encephalopathy, seizures, etc. are reported with intravenous tacrolimus.
Posterior reversible encephalopathy syndrome (PRES)	PRES manifests with seizures, blurring of vison, and altered sensorium. It is a rare neurologic side effect of the CNIs.
Metabolic abnormalities	Impaired glucose tolerance, diabetes mellitus, hyperlipidemia, hypokalemia, hypomagnesemia can occur during therapy with the CNIs. All these metabolic effects are less in tacrolimus.
Hyperuricemia	There is an increased risk of hyperuricemia and new-onset gout with use of CNIs.
Gingival hyperplasia	Cyclosporine (not tacrolimus) causes gingival hyperplasia and hirsutism
Calcineurin inhibitor pain syndrome (CIPS)	A syndrome presenting with symmetrical pain in both the lower limbs, pruritus without rash has been reported in the context of hematopoietic stem cell transplant (HSCT) and organ transplantation. CIPS typically occur early after starting CNIs in HSCT and after 6 weeks of therapy in solid organ transplant.

Table 4.10.2: Dosing, administration, and monitoring of calcineurin inhibitors

Dosing (*for rheumatology indications*)	Cyclosporine is 2.5–4 mg/kg/day orally Tacrolimus is 0.075 mg/kg/day or 1–3 mg/day orally Voclosporin is 23.7 mg twice a day (dose in lupus nephritis) orally. No dose adjustment is required when the eGFR is >60 mL/min/1.73 m^2. When eGFR is <60 mL/min/ 1.73 m^2, and there is 20–30% fall from baseline reduce dose by 9.7 mg BD, when the fall is >30% discontinue the dose and reassess GFR after 2 weeks.
Administration	All CNIs should be administered preferably on an empty stomach at 12-hour intervals. It is recommended to take CNIs at a consistent time of the day.
Monitoring	Serum creatinine and blood pressure should be checked at baseline for all patients on at least two occasions. This is followed by monitoring every 2 weeks for 3 months and every 4 weeks thereafter. If the serum creatinine has acutely increased, a search should be done for other causes of acute kidney injury (AKI), if none is found then the AKI is attributed to CNI acute nephrotoxicity and dose is decreased. Therapeutic drug (blood) levels are recommended especially in transplant recipients and autoimmune disorders, because the therapeutic index is narrow. Target blood concentrations varies by indications. Blood concentrations should be checked two to three days after starting the medication. Blood levels of cyclosporine are monitored using 12-hour trough or two-hour post-dose and tacrolimus are monitored using 12- and 24-hour trough.
Key drug interactions	*Drugs that increase CNIs blood levels:* Allopurinol, antimalarials, MTX, high dose methylprednisolone, bosentan, clarithromycin, fluconazole, veerapamil, amlodepine, etc. *Drugs that decrease CNIs blood levels:* Sulfasalazine, rifampin, isoniazid, phenytoin, carbamazepine, barbiturates, etc. *Drugs that enhances nephrotoxicity:* Aminoglycosides, amphotericin B, ciprofloxacin.

pressure, blood glucose and renal functions has to be carefully monitored during pregnancy.

CONTRAINDICATIONS

Hypersensitivity to CNIs, concurrent malignancy, uncontrolled hypertension and infection are contraindications for the use of CNIs.

CONCLUSION

CNIs possess suppressive effects on both cell-mediated and humoral immune responses and represents a suitable option in several autoimmune and inflammatory rheumatic diseases.

LEARNING POINTS

- Cyclosporine and tacrolimus are inhibitors of calcineurin that is responsible for nuclear translocation and activation of NFAT transcription factors.
- The CNIs are associated with many adverse events, but the newer agent voclosporin has a better safety profile
- Being potent inhibitors of T cell activation, their uses extends across all spectrum of autoimmune rheumatic diseases
- Tacrolimus is particularly useful in refractory lupus nephritis.
- Voclosporin added to MMF and low dose steroid is superior to MMF and low dose steroid alone in lupus nephritis
- Cyclosporine is useful in macrophage activation syndrome associated with soJIA.

FURTHER READING

1. Azzi JR, Sayegh MH, Mallat SG. Calcineurin inhibitors: 40 years later, can't live without. J Immunol. 2013;191:5785–91.

2. Hiramatsu Y, Yoshida S, Kotani T, et al. Changes in the blood level, efficacy, and safety of tacrolimus in pregnancy and the lactation period in patients with systemic lupus erythematosus. Lupus. 2018;27:2245–52.
3. Jasper C A Broen, Jacob M van Laar. Mycophenolate mofetil, azathioprine and tacrolimus: mechanisms in rheumatology. Nat Rev Rheumatol. 2020;16:167–178.
4. Kakihana K, Ohashi K, Murata Y, et al. Clinical features of calcineurin inhibitor-induced pain syndrome after allo-SCT. Bone Marrow Transplant. 2012;47:593–5.
5. Li Y, Palmisano M, Sun D, et al. Pharmacokinetic Disposition Difference Between Cyclosporine and Voclosporin Drives Their Distinct Efficacy and Safety Profiles in Clinical Studies. Clin Pharmacol. 2020; 12:83–96.
6. Naesens M, Kuypers DR, Sarwal M. Calcineurin inhibitor nephrotoxicity. Clin J Am Soc Nephrol. 2009;4:481–508.

Tumor Necrosis Factor-α Inhibitors

Ved Chaturvedi, Molly Mary Thabah

INTRODUCTION

Tumor necrosis factor α (TNF-α) is found in high concentrations in rheumatoid joints and in the sacroiliac joints of spondyloarthritis (SpA) patients. Blocking TNF-α by recombinant monoclonal antibodies (mAb) leads to rapid control of disease activity in rheumatoid arthritis (RA). There are currently five such mAb disease-modifying anti-rheumatic drugs (bDMARD) that block TNF-α also called TNF inhibitors (TNFi). These are etanercept, infliximab, adalimumab, golimumab, and certolizumab pegol (Table 4.11.1).

MECHANISM OF ACTION

The binding of TNF-α to its receptors leads to the activation of several signaling pathways, including transcription factor activation (nuclear factor-κB), proteases (caspases), and protein kinases, further activating neutrophils, B cells and endothelial cells. Monoclonal antibodies that target TNF-α are able to prevent the cytokine inflammatory cascade resulting in amelioration of inflammation. TNFi are FDA approved for a variety of autoimmune inflammatory rheumatic diseases (Table 4.11.2).

Table 4.11.1: A summary of the structure, mechanism of action and dose of TNF inhibitors

TNF inhibitor	*Structure*	*Mechanism of action*	*Dose*
Etanercept	Etanercept is a fusion protein made up of the Fc portion of human IgG1 and two identical chains of the extracellular human TNF-receptor p75	Etanercept binds to both soluble and membrane bound TNF-α preventing it from interacting with its receptor. It also binds to TNF-β (lymphotoxin). It does not cause apoptosis of TNF expressing cells.	25 mg subcutaneously twice a week or 50 mg subcutaneously once a week
Infliximab	A mouse-human IgG1 monoclonal antibody (mAb) to TNF-α with a predominance of human amino acid sequences (70%).	Binds to soluble and membrane-bound TNF-α and inhibits TNF-α–receptor interactions. Causes apoptosis of TNF-α expressing cells.	Rheumatoid arthritis (RA): 3 mg/kg/dose at 0, 2, 6 weeks and thereafter every 8 weeks. (Premedication with 100 mg of methylprednisolone is preferred by a few to prevent anaphylaxis) Axial SpA/ankylosing spondylitis: 5 mg/kg IV infusion at 0, 2, and 6 weeks, then every 8 weeks

(Contd.)

Table 4.11.1: A summary of the structure, mechanism of action and dose of TNF inhibitors *(Contd.)*

TNF inhibitor	*Structure*	*Mechanism of action*	*Dose*
Adalimumab	Fully human IgG1κ monoclonal antibody to TNF-α	Same as infliximab	40 mg subcutaneously once in two weeks
Golimumab	Golimumab is a fully human IgG1κ mAb to TNF-α.	Golimumab inhibits TNF by binding to both soluble and transmembrane TNF	50 mg subcutaneously once a month
Certolizumab pegol	Fab fragment of fully human monoclonal antibody to TNF fused with 400 kilodalton Peg moiety.	Binds with high affinity to soluble and membrane-bound TNF-α. Does not cause apoptosis of TNF-α expressing cells, and also does not cause complement or antibody-mediated cytotoxicity.	200 mg subcutaneously at 0, 2, and 4 weeks, then 200 mg subcutaneously once in two weeks

Table 4.11.2: Indications for TNF inhibitors (TNFi) in immune-mediated rheumatic disease

Indications	*TNFi*	*Comments*
Active rheumatoid arthritis whether early, advanced, or refractory disease.	Etanercept, infliximab, adalimumab, golimumab and certolizumab pegol are all effective	TNFi is always used in combination with methotrexate.
Active axial SpA/ankylosing spondylitis and non-radiographic SpA	Infliximab, etanercept, adalimumab, golimumab and certolizumab pegol are all effective	Patients with shorter disease duration, younger patients, higher baseline disease activity, and high inflammatory markers will respond better
Psoriatic arthritis, enthesitis, and dactylitis	Infliximab, adalimumab, etanercept, certolizumab, and golimumab are effective	TNFi may worsen preexisting psoriasis skin lesions or induce psoriatic lesions. The longest retention is for infliximab and etanercept.
Juvenile idiopathic arthritis (JIA) inadequate response to methotrexate.	Etanercept, adalimumab, and golimumab are effective and approved for use in polyarticular JIA. Extended oligoarticular, persistent oligoarticular, psoriatic arthritis, and enthesitis related JIA also respond well to etanercept. Systemic JIA responded poorly to etanercept.	Registry data from the Netherlands show the longterm efficacy of etanercept in JIA. Those patients with low baseline disability, usage of DMARDs before etanercept, and younger age at onset of JIA had excellent responses.
Arthritis dominant adult-onset still's disease (AOSD) who have not responded to glucocorticoids and methotrexate, and when anakinra is unavailable.	Infliximab, etanercept, and adalimumab are tried in arthritis dominant AOSD.	Only 11% of AOSD will achieve remission with TNFi

(Contd.)

Table 4.11.2: Indications for TNF inhibitors (TNFi) in immune-mediated rheumatic disease (*Contd.*)

Indications	*TNFi*	*Comments*
Severe and refractory cutaneous polyarteritis nodosa	Infliximab and etanercept were reported to be helpful	Cutaneous polyarteritis nodosa that is refractory to standard therapy with steroids, azathioprine, methotrexate, and cyclophosphamide may respond to TNFi
Deficiency of adenosine deaminase 2 syndrome	TNFi (infliximab, etanercept, and adalimumab) are first-line agents in controlling inflammation of this monogenic vasculitis syndrome.	Hematopoietic stem cell transplant is the definitive treatment in patients with hematological manifestations.

INDICATIONS

Rheumatoid Arthritis

TNFi are indicated in active rheumatoid arthritis (RA) when conventional synthetic DMARD (csDMARD) has failed, or an inadequate response to csDMARDS and in presence of poor prognostic factors such as erosive joint disease, rheumatoid factor, anticitrullinated peptide antibodies, functional limitation, and extra-articular disease.

Benefits of Therapy with TNFi in RA

All five TNFi reduce disease activity, improve functional ability and health-related quality of life, prevent bone erosions and improve bone mineral density. In some proportions of patients, treatment with TNFi results in remission defined by a disease activity score of 28 joint (DAS28) of <2.6. It is important that disease activity and functional status are assessed periodically and compared with previous results to determine the drug's efficacy.

The effectiveness of TNFi spans the spectrum of RA: early active RA, advanced RA (even with a median disease duration of 9–10 years), and refractory and erosive RA. Though more recent data indicate that by using a strategy of tight control, csDMARD can produce as much benefit as a biological agent, in this context it is worthwhile to mention that in the BeST trial, there is clear superiority of combination therapy with infliximab in achieving early remission, this translates to early achievement of better functional ability and health-related QOL.

Etanercept and methotrexate (MTX) combination results in inhibited radiographic progression and improved radiographic outcomes of RA. Efficacy is also sustained in patients who complete 5 years of etanercept, even in those who decreased or discontinued use of MTX or corticosteroids.

How Long should TNFi be Continued in RA?

Since treatment with TNFi incurs a significant economic burden, patients and doctors often asks the question as to when to stop the therapy? Is it safe to continue TNFi for the long-term? To answer this question, studies show that some patients have received TNFi safely for as long as seven years. A long-term follow-up study of active refractory and erosive RA shows that at seven years about 30% are still on infliximab, 61% patients are in low disease activity (DAS28 <3.2) state and 45% achieved remission (DAS28 <2.6) with infliximab. The major reasons for infliximab discontinuation are adverse events and secondary lack of efficacy.

Axial Spondyloarthritis

TNFi are indicated in axial radiographic and non-radiographic SpA when the Bath ankylosing spondylitis disease activity index (BASDAI) is >4 or Ankylosing Spondylitis Disease Activity Score (ASDAS) >2.1, and there is no response to NSAIDs for at least 4 weeks.

An ASDAS improvement of >1.1 or BASDAI >2 is an indication to continue TNFi. Whereas a lack of improvement is an indication to switch TNFi or change to an IL-17 inhibitor. Once an inactive ASDAS score (a surrogate marker of remission) is reached it is time to taper TNFi.

Benefits of TNFi in Axial SpA

TNFi reduces disease activity, and improves function measured by Bath ankylosing spondylitis functional index (BASFI). Etanercept helps control enthesitis in early axial SpA and ankylosing spondylitis (AS). More than 85% of etanercept treated patients have an improvement in MRI sites of inflammation. TNFi retard radiographic progression.

How Long should TNFi be given in Axial SpA?

Long-term extension of trials shows that the Assessment in SpondyloArthritis International Society (ASAS) partial remission is achieved by 44% of patients at week 192. In the real-world scenario, ASAS partial remission is achieved by 50% and 70% at 12 and 24 months respectively, with continued use of TNFi. But due to the cost involved, loss of efficacy, and the emergence of adverse effects, the retention rate of patients with axial SpA patients on TNFi in the real world is about 30% at 5 years.

In the author's clinical practice TNFi (infliximab or etanercept) is given till a clinically inactive disease (measured by BASDAI) is attained. This is followed by a gradual increase in dosing interval and/or on-demand administration. For example, if etanercept was given every week it is tapered to once a month dosing. With regards to infliximab, a maintenance regimen of 3 mg/kg (low dose infliximab) every 2 months is able to maintain improvement in many cases. It is still not known when to completely stop treatment.

In AS who will Respond to TNFi?

It has been consistently shown that those with a shorter duration of disease, younger patients, those with higher baseline BASDAI, and those with high CRP and ESR are more likely to achieve a good clinical response to TNFi.

ADVERSE EFFECTS, VARIOUS CONSIDERATIONS AND CONTRAINDICATIONS (TABLE 4.11.3) TO TNFI

Infections

a. **Tuberculosis:** TNFi results in impairment of granuloma formation, so there is a high risk for reactivation of tuberculosis. The risk is highest with adalimumab and least with etanercept. Active screening for tuberculosis by a good history, tuberculin skin test, and plain chest radiographs are prerequisites prior to TNFi therapy. If the chest radiographs look suspicious it is better to advise CT chest to rule out active tuberculosis. Latent tuberculosis infection should be treated preferably for a month before initiating TNFi. In the case of active tuberculosis, the patient must complete at least the intensive phase before beginning TNFi. One practical way to decrease the occurrence of tuberculosis as seen in the authors' experience is not to give loading dose of infliximab.

Table 4.11.3: Contraindications to TNF inhibitors (TNFi)

1. History of hypersensitivity reaction to the agent.
2. Active infection or sepsis.
3. Active malignancy.
4. Heart failure NYHA class III or IV.
5. Concomitant use with another biological agent is contraindicated.
6. Cirrhosis of liver Child–Pugh class B and C.
7. Use TNFi in pregnancy cautiously. Avoid TNFi during the last trimester, as they cross the placenta and can cause immunosuppression of the neonate, also live vaccines are not to be given during the first six months of life. Certolizumab is safe as it doesn't cross the placenta.

b. **Chronic hepatitis:** Hepatitis B virus (HBV) can reactivate, so prior to initiating TNFi apart from HBsAg also ask for IgM and IgG anti-HBc to rule out recent HBV and occult HBV respectively. Chronic hepatitis B (including occult HBV) must be treated with entecavir or tenofovir and TNFi can be resumed concurrently. TNFi is also safe for chronic HCV infection. But patients who are Child–Pugh class B and C should not receive TNFi.
c. **Slow viruses:** Prolonged suppression of the immune response may allow for the reactivation of slow viruses such as the JC polyomavirus, which can cause progressive multifocal leukoencephalopathy (PML). The occurrence of PML is very uncommon and most studies are limited to case reports. In rheumatology, rituximab is associated with the highest risk of PML.
d. **Sepsis:** Many of the usual signs of sepsis may be suppressed in patients treated with TNF

inhibitors, since their ability to mount anti-inflammatory responses may be seriously compromised.

Cancer Risk with TNFi

The risk for lymphoma and solid organ malignancy in RA patients receiving TNFi is not different from biological naïve RA patients. The reduction of inflammation in RA patients due to biologics have led to a significantly decreased risk of mortality and cardiovascular events.

Congestive Heart Failure

TNFi are contraindicated in patients with NYHA Class III or IV heart failure, because initial studies in patients with RA and heart failure showed poor cardiac outcomes and mortality. However, there does not seem to be an increased incidence of new congestive heart failure among individuals who receive TNFi.

Drug-induced Lupus

Antinuclear antibody (ANA) and anti-dsDNA antibodies are known to develop in up to 50% of patients who receive TNFi, but clinical drug-induced lupus is rare. Anti-TNF induced lupus has more cutaneous, renal, and cerebral manifestations compared to the usual drug-induced lupus. Symptoms usually resolve soon after discontinuation of the TNFi.

Immunogenicity of TNFi

Serum antibodies to infliximab called human antichimeric antibody (HACA) can be detected in up to 17% of all infliximab treated patients. However, concomitant MTX is associated with lower incidences of HACA. The EULAR recommendation is that in RA, TNFi is to be used along with MTX.

Demyelinating Disorders

Demyelinating events such as optic neuritis, transverse myelitis, acute inflammatory demyelinating polyneuropathy, etc. have been reported in patients while on TNFi. It is still elusive whether it is mere coincidence or an adverse event of TNFi. Nevertheless, it is prudent to immediately discontinue TNFi if such events occur and to use TNFi cautiously in patients with an underlying demyelinating disorder.

TNFi during Pregnancy and Lactation

TNFi can be given during pregnancy if the situation warrants it. Registry data show that the occurrence of pre-term births, spontaneous abortion, and congenital defects with the use of TNFi in pregnancy are similar to disease matched controls. There are no specific birth-defect patterns. All TNFi (except certolizumab pegol) cross the placenta, especially in the last trimester and can cause immunosuppression in the newborn. So neonates who have been exposed to TNFi in utero should not receive live vaccines in the first 6 months of life. TNFi can also be given during lactation, as only very small amounts are secreted in the breast milk.

TNF in Renal Impairment

TNFi being immunoglobulins and proteins are not excreted by the kidneys. There are case series that have demonstrated the safety of TNFi in RA with chronic kidney disease (CKD). Etanercept in RA patients on maintenance hemodialysis is also safe. So, TNFi can be given in the presence of renal impairment or CKD if the situation warrants it, but in practice, we generally avoid TNFi in renal impairment as the risks of infections are higher in this group of patients.

LEARNING POINTS

- TNFi are indicated in RA when csDMARD have failed or when there is an inadequate response to csDMARDS
- They are drugs of choice in the management of SpA. Because of the high cost involved TNFi is given till a partial remission is achieved, this is followed by an on-demand administration.
- Active screening for tuberculosis should be performed before administration of TNFi
- TNFi (except certolizumab) should be avoided in the last trimester of pregnancy.

FURTHER READING

1. Smolen JS, Aletaha D, Koeller M, et al. New therapies for the treatment of rheumatoid arthritis. Lancet. 2007; 370:1861–74.

2. Vander Cruyssen B, Durez P, et al. Seven-year follow-up of infliximab therapy in rheumatoid arthritis patients with severe long-standing refractory disease: attrition rate and evolution of disease activity. Arthritis Res Ther 2010;12:R77.
3. Maxwell LJ, Zochling J, Boonen A, et al. TNF-alpha inhibitors for ankylosing spondylitis. Cochrane Database Syst Rev. 2015;(4):CD005468.
4. Yu CL, Yang CH, Chi CC. Drug survival of biologics in treating ankylosing spondylitis: a systematic review and meta-analysis of real-world evidence. Bio Drugs. 2020; 34:669–79.
5. Davies R, Gaynor D, Hyrich KL, Pain CE. Efficacy of biologic therapy across individual juvenile idiopathic arthritis subtypes: A systematic review. Semin Arthritis Rheum. 2017;46:584–93
6. Malaviya AN, Kapoor S, Garg S, et al. Preventing tuberculosis flare in patients with inflammatory rheumatic diseases receiving tumour necrosis factor-alpha inhibitors in India—An audit report. J Rheumatol. 2009; 36:1414–20.

Chapter 4.12

Costimulatory Blockers

Aishwarya Gopal, Chengappa KG

INTRODUCTION

The adaptive immune system plays a major role in the pathogenesis of several autoimmune inflammatory diseases (AIRDs). Even though the exact pathophysiology of the majority of AIRDs are not known, therapeutics targeting immune system have shown reasonable success in managing these diseases. These therapeutic agents are designed based on the general understanding of immune pathway activation. The adaptive arm of the immune system is activated by a series of three signals. The first signal is the interaction between antigen-loaded major histocompatibility complex (MHC) on antigen presenting cells and the T cell receptor (TCR). This is followed by signals from supporting receptor interactions, commonly known as costimulation (signal 2). This is then complemented by a signal 3, in the form of cytokines released by the same cells or by the cells in the surrounding area. Majority of the current day biological or targeted synthetic agents are based on the inhibition of the signal 3. This approach has been hugely successful in AIRDs, but carries significant risk of adverse events given the marked immunosuppression it causes. On the other hand blocking signal 2 (costimulation) has a potential to modulate the immune system and generate regulatory immune cells. Thus, immunomodulation by pharmacologically activating or inhibiting the signal 2 seems to be an exciting and safe therapeutic strategy. Currently this strategy has been tried in several autoimmune rheumatic diseases, solid organ transplants and malignancies.

COSTIMULATION IN T CELLS

Following antigen presentation, several cell-surface proteins (costimulatory ligands) on antigen presenting cells (APCs) engage with their complementary receptors on naive T cells to form signal 2. The costimulatory ligands and their receptors are depicted in Figure 4.12.1. For example CD40 on the APC binds to its T-cell ligand CD40L following which there is an upregulation of B7 molecules (CD80/CD86) and other co-stimulatory molecules on the APC, these upregulated molecules interact with CD28, which is expressed constitutively on T cells causing T cells to become activated.

Inhibitory receptors, which switch off the system to prevent uncontrollable activation, are likewise activated by costimulatory pathways. The ligands for inhibitory receptors are the same as those for stimulatory receptors. As a result, ligand competition is another mechanism for fine-tuning T-cell activation. The cytotoxic T-lymphocyte antigen-4 (CTLA-4) is an inhibitory receptor contained in intracellular vesicles of the resting T-cell and is produced on the cell surface 48–72 hours after T-cell activation. CTLA-4 has a stronger affinity for CD80 and CD86 than for CD28. T cell activation is slowed when CTLA-4 binds to CD80/CD86.

Another co-stimulatory receptor is OX40 (also called CD134 and TNFRSF4). Most CD4+ and CD8+ T lymphocytes express OX40, which produces a strong positive costimulatory signal. Resting memory T cells do not express OX40, but after TCR activation, its expression is rapidly increased.

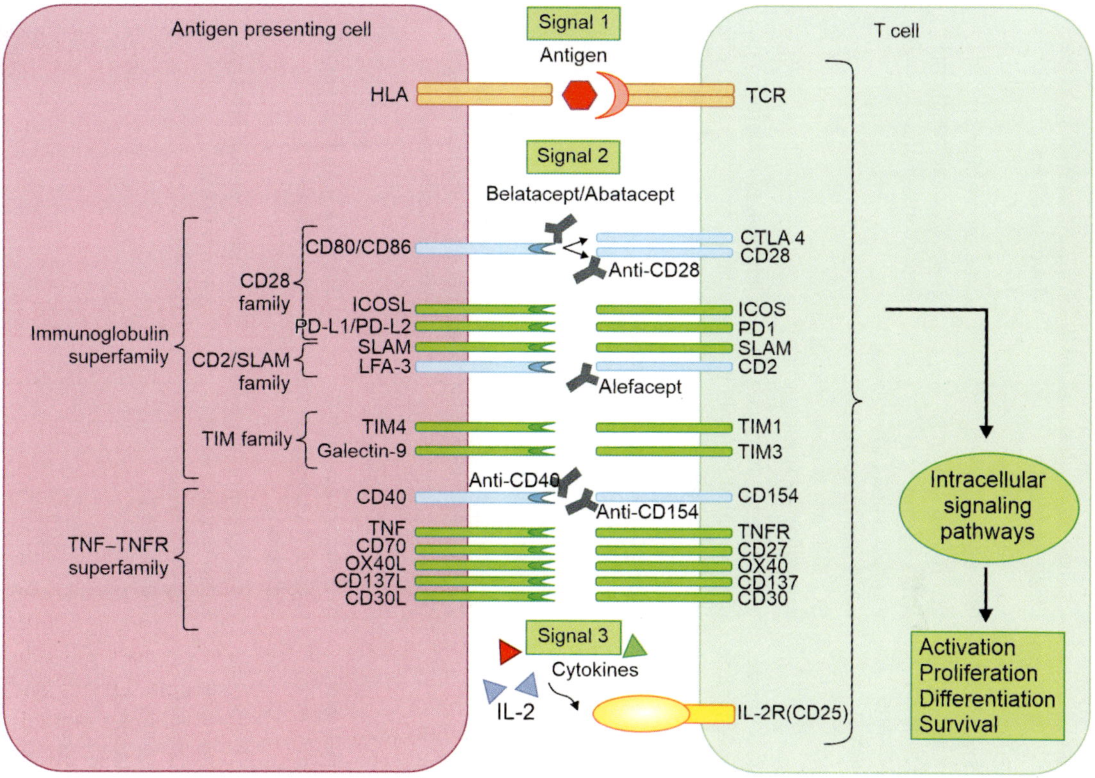

Fig. 4.12.1: Co-stimulation in T cells and antigen-presenting cells: T-cell activation signals 1, 2, and 3 are depicted in this Figure. After alloantigen detection, costimulatory molecules on T cells and antigen-presenting cells interact to activate or inhibit T cells during signal 2. The immunoglobulin superfamily and the TNF/TNFR superfamily are two key categories of costimulatory molecules. Agents that interfere with costimulatory molecules on T cells and antigen-presenting cells have been developed.

CTLA 4: Cytotoxic T lymphocyte protein 4; *HLA:* Human leukocyte antigen; *ICOS:* Inducible T-cell costimulatory; *PD:* Programmed death; *SLAM:* Signalling lymphocytic activation molecule; *TCR:* T-cell receptor; *TIM:* T cell/transmembrane, immunoglobulin, and mucin; *TNF:* Tumour necrosis factor; *TNFR:* Tumour necrosis factor receptor.

Inhibition of OX40 may be able to suppress effector T-cell responses while simultaneously encouraging optimum regulatory T-cell activity. Tables 4.12.1 and 4.12.2 summarize various costimulatory blockers and their clinical effects.

COSTIMULATION IN T FOLLICULAR HELPER (Tfh) CELLS AND B CELLS

T helper cells that aid in the humoral response of germinal centre B cells are Tfh cells. The co-stimulatory molecules ICOS (Inducible T-cell Costimulator; CD278) and programmed cell death-1 (PD-1) are expressed by Tfh cells. The co-stimulatory ligands and their receptors on B cells and Tfh cells are depicted in Figure 4.12.2.

T-cell activation, differentiation, proliferation, and effector activities are all enhanced by ICOS costimulation. In addition, ICOS has been linked to the induction of T follicular helper cells, which are important in T-cell-dependent humoral responses. Lack of ICOS signaling severely impairs T-cell-dependent B-cell responses, including impaired germinal centre development and immunoglobulin class switching. Another important marker that identifies the Tfh phenotype is PD-1. It aids in Tfh formation and germinal center localization. These costimulatory blockers are being tried in various autoimmune diseases as well as have approved indications as immune check point inhibitors in cancer chemotherapy (Tables 4.12.1 and 4.12.2).

Table 4.12.1: Costimulatory blockers and their approved indications, dosing and adverse effects

Drug	*Target*	*Pathway involved*	*Effect on immune response*	*Clinical use*	*Dose and route*	*Adverse effect*
Abatacept	CD80/86	CTLA-4 (CD152)/ CD80/CD86	Inhibits T cell dependent antibody responses	Approved for rheumatoid arthritis, juvenile idiopathic arthritis (JIA), psoriatic arthritis, stem cell and renal transplantation	IV: <60 kg–500 mg 60–100 kg–750 mg >100 kg–1 g Every 4 weeks after three initial doses every 2 weeks SC: 125 mg weekly with or without an IV loading dose	Infusion reactions Anaphylactoid reactions Risk of infections
Belatacept	CD80/86	CTLA-4 (CD152)/ CD80/CD86	Inhibits T cell dependent antibody responses	Approved for renal transplantation to prevent acute rejection	Initial phase: 10 mg/kg on day 1 (day of transplant, prior to implantation) and on day 5 , followed by 10 mg/kg at the end of week 2, week 4, week 8, and week 12 following transplantation Maintenance phase: 5 mg/kg every 4 weeks	Diarrhea, peripheral edema, anemia, hypertension, infections
Alefacept	CD2	LFA3/CD2	Interferes with T cell immune responses, also causes apoptosis of memory effector T cells	Moderate to severe plaque psoriasis	Weekly application of either 7.5 mg IV or 15 mg IM for a course of 12 weeks	Pharyngitis, dizziness, cough, pruritus, myalgia, injection site reactions
Ipilimumab	CTLA-4	CTLA-4 (CD152)/ CD80/CD86	Downregulates T cell immune response	Approved for melanoma, colorectal cancer*, renal cell carcinoma*	1–3 mg/kg every 3–6 weeks (depends on the indication)	Diarrhea, pruritus, weight loss, fatigue
Nivolumab	PD-1	PD-1 (CD279)/ PD-L1 or PD-L2	Increases immune cell proliferation Improves antitumor surveillance system	Bladder cancer, colorectal cancer, head and neck cancer, hepatocellular carcinoma Hodgkin's lymphoma, melanoma, non-small cell lung cancer, renal cell carcinoma	3 mg/kg every two weeks. Dose ranging varies depending upon the malignancy	Immune related adverse events (irAE[$])

(Contd.)

Table 4.12.1: Costimulatory blockers and their approved indications, dosing and adverse effects *(Contd.)*

Drug	*Target*	*Pathway involved*	*Effect on immune response*	*Clinical use*	*Dose and route*	*Adverse effect*
Cemiplimab	PD-1	PD-1 (CD279)/ PD-L1 or PD-L2	Increases immune cell proliferation Improves antitumor surveillance system	Cutaneous squamous cell carcinoma	350 mg IV every 3 weeks	Immune related adverse events (irAE$)
Atezolizu-mab	PD-L1	PD-1 (CD279)/ PD-L1	Increases immune cell proliferation improves antitumor surveillance system n	Bladder cancer, breast cancer, non-small cell lung cancer	840 mg IV q2 weeks or 1200 mg IV q3 weeks or 1680 mg IV q4 weeks	Immune related adverse events (irAE$)
Avelumab	PD-L1	PD-1 (CD279)/ PD-L1	Increases immune cell proliferation Improves antitumor surveillance system	Bladder cancer, Merkel cell carcinoma	800 mg IV q2 weeks	Immune related adverse events (irAE$)
Durvalumab	PD-L1	PD-1 (CD279)/ PD-L1	Increases immune cell proliferation Improves antitumor surveillance system n	Bladder cancer, non-small cell lung cancer	Weight >30 kg: 10 mg/kg IV q2 weeks OR 1500 mg IV q4 weeks Weight <30 kg: 10 mg/kg IV q2 weeks	Immune related adverse events (irAE$)

*In combination with Nivolumab

$ Immune-related adverse events (irAEs) are a distinct spectrum of ICI side effects that resemble autoimmune responses and affect nearly every organ of the body, with the skin, gastrointestinal tract, lung, endocrine, musculoskeletal, and other systems being the most typically affected.

Table 4.12.2: Other drugs in the investigational stage

Pathway	*Drug*	*Target*	*Effect on immune response*	*Investigational use*
CD 28/CD80–86	Lulizumab	CD28	Inhibits T cell dependent antibody responses	Phase I/II studies in renal transplant, SLE
CD 28/CD80–86	FR104	CD28	Inhibits T cell dependent antibody responses	Phase I study in renal transplant
CD 28/ CD80–86	ASP2409	CD86	Inhibits T cell dependent antibody responses	Phase I study in renal transplant
ICOS (CD278)/ ICOSL	Prezalumab (AMG 557)	ICOS-L	Impairs Tfh dependent GC formation	Phase I study in SLE, Phase II study in primary Sjögren syndrome
ICOS (CD278)/ ICOSL	MEDI-570	ICOS	Impairs T cell proliferation, impairs Tfh dependent GC formation	Phase I study in SLE
CD40/CD40L	Iscalimab (CFZ5333)	CD40	Prevents clonal proliferation of B cells as well as impairs GC reaction	Positive phase II study in kidney allograft transplantation, dose range-finding study ongoing Positive phase II study in primary Sjögren's syndrome Ongoing phase II studies in lupus nephritis and hidradenitis suppurativa Completed phase II studies in Graves' disease and myasthenia gravis
CD40/CD154	Ruplizumab (BG9588)	CD154	Blocks GC and production of high affinity antibodies	Investigated in SLE. Terminated due to life threatening thromboembolism
CD40/CD154	Dapirolizumab (CDP7657)	CD154	Blocks GC and production of high affinity antibodies	Discontinued after negative phase II study in SLE
CD40/CD154	MEDI4920	CD154	Blocks GC and production of high affinity antibodies	Completed phase I study in healthy volunteers and rheumatoid arthritis Ongoing phase II study in kidney allograft transplantation
CD40/CD154	Bleselumab (ASKP1240)	CD40	Blocks GC and production of high affinity antibodies	Negative results in phase II study in kidney allograft transplantation
CD40/CD154	Letolizumab	CD40L	Blocks GC and production of high affinity antibodies	Open-label phase II study completed in immune thrombocytopenic purpura. Ongoing phase II study in GVHD
OX40(CD134)/ OX40L	IBI101	OX40L	Agonism-source of survival signal for T cells and enables the development of memory T cells	Phase Ia/Ib Trial in advanced solid tumors

CD: Cluster of differentiation; *CTLA-4:* cytotoxic T-lymphocyte–associated antigen 4

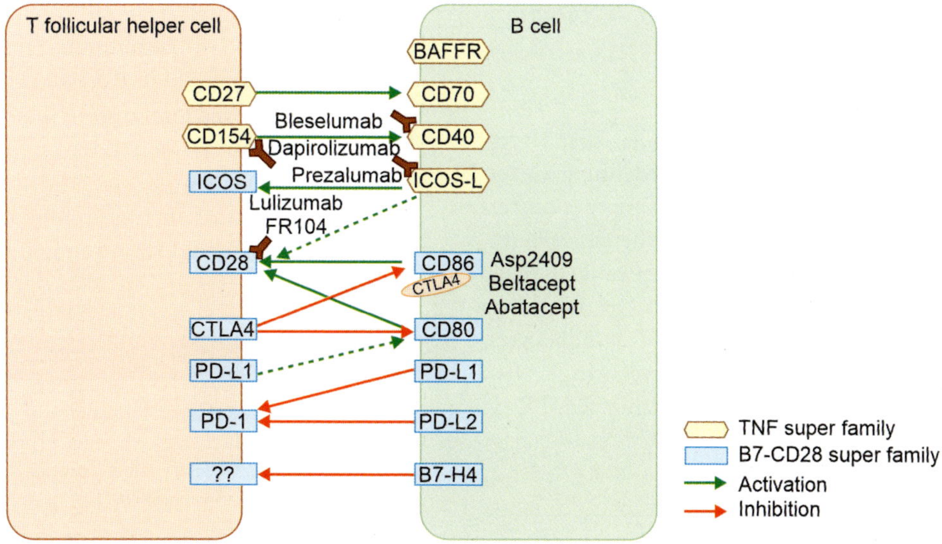

Fig. 4.12.2: Costimulation in B cells and T follicular helper (Tfh) cells. (a) To illustrate the complexity of their connections, costimulatory molecule expression and interaction patterns between T follicular helper (Tfh) and B cells are depicted. The TNF superfamily is represented by yellow molecules, while the B7 family is represented by blue molecules. Interactions that are green arrows are stimulatory, whereas those that are red are inhibitory. Some drugs that target these interactions also are shown.

BAFFR: B-cell– activating factor receptor; *BCR:* B cell receptor; CTLA-4: Cytotoxic T lymphocyte antigen-4; *ICOS:* Inducible T-cell costimulator; *ICOS-L:* ICOS ligand; *MHC:* Major histocompatibility complex; *PD-1:* Program death 1; *PD-L1:* PD-1 ligand; *TCR:* T-cell receptor.

CLINICAL IMPLICATIONS

Costimulation blockade therapy using biologicals enables precise immune response targeting while avoiding nonimmune side effects.

COSTIMULATORY BLOCKADE IN AUTOIMMUNE DISEASES

In the context of autoimmunity, CTLA4-Ig suppresses antibody responses in humans. Abatacept is a CTLA4 fusion protein made up of extracellular domain of human CTLA-4 protein and the Fc region of human IgG1 (CTLA4-Ig). Abatacept was the first CTLA4–Ig molecule to be developed, and a phase I trial in psoriasis vulgaris generated lot of interest because almost 50% patients had persistent improvement in their clinical symptoms by 50% or more. It was USFDA approved for active rheumatoid arthritis in 2005 after successful phase 3 trial. The efficacy of Abatacept has also been found in juvenile idiopathic arthritis, the majority of children exhibited a significant reduction in disease activity. Besides these indications, Abatacept has also been used with limited benefit for off-label indications and on an experimental basis in systemic sclerosis, systemic lupus erythematosus, inflammatory myositis, giant cell arteritis, Sjogren's disease, and ANCA associated vasculitis.

Organ Transplantation

Before and after transplantation, antihuman leukocyte antigen (HLA) donor-specific antibodies (DSAs) are likely to cause antibody mediated rejection (AMR) in sensitized kidney allograft recipients. The formation of donor specific antibodies (*de novo*) must be inhibited or limited in order to prevent acute/chronic AMR and thus have a successful transplant outcome.

In the past decade several drugs that block costimulation and T cell activation have been evaluated in kidney transplant recipients. Belatacept is a molecule that inhibits the interaction between the antigen CD28 and CD80/86. It is the only costimulation blocker currently approved to prevent kidney transplant rejection. When compared to calcineurin inhibitors belatacept is well tolerated and linked to improved allograft function (Table 4.12.1).

Cancer Therapy

Immune checkpoint inhibitors (ICIs) that target the CTLA4 or PD-1 pathways are redefining cancer treatment, with clinical success in a variety of cancer types. ICIs attempt to strengthen the surveillance system of anergized T cells and reawaken their anticancer and cytolytic function by blocking the inhibitory pathway between T lymphocytes and tumour cells or antigen-presenting cells. Table 4.12.1 summarizes the authorised PD-1 pathway blockers.

LEARNING POINTS

- The adaptive arm of the immune system is activated by a series of three signals.
- Currently used biologic therapy in autoimmune rheumatic diseases is based on blocking signal 3
- Costimulation (signal 2) blockade has a potential to modulate the immune system and generate regulatory immune cells, and has wide applications in autoimmunity, cancer treatment, and prevention of renal allograft rejection
- An example of application of costimulation blockade molecules in autoimmune diseases is abatacept which is useful in RA and JIA
- Belatacept is approved for the prevention of renal allorgaft rejection
- Examples of costimulation and immune checkpoint inhibitors in cancer treatment are ipilimumab that targets CTLA4 and Nivolumab that targets PD-1

FURTHER READING

1. Nakajima M, Tamada K. Cancer Immunotherapy Targeting Co-signal Molecules. In: Azuma M, Yagita H, editors. Co-signal Molecules in T Cell Activation: Immune Regulation in Health and Disease, Springer; 2019.
2. Edner NM, Carlesso G, Rush JS, et al. Targeting co-stimulatory molecules in autoimmune disease. Nat Rev Drug Discov. 2020;19:860–83.
3. van der Zwan M, Hesselink DA, van den Hoogen MWF, et al. Costimulation Blockade in Kidney Transplant Recipients. Drugs. 2020;80:33–46.
4. Leibler C, Thiolat A, Elsner RA, et al. Costimulatory blockade molecules and B-cell-mediated immune response: current knowledge and perspectives. Kidney Int. 2019; 95:774–86.

Chapter 4.13

Rituximab

Padmanabha Shenoy, Kaveri K Nalianda

INTRODUCTION

Presence of autoantibodies namely rheumatoid factor (RF) and anticitrullinated peptide antibodies (ACPA) in rheumatoid arthritis (RA) attests to the role of B cell in the pathogenesis of RA. Similarly systemic lupus erythematosus (SLE) and primary Sjögren's syndrome are both characterized by the production of antibodies against self-antigens. ANCA-associated vasculitis (AAV) also has antibodies against myeloperoxidase and proteinase-3 present inside neutrophils. ANCA also increases survival of autoreactive B-lymphocytes by causing neutrophils to release B cell activating factor (BAFF). Thus B-cell depletion with monoclonal antibodies that are directed toward the B cell receptor would lead to reduction in autoantibody titers.

MECHANISM OF ACTION

CD-20 is a nonglycosylated phosphoprotein expressed on mature B-cells but is absent in the precursor stem cells and antibody generating plasma cells. Rituximab (RTX) is a chimeric anti-CD20 monoclonal antibody comprisitng 20% murine and 80% human sequence in its protein structure. Originally developed for the treatment of B-cell non-Hodgkin's lymphoma (NHL), it has potent cell lytic properties. It is effective in the treatment of autoimmune inflammatory rheumatic diseases by modulating the immune system by many mechanisms (Table 4.13.1).

INDICATIONS

Rheumatoid Arthritis (RA)

Indications of RTX in RA

- Active severe RA with intolerance or inadequate response to one or more tumor necrosis factor alpha inhibitors (TNFi)
- First-line biologic disease modifying anti-rheumatic drug (bDMARD) in those with contraindications to TNFi.
- RA with interstitial lung disease
- RA with systemic vasculitis

Several trials (Table 4.13.2) have proven the efficacy of RTX in RA. Meta-analysis data show that RTX is more beneficial in seropositive RA as compared to seronegative.

Table 4.13.1: Mechanism of action of rituximab
Rituximab kills B cells by a combination of three possible mechanisms:
1. Complement dependent cytotoxicity (CDC)
2. Antibody-dependent cell mediated cytotoxicity (ADCC)—This is the dominant mechanism. B-cell destruction is caused by Fc-gamma receptors-bearing NK cells after the binding of rituximab to CD-20
3. Apoptosis—Cross-linking of multiple CD-20 molecules and activation of caspase3, leading to induction of apoptosis and cell death

Table 4.13.2: Summary of key clinical trials that proved the efficacy of rituximab (RTX) in rheumatoid arthritis (RA)

Trial name year	*Patient population*	*RTX dose and interval*	*Background therapy*	*Primary end point*	*Results*
DANCER 2006	*N* = 465 Inadequate responders to MTX or TNFi	Group 1: 1 g IV, 2 weeks apart Group 2: 500 mg IV, 2 weeks apart Group 3: Placebo	MTX	ACR 20 response at 24 weeks	ACR 20 response was 54%, 55%, and 28% in groups 1, 2 and 3, respectively. $P < 0.001$ Similar trend in ACR 50, 70
REFLEX 2006	*N* = 520 Incomplete responders to one or more TNF-i	Group 1: RTX 1g IV 2 weeks apart Group 2: Placebo	MTX	ACR 20 response at week 24	RTX + MTX gp: ACR20 51% Placebo + MTX: ACR20 18% $P < 0.0001$
MIRROR 2010	*N* = 378 MTX and TNFi inadequate responders	Group 1: RTX 500 mg × 2. Repeat at week 24 Group 2 : RTX 500 mg × 2. At week 24, RTX 1 g × 2 Group 3: RTX 1 g × 2 At week 24, RTX 1 g × 2	MTX and oral GC <10 mg/day	ACR 20 response at week 48	At week 48, ACR 20 responses were not statistically significant between dose regimes. ACR 50, 70 similar. Group 3: higher proportion of patients maintained clinical response to treatment at week 48
SERENE 2010	*N* = 512 Inadequate MTX responders and naïve to biologics	Group 1: RTX 500 mg × 2 Group 2: RTX 1 g × 2 Group 3: Placebo	MTX	ACR 20 response at 24 weeks	ACR 20 was 54%, 51%, and 23% respectively in groups 1,2, and 3, $p < 0.0001$ Weeks 24–48: further improvements in the RTX arms compared to placebo
IMAGE 2011	755 patients MTX naïve early RA	Group 1: MTX alone Group 2: RTX 500 mg × 2 Group 3: RTX 1 g × 2	MTX	Change in joint damage at week 52	Reduction in progression of joint damage ($p = 0.0004$) and improvement in ACR 50 (65% vs 42%; $p<0.0001$) in the RTX 1 g × 2 + MTX compared with MTX alone
ORBIT 2016	295 patients Inadequate response to csDMARDs. Naïve to biologics	Group 1: RTX 1 g × 2 and repeated after 26 weeks if DAS 28 ESR >3.2 Group 2: Adalimumab or etanercept		Change in DAS 28-ESR between 0 and 12 months	At 12 months, DAS 28 ESR –2.6 in RTX and 2.4 in TNFi group. RTX non inferior to TNFi in active RA naïve to biologics

MTX: Methotrexate; *TNFi:* Tumor necrosis alpha inhibitors; *ACR:* American College of Rheumatology; *GC:* Glucocorticoid; *DAS 28:* Disease activity score 28 joints

Dose of RTX in RA

- The usual dose of RTX in RA is 1 g at 0 and 15 days. Methotrexate (MTX) is given concomitantly.
- Recent meta-analyses show that a lower RTX dose, i.e. 500 mg × 2 is as efficacious as the standard dose of 1 g × 2.
- In the authors' experience even lower doses of RTX are effective, such that active RA (seropositive) who have failed cs-DMARDs or TNF-i were treated with a single dose of RTX 500 mg. Those who fail to show EULAR response at 6 weeks were given another 500 mg. At 6 months, 90% of patients had achieved a good to moderate EULAR response.

SLE

The indications of RTX in SLE (EULAR recommendations)

- Severe extrarenal or renal lupus
- Those who are refractory or intolerant or with contraindications to standard immunosuppressive agents and/or belimumab.

Open label and cohort studies have demonstrated RTX's efficacy in arthritis, vasculitis, cutaneous, neuropsychiatric, autoimmune hemolytic anemia (AIHA), and immune thrombocytopenia. Those patients with high anti-ds-DNA titers respond better. However, trial data, namely the EXPLORER and LUNAR trials (Table 4.13.3) showed the contrary.

AAV

RTX in AAV is beneficial both for induction and maintenance of remission. More specifically the indications are:

- As a remission induction agent in active severe GPA and MPA, especially in PR3 positive cases.
- It is also a preferred agent for remission induction in relapsing cases.
- It is also recommended as first choice therapy to maintain remission of AAV.

The RAVE and RITUXVAS trials (Table 4.13.4) demonstrated its efficacy in induction of remission, while its effectiveness to maintain remission was established in the MAINRITSAN trials (Table 4.13.5). Though patients with severe renal insufficiency and pulmonary hemorrhage were excluded in the RTX-based RCTs, RTX was effective in treating these manifestations in several uncontrolled studies.

As EGPA patients were not included in RAVE and RITUXVAS, the effectiveness of RTX in EGPA has not been evaluated in RCT, though open label studies have demonstrated its efficacy in relapsing/refractory EGPA patients. The results of an RCT comparing RTX to cyclophosphamide in EGPA (REOVAS) is awaited.

Systemic Sclerosis (SSc)

The indications of RTX in SSc are:

- Diffuse cutaneous SSc (dcSSc) to decrease skin fibrosis
- It is increasingly used in active ILD.

Primary Sjögren's Syndrome (pSS)

The indications of RTX in Sjögrens syndrome are:

- Severe systemic disease that is refractory to conventional therapies. Global response rates of 60–100% are observed in manifestations such as cryoglobulinemic vasculitis. Improvements are noted in glandular functions, arthritis, hematological, ESSDAI, and reductions in prednisolone dose.
- RTX also leads to improvement in fatigue as shown in earlier studies and the TEARS study. But the TRACTISS study (an RCT) found no significant benefit of RTX in fatigue.

Overall RTX has a stabilizing effect on dry eyes, tear production, and salivary gland function, but there is definite improvement in histology of salivary glands.

Idiopathic Inflammatory Myositis (IIM)

The indications of RTX in idiopathic inflammatory myositis are:

- Those who are refractory to standard therapy

The rituximab in myositis (RIM) trial is an RCT of RTX carried out in refractory adult polymyositis, and adult and juvenile dermatomyositis, where RTX was given either early or late against a background of immunosuppressive treatment and glucocorticoids. The primary end point that was time to achieve the International Myositis Assessment and Clinical Study preliminary definition of improvement was similar in RTX and placebo. But

Table 4.13.3: Summary of key clinical trials that examined the efficacy of rituximab (RTX) in systemic lupus erythematosus (SLE)

Study	*Population*	*RTX dose and interval*	*Background therapy*	*Primary Endpoint*	*Follow up*	*Results*
EXPLORER 2010	*N* = 257 Moderate to severe active extrarenal SLE	RTX vs Placebo RTX 1 g on days 1, 15, 168, and 182	Oral GC + MTX or AZA or MMF	Major or partial clinical response	52 weeks	No difference in primary endpoints, but a significant decrease in dsDNA level in RTX group, post hoc analysis more patients in RTX achieved low disease activity without BILAG-A flares
LUNAR 2012	*N* = 144 Class III or IV lupus nephritis	RTX vs Placebo RTX 1 g on days 1, 15, 168, and 182	Oral GC + MMF	Renal response	52 weeks	Renal response rates were similar. Declining proteinuria, glucocorticoid sparing effect and decreased necessity for rescue therapy with cyclophosphamide in RTX group. Complete depletion of B-lymphocytes following RTX was associated with greater likelihood of complete renal remission at 78 weeks
RITUXILUP 2013 Prospective observational study	*N* = 50 Class III, IV, V lupus nephritis	1 g of RTX and 500 mg methylprednisolone on days 1 and 15	No background GCs. ARBs and ACE inhibitors were given, and MMF as maintenance	Complete and partial biochemical remission	52 weeks	About 90% patients achieved complete or partial remission by a median of 37 weeks. Half the patients had achieved complete remission at week 52

GCs: Glucocorticoids; *MTX:* Methotrexate; *AZA:* Azathioprine; *MMF:* Mycophenolate mofetil

Table 4.13.4: Summary of key clinical trials that showed the efficacy of rituximab (RTX) in remission induction in ANCA-associated vasculitis (AAV)

Study	*Population*	*RTX dose and interval*	*Background therapy*	*Primary Endpoint*	*Results*
RITUXVAS 2010	*N* = 44, newly diagnosed generalised GPA/MPA with renal involvement	RTX 375 mg/m^2 IV weekly × 4 (patients also received IV CYC 15 mg/kg × 2 at weeks 0 and 3) compared to CYC 15 mg/kg IV × 3–6 months and then AZA	Standard gluco-corticoid regimen	Sustained remission rates at 12 months and severe adverse events	At 12 months sustained remission 76% in the RTX vs 82% in CYC ($p = 0.68$)
RAVE 2010	*N* = 197, newly diagnosed or severe relapsed GPA/ MPA with positive ANCA	RTX: 375 mg/m^2 IV q week × 4 compared to oral CYC: 2 mg/kg/ day × 3–6 months until remission and then AZA (2 mg/kg/day)	Glucocorticoids tapered off	Remission without the use of prednisolone at 6 months	At 6 months RTX noninferior to CYC for remission induction. RTX superior to CYC for relapsing disease and PR3-positive patients at 6 months
RAVE—long-term (2013)					At 18 months, RTX noninferior to CYC for remission (BVAS = 0)

GPA: Granulomatosis with polyangiitis; *MPA:* Microscopic polyangiitis; *CYC:* Cyclophosphamide; *AZA:* azathioprine; *ANCA:* Anti-neutrophil cytoplasmic antibodies

Table 4.13.5: Summary of key clinical trials that showed the efficacy of rituximab (RTX) in maintenance of remission in ANCA-associated vasculitis (AAV)

Study	*Population*	*Treatment*	*Primary endpoint*	*Results*
MAINRITSAN-1 (2014)	*n* = 115, newly diagnosed GPA/MPA/renal limited AAV–in complete remission after CYC–GC regimen	RTX vs AZA RTX: 500 mg IV at days 0 and 14 and then at 6, 12, and 18 months AZA: 2 mg/kg/day for 12 months, 1.5 mg/kg/day for 6 months, and then 1 mg/kg/day for 4 months (total: 22 months)	Rate of major relapse at 28 months	Fewer major relapses in the RTX group (5%) compared to AZA (29%)
MAINRITSAN-2 (2018)	*n* = 162, newly diagnosed or relapsing severe GPA or MPA in complete remission after induction therapy with RTX or CYC and GC	Fixed biannual RTX vs individually tailored regimens Fixed: 500 mg IV at days 0 and 14 and then at 6, 12, and 18 months Individualized: 500 mg IV at randomization and then reinfusion only if reappearance of ANCA or CD19 or increased titre of ANCA; measured every 3 months, until month 18	Number of relapses at month 28	AAV relapse rates did not differ significantly between individually tailored (17.3%) and fixed-schedule rituximab (9.9%) regimens
MAINRITSAN-3 (2020)	*N* = 97, newly diagnosed or relapsing severe MPA or GPA in complete remission following the completion of MAINRITSAN-2 trial and 18 months maintenance regimen	RTX vs placebo infusion every 6 months for 18 months–at inclusion , months 34, 40 and 46	Relapse free survival at month 28	Relapse-free survival rates superior with extended RTX maintenance therapy compared to standard maintenance
RITAZAREM (2019)	*n* = 170, following induction therapy with RTX + GC, maintenance therapy in relapsing GPA or MPA	RTX vs AZA RTX: 1g IV every 4 months × 5 doses AZA: 2 mg/kg/day	Time to disease relapse	RTX was found to be superior to AZA in lower relapse rates

GPA: Granulomatosus with polyangiitis; *MPA:* Microscopic polyangiitis; *CYC:* Cyclophosphamide; *AZA:* Azathioprine

83% participants had the definition of improvement by week 44. Further in those with dermatomyositis improvements of skin rashes and pulmonary functions were also observed. Open label studies and case series have also found that close to 78% refractory patients improve with RTX. Despite a lack of formal recommendations there is a general consensus among clinicians that RTX is useful in refractory IIM.

IgG4-related Disease (IgG4-RD)

Case reports and case series have reported the efficacy of RTX in the treatment of IgG4-RD. In an open label pilot trial (Carruthers 2015), 97% of participants showed a good response at 6 months, and at 1 year close to 40% remained in remission. A French multicenter study showed that RTX in IgG4-RD is effective in induction, treatment of relapse, and has steroid sparing effect.

ADVERSE EFFECTS

RTX is safe. But there is a risk of infusion related adverse effects, so it should be administered in environments where full resuscitation facilities are available. Premedicate with IV corticosteroids. Safety concerns while administering RTX is summarized in Table 4.13.6. The contraindications, use in pregnancy and lactation are summarized in Table 4.13.7.

CONCLUSION

RTX is an important therapeutic agent in autoimmune diseases.

Table 4.13.6: Adverse effects, safety considerations and practical concerns while administering rituximab

Adverse effects	*Manifestations*	*Management*
Infusion-related reactions, highest frequency in 1st infusion	Nausea, rash, hypotension, hypertension, fever, urticaria, angioedema, bronchospasm, anaphylaxis	Rituximab stopped and provided supportive care. If adverse reactions are mild, infusion can be resumed at a lower rate
Serum sickness is rare but can occur, it is immune complex mediated, usually occurs 8–13 days after the first rituximab infusion or some days after retreatment	Fever, rash, arthralgia, lymphadenopathy, hematuria, proteinuria. Can be associated with HACA (human anti chimeric antibodies). Incidence of HACA ranges from 2.7–7.1%	Short course of corticosteroids and antihistamines
Infections	Urinary tract and respiratory infections are most common. Progressive multifocal leukoencephalitis (PML) are reported. The true incidence of PML in RA treated with rituximab is uncertain and though the risk PML is considered to be small, so vigilance is advised	Appropriate antibiotic therapy is given for infection Screening for hepatitis B, C, and HIV should be carried out
Tuberculosis	No increase in frequency of TB in rituximab treated patients	Screening for tuberculosis is not currently considered necessary prior to starting rituximab
Hypogammaglobulinemia	Repeated courses of rituximab can lead to low IgM and IgG levels. Serum IgG <6 g/L prior to rituximab is associated with a higher risk of serious infections	Immunoglobulin concentrations should be quantified before and after each rituximab treatment, particularly in patients with the risk factors: Chronic lung disease, history of malignancy and older age
Malignancy	No increase in the risk of malignancy	

Table 4.13.7: Vaccination, pregnancy and lactation, and contraindications to rituximab

Vaccines	*Pregnancy*	*Lactation*	*Contraindications to rituximab*
Vaccination is given 4 weeks before or 6 months after rituximab • Annual vaccination against seasonal influenza • Pneumococcal vaccination (PCV-13 first 8 weeks later PPV-23, the latter to be given every 5 years) • Live vaccines contraindicated	Rituximab is discontinued months before conception	Though the amount secreted in breast milk is very low, it is advised to use with caution during lactation	• Active severe infection • Severe heart failure • Other significant controlled cardiac disease • Severely immunocompromised patients • Pregnancy • Preexisting hypogamma-globulinemia • Hypersensitivity to murine proteins

LEARNING POINTS

1. Rituximab is a valuable treatment agent in RA, AAV, refractory lupus, myositis, and systemic sclerosis.
2. It has a good safety profile.
3. An increased risk of infection should always be borne in mind along with the contraindications of use while initiating treatment.
4. Women in child bearing age must be counseled to take contraceptive measures while on rituximab. Pregnancy must be planned, and rituximab must be stopped 6 months before conception. In life threatening situations Rituximab can be given in the first and second trimester of pregnancy.

FURTHER READING

1. Ebbo M, Grados A, Samson M, et al. Long-term efficacy and safety of rituximab in IgG4-related disease: Data from a French nationwide study of thirty-three patients. PLoS One 2017; 12(9): e0183844.
2. Fanouriakis A, Bertsias G. Changing paradigms in the treatment of systemic lupus erythematosus. Lupus Sci Med; 2019;6,e000310.
3. Fox RI, Fox CM, Gottenberg JE, et al. Treatment of Sjögren's syndrome: current therapy and future directions. Rheumatology (Oxford). 2021; 60:2066-74.
4. Montoya GL, Villota- Eraso C, et al. Lessons for rituximab therapy in patients with rheumatoid arthritis. Lancet Rheumatol 2020; 2 (8): E497–E509.
5. Oddis CV, Reed AM, Aggarwal R, et al. Rituximab in the treatment of refractory adult and juvenile dermatomyositis and adult polymyositis: a randomized, placebo-phase trial. Arthritis Rheum. 2013;65:314–324.
6. Raffray L, Guillevin L. Rituximab treatment of ANCA-associated vasculitis. Expert Opin Biol Ther. 2020; 20:899–910.
7. Roofeh D, Lescoat A, Khanna D. Treatment for Systemic Sclerosis -associated interstitial lung disease. Curr Opin Rheumatol 2021, 33:240–8.

IL-6 Inhibitors

Sundeep Kumar Upadhyaya

INTRODUCTION

Interleukin 6 (IL-6) was discovered by Tadamitsu Kishimoto of Osaka University in 1973. IL-6 is a proinflammatory cytokine secreted by macrophages, dendritic cells, T-cells and it induces an acute phase response through the production of C-reactive protein (CRP) from the liver. IL-6 mediated inflammation is of clinical significance in rheumatoid arthritis (RA), large vessel vasculitis both Takayasu's arteritis and giant cell arteritis, in Castleman's disease, a lymphoproliferative disorder. More recently in the year 2020, IL-6 inhibition is found to have mortality benefit in the treatment of severe acute respiratory syndrome coronavirus 2 (SARS-Cov2) disease 2019 (COVID-19).

MECHANISM OF ACTION

IL-6 signaling occurs through its IL-6 receptor (IL-6R). The IL-6R has a cytokine-binding chain and a signal transducing chain (gp-130). Binding of IL-6 to its receptor leads to formation of a complex hexameric complex of IL-6 receptor (IL-6R), gp 130, and IL-6, with downstream activation of the JAK-STAT-3 pathway, and is a major contributor to the inflammation (Fig. 4.14.1).

Inhibition of IL-6 activity can be achieved either by blocking its receptor IL-6R or by directly blocking IL-6. Monoclonal antibodies that block IL-6R are tocilizumab and sarilumab. While siltuxizumab and clazakizumab are monoclonal antibodies to IL-6. Table 4.14.1 gives a summary of monoclonal antibodies to IL-6R and IL-6.

INDICATIONS

IL-6 Inhibitors in Rheumatoid Arthritis (RA)

Large randomized controlled trials have demonstrated that tocilizumab is effective and safe in RA that is refractory to csDMARDs. In such patients, it leads to significant reduction in symptoms, signs, improvement in laboratory parameters, health-related quality of life, and functional improvements. Tocilizumab also leads to retardation of radiographic progression much more when compared to adalimumab. It is also approved for treatment of early treatment naive RA with or without methotrexate.

One advantage of tocilizumab is it can be given as monotherapy, when there is contraindication to methotrexate. Sarilumab, another monoclonal to IL-6R, is also effective and safe in RA.

Monoclonal antibodies to IL-6 namely sirukumab, olokizumab and clazakizumab, have undergone trials in RA, of which sirukumab and olokizumab have shown therapeutic benefits, but trials for clazakizumab are terminated.

IL-6 Inhibitors in Juvenile Idiopathic Arthritis (JIA) and Adult Onset Still's Disease (AOSD)

IL-6 has a prominent role in systemic onset JIA (SoJIA). Many of SoJIA's clinical features such as spiking fevers, anemia, high inflammatory markers, joint destruction, and growth retardation are explained by high IL-6 levels. Tocilizumab is successfully employed for treatment of SoJIA, and results in resolution of symptoms and signs, with the

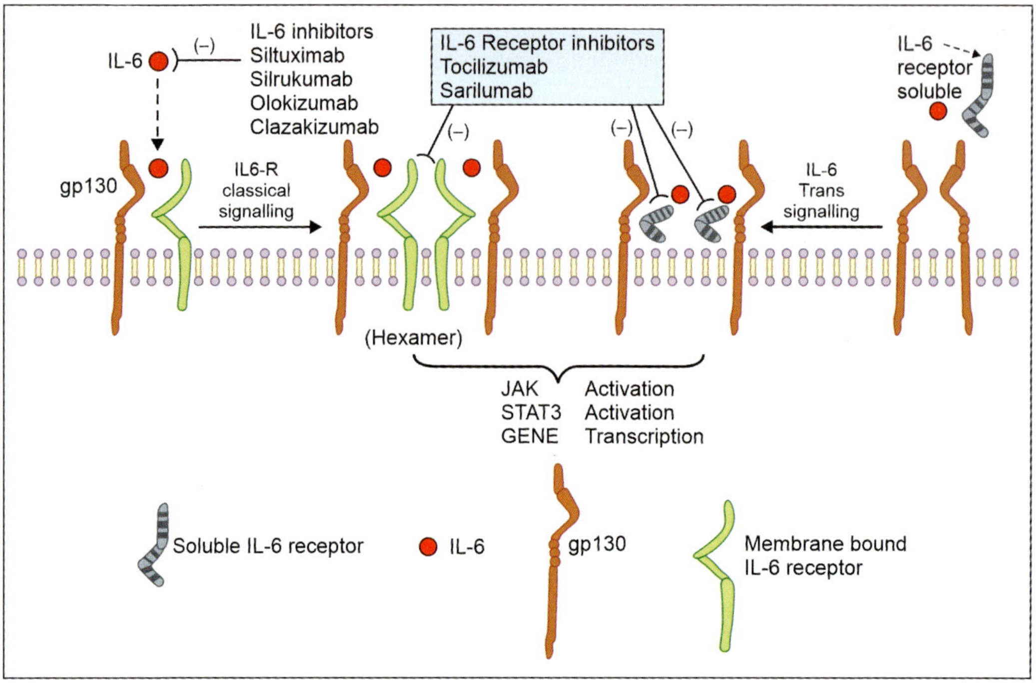

Fig. 4.14.1: IL-6 signaling: IL-6 can activate transcription through two mechanisms. The first is the classical signaling where IL-6 directly engages with membrane bound IL-6 receptor, which is mostly found on immune cells. This signaling is mostly for immune-regulation and is protective. The second mechanism is through the binding of IL-6 to the proteolytically cleaved, free soluble IL-6 receptor, also called the trans signaling. The trans-signaling is responsible for the proinflammatory effects all across body tissues and is pathogenic for RA and other diseases discussed in the text.

Both mechanisms involve the engagement of IL-6 bound to the IL-receptor (membrane or soluble) with gp130 (glycoprotein 130). The complex of IL-6, IL-6 receptor and GP 130 dimerizes to form a hexamer, which through JAK and then STAT activation, induces gene transcription. It is believed that the selective inhibition of soluble IL-6 receptor will have greater anti-inflammatory effect and less of immune-dysregulation.

Table 4.14.1: A summary of monoclonal antibodies (Mab) directed against Interleukin- 6 receptor (IL-6R) and IL-6

Name of Mab	*FDA approved indication*	*Remarks*	*Dose*
Mab that target IL-6 receptor			
Tocilizumab	Rheumatoid arthritis Systemic sclerosis associated ILD Giant cell arteritis (GCA) Takayasu arteritis (TAK) Polyarticular JIA Systemic onset JIA (SoJIA) Cytokine release syndrome (CRS)	Tocilizumab is one biologic DMARD that can be used as monotherapy in RA. In GCA, TAK, SoJIA, and adult onset Still's disease it has good glucocorticoid sparing effect	8 mg/kg every 4 weeks IV 162 mg every week SC if >100 kg, 162 mg every 2 weeks SC if <100 kg
Sarilumab	Rheumatoid arthritis	Limited efficacy in SLE, ankylosing spondylitis, Crohn's Disease. Tried in SARS-CoV2 disease	200 mg every 2 weeks SC

(Contd.)

Table 4.14.1: A summary of monoclonal antibodies (Mab) directed against Interleukin- 6 receptor (IL-6R) and IL-6 *(Contd.)*

Name of Mab	*FDA approved indication*	*Remarks*	*Dose*
Mab that target IL-6			
Sirukumab	None	Phase 3 trial shows efficacy in RA	50 mg every 4 weeks SC Or 100 mg every 2 weeks SC
Olokizumab	None	Phase 3 trial shows efficacy in RA	64 mg every 2–4 weeks SC
Clazakizumab	None	Phase 3 trial ongoing for late ABMR kidney transplant Tried in psoriatic arthritis, non-small cell lung cancer, head and neck cancer	25 mg every 4 weeks SC
Siltuximab	HIV-negative and HHV-8 negative multicentric Castleman's disease	Failed in multiple myeloma. Clinical trials ongoing for COVID-19	11 mg/kg IV every 3 weeks

ABMR: Antibody-mediated rejection; *CRS:* Cytokine release syndrome; *FDA:* Food and Drug Administration; *HIV:* Human immunodeficiency virus; *HHV-8:* Human herpesvirus 8; *IL:* Interleukin; *ILD:* Interstitial lung disease; *IV:* Intravenous; *JIA:* Juvenile idiopathic arthritis; *RA:* Rheumatoid arthritis; *SC:* Subcutaneous

added advantage of steroid sparing effect. Sarilumab is tried in SoJIA and polyarticular JIA as well.

Similarly tocilizumab is a useful agent in the management of AOSD (with predominant chronic arthritis). It has a steroid sparing effect. It is increasingly recognized that AOSD with chronic articular form responds well to tocilizumab, while the systemic predominant form responds to IL-1 inhibition (anakinra).

IL-6 Inhibitors in Large Vessel Vasculitis

Takayasu's arteritis (TAK) and giant cell arteritis (GCA) are large vessel vasculitis where IL-6 inhibition is effective. The conventional treatment for TAK is glucocorticoids and methotrexate or cyclophosphamide. However about one fourth do not respond to conventional treatment. In such refractory cases intravenous tocilizumab has been shown to lead to clinical remission in as many as 70% as defined by improvements in ESR, CRP, and decrease in the Indian Takayasu Activity Score (ITAS), with an impressive glucocorticoid sparing effect.

Similarly in GCA, the giant cell arteritis actemra (GiACTA) trial showed that tocilizumab 162 mg subcutaneous injection every week for a duration of 1 year combined with glucocorticoid taper has been shown to lead to clinical remission and significant glucocorticoid sparing effect. It has also been shown that tocilizumab leads to a drug free remission in a sizable number of patients on a two year-follow-up.

IL-6 Inhibitors in Systemic Lupus Erythematosus (SLE)

Initial studies in 2011 have shown that tocilizumab improved arthritis and reduced antibody levels in SLE patients, but further trials with sirukimab failed, hence further studies have not been done.

IL-6 Inhibitors in Systemic Sclerosis (SSc)

Earlier reports showed that tocilizumab leads to reduction in skin thickening. But an adequately powered RCT that evaluated tocilizumab in SSc with disease duration <60 months found that skin scores did not change significantly between tocilizumab and placebo group. However, lung functions seem to remain stable and did not worsen. In this trial, the dose of tocilizumab was 162 mg given subcutaneously every week for 48 weeks.

IL-6 Inhibitors in

Tocilizumab is FDA approved for treatment of CRS caused by chimeric antigen receptor T-cell infusion.

A much newer indication is in treatment of severe COVID-19. Highly elevated IL-6 and CRP signifies hyperinflammation and CRS in COVID-19.

Tocilizumab has been shown in multiple observational studies to have a mortality benefit in moderate to severe COVID-19. In these observational studies, the typical indication for tocilizumab in COVID-19 would be a patient with moderate disease, i.e. on oxygen therapy of at least 3 L/minute, or severe disease ie on mechanical ventilation, and also those patients at high risk to progression of CRS defined as having high CRP. However, it is the REMAP-CAP trial that showed that critically ill patients in the intensive care unit who within 24 hours of organ support received tocilizumab had a significantly higher number of organ support free days, and higher 90-day survival period. The dose of tocilizumab in COVID-19 is 8 mg/kg as a single dose up to a maximum of 800 mg given by intravenous infusion.

IL-6 Inhibitors in Castleman Disease

Multicentric Castleman disease is a lymphoproliferative disorder that is characterised by hyperinflammation and hypercytokinemia. Clinically the presentation is with lymphadenopathy, fever, anemia, hepatomegaly, splenomegaly, high CRP, low albumin, high IL-6 levels etc with a characteristic histological picture in the lymph node. It is caused by human herpesvirus 8 (HHV8) and HIV or can be idiopathic. Both tocilizumab and siltuximab are preferred biological agents to treat idiopathic multicentric Castleman disease.

ADVERSE EFFECTS

From clinical trials data, we know that the tocilizumab is safe; most adverse events are mild and moderate. In the AMBITION trial, most common adverse effects with tocilizumab as compared to methotrexate are skin and soft tissue infections (34% vs 37%), transaminitis <3 times upper limit of normal (1% vs 2.5%), hypercholesterolemia (13% vs 0.4%), and transient neutropenia (3% vs 0.4%). Gastrointestinal symptoms were also equal, and no increased risk of perforation. Having a monitoring plan (Table 4.14.2) will help detect complications earlier.

Table 4.14.2: Monitoring a patient who is on tocilizumab

Liver function tests: AST and ALT are monitored every month for the first six months. If AST or ALT >5 times upper limit of normal (ULN), stop tocilizumab till transaminitis resolves. If AST or ALT between 3 to 5 times, withhold further infusions. If <3 times, continue as usual
Complete blood counts: Every month for the first months. Stop tocilizumab if there is neutropenia
Lipid profile: Hypercholestrolemia is a common occurrence. Statins are usually not indicated, unless there are cardiovascular indications
Skin and soft tissue infections: Infection risks are not greater when compared to anti-TNF users. Use tocilizumab cautiously in diabetics, elderly, and whenever there is a higher risk of having skin and soft tissue infections. Tuberculosis is not seen to occur among tocilizumab users, as compared to anti-TNF users

LEARNING POINTS

1. IL-6 inhibition is vital for control of disordered uncontrolled inflammation and damage.
2. IL-6 inhibition is important in the management of RA, large-vessel vasculitis, SoJIA, polyarticular JIA, AOSD.
3. Newer indications are cytokine release syndrome due to COVID-19, and CAR-T cell immunotherapy as well as in some cancers and transplant scenarios.

FURTHER READING

1. Choy EH, De Benedetti F, Takeuchi T, et al. Translating IL-6 biology into effective treatments. Nat Rev Rheumatol. 2020;16:335–45.
2. Hata H, Sakaguchi N, Yoshitomi H, et al. Distinct contribution of TNF alpha, IL-6 and IL-1 to spontaneous T-cell mediated autoimmune arthritis in mice. J Clin Invest. 2004;114:582–8.
3. REMAP-CAP Investigators, Gordon AC, Mouncey PR, et al. Interleukin-6 Receptor Antagonists in Critically Ill Patients with COVID-19. N Engl J Med. 2021; 384:1491–502.
4. Sasai M, Saeki Y, Ohshima S, et al. Delayed onset and reduced severity of collagen-induced arthritis in interleukin-6-deficient mice. Arthritis Rheum. 1999; 42:1635–43.
5. Tanaka T, Narazaki M, Kishimoto T. IL-6 in inflammation, immunity, and disease. Cold Spring Harb Perspect Biol. 2014 Sep 4;6(10):a016295. doi: 10.1101/cshperspect.a016295.

IL-17/23 Inhibitors

Neha Arora, Sumeet Agrawal

INTRODUCTION

Interleukin (IL) 17 and IL-23 are proinflammatory cytokines that are involved in the pathogenesis of psoriasis, psoriatic arthritis (PsA), and axial spondyloarthritis (axSpA). The pathogenesis of psoriasis and PsA (Fig. 4.15.1) involves a combination of genetic and environmental triggers (Table 4.15.1).

IL-17 AND IL-23 IN PSORIASIS AND SpA

There is good evidence to show that IL-17 is a driver of inflammation in psoriasis and PsA. Levels of IL-17 are markedly increased in synovial fluid of patients with PsA, IL-17 is over expressed in skin of patients with psoriasis. In axSpA patients, IL-17 is found to be increased in subchondral biopsy samples. Moreover misfolding of HLA-B27 in SpA also can trigger and activate the IL-17/23 pathway.

IL-17 causes stimulation of osteoclastogenesis, chondrocyte activation, fibrogenesis, angiogenesis, stimulation of proinflammatory cytokines and

Table 4.15.1: Triggers for psoriatic arthritis

Genetic	*Environmental*
HLA-B13	Physical trauma
HLA-B17	Infection
HLA-B57	Obesity
HLA CW*0602	Smoking
HLAB08	

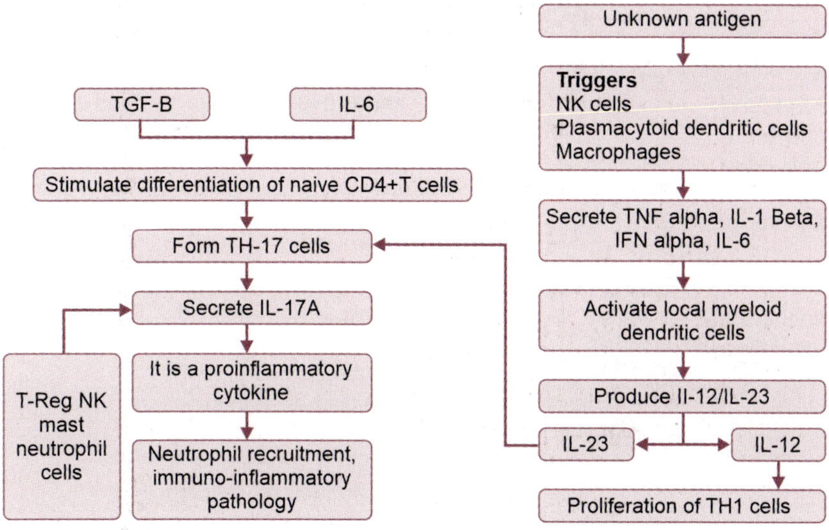

Fig. 4.15.1: IL-17/23 in the pathogenesis of psoriasis

metallomatrix proteinases (MMP) production leading to joint inflammation and damage.

The main cells that produce 1L-17 are the Th17 subset of the CD4+ T cell, gamma-delta T cells, CD8+ T cells, and innate lymphoid cells (ILCs). The various isoforms of IL-17 include 1L-17A, IL-17E, IL-17F, IL-17C. Differentiation of Th17 T cells is sustained by upstream IL-23.

IL-17 INHIBITORS

Indications

Both IL-17 and IL-23 inhibitors are effective therapeutic targets in psoriasis and PsA, but in SpA only IL-17 inhibitors are found to be effective for reasons yet unclear. The IL-17 inhibitors that are in clinical use are secukinumab, ixekizumab, brodalumab and bimekizumab (Table 4.15.2).

Table 4.15.2: IL-17 inhibitors: Indications, dose, and adverse effects

Monoclonal antibody	*Indications*	*Dose*	*Adverse effect*
Secukinumab Human IgG1k anti-IL-17A monoclonal antibody	PsA. Moderate-to-severe plaque psoriasis. Radiographic axial SpA or ankylosing spondylitis intolerant or not responding to TNF inhibitors	PsA: 150 mg (subcutaneous) at 0, 1, 2, 3 and 4 weeks, followed by monthly. Psoriasis: The initial dose is 300 mg (subcutaneous injection) at 0, 1, 2, 3 and 4 weeks, followed by 300 mg monthly. Ankylosing spondylitis: 150 mg every four weeks, with or without loading dose	Nasopharyngitis, diarrhea, upper respiratory tract infection (URTI). Serious adverse events are rare
Ixekizumab Humanized IgG4 anti-IL-17A monoclonal antibody	Radiographic axial SpA/ ankylosing spondylitis, non-radiographic SpA not responding to NSAIDs or intolerant to TNF inhibitors or not responding to TNF inhibitors. Moderate-to-severe plaque psoriasis.	160 mg at week 0, followed by 80 mg subcutaneous injection at weeks 2, 4, 6, 8, 10 and 12 and then 80 mg every 4 weeks thereafter. Administered alone or in combination with a conventional DMARD	Nasopharyngitis, candidal infection can occur. Serious adverse events are rare
Brodalumab Human IgG2 IL-17A receptor antagonist monoclonal antibody, block's activity of IL-17A, 17A/F, 17E	PsA	140 or 210 mg subcutaneous every 2 weeks	Nasopharyngitis, URTI, and injection site erythema. Neutropenia, candidal infection, depression and suicide have been reported in trials
Bimekizumab Humanized monoclonal antibody directed toward IL-17A and IL-17F	Tried for moderate to severe plaque psoriasis, PsA, and ankylosing spondylitis, hidrenadenitis supparativa	320 mg at weeks 0 and 4, followed at week 16 by bimekizumab 320 mg results in greater skin clearance than secukinumab. PsA 160 mg (with or without 320 mg loading dose) every 4 weeks	Nasopharyngitis, oral candidiasis, URTI are observed

PsA: Psoriatic arthritis; *SpA:* spondyloarthritis

PsA: Overall they improve peripheral arthritis, enthesitis, dactylitis, and inhibit progression of radiographic damage. Improve psoriasis disease activity. Their efficacy in PsA is comparable to TNF inhibitors.

Psoriasis: Their efficacy in psoriasis is greater than that of TNF inhibitors.

AxSpA: They are effective in axSpA/ankylosing spondylitis, but ineffective or minimally effective in rheumatoid arthritis (RA) and inflammatory bowel disease (IBD) and even worsening of uveitis and flare in IBD.

Other IL-17 Inhibitors are netakimab. Clinical trials are underway to evaluate efficacy in ankylosing spondylitis. Anti-IL-17A/F nanobody or MSB-0010841 or sonelokimab is a novel drug candidate targeting IL-17. Also promising and in the pipeline is the dual anti-IL-17 and TNFα inhibitors. Fynomers are small binding proteins whose fusion to antibodies allows production of fully human anti-TNF and anti-IL-17A antibodies. One such clinical stage product inhibiting both TNF and IL-17 is FynomAb COVA 322

Adverse Effects

Secukinumab can cause nasopharyngitis, diarrhea, upper respiratory tract infection (URTI). Adverse events with brodalumab is nasopharyngitis, URTI, and injection site erythema. Others like neutropenia, candidal infection, depression and suicide have been reported in trials.

IL-23 INHIBITORS

Indications

The IL-23 inhibitors are guselkumab, tildrakizumab, risankizumab, ustekinumab, and mirikizumab (Table 4.15.3). In psoriasis, guselkumab, tildrakizumab, rizankizumab, ustekinumab, and more recently mirikizumab are all effective. In inflammatory bowel disease ustekinumab is effective in Crohn's disease.

Adverse Effects

Tildrakizumab: Most vcommon adverse effects are nasopharyngitis and headache.

Table 4.15.3: IL-23 inhibitors: Indications, dose, and adverse effects

Monoclonal antibody	*Indication*	*Dose*	*Adverse effects*
Ustekinumab Human IgG1k monoclonal antibody against p40 subunit of IL12 and IL-23	PsA, plaque psoriasis, Crohn's disease, ulcerative colitis	PsA: 45 mg subcutaneous at weeks 0 and 4, then every 12 weeks	Nasopharyngitis, diarrhea, depression, injection site erythema
Guselkumab Human monoclonal antibody against P19 subunit of IL-23	PsA, plaque psoriasis	100 mg subcutaneous at weeks 0 and 4 then every 8 weeks	Infections, upper respiratory tract infections (URTI)
Tildrakizumab Humanized monoclonal antibody targeting P19 subunit of IL-23	Plaque psoriasis	200 mg subcutaneous at weeks 0 and 4 then every 12 weeks	URTI, injection site reactions, headache
Risankizumab Humanized monoclonal antibody targeting P19 subunit of IL-23	Plaque psoriasis, PsA. Awaiting approval for Crohn's disease and ulcerative colitis	180 mg subcutaneous at weeks 0, 4, and then every 12 weeks	URTI, nasopharyngitis, and headache
Mirikizumab Humanized monoclonal IgG4 antibody against p19 subunit of Il-23.	Currently in Phase III trials for ulcerative colitis		

PsA: Psoriatic arthritis

Table 4.15.4: Key differences between IL-17 and IL-23 inhibitors

IL-17 inhibitors	*IL-23 inhibitors*
1. More effective quickly, with 50% reduction in PASI scores as early as 1.8 weeks	1. Take months to reach their peak efficacy
2. Require more frequent injection, maintenance treatment as often as 2–4 weeks	2. Require injections as infrequently as every 3 months
3. Slow down radiographic progression of joint disease	3. Finding not yet shown by IL-23 Ab
4. IL-17 blockade can exacerbate Crohn's disease	4. IL-23 blockade can improve Crohn's disease

Table 4.15.5: Role of IL-17 inhibitors beyond psoriasis, psoriatic arthritis, and axial spondyloarthritis

Preclinical data indicate efficacy in:

- Oral lichen planus
- Alopecia areata
- Pyoderma gangrenosum
- Palmoplantar pustulosis
- Systemic lupus erythematosus
- Systemic sclerosis
- Mixed connective tissue disease
- Pemphigus vulgaris
- Pemphigoid
- Dermatitis herpetiformis
- Atopic dermatitis
- Chronic periodontitis

Risankizumab: Common adverse effects are non-dose dependent URTI, nasopharyngitis and headache.

There are some differences between IL-17 and IL-23 inhibitors (Table 4.15.4) in terms of onset of action, dosing schedule. One important clinical difference is that IL-23 inhibitors are ineffective in axSpA, but are effective in IBD. On the other hand, IL-17inhibitors are effective in axSpA, but they exacerbate uveitis and causes flare of IBD.

Apart from psoriasis, PsA, and axSpA inhibitors of the IL-17/23 axis might also be useful in other inflammatory, autoimmune conditions as listed in Table 4.15.5. To conclude IL-17/23 inhibitors are effective, safe new therapeutic options in psoriasis, PsA, and axSpA.

LEARNING POINTS

1. IL-17/23 axis has a prominent role in the pathogenesis of psoriasis, PsA, SpA, IBD and rheumatoid arthritis.
2. The IL-17/23 inhibitors have revolutionized management of psoriasis with an achievement of psoriasis area severity index (PASI) 90–100.
3. In psoriasis ixekizumab, brodalumab, and risankizumab are more effective as compared to ustekinumab.
4. IL-17 inhibitors are very effective in axial SpA/ ankylosing spondylitis, whereas IL-23 blockade is ineffective.
5. Il-17 inhibitors exacerbate uveitis and inflammation in IBD, whereas IL-23 is found to be effective.
6. IL-17/23 blockade is ineffective in RA.

FURTHER READING

1. Fauny M, Moulin D, D'Amico F, et al. Paradoxical gastrointestinal effects of interleukin-17 blockers. Ann Rheum Dis. 2020;79:1132–8.
2. Kirkham BW, Kavanaugh A, Reich K. Interleukin-17A: a unique pathway in immune-mediated diseases: psoriasis, psoriatic arthritis and rheumatoid arthritis. Immunology. 2014;141:133–42.
3. Raychaudhuri SK, Saxena A, Raychaudhuri SP. Role of IL-17 in the pathogenesis of psoriatic arthritis and axial spondyloarthritis. Clin Rheumatol. 2015;34:1019–23.
4. Sbidian E, Chaimani A, Garcia-Doval I, et al. Systemic pharmacological treatments for chronic plaque psoriasis: a network meta-analysis. Cochrane Database Syst Rev. 2017;12(12):CD011535.

Janus Kinase Inhibitors

Rohini Handa

INTRODUCTION

Targeted treatments have transformed the therapeutic landscape of rheumatology. In contrast to conventional disease-modifying antirheumatic drugs (DMARDs), these agents target specific cytokines, receptors, cells or intracellular pathways (Fig. 4.16.1). Janus kinase (JAK) initially named "just another kinase" were one of the several kinases discovered in a PCR-based screening. JAK is a family of intracellular tyrosine kinases that possess two near-identical phosphate-transferring domains. One domain exhibits the kinase activity, while the other catalytically inactive pseudo-kinase domain negatively regulates the kinase activity of the first. This led to their renaming as Janus kinase in reference to the two-faced Roman god of gateways. Cytokines on binding to their receptors lead to activation of JAKs which phosphorylate the receptors, thereby signaling pathways especially the signal transducer and activator of transcription (STAT) family are activated. Therefore, the JAK inhibitors by interfering with cytokine-induced signal transduction pathways and are able to inhibit a host of inflammatory cascade that so characterises many inflammatory and immune mediated diseases.

How Do JAK Inhibitors Differ from Biologics?

JAK inhibitors are small molecules, orally administered. The salient differences from biologics are spelt out in Table 4.16.1.

JAK INHIBITORS IN RHEUMATOLOGY

As of date, five JAK inhibitors are approved for use in rheumatology (Table 4.16.2). It is to be noted that not all drugs are approved in all countries. Except for tofacitinib and upadacitinib, the current approval for JAK inhibitors in rheumatology is for rheumatoid arthritis (RA).

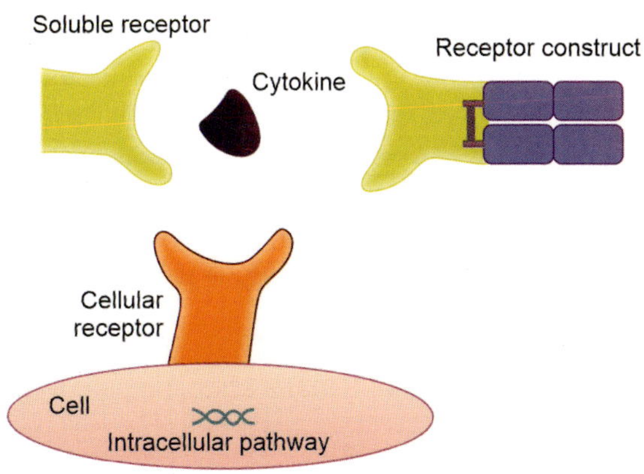

Cytokines	• Infliximab, adalimumab, golimumab, secukinumab, ixekizumab
Receptor constructs	• Etanercept, rilonacept
Receptor	• Tocilizumab, anakinra, brodalumab
Cells	• Rituximab
Intracellular pathways	• JAK inhibitors, apremilast

Fig. 4.16.1: Targeted treatments: Agents and targets

Table 4.16.1: Differences between biologics and JAK inhibitors

Properties	*Biologics*	*JAK inhibitors*
Structure	Complex proteins	Small molecules with a simple structure
Target	Extracellular	Intracellular
Manufacturing process	Requires living systems such as a microorganism, or animal cells and recombinant DNA technology	Chemical synthesis
Cost of manufacture	High	Low
Immunogenicity	Major concern. Can cause adverse effects and attrition of therapeutic response	Absent
Storage	Cold chain required	No special requirements
Administration	Parenteral	Oral
Term used for copy molecules	Biosimilars	Generics
Demonstrating equivalence to reference product	Complex, multi-step process that requires rigorous analytical characterization, animal studies, human pharmacologic and immunogenicity data, and clinical trials. The process defines the product	Bioequivalence is demonstrated through relatively simple analyzes such as blood level testing. Human clinical trials not required

Table 4.16.2: Approved JAK inhibitors and indications

Tofacitinib	→	RA, PsA, UC, polyarticular JIA (>2 years)
Baricitinib	→	RA
Upadacitinib	→	RA, non-radiographic axial SpA and AS
Filgotinib*	→	RA
Peficitinib**	→	RA

*Filgotinib is approved by EMA and PMDA Japan. Not approved by FDA

**Peficitinib is approved by PMDA Japan and not by EMA and FDA

FDA: Food and Drug Administration, *USA:* EMA: European medicines agency; *PMDA:* Pharmaceuticals and Medical Devices Agency, Japan.

RA: Rheumatoid arthritis; *PsA:* Psoriatic arthritis; *UC:* Ulcerative colitis; *JIA:* Juvenile idiopathic arthritis; *SpA:* spondyloarthritis; *AS:* ankylosing spondylitis

INDICATIONS OF JAK INHIBITORS

Rheumatoid Arthritis

In general, JAK inhibitors are indicated in moderately to severely active RA who have had an inadequate response to methotrexate or are intolerant to methotrexate. While clinical trials have included methotrexate naïve patients, current guidelines and recommendations do not recommend first line use in treatment-naïve patients. JAK inhibitors can be used alone (monotherapy) or in combination with methotrexate or with other nonbiologic DMARDs. Combinations of JAK inhibitors or combination with biologic DMARDs is not recommended. Similarly, it is not recommended to use a JAK inhibitor in combination with other immunosuppressive agents such as azathioprine and cyclosporine for fear of profound immunosuppression. JAK inhibitors can be combined with corticosteroids.

Psoriatic Arthritis (PsA)

Of the various JAK inhibitors, only tofacitinib is approved for the treatment of adult patients with active PsA who have had an inadequate response or intolerance to methotrexate or other DMARDs. Of note, tofacitinib despite its approval in PsA and benefit in skin clearing, is still not approved for psoriasis.

Polyarticular Juvenile Idiopathic Arthritis (PolyJIA)

Tofacitinib oral solution or tablets are indicated in children with active polyJIA who are 2 years and older.

Other Immunoinflammatory Conditions

Tofacitinib in higher doses (10 mg twice daily or 22 mg once daily) is approved for treatment of adult patients with moderately to severely active ulcerative colitis (UC) who have had an inadequate response or lost response or were intolerant or to conventional therapy or a biologic agent. After the induction phase of 8 (maximum 16) weeks, the maintenance dose recommended is 5 mg twice daily or 11 mg once daily. For those patients with loss of response during maintenance treatment, the dose of 10 mg twice daily or 22 mg once daily may be considered and limited to the shortest duration. The lowest effective dose needed to maintain response is continued. JAKinibs are also being tried in other conditions like ankylosing spondylitis, lupus, Crohn's disease, etc. Topical JAK inhibitors are being trialled in psoriasis, atopic dermatitis, alopecia areata, and vitiligo. The use of JAK inhibitors like ruxolitinib for polycythemia vera, myelofibrosis, etc. is beyond the scope of this article.

JAK SELECTIVITY

Tofacitinib mainly inhibits JAK1 and JAK3 while inhibiting JAK-2 to a lesser degree. Baricitinib inhibits JAK 1 and 2. Filgotinib and upadacitinib are JAK 1 inhibitors while peficitinib is a pan JAK inhibitor. Selectivity for JAK1 drives efficacy in RA while inhibition of JAK2 and JAK3 may contribute to adverse events. JAK selectivity is determined by the ratio and difference between IC50s (concentration needed to inhibit 50% of activation) for different JAK isoforms. A low IC50 value implies higher potency. However, JAK isoform selectivity of JAKinibs is relative since it is dose and tissue dependent. At the present there is no evidence one JAK inhibitor is safer or more efficacious clinically, functionally or structurally than another JAK inhibitor.

HOW TO INITIATE AND MONITOR JAK INHIBITORS?

Like all targeted treatments, initiation of JAK inhibitors requires clinical examination, complete blood counts, renal function tests, liver enzymes, baseline lipid levels, and screening to rule out hepatitis B, hepatitis C, and tuberculosis. Where appropriate, HIV screening should be carried out. Ideally, vaccinations like pneumococcal, influenza, etc. should be completed before the start of treatment. Monitoring entails measurement of full blood count, renal function, and aminotransferases at one and three months. Subsequent monitoring every 3–4 months or earlier is dictated by the patient's clinical condition.

Drug Interactions and Dose Adjustments in Renal/Hepatic Disease

Tofacitinib is metabolised in the liver by cytochrome P (CYP) 450. Rifampicin increases hepatic metabolism of tofacitinib and upadacitinib that may require a dose increase of these JAKinibs, a point that assumes importance in RA patients being treated for latent or active tuberculosis. Concomitant ketoconazole reduces tofacitinib and upadacitinib metabolism necessitating a dose reduction. Baricitinib is 70% renally excreted while filgotinib, upadacitinib and peficitinib are metabolised by the liver primarily (Table 4.16.3). JAK inhibitors should not be used in patients with advanced liver disease (Child–Pugh C). Similarly, in those with severe renal disease, i.e. creatinine clearance (CrCl) <30 mL/min tofacitinib requires a reduction in dose to 5 mg once daily. The dose of baricitinib is reduced to 2 mg daily if the CrCl is between 30 and 60 mL/min. Baricitinib is not recommended if CrCl is <30 mL/min. Dosage reduction is currently not recommended for filgotinib, peficitinib and upadacitinib in renal disease.

ADVERSE EFFECTS

The safety profile of JAK inhibitors compares with the biologic drugs used for immune-mediated inflammatory diseases. The data is gleaned from extension studies of RA cohorts. It is unclear if the adverse events in different diseases will differ.

Laboratory pertubations during treatment with tofacitinib, the most well studied JAKinib, include increase in hemoglobin, decrease in neutrophils, lymphocytes, and platelets, as well as increased transaminases and serum creatinine levels. These abnormalities are generally mild and reversible. Neutropenia and lymphopenia are class effects. Baricitinib, peficitinib and upadacitinib may have a greater decrease in hemoglobin levels because of the effect of on JAK2. However, this is dose-dependent

Table 4.16.3: JAK inhibitors: Fact file for clinicians

Agent	*JAKs targeted*	*Usual oral dose*	*Use in hepatic and renal impairment*	*Some key trials*
Tofacitinib	JAK1, JAK2, JAK3	5 mg BD or 11 mg ER OD	Metabolism by kidney 30% and liver 70%. Reduce dose in patients with moderate liver dysfunction or severe renal impairment	ORAL-Solo, Scan, Standard, Step, Sync, Start, Strategy, Sequel
Baricitinib	JAK1, JAK2	2–4 mg OD	Renal elimination principal clearance mechanism. Less than 10% undergoes hepatic metabolism. No dose adjustment necessary in mild or moderate hepatic impairment. Do not use in patients with severe hepatic impairment or patients with CrCl <30 mL/min	RA-BEGIN, BUILD, BEAM, BALANCE, BEYOND, BEACON
Upadacitinib	JAK1	15 mg OD	No dose adjustment is required in patients with mild, moderate or severe renal impairment. No dose adjustment is required in patients with mild (Child–Pugh A) or moderate (Child–Pugh B) hepatic impairment. Not recommended for use in patients with severe hepatic impairment (Child–Pugh C)	SELECT-BEYOND, NEXT, Monotherapy, CHOICE, COMPARE, EARLY
Filgotinib	JAK1	200 mg OD	No dose adjustment required in mild renal impairment (creatinine clearance [CrCl] ≥ 60 mL/min). A dose of 100 mg of filgotinib once daily is recommended for patients with moderate or severe renal impairment (CrCl 15 to <60 mL/min). No dose adjustment is required in mild or moderate hepatic impairment (Child–Pugh A or B). Not studied in severe hepatic impairment (Child–Pugh C). Do not use in these patients	FINCH 1–4, DARWIN 1–3
Peficitinib	JAK1, JAK2, JAK3 and Tyk 2	100–150 mg OD	Metabolism mainly hepatic. Reduce dose in moderate liver dysfunction	RAJ-1-4, RA 21, 22, 25

JAK: Janus kinase; *OD:* Once daily; *BD:* twice daily; *ER:* Extended release

and rarely clinically significant. The effect of filgotinib on hemoglobin is similar to tofacitinib.

Opportunistic infections, including tuberculosis, represent the most critical adverse events. The incidence rate for severe infections with JAK inhibitors is approximately 2.5–3.8 per 100 patient-years. There is a higher risk of herpes zoster especially in Japanese and Korean patients in comparison to biologics. Zoster reactivation rates are 9 in Japan and South Korea, 3–4 in western Europe and USA per 100 patient-years compared with 2–3 per 100 patient-years for anti-TNFs. Zoster reactivation is a class effect of JAK1 inhibitors. One plausible explanation is the downregulation of interferons and IL-15 responsible for viral elimination. The zoster is generally mild and limited to a single dermatome. Of note, filgotinib clinical trials did not show increased zoster. However, large registry data and real-world experience is awaited. As with biologics, the frequency of TB parallels the background prevalence in the country. The overall risk of malignancy is not increased, other than non-melanoma skin cancer (NMSC). The risk of NMSC may be increased necessitating regular dermatologic screening in countries like Australia which have increased NMSC risk.

Increase in LDL and HDL levels are observed in the first few months which stabilise subsequently. The LDL: HDL cholesterol ratio remains stable without an apparent increase in major adverse cardiovascular events (MACE). The tofacitinib dose approved for RA (5 mg twice daily dose) has not been associated with an increased risk of thrombosis (venous thromboembolism/pulmonary embolism [VTE/PE]). The FDA in 2019 added a boxed warning for the 10 mg twice-daily dose that is approved for UC. The ORAL Surveillance study, a post-marketing safety study, evaluated the safety of tofacitinib (5 mg twice daily and 10 mg twice daily) versus a TNF inhibitor in 4,362 patients with RA aged ≥50 years with at least one additional cardiovascular risk factor. The study failed to meet its co-primary endpoints, i.e. non-inferiority of tofacitinib compared to a TNF inhibitor with regards to cardiovascular events and cancer. The secondary end points such as pulmonary embolism, mortality, etc. are not yet available. A recent meta-analysis of VTE risk with JAK inhibitors did not provide evidence that VTE risk for JAK inhibitors are increased.

Filgotinib was approved in September 2020 for medical use in Japan and the European Union. However, FDA approval was withheld due to reports of testicular toxicity and reduced sperm count. Studies evaluating testicular safety of filgotinib in men with IBD (the MANTA study), and in men with active RA, ankylosing spondylitis, nonradiographic axial spondyloarthritis, and PsA (the MANTA-RAy study) are ongoing.

Pregnancy, Breastfeeding, and Fatherhood

JAKinibs are contraindicated during pregnancy and breastfeeding. It is recommended to discontinue the dose at least four weeks before contemplating pregnancy. Men and women in the reproductive age group using JAKinibs should use effective contraception.

GENERICS OF JAK INHIBITORS

The availability of tofacitinib generics in India is a double-edged sword. On one hand we have expanded access to an important drug. On the other hand, injudicious use as first-line agents and without appropriate screening is fraught with serious consequences.

CONCLUSION

JAK inhibitors represent a novel class of drugs for immunoinflammatory rheumatic diseases. The advent of new agents in this group is likely to change the existing treatment paradigms. Better understanding of the molecular basis of JAK/STAT inhibition, well designed clinical trials, long-term extension studies, real world registry data, rigorous post-marketing surveillance, and robust regulatory oversight are needed in equal measure to harness the full potential of these drugs.

LEARNING POINTS

1. JAK inhibitors are targeted treatments that block the JAK/STAT pathway which is important in the pathogenesis of many immune-mediated diseases.
2. Being small molecules, they are orally administered, easy to manufacture and store, and circumvent the immunogenicity encountered in case of biologics.
3. JAK inhibitors are approved for use in RA. Some agents like tofacitinib are approved for use in PsA, polyarticular JIA, and ulcerative colitis. Newer agents and additional indications are likely in the future.
4. JAK inhibitors may be used as monotherapy or in combination with methotrexate/other conventional synthetic DMARDs, and corticosteroids.
5. Current consensus does not recommend use in methotrexate naïve patients.
6. JAK inhibitors should not be combined with biologic DMARDs.
7. Increased risk of herpes zoster is seen with JAK inhibitors.
8. Venous thromboembolism may be a concern with JAK inhibitors in higher doses.

FURTHER READING

1. Kerschbaumer A, Smolen JS, Nash P, et al. Points to consider for the treatment of immune-mediated inflammatory diseases with Janus kinase inhibitors: a systematic literature research. RMD Open 2020;6:e001374. doi:10.1136/rmdopen-2020-001374.
2. Nash P, Kerschbaumer A, Dörner T, et al. Points to consider for the treatment of immune-mediated inflammatory diseases with Janus kinase inhibitors: a consensus statement. Ann Rheum Dis. 2021;80:71–87.
3. Yates M, Mootoo A, Adas M, et al. Venous Thromboembolism Risk With JAK Inhibitors: A Meta-Analysis. Arthritis Rheumatol. 2021;73:779-88.

Chapter 4.17

Intravenous Immunoglobulins and Plasma Exchange in Rheumatic Diseases

Anna C Das, Chengappa KG, Vir Singh Negi

INTRAVENOUS IMMUNOGLOBULINS

Introduction

Intravenous immunoglobulin (IVIg) therapeutic preparations are derived from pooled plasma of several thousand (15,000–60,000) healthy individuals using cold alcohol fractionation, polyethene glycol precipitation and ion-exchange chromatography followed by viral inactivation/ elimination. The immunoglobulin contents of IVIg are similar to that found in normal plasma, with IgG1 being the predominant subclass. It contains antibodies with a wide range of specificities against various infectious agents, autoantigens, and autoantibodies. Therapeutic immunoglobulin preparations are available in subcutaneous and intramuscular formulations.

Mechanism of Action and Properties

Since IVIg comprises pooled immunoglobulins, it can target both cellular elements (innate and adaptive immune cells, endothelial cells) and soluble factors (cytokines, chemokines, complements and pathogenic antibodies) of the immune system. The precise mechanism of therapeutic benefit in each of the indications depends on the cells and signaling pathways unique to the disease and the dosage of IVIg administered. In general, the action of IVIg can be understood under two broad headings: immunomodulatory and replacement actions.

In immunomodulatory doses, the predominant action is Fc and F(ab')2 mediated (Fig. 4.17.1). For replacement doses in primary immunodeficiency diseases (PID) or secondary immunoglobulin deficiency, the mechanism of action is to provide sufficient levels of functional antibodies to prevent infections. Since IVIg is a blood product, the World Health Organization (WHO) has set specific quality standards for its production:

- IVIg should be a concentrate extracted from the plasma of a minimum of 1,000 healthy donors
- It should be clear on visual inspection
- Have a pH of 4–6 and osmolality >240 mosmol/kg
- The total protein concentration should be >30 g/L with a polyvalent globulin content of >95% and <3% immune aggregates
- Should have passed viral marker test, bacterial sterility test and endotoxin assay
- Should be free of IgG anti-iso-hemagglutinins (anti-A, anti-B IgG antibodies)

Clinical Indications

The approved indications for IVIg includes replacement therapy in primary and secondary immunodeficiencies and immunomodulatory therapy in autoimmune diseases such as immune thrombocytopenia, Kawasaki disease, autoimmune demyelinating neuropathies, inflammatory myositis, systemic lupus erythematosus (SLE) and antineutrophil cytoplasmic antibody (ANCA) associated vasculitis (Table 4.17.1). In addition to these, IVIg has also been used with potential benefit in toxic epidermal necrolysis (TEN) and Stevens-Johnson syndrome (SJS).

Adverse Events

Adverse reactions to IVIg are related to the rate of infusion, presence of infective contaminants

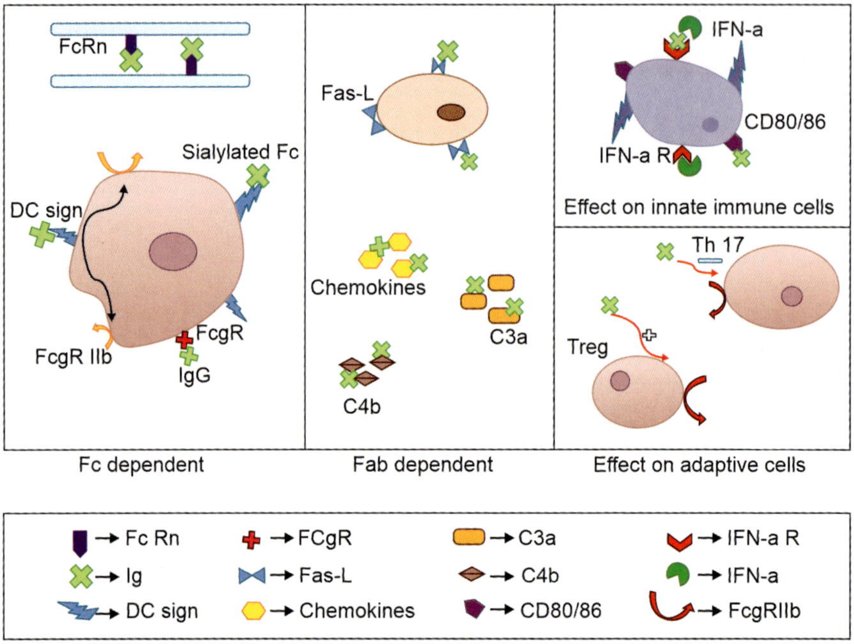

Fc dependent actions include:

1. Blocking FcγR on phagocytic cells—prevents ingestion and depletion of antibody-coated cells (e.g. ITP, AIDP).
2. Saturation of FcRn—IVIg produces a state of hypergammaglobulinemia, accelerating the catabolism of pathogenic IgG (e.g. APS, myasthenic crisis).

F(ab')2 dependent actions include:

1. Neutralization of cytokines.
2. Blocking anti-idiotypic antibodies against toxins and superantigens (e.g. toxic shock syndrome), dsDNA/histone BCRs (SLE).
3. Binding to complement components (C3b, C4b, MAC) and preventing attachment to tissue targets (e.g. dermatomyositis).
4. Blockade of Fas ligand mediated apoptosis by anti-Fas antibodies (e.g. toxic epidermal necrolysis).

Effect on immune cells:

Innate immune cells:

1. Inhibits type I interferon mediated differentiation of dendritic cells (e.g. SLE).
2. Induces inhibitory FcγRIIB on effector macrophages (sialylated CH2 domain binding to CLR on dendritic cells).
3. Downregulates costimulatory molecules on dendritic cells.

Adaptive immune cells:

1. Expansion of Treg cells (multiple sclerosis).
2. Inhibition of Th17 cells (dermatomyositis).

Fig. 4.17.1: Mechanism of action of IVIg

FcRn: Neonatal Fc Receptor; *Ig:* Immunoglobulins; *DC sign:* Dendritic cell-specific intercellular adhesion molecule-3 grabbing non-integrin; *FcgR:* Fc gamma Receptor; *Fas-L:* Fas ligand; *IFN-a:* Interferon alpha; *IFN-aR:* Interferon alpha Receptor; *Treg:* T regulatory cells.

and concentration of lyophilized components. Headache is the most common rate related side effect (5–20%). The stabilizers used in IVIg preparation may worsen preexisting conditions. For instance, maltose and glucose as stabilizers can cause hyperglycemia and worsen blood glucose

Table 4.17.1: Indications for intravenous/ subcutaneous immunoglobulins in diseases with autoimmune basis

Therapeutic modality	*Disease*	*Dosage*	*Special considerations*
IVIg	Immune thrombocytopenia	Children: 0.8–1 g/kg Adults: 1 g/kg as one time dose	
	Kawasaki disease	2 g/kg (to repeat if relapses within 48 hours)	To be given within 10 days of onset of fever
	Dermatomyositis (steroid-resistant/aggressive)	2 g/kg over 2–3 days	In steroid-resistant or refractory JDM Currently approved for use in adults with dermatomyositis
	AIDP	0.4 g/kg/day over 5 days	Start within 2 weeks for severe disease Risk of thromboembolism with daily dose >35 g
	CIDP	0.4 g/kg/day over 5 days	Repeat every 2–8 weeks Preferred in children
	Systemic vasculitis (ANCA associated vasculitis)	0.5 g/kg/d × 4 days/ month–6 months	In relapsed disease to prevent further relapses
	Catastrophic antiphospholipid antibody syndrome	2 g/kg given after last sitting of TPE	In combination with TPE and immunosuppressive agents
	SLE	2 g/kg over 4–5 days	Myocarditis, polyneuropathy, bone marrow suppression, multiorgan disease
	Myasthenia gravis	0.4 g/kg/d × 4–5 days	Moderate-severe disease within two weeks Myasthenic crisis Juvenile myasthenia Preoperative
	Multiple sclerosis	0.15–0.2 g/kg monthly	To reduce pregnancy/postpartum relapses
	Immunodeficiency disorders. 1. Agammaglobulinemia due to absent B cells. 2. Hypogammaglobulinemia with poor antibody function. 3. IgG subclass deficiency with recurrent infections. 4. Post B cell depletion therapy-induced hypogammaglobulinemia.	0.4–0.6 g/kg month	Maintain trough IgG levels at 0.8–1 mg/dL. Aim for a dose that prevents recurrent infections
SCIg	Immunodeficiency disorders	100–200 mg/kg per week-for newly started	Maintenance Ig infusion: IV to SC conversion: Multiply total monthly dose of IVIg × 1.37 for 16% preparations. X 1.53 for 20% formulation. Divide by total injections to be given each month

IVIg: Intravenous immunoglobulin; *JDM:* Juvenile dermatomyositis; *AIDP:* Acute inflammatory demyelinating polyneuropathy; *CIDP:* Chronic inflammatory demyelinating polyneuropathy; *TPE:* Therapeutic plasma exchange; *SLE:* Systemic lupus erythematosus; *ANCA:* Antineutrophil cytoplasmic antibodies

levels. Sodium and albumin content and the use of sucrose stabilizers can precipitate cardiac and renal failure.

All the adverse events of IV and SCIg, risk factors and preventive measures are summarized in Table 4.17.2.

Table 4.17.2: Adverse effects of intravenous immunoglobulins (IVIg) and subcutaneous immunoglobulins (SCIg)

Adverse events	*Risk factor*	*Manifestation*	*Mechanisms*	*Prevention and treatment strategies*
		IVIg		
Inflammatory reactions	Fast infusion rate Allergic or anaphylactic reactions IgA deficiency	Mild reactions* Moderate reactions‡ Severe reactions§	Anaphylactoid reactions Immune complex formation Anti-complement activity Fc receptormediated release of prostaglandins, platelet-activating factor, and cytokines from macrophages and leukocytes Vasoactive contaminants Development of anti-IgA antibodies that react with the IgA molecules in the IVIg preparation	Slow infusion rate as per body weight Product substitution Prophylactic steroids Antihistamines, or anti-inflammatory agents (not very useful) Cautious use of IVIg containing low levels of IgA
Thromboembolic events	Age >60 years High dose Fast infusion rate Hypertension Coronary heart disease Type 1 diabetes Hyperlipidemia	Coronary artery disease Transient ischemic attack Stroke Peripheral thromboembolism	Hyperviscosity Contamination with clotting factors Vasospasm Formation of platelet–leukocyte aggregates	Slower infusion rate Prophylaxis Early treatment of high-risk patients
Renal complications	Age >60 years Type 1 diabetes Renal disease Sepsis Paraproteinemia Nephrotoxic agents Stabilizers in IVIg (sucrose, maltose, glucose)	Acute renal failure Mild alteration in renal function	Osmotic injury	Adequate hydration Use of correct dose Periodic monitoring of renal function Use of sugar-free stabilizers

(*Contd.*)

Table 4.17.2: Adverse effects of intravenous immunoglobulins (IVIg) and subcutaneous immunoglobulins (SCIg) *(Contd.)*

Adverse events	*Risk factor*	*Manifestation*	*Mechanisms*	*Prevention and treatment strategies*
IVIg				
Hemolysis	High dose Blood group other than O Multiparous women	Intravascular hemolysis	Passive transfer of ABO isohemagglutinins to non-O blood group patients Underlying inflammatory state	Blood type cross-matching Determination of anti-A and anti-B antibody titer before infusion Posttransfusion testing for hemolysis within 36 hours
Acute meningeal inflammation	Fast infusion rate History of migraine Single high dose of IVIg	Aseptic meningitis	Release of inflammatory cytokines Presence of ANCA-like immunoglobulins	Anti-inflammatory agents
SCIg				
Local reactions	Initiation of SCIg therapy	Swelling, redness, and itching or burning sensation Headache, vomiting, pain, and fatigue	Local irritant effect	Symptomatic management Monitoring to ensure no long-term changes such as fat necrosis or fibrosis

*Mild reactions include headache, fever, chills, nausea, emesis, hypotension and muscle cramps.

‡Moderate reactions include worsening of mild reactions necessitating discontinuation of the infusion.

§Severe reactions include persistence or worsening of moderate reactions or appearance of new symptoms such as tightness of the throat or chest (anaphylaxis), severe chills and rigour, breathlessness, dizziness, fainting or collapse.

ANCA: Antineutrophil cytoplasmic antibody; *IVIg:* Intravenous immunoglobulin; *SCIg:* Subcutaneous immunoglobulin.

Contraindications

Though IVIg is safe, in certain situations it can precipitate life-threatening complications. Some of the contraindications to the use of IVIg are as follows:

- Selective IgA deficiency: This can result in anaphylaxis due to the presence of anti-IgA-IgE antibodies. Consider switching to SCIg in such individuals.
- History of anaphylaxis during previous infusions.
- Creatinine clearance of <10 mL/min will result in volume overload.
- Known cases of hyperviscosity syndromes due to the risk of thromboembolic events.

Dosage and Administration

IVIg products come in solution with concentrations ranging from 5 to 12%. The dose is 1–2 g/kg

Table 4.17.3: Infusion rates for IVIg in pediatric and adult patients

	IVIg 5–6%	*IVIg 10–12%*
Pediatrics	0–15 minutes 0.5 mL/kg/hour 15–45 minutes 1 mL/kg/hour 45–75 minutes 2 mL/kg/hour Remainder of infusion 4 mL/kg/hour	0–15 minutes 0.25 mL/kg/hour 15–45 minutes 0.5 mL/kg/hour 45–75 minutes 1 mL/kg/hour Remainder of infusion 2 mL/kg/hour
Adults (infusion rate is independent of total dose/ volume/ concentration)	10 mL/hour for 10 min 20 mL/hour for 20 min 50 mL/hour for 20 min 100 mL/hour for 1 hour 200 mL/hour until the infusion is completed	10 mL/hour for 10 min 20 mL/hour for 20 min 50 mL/hour for 20 min 100 mL/hour for 1 hour 200 mL/hour until the infusion is completed

divided over 4–5 days (400 mg/kg/day) for immunomodulatory indications and 400–600 mg/kg every 3–4 weeks for maintenance in PID. The recommended infusion rates are given in Table 4.17.3.

Premedication, as mentioned below, may be required for those receiving IVIg for the first time and those who had experienced headache, flushing or fever during initial infusions.

- Acetaminophen: up to 1 g P/O.
- Ibuprofen: up to 800 mg P/O.
- Diphenhydramine: 1 mg/kg P/O, IV or IM.
- Hydrocortisone: 100 mg IV.
- Prehydration with 0.9% saline 10–20 mL/kg in patients with thrombotic risk such as those with paraproteinemia.

THERAPEUTIC PLASMA EXCHANGE

Introduction

Plasma is the liquid part of the blood which constitutes 55% of total blood volume and comprises water (95%), serum proteins (6–8%), along with solutes like nutrients, gases and metabolic wastes (1%). Its function is to transport proteins, electrolytes, hormones, growth factors, nitrogenous waste products, and maintain blood pressure. Therapeutic plasma exchange (TPE) is a procedure that is used in emergent life-threatening conditions where the plasma component of an individual is wholly replaced to achieve rapid stabilization of disease.

Mechanism of Action and Procedure

By altogether exchanging the plasma of an individual with a physiologically similar component, TPE is expected to temporarily remove the immune complexes and cytokines responsible for the disease.

There are two steps in plasmapheresis: (Fig. 4.17.2)

1. Cell separation—using a centrifugation-based cell separator.
2. Membrane filtration—passage of plasma water, molecules, and proteins across a semipermeable membrane. Standard plasma filters allow molecules of 15–980 kDa to pass-through.

Most plasma exchange protocols remove 2–4 L (30–40 mL/kg = 1 plasma volume) of plasma over a 2–3-hour period. The fluid volume usually exchanged in each TPE session is 100–150% of the patient's plasma volume. Each 1–1.5 plasma volume exchange removes 60–70% of pathogenic antibodies or immune complexes in plasma.

Indications

There are four category definitions for therapeutic plasma exchange provided by the American Society for Apheresis:

- Category I: Apheresis is first-line therapy alone or with other modes.
- Category II: Apheresis is second line alone or with other modes.
- Category III: Optimum role of apheresis is not established.
- Category IV: Apheresis is ineffective or harmful.

Rheumatological indications (Category I and II) for TPE are summarized in Table 4.17.4. Plasma exchange is used in conjunction with corticosteroids

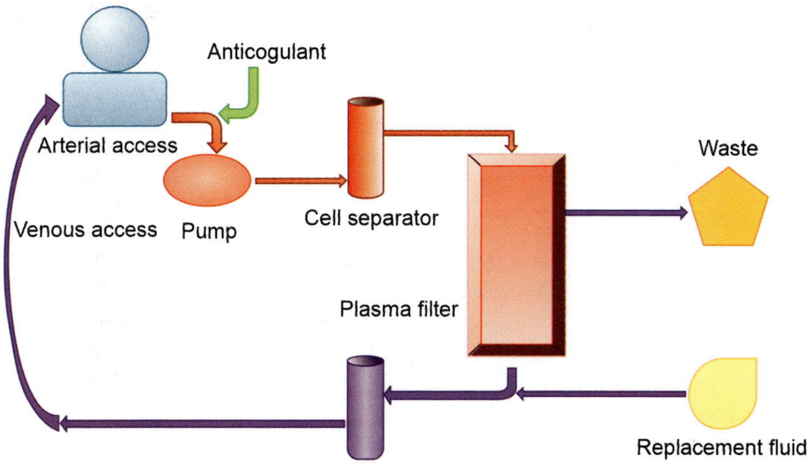

- In TPE, the patients' blood is passed through a cell separator, separating plasma from cellular components.
- The separated plasma is discarded and is replaced with equal volumes of either a colloid (albumin and/or fresh frozen plasma) or a combination of crystalloid-colloid solution.
- Cellular components are reinfused into the patient along with the replacement fluid.

Fig. 4.17.2: Procedure of therapeutic plasma exchange

and/or cytotoxic therapy to reduce the risk of rebound flare. One volume exchange removes 55–65% of pathological factors; a second exchange will remove a further 20–25% and a third exchanges an additional 10%. The target is to reduce the pathological factors to <10% of their pretreatment concentration.

Precautions

Certain drugs like mycophenolate, when given <4 hours before TPE, rituximab (<12 hours), and cyclophosphamide (<24 hours), can be removed by TPE. Hence, enough time between the administration of these drugs and scheduling TPE must be planned. Baseline blood counts, electrolytes (calcium, magnesium, potassium), clotting parameters and hematocrit must be checked.

Plasma exchange with albumin or saline causes a transient fall in blood clotting factors and mild prolongation of prothrombin and activated partial thromboplastin times, which recovers in 4–24 hours. Factor VIII, IX and VWF return to baseline in 4 hours, whereas fibrinogen takes 72 hours to return to 65% of baseline. To reduce the risk of bleeding, 1–2 units of fresh frozen plasma must be a part of the replacement solution.

Adverse Events

- Bleeding tendency—monitor INR/aPTT
- Hypogammaglobulinemia—IVIg 0.4 g/kg single dose can be given.
- Hypotension
- Hypoglycemia
- Hypothermia
- Hypocalcemia
- Fluid overload
- Allergic/anaphylactic reactions.
- Metabolic alkalosis (FFP replacement)
- Metabolic acidosis (albumin replacement)

The benefits and harms of TPE depend on the timing of the procedure with respect to the onset of illness, the volume of fluid exchanged, type of replacement solution and frequency of plasma removal. The technique induces significant immunosuppression by removing circulating immune factors. Hence, TPE should be judiciously used only when the benefits outweigh the risks of the procedure.

Table 4.17.4: Indications for therapeutic plasma exchange in diseases with autoimmune basis

Therapeutic modality	*Disease*	*Dosage*	*Special considerations*
Therapeutic plasma exchange (TPE)	Thrombotic thrombocytopenic purpura associated with rheumatic diseases	150% PV daily until Platelet count >1.5 lakh/mm^3 for >2 days	FFP better than albumin SD-FFP is preferable Rituximab 375 mg/m^2 after TPE session
	Catastrophic antiphospholipid syndrome	150% PV daily–6 exchanges over 10–15 days	Anticoagulation + pulse MP before TPE IVIg immediately after TPE (Days 2, 6, 10)
	SLE—Diffuse alveolar hemorrhage (DAH), NPSLE with coma, TTP	150% PV daily–5 exchanges over 10 days	Steroids/Rituximab/IV CYC after TPE
	ANCA associated vasculitis–DAH, rapidly progressive crescentic glomerulonephritis	100% PV–7 exchanges over 10 days	Pulse MP prior to TPE, IV CYC after TPE
	Antiglomerular basement membrane disease	100% PV–10 exchanges over 14 days	Pulse MP prior to TPE, IV CYC after TPE
	Cryoglobulinemic vasculitis	100% PV–5 exchanges over 10 days	Pulse MP prior to TPE, IV CYC after TPE
	Demyelinating polyneuropathies	100% PV daily initially–5 exchanges	IV CYC 1 g/m^2 after TPE
	Myasthenia gravis	100% PV daily /alternate days × 5	TPE better than IVIg in MuSK–MG
	Severe cold agglutinin autoimmune hemolytic anemia	100% PV daily initially–5 exchanges	Albumin replacement is recommended

TPE: Therapeutic plasma exchange; *SLE:* Systemic lupus erythematosus; *PV:* Plasma volume; *FFP:* Fresh frozen plasma; *SD-FFP:* Single donor fresh frozen plasma; *MP:* Methylprednisolone; *DAH:* Diffuse alveolar hemorrhage; *NPSLE:* Neuropsychiatric systemic lupus erythematosus; *TTP:* Thrombotic thrombocytopenic purpura; *ANCA:* Antineutrophil cytoplasmic antibodies; *IV CYC:* Intravenous cyclophosphamide; *MuSK-MG:* Muscle-specific kinase-myasthenia gravis

LEARNING POINTS

1. Commercial immunoglobulin preparations are made from the pooled plasma of minimum 1,000 healthy donors with an immunoglobulin composition similar to that of normal human plasma.
2. It has immunomodulatory and replacement action; the former affecting cellular, humoral and cytokine elements of the immune system.
3. It can cause local and systemic adverse effects which needs to be monitored during and after administration.
4. Plasma exchange is an immunosuppressive technique where the entire plasma of the subject is removed to achieve rapid reduction in circulating immune complexes.
5. TPE aims to achieve reduction of pathological factors to <10% of their pre treatment concentration.

FURTHER READING

1. Bayry J, Negi VS, Kaveri SV. Intravenous immunoglobulin therapy in rheumatic diseases. Nat Rev Rheumatol. 2011; 7:349–59.
2. Perez EE, Orange JS, Bonilla F, et al. Update on the use of immunoglobulin in human disease: A review of evidence. J Allergy Clin Immunol. 2017; 139(3, Supplement):S1–46.
3. Padmanabhan A, Connelly-Smith L, Aqui N, et al. Guidelines on the Use of Therapeutic Apheresis in Clinical Practice–Evidence-Based Approach from the Writing Committee of the American Society for Apheresis: The Eighth Special Issue. J Clin Apheresis. 2019; 34:171–354.

Section

V

DISEASE OUTCOME MEASURES

Chapter 5.1

Outcome Measures in Rheumatologic Disorders: Introduction and General Principles

Sapan Pandya

INTRODUCTION

Some of the fundamental problems with chronic diseases as in rheumatology are a poorly understood natural disease course, difficulties in differentiating disease flares from infections, activity from damage, and higher stakes due to costly intervention (e.g. biologics), and financial constraints (considering life-long therapies). Individual healthcare providers would have their own experiences, coupled with patient heterogeneity, different brands, socio-economic issues, habits of patients, and their own core competence–these are innumerable variables that could affect the decision of choice as regards which is better–the old or the new?

Therefore *outcome assessment is the measurement of these in a standardized and validated manner—the way by which consequences of diseases and health care management decisions are evaluated.* Process measures include histological, biochemical, or imaging procedures whereas outcome measures reflect the suffering or loss of health experienced by patients as a consequence of the disease.

Outcome measures (OM) can also be divided into two categories–observer dependent (rated by the evaluator e.g. swollen joint count, tender joint count, grip strength etc) or observer independent (self reported, e.g. visual analogue scales VAS for pain, global disease, etc.) OR qualitative/quantitative.

What are The Domains? What is a 'Filter'?

A simple definition of an outcome measure domain is an attribute that patients feel is important and can be measured. The next question is what is to be measured? The OMERACT's (Outcome Measures in Rheumatoid arthritis Clinical Trials) initial definition of the core domains relied on the Fries's paradigm (5Ds–Death, Disability, Discomfort, Drug, and Dollar). Put simply, they define disease consequences in terms of mortality or survivorship and morbidity or impact of disease, and the symptom severity on health-related quality of life. The PROMIS (Patient Reported Outcome Measurement Information Systems Initiative) is an NIH initiative using computer adaptive testing to question patients where answers to initial questioning give rise to subsequent questions.

There are some common attributes that an outcome measure must meet. These are ethicality (risk involved must be weighed against any new information that would be gained), validity (measures what it is supposed to measure), reliability (measure yields same result on repeated usage), and responsiveness (detects minimal change). Each of the domains must go through the three filters of truth, discrimination, and feasibility. The last one includes harmful effects of drugs also.

What are the Common Outcome Measures that Should be Included in Clinical Trials ?

Disease specific outcome measures would differ but there are common ones that need to be assessed, e.g. pain, disability, handicap etc. Organizations like the OMERACT, ACR, IMMPACT (Initiative on Methods, Measurement and Pain Assessment in Clinical Trials) have come out with consensus on the core sets, domains, instruments, and responder criteria to be included in trials. Over the last decade, with the advent of EHR (Electronic Health Records), patient responses to PROMS are being captured in an electronic format.

Pain can be measured in terms of Likert scale, visual analog scale (VAS), ladder scale, chromatic continuous scale, pain face scale etc but VAS is by far the one most commonly used. Other domains are *impairment*, e.g. swollen and tender joint count; *disability* can be physical, social or emotional, e.g. HAQ, WOMAC, hand grip; *handicap*, e.g. Disease Repercussion Profile; *global assessments*—both patients' and physicians. One has to mention what is being gauged—overall disease or symptom and also the time frame–last one week or one month. The physician or evaluator's global assessment generally has greater insight into disease status due to available lab tests, imaging results, etc. Psychosocial issues—Depression can be measured using validated scales like the Beck depression inventory–depression contributes to pain and has to be differentiated from inflammatory pain. Fatigue and sleep—using validated fatigue scales and sleep scales eg Pittsburgh Sleep Quality Index. These are patient-reported scales which are easier to perform in rheumatology patients than sleep studies due to difficult ambulation in many.

Composite indices like DAS28 in RA are useful to assess disease activity at that point of time and takes into consideration patient related, evaluator related, and laboratory parameters of the patient.

Treatment related OM like adverse reactions are very relevant to drug trials. Systems like COSTART and WHOARD grade adverse effects as none, possible, probable and definite. Concomitant therapy: rescue therapy, pill counts, keeping a diary, etc. self management interventions: psychoeducational–patients are taught to learn to self manage, and economic issues: both direct, e.g. labs, imaging, consultations etc and indirect–work loss have also been included in the list for drug trials. The *patients' perspective* is gaining more and more importance over the years, e.g. fatigue was listed into the list of outcome measures only after the involvement of patients.

What are the Problems Unique to our Country in Relation to Applying Outcome Measures?

These could be both patient related and healthcare worker related. The former include issues like lack of education to understand these, different languages (need to be validated in each), cultural inability to interpret health status into a number, lack of willingness to do so due to more urgent priorities, economic constraints making it irrelevant to measure, very few patient advocacy groups, etc. The latter includes lack of willingness, lack of time in a busy OPD, lack of trained manpower for the same, inability to put down health status into a number, only a few into international collaborations, etc.

Possible solutions could be—representation of Indian patients/ patient groups in the ethics committees and international workshops, adaptations of the OM to suit our needs and as per our socio-economic milieu, short less time consuming questionnaires to be validated since the burden is huge and using Likert scale more often that our patients are able to use.

LEARNING POINTS

- We should be using outcome measures in our clinics, so as to be more objective in our assessments and remove subjective biases.
- To convert narratives into scales so that we can not only know how individual patients respond longitudinally and we could plan 'treat to target' in them but also compare populations in clinical trials as well as real life where it actually matters.
- However all outcome measures may not be applicable in our settings because of language and cultural barriers.
- But many outcome measures are useful, for example, the CDAI and DAS28 in rheumatoid arthritis. These tools help us monitor disease and damage, and adjust treatment.

FURTHER READING

1. Boers M, Beaton D, Shea B, et al. OMERACT Filter 2.1: Elaboration of the conceptual framework for outcome measure in health intervention studies. J Rheumatol 2019:46:1021–7.
2. Boers M, Brooks P, Strand CV, et al. The OMERACT filter for outcome measures in Rheumatology. J Rheumatol. 1998;25:198–9.
3. Bombardier C, Tugwell P, Sinclair, et al. Preferences for endpoint measures in clinical trials: result of structured workshops. J Rheumatol. 1982;9:798–801.
4. Kirwan J, Minnock P, Adebajo A, et al. Patient Perspective Workshop: fatigue as a recommended patient-centred outcome measure in rheumatoid arthritis. J Rheumatol. 2007 34:1174–77.
5. Ravindran V. Rheumatology outcome measures in principle and practice in India: So near and yet so far. Indian J Rheumatol. 2013;8:8–10.

Outcome Measures in Rheumatoid Arthritis

S Kartik, Abhishek Kumar

INTRODUCTION

Rheumatoid arthritis (RA) is systemic autoimmune disease characterized by synovitis and deforming erosive arthritis in untreated patients. In addition to symmetrical polyarthritis, a host of extra-articular manifestations also affect the individual's daily function that in turns affects the quality of life. So, a comprehensive disease burden estimation in RA also entails assessment of function and quality of life apart from measuring the number of joints that are affected, global assessment of the disease both by physician and patient, and inflammatory markers. In RA pain is typically measured with a visual analogue scale (VAS). Thus, outcome measures in RA are in three domains:

1. Disease activity
2. Radiographic damage
3. Health status.

DISEASE ACTIVITY

The key components of a basic assessment of RA disease activity take into account the following.

Joint count: A patient's swollen and tender joints reflect active disease. Hence, counting the number of swollen joints (SJC) and tender joints (TJC) are used for assessing RA disease activity. It is standard practice to assess only 28-joints that includes both hands proximal interphalangeal (PIP), metacarpophalangeal (MCP), both wrists, elbows, shoulders, and knees while excluding the hip joints, ankles, and joints of the feet. The 28-joint count is convenient to perform in the outpatient setting compared to the 68-joint count that was used in previous times.

Patient and physician (or evaluator) global assessment: The patient's global assessment (PGA) is his or her assessment of how the disease affects them in totality beyond the joint pain and swelling. Physician global assessment (PhyGA) relate the individual patient's disease in comparison to all the other patients seen by the physician. The use of both measures averages the possible discordance in both.

Inflammatory Markers

Erythrocyte sedimentation rate (ESR) and C-reactive protein (CRP) are readily available tests, and their addition improves the objectivity of the disease activity measurement.

Composite Indices to Assess RA Disease Activity

Disease activity score (DAS): A combination of the above mentioned parameters results in a composite score for disease activity. The DAS is statistically derived; the original variables included 68 TJC, 68 SJC, and overall health assessment of the patient. Subsequently the original DAS was modified, and the number of joints evaluated was reduced to 28 (DAS-28). By adding ESR or CRP, we have DAS-28 ESR and DAS-28 CRP. The DAS score is a continuous measure of disease activity and helps physicians to adjust treatment to achieve a pre-specified target of disease control (Table 5.2.1). DAS score calculator is available on the internet.

The simplified disease activity index (SDAI) was introduced in 2003. It is a simple sum of the TJC, SJC, PGA, PhyGA, and CRP in mg/dL.

Table 5.2.1: Tools to assess disease activity in rheumatoid arthritis

Activity score	*Remission*	*Low*	*Moderate*	*High*	*Comments*
Disease activity score 28 joints (DAS28), DAS28 ESR, DAS28 CRP Calculated using a calculator or web-based calculator with SJC, JTC, patient global assessment of health. Range is 0–10	<2.6	2.6–3.2	>3.2–5.1	>5.1	Widely used. Incorporated in patient-reported outcomes measures for self-monitoring. A significant proportion of patients classified as remission will still have at least two SJCs.
Simplified disease activity index (SDAI) SDAI = SJC + TJC + PGA + EGA + CRP Range is 0–86	0.3.3	3.4–11	11.1–26	26.1–86	A score >15 has best sensitivity and specificity compared to a clinical decision to change DMARD because of inadequate response
Clinical disease activity index (CDAI) CDAI = SJC + TJC + PGA + EGA Range is 0–76	0–2.8	2.9–10	10.1–22	22.1–76	Only clinical parameters are required.
RAPID3 (routine assessment of patient index data 3) Pain VAS + multi-dimensional HAQ + PGA Range is 0–30	</=3	3.1–6	6.1–12	>12	There is no joint count. RAPID3 scores correlate with DAS28 and CDAI

SJC: Swollen joint count; *TJC:* Tender joint count; *PGA:* Patient global assessment of disease activity; *EGA:* Evaluator global assessment of disease activity; *CRP:* CRP in mg/dL

Table 5.2.2: EULAR criteria for response (primarily used in clinical trials) based on DAS28

Remission: DAS 28<2.6

Good response: DAS 28 ≤3.2 and improvement >1.2

Moderate response: DAS 28 is between 3.2 and 5.1 or DAS 28 improvement >0.6 to 1.2 and DAS 28 ≤3.2 or DAS 28 improvement >1.2 but DAS 28 >5.1

No response: DAS 28 improvement <0.6 or DAS 28 improvement is between 0.6 and 1.2 but DAS 28 >5.1

Clinical disease activity index (CDAI) omits acute-phase reactants as a variable. It is a sum of SJC, TJC, PGA, and PhyGA. The CDAI performs equally well compared to SDAI and DAS-28.

The score range and cut-off to classify low, moderate, and high disease activity are given in Table 5.2.1, while Table 5.2.2 shows the utility of DAS28 as response measures in clinical trials.

https://www.das-score.nl/das28/DAScalculators/dasculators.html

RADIOGRAPHIC ASSESSMENT

The Sharp/van der Heijde (SvH) Score

Radiographic erosion of bone is a measurement of damage caused by RA, and it is most commonly measured by the van der Heijde modification of the Sharp Scoring system. This scoring incorporates joint space narrowing and erosions in high-resolution plain radiographs of the hands and feet.

Magnetic resonance imaging (MRI) and ultrasonography are being increasingly used to assess both active inflammation by looking for vascularity and damage by looking at erosions and cartilage thickness.

FUNCTION

The Health assessment questionnaire (HAQ) provides essential information about the patient's functional status. It is a widely used disability measure and is validated and adapted for use in India also. The HAQ disability index (HAQ-DI) has 8 categories of function. These are arising, reaching, gripping, dressing and grooming, hygiene, eating, walking, and common daily activities. The Multidimensional HAQ (MDHAQ) is a modification of HAQ. It gives a broader assessment of disability by measuring morning stiffness, fatigue, psychological distress. It also reviews medications and assessment of other systems.

Patient Reported Outcomes Measures (PROMs)

1. **The routine assessment of patient index data 3 (RAPID3)** is a patient self-reported questionnaire consisting of three items: Pain, PGA, and function (HAQ).
2. **The RA disease activity index (RADAI)** is a self-reported questionnaire of five items: Global disease activity (current and past), joint count assessed by the patient, and morning stiffness. RADAI takes only 3 minutes to complete, and patients can score themselves at home or in the waiting hall.
3. **Patient activity score (PAS)** and its modification PAS-II uses HAQ-DI, pain VAS, and PGA.

CONCLUSION

Outcome measures in RA included the DAS28, SDAI, CDAI for disease activity, the van der Heijde scoring for radiographic damage, and the HAQ-DI for measuring disability. These outcome measures are increasingly applied in clinical practice to optimise treatment.

LEARNING POINTS

- Outcome measures in RA can be grouped as those to assess disease activity, damage, and patient functioning.
- Composite measures include the DAS28 ESR/CRP, SDAI, CDAI. These are validated disease measures, they aid clinical treatment decisions, and are used in clinical trials too
- PROMs such as RAPID3 correlate with DAS28 and CDAI.

FURTHER READING

1. Anderson JK, Zimmerman L, Caplan L, Michaud K. Measures of rheumatoid arthritis disease activity: Patient (PtGA) and Provider (PrGA) Global Assessment of Disease Activity, Disease Activity Score (DAS) and Disease Activity Score with 28-Joint Counts (DAS28), Simplified Disease Activity Index (SDAI), Clinical Disease Activity Index (CDAI), Patient Activity Score (PAS) and Patient Activity Score-II (PASII), Routine Assessment of Patient Index Data (RAPID), Rheumatoid Arthritis Disease Activity Index (RADAI) and Rheumatoid Arthritis Disease Activity Index-5 (RADAI-5), Chronic Arthritis Systemic Index (CASI), Patient-Based Disease Activity Score With ESR (PDAS1) and Patient-Based Disease Activity Score without ESR (PDAS2), and Mean Overall Index for Rheumatoid Arthritis (MOI-RA). Arthritis Care Res (Hoboken). 2011;63 Suppl 11:S14–S36.
2. Aletaha D, Nell VP, Stamm T, et al. Acute phase reactants add little to composite disease activity indices for rheumatoid arthritis: validation of a clinical activity score. Arthritis Res Ther 2005;7:796–806.
3. Kumar A, Malaviya AN, Pandhi A, Singh RR. Validation of an Indian version of the Health Assessment Questionnaire in patients with rheumatoid arthritis. Rheumatology 2002;41:1457–9.
4. Pincus T, Yazici Y, Bergman M, et al. A self-report questionnaire Routine Assessment of Patient Index Data (RAPID) score as a guide to a 'continuous quality improvement'. Clin Exp Rheumatol 2006, 24 (6 Suppl 43):S-60–5.
5. Pincus T, Swearingen C, Wolfe F. Toward a Multi. Dimensional Health Assessment Questionnaire (MDHAQ): assessment of advanced activities of daily living and psychological status in the patient-friendly health assessment questionnaire format. Arthritis Rheum 1999;42:2220–30.
6. Smolen JS, Breedveld FC, Schiff MH, et al. A simplified disease activity index for rheumatoid arthritis for use in clinical practice. Rheumatology (Oxford) 2003;42: 244–57.

Outcome Measures in Systemic Lupus Erythematosus

Taral Parikh, Avinash Jain

INTRODUCTION

Outcome measures for systemic lupus erythematosus (SLE) include disease activity, damage, drug-related adverse events, quality of life, and economic impact.

DISEASE ACTIVITY

Tools to assess activity include the SLE disease activity index (SLEDAI) and the British Isles Lupus Assessment Group (BILAG). Both are simple to use and have been validated. There are other indices as well (Figure 5.3.1). All except BILAG give a composite score of disease activity. A single composite score allows the clinician to monitor patients' overall progress. The major limitation of a composite score is inability to reflect differences in disease activity from one organ system to another. Other drawbacks of composite scores (for example SLEDAI) are that multiple mild

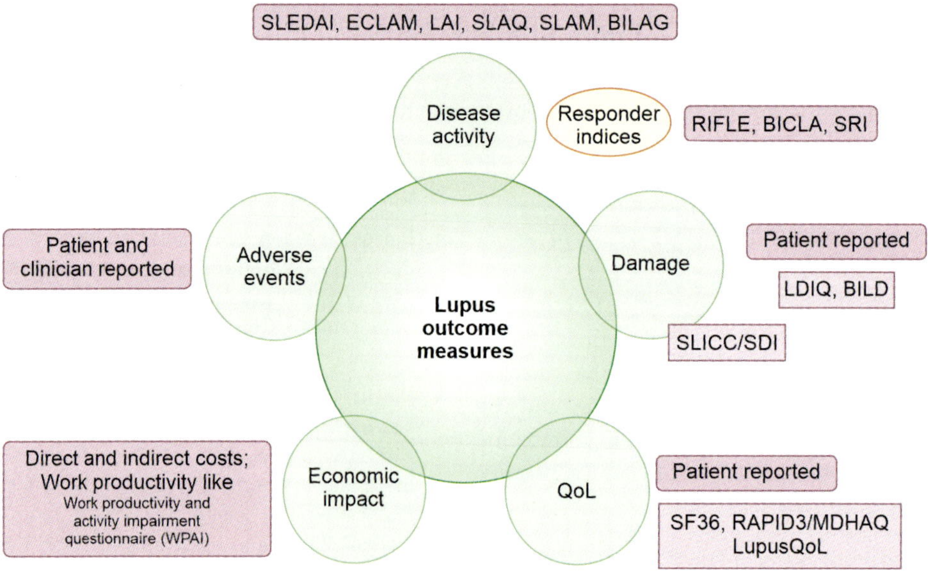

Fig. 5.3.1: Outcome measures in systemic lupus erythematosus (SLE)

BICLA: BILAG based composite lupus assessment; *BILAG:* British isles lupus assessment group; *BILD:* Brief index of lupus damage; *ECLAM:* European consensus lupus activity measure; *LAI:* Lupus activity index; *LDIQ:* Lupus damage index questionnaire; *LupusQoL:* Lupus quality of life; *MDHAQ:* Multidimensional health assessment questionnaire; *RAPID3:* Routine assessment of patient index data 3; *RIFLE:* Responder index for lupus erythematosus; SF36: Short form 36; *SLAM:* Systemic lupus activity measure; *SLAQ:* Systemic lupus erythematosus activity questionnaire; *SLEDAI:* Systemic lupus erythematosus disease activity index; *SLICC/SDI:* Systemic lupus international collaborating clinics/American College of Rheumatology-damage index; *SRI:* SLE responder index manifestations and one major organ involvement will result in the same score.

SLEDAI

SLEDAI is a widely accepted tool, it has good predictive value for damage and mortality, has good sensitivity to change, and validated in childhood-onset lupus. SLEDAI measures disease activity using 24 descriptors. Major organ manifestations namely central nervous system involvement, vasculitis, psychosis are given higher weightage (score of 8) as compared to skin (rash and alopecia 2 each) and joints (score of 4). For more details, refer to references 1 and 2.

SELENA-SLEDAI and SLEDAI-2K differ from the original SLEDAI, as they record persistent disease in few domains (proteinuria, rash, alopecia and mucosal ulcers). Unlike SLEDAI which records disease activity 10-day before evaluation, both SELENA SLEDAI and SLEDAI2K measure in the preceding 30 days. Another modification, SLEDAI–2KG, was developed that adds a weighted score for glucocorticoids to SLEDAI-2K. For, example, the use of a prednisolone-equivalent dose of less than 5 mg gets a score of zero whereas a dose of 37.5 mg or more gets an additional score of 8.

CASE-BASED EXAMPLE

A 32-year-old female patient a known case of lupus who was doing well till two months ago has presented now with persistent oral ulcer for 2 months, acute cutaneous lupus erythematosus (ACLE) rash, fever, and thrombocytopenia for 8 days. What will be the SLEDAI, and SLEDAI-2K scores?

Manifestations that are persistent but active will count in SLEDAI-2K but not in SLEDAI. So, in this case SLEDAI score is 4 whereas SLEDAI-2K is 6. Based on SLEDAI scores, the disease is called inactive, mild, moderate, high and very high if SLEDAI scores are 0, 1–5, 6–10, 11–19 and >19 respectively.

BILAG

BILAG and its revised version BILAG 2004 measures disease activity in individual organ systems. In this scoring system 86 items (over the past 4 weeks) in nine organ systems are scored and compared with the previous month. The items in BILAG and BILAG 2004 are scored as improved, same, worse, or new. The final scores are converted into categories A, B, C, D, and E (Table 5.2.1). Based on these categories the clinician can make a therapeutic decision.

MEASURES OF CHANGE IN DISEASE ACTIVITY

The Composite Responder Indices

They are designed to identify patients who have improved or not with treatment (Table 5.3.2).

Table 5.3.1: Assessment of activity of SLE by the BILAG and BILAG-2004

Grade	*Disease severity*	*Numerical scores*	*Definition*
A- Active	Severe	12	Severe disease resulting in an increase in prednisone of more than 20 mg/day and/or addition of immunosuppressant
B- Be aware	Moderate	8	This category means that the disease is less active, needs prednisone in low dose and/or symptomatic management with NSAIDs and/or antimalarial
C- Contentment	Mild	1	This is mild disease needing only symptomatic treatment or the disease is stable and maintained on current therapy
D- Discount	Inactive but previously affected	0	An organ system has been involved earlier, with no current activity in it
E- No evidence	Inactive with no previous involvement	0	No current or previous involvement in that organ system

Table 5.3.2: Composite indices of response (outcome) to treatment primarily for research

Responder index	*Definition of response*
Responder index for DHEA trials	There should be no treatment failures There has to be an improvement in one of the commonly used disease activity index (SLEDAI or SLAM) with no worsening in the other Improvement in physician global assessments (PGA) or KFSS with no worsening in the other
RIFLE	Complete response is basically a resolution of abnormal features in specific organs that includes skin and mucosal, kidney, joints/muscles, and nervous system Partial response is an improvement of disease in an organ but not fully resolved. No response if there is no response at all Not present signs/symptoms are absent
SLE responder index	No early drop outs, or new medications or increased dose of medications SELENA-SLEDAI ≥4 point reduction No new BILAG A or more than 2 new BILAG B No PGA deterioration from baseline by more than 0.3 points
BICLA (BILAG–based Composite Lupus Assessment)	A organ with baseline BILAG A is reduced to B, C, or D. Whereas in those with baseline B the scores have reduced to to C or D No new BILAG A or 2 new BILAG B No worsening in PGA scores (<10% worsening relative to baseline) or baseline SLEDAI No treatment failure

SLEDAI: SLE disease activity index; *SLAM:* SLE assessment measure; *PGA:* Patient global assessment; *KFSS:* Krupp fatigue severity scale; *RIFLE:* Response index for lupus erythematous; *BILAG:* British isles lupus assessment group

Within each index, "responses" require that patients not be "treatment failures". SLEDAI measure some items on an "all-or-none" basis, thus is unable to identify partial improvement in disease activity. The SLEDAI-2K Responder Index-50 was developed to detect 50% improvement in SLEDAI-2K.

ORGAN-SPECIFIC INDICES

Outcome Measures—Lupus Nephritis

Clinical trials have used different renal outcome measures. To measure outcome in lupus nephritis the SLE International Collaboration Clinics (SLICC) group proposed a definition, whereby complete remission is defined as proteinuria <300 mg/day, with no active sediment, serum biomarkers including albumin, and creatinine should be in normal range, and creatinine clearance should be less than 15% above baseline. A proteinuria >300 mg/day but <2.9 g/day, serum albumin more than 3 g/dL and stable kidney function, denotes partial remission.

Cutaneous Outcome Measures

The Cutaneous LE disease Area and Severity Index (CLASI) measures cutaneous damage and activity. It includes erythema, scale or hypertrophy, non-scarring alopecia, mucosa involvement, etc.

FLARE

A flare is defined as 'increase in disease activity (that is measurable) in one or more organ systems involving new or worse clinical manifestations and/or laboratory parameters.' Outcome measures commonly used to define flares are SELENA-SLEDAI and BILAG.

SELENA-SLEDAI FLARE INDEX

Mild or moderate flares are defined as new or worsened clinical features with:

a. Change in SELENA/SLEDAI score >3 points
b. Increase of prednisone dose but <0.5 mg/kg/ day
c. Patient global assessment (PGA) –1.0 to 2.5 [range- 0 to 3 visual analogue scale (VAS)]

Definition of severe flares is:

a. SELENA-SLEDAI score >12 or
b. Clinical manifestations (nephritis, neuropsychiatric, myositis, thrombocytopenia, anemia) leading to twofold increase in steroid dose or requiring an increment to prednisolone of >0.5 mg/kg/day or hospitalization
c. New cyclophosphamide, azathioprine, or methotrexate, or hospitalization due to disease
d. PGA >2.5

BILAG definition of flare: Flares can also be defined using BILAG index

Severe flares: A patient with an 'A score' in any domain with items being labelled as new or worse

Moderate flare: A patient with ≥2 'B scores' with items being labelled as new or worse

Mild flare: A patient with 1 'B score' or 3 or more 'C scores' due to items that are either new or worse

REMISSION IN SLE

Definition of complete remission needs absence of both clinical and laboratory features. Serologically active and clinically quiescent (SACQ) is defined as high dsDNA and/or low complements but no active clinical manifestations. There are organ-specific definitions which talk about partial, complete remission and prolonged remission.

Lupus Low Disease Activity State (LLDAS) is termed as:

a. SLEDAI-2K score of 4 or less, with no activity in major organ.
b. No new SLE features.
c. PGA should be 1 or less, and
d. Prednisolone dose ≤7.5 mg/d with stable dose of immunosuppressant. A low disease activity state is a reasonable target whenever aiming at treat-to-target strategy.

MEASUREMENT OF DAMAGE

The Systemic Lupus International Collaborating Clinics/American College of Rheumatology-Damage Index (SLICC/SDI) measures damage from disease activity, treatment, and comorbidities which have been present for 6 months or more (42 items, 12 domains). Lupus Damage Index Questionnaire (LDIQ) is a tool incorporating 56-item from SDI. Brief Index of Lupus Damage (BILD) is abbreviated version with 28 items. Both are self-reported.

HEALTH-RELATED QUALITY OF LIFE

The definition of health-related quality of life (QoL) includes the impact of disease on various aspects of health including physical, social, psychological, and mental domain. The generic validated QoL measures include Short Form 36-Item Survey (SF-36), multidimensional health assessment questionnaire/ Routine Assessment of Patient Index Data (MDHAQ/RAPID3). LupusPRO measures QoL for SLE patients. It is also available in many Indian languages. The Lupus Impact Tracker derived from the LupusPRO items is shorter and easier to use.

The Krupp Fatigue Severity Scale (KFSS) and the FACIT—Fatigue (FACIT-F) measure fatigue.

There are tools available to measure adverse events, as well as economic impact of disease.

LEARNING POINTS

- SLEDAI, SELENA-SLEDAI, and BILAG scoring system are widely in SLE, both in the clinics and research.
- A disease flare can be objectively measured using SELENA-SLEDAI and BILAG
- A lupus low disease activity state (LLDAS) is an achievable target.
- Definitions of renal response to treatment ie complete remission and partial remission aids the clinician to adjust treatment appropriately
- Being a multisystem heterogeneous disease there is no single instrument that will adequately capture all aspects of the disease.

FURTHER READING

1. Bombardier C, Gladman DD, Urowitz MB, et al. Derivation of the SLEDAI. A disease activity index for lupus patients. Arthritis Rheum. 1992;35:630–40.
2. Castrejon I, Tani C, Jolly M, Huang A, Mosca M. Indices to assess patients with systemic lupus erythematosus in clinical trials, long-term observational studies, and clinical care. Clin. Exp. Rheumatol. 2014;32:S-85-95.
3. Gladman D, Ginzler E, Goldsmith C, et al. The development and initial validation of systemic lupus international collaborating clinics/American college

of rheumatology damage index for systemic lupus erythematosus. Arthritis Rheum. 1996;39:363–9.

4. Isenberg DA, Rahman A, Allen E, et al. BILAG 2004. Development and initial validation of an updated version of the British Isles Lupus Assessment Group's disease activity index for patients with systemic lupus erythematosus. Rheumatology (Oxford) 2005;44: 902–6.
5. Petri M, Kim MY, Kalunian KC, et al.: OC-SELENA Trial. Combined oral contraceptives in women with systemic lupus erythematosus. N Engl J Med. 2005;353: 2550–8.
6. Touma Z, Gladman DD, Ibañez D, et al. Development and initial validation of the systemic lupus erythematosus disease activity index 2000 responder index 50. J Rheumatol. 2011; 38:275–84.

Chapter 5.4

Outcome Measures in Spondyloarthritis

Bhowmik Meghnathi, Isha Sood

INTRODUCTION

Outcome measures in spondyloarthritis (SpA) include disease activity, damage, function, and quality of life. The Ankylosing Spondyl Arthritis International Society (ASAS) is dedicated to SpA research, work from this group led to the classification of AS into axial-SpA and peripheral SpA, and the development of core set outcome measures to assess response to treatment in clinical trials.

The Bath indices developed by Calin et. al., are widely accepted in clinical practice and continue to remain an integral part of recent outcome measures in SpA.

DISEASE ACTIVITY

BASDAI and ASDAS

The Bath ankylosing spondylitis disease activity index (BASDAI) is a patient symptom-based measure of disease severity or activity. An inflammatory marker CRP or ESR was added to make it more objective. Hence ASAS disease activity score (ASDAS) came into place. Thus BASDAI and ASDAS ESR or CRP are two indices used to assess disease activity in SpA (Tables 5.4.1 and 5.4.2).

Table 5.4.1: Bath Ankylosing Spondylitis Disease Activity Index (BASDAI) scoring

Each question in BASDAI relates to how they have felt in the past one week.		Score of 0–10
Q1.	How would you describe the overall level of fatigue/tiredness you have experienced?	0–10
Q2.	How would you describe the overall level of AS neck, back or hip pain you have had?	0–10
Q3.	How would you describe the overall level of pain/swelling in joints other than the neck, back or hips?	0–10
Q4.	How would you describe the overall level of discomfort you have had from any tender areas to touch or pressure?	0–10
Q5.	How would you describe the overall level of morning stiffness you have had from the time you wake up?	0–10
Q6.	How long does your morning stiffness last from the time you wake up?	0–10
Calculating the BASDAI score		Final BASDAI score
A. Add scores for questions 1–4		
B. Calculate the mean for questions 5 and 6		
C. Add A and B and divide by 5		
The higher the BASDAI score, the more severe the patient's disability due to their AS		

Data from Garrett et al. J Rheumatol 1994;21:2286–91.

Table 5.4.2: ASDAS: Ankylosing Spondylitis Disease Activity Score

ASDAS		*Score*
Calculated using ASDAS Calculator app. Below are the 5 questions		
Q1.	Back Pain (BASDAI Question 2) [0–10]	0–10
Q2.	Peripheral pain/swelling (BASDAI Question 3) [0–10]	0–10
Q3.	Duration morning stiffness (BASDAI Question 6) [0–10]	0–10
Q4.	Patient global [0–10]	0–10
Q5.	C-reactive protein in mg/lL or mg/dL or erythrocyte sedimentation rate (ESR) in mm/hour	CRP value ESR Value
If CRP is below the limit of detection or is <2 mg/L (<0.2 mg/dL), the fixed value of 2 mg/L (0.2 mg/dL) will be entered		
ASDAS score	**Disease activity states**	
<1.3	Inactive disease	
1.3 to <2.1	Low disease activity	
2.1 to <3.5	High disease activity	
> = 3.5	Very high disease activity	
ASDAS Improvement criteria		
Improvement > =1.1	Clinically important improvement'	
Improvement > =2.0	Major improvement	
ASDAS Clinical deterioration		
Worsening of ASDAS score by atleast 0.9 (> = 0.9 increase in ASDAS)	"Clinically important worsening" in axSpA for use in trials.	

Data from Sieper, J et al. Ann Rheum Dis.2009,68:ii1–ii44; 2. Molto A et al. Ann Rheum Dis. 2018;77(1).

Both BASDAI and ASDAS are used as targets when deciding change in treatment using biologic agents.

SPINAL MOBILITY

Bath ankylosing spondylitis metrology index (BASMI) measures the AS patient's spinal mobility. There are five components: lateral flexion, lumbar flexion (modified Snober's test), tragus to wall distance, cervical rotation, and maximal inter malleolar distance. The original BASMI is a continuous scale from 0 to 10. Spinal mobility impairment as per BASMI can be categorized as mild, moderate, or severe (Table 5.4.3).

ASAS has recommended five measures to assess spinal mobility (Table 5.4.4). Four out of these are BASMI components: lateral flexion, lumbar flexion, cervical rotation, and occiput to the wall (instead of tragus to the wall).

Table 5.4.3: BASMI: 3-point answer scale

Measure	*0 (Mild)*	*1 (Moderate)*	*2 (Severe)*
Lateral lumbar flexion (cm)	>10 cm	5–10 cm	<5 cm
Tragus to wall distance (cm)	<15 cm	15–30 cm	>30 cm
Lumbar flexion (modified Schober) (cm)	>4 cm	2–4 cm	<2 cm
Maximal intermalleolar distance (cm)	>100 cm	70–100 cm	<70 cm
Cervical rotation (°)	>70°	20–70°	<20°

Table 5.4.4: ASAS recommended measures of spinal mobility

Chest expansion	Chest expansion is measured in fourth intercostal space anteriorly. The difference between maximum inspiration and expiration is measured and the better of the two tries is taken as final. In population based studies an increase of 2.2 cm in chest expansion was considered normal.
Modified Schober's test	Also known as anterior spinal flexion. In the modified Schober's test the patient stands erect and a horizontal imaginary line is placed connecting two posterior superior iliac spines. A second mark is placed 10 cm vertically above this line and a third line is placed 5 cm below the first line. The patient bends forward maximally and the distance between the two marks is measured which now increases. The better of the two tries is taken as final value. Moll and Wright proposed normal ranges for modified Schober's between 3.4 and 5.5 cm for various age and gender based on 237 unaffected relatives of psoriasis patients.
Occiput to wall distance	The patient stands straight with heel and back touching the wall at a usual carrying angle. The patient should make an effort so that the head touches the wall. The distance between the occiput and wall (measured twice, with better of two tries recorded) is measured in cm for which a normal value is zero.
Cervical rotation	The patient sits straight with chin at a normal carrying angle. A goniometer is placed at the top of the head in line with the patient's nose. The patient first rotates the neck maximally to the left and then right, and the goniometer is followed along with it. The angle between the first sagittal plane and the new plane after rotation is measured in degrees on both sides. The average for the left and the right side is recorded in degrees.
Lateral spinal flexion	Patient is asked to stand straight with their heel and back resting against the wall. A mark is placed on the right thigh first at the level of the patient's middle finger. The patient is then asked to bend sideways to the right as far as possible without bending the knee or lifting the heel and the second mark is placed again at the level of the middle finger. The distance between the two marks is recorded in cm. This is done twice and a better of two tries is recorded. This is again repeated on the left side. The mean of left and right is the lateral spinal flexion.

PHYSICAL FUNCTION

BASFI, and HAQ-S

The Bath ankylosing spondylitis functional index (BASFI) measures spinal function. Similar to BASDAI, it is a patient-based measure of function. The BASFI uses 8 questions related to functional anatomy and 2 questions about a patient's ability to cope with daily life. The Dougados functional index (DFI) is another tool to measure spinal function in SpA, but it is no longer used.

The health assessment questionnaire for AS (HAQ-S).

RADIOGRAPHIC PROGRESSION

BASRI and mSASS

The radiological index (BASRI) is less frequently used in clinical practice. The modified Stokes ankylosing spondylitis scores (mSASS) is an alternative tool available to score plain radiographs to look for radiographic progression of AS mostly in clinical trials.

All the four indices BASDAI, BASMI, BASFI, and BASRI are validated for reliability, reproducibility, and sensitivity to change. They can be scored using a free online web-based calculator.

PERIPHERAL JOINTS ASSESSMENTS

Peripheral joint assessment in SpA is done using 44 joint counts with scores as 0 (absent) to 1 (synovitis present) as illustrated in (Fig. 5.4.1).

Enthesitis Indices

Table 5.4.5 summarizes all the enthesitis indexes. ASAS does not recommend the use of enthesitis indices in daily clinical practice.

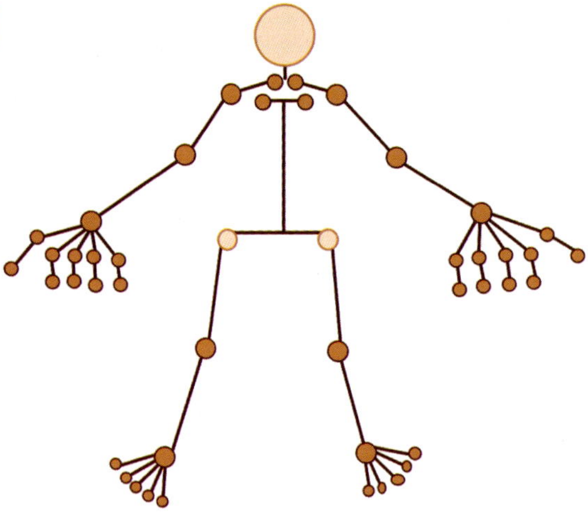

Fig. 5.4.1: Peripheral 44-joint count in SpA.

Table 5.4.5: Enthesis indices		
Enthesitis index	*Entheseal sites*	*Score range*
Manders enthesis index	66 sites	0–90
San Francisco enthesitis index (SFI)	17 sites	0–51
Maastricht ankylosing spondylitis enthesitis score (MASES)	13 sites	0–13
Berlin enthesitis index (BEI)	12 sites	0–12
Spondyloarthritis Research Consortium of Canada (SPARCC) enthesitis index	16 sites	0–16
Leeds enthesitis index (LEI)	6 sites	0–6

Quality of Life (QoL)

The AS-QoL measures the impact that AS has on the patient's health-related quality of life. It can be accessed at *https://asas.org*

The ASAS Core Domain Set for Ankylosing Spondylitis

The ASAS core set of outcome measures (Table 5.4.6) defined in 1999 are a minimum set of variables that need to be collected when considering clinical trials with nonsteroidal anti-inflammatory drugs (NSAIDs), physical therapy, and/or biological agents. These core set measures are applicable to the entire spectrum of SpA.

The core set has been updated in 2020–2021 a collaborative effort of ASAS and OMERACT. These core domain sets are meant for application in research settings and are not mandatory for observation al studies or clinical practice. The major changes are:

- Terminology for AS was replaced by ax-SpA.
- Included extramuscular domains such as uveitis, inflammatory bowel disease, and psoriasis.

Table 5.4.6: ASAS core domains set for SpA		
	Domain	*Instrument*
1	Physical function	BASFI
2	Spinal mobility	Chest expansion Modified schober test Occiput to wall Cervical rotation BASMI or lateral spinal flexion
3	Patient global assessment "How active was your spondyloarthritis on an average during last week?"	NRS/VAS (last week)
4	Fatigue "How would you describe the overall level of fatigue/tiredness you have experienced?"	Fatigue question on BASDAI
5	Pain How much pain in your spine due to AS do you have? How much pain in your spine due to AS do you have at night?	NRS/VAS for Pain (last week)

(Contd.)

Table 5.4.6: ASAS core domains set for SpA *(Contd.)*

	Domain	*Instrument*
6	Spinal stiffness "How long does your morning stiffness last from the time you wake up?" Three anchors are used for rating are 0-hour, 1 hour, and 2 or more hours. NRS preferred over VAS.	NRS/VAS (Last week)
7	Acute phase reactants	ESR or CRP
8	Peripheral joint/enthesis	No. of swollen joint count (44 joints) Validated enthesitis score like MASES
9	Spinal radiographs	Lateral lumbar and spinal radiograph

AS: Ankylosing spondylitis; *BASDAI:* Bath ankylosing spondylitis disease activity index; *BASFI:* Bath ankylosing spondylitis functional index; *BASMI:* Bath ankylosing spondylitis metrology index; *MASES:* Maastricht ankylosing spondylitis enthesis score; *NRS:* Numerical rating scale 0–10; *VAS:* Visual analog scale 0–100.

Table 5.4.7: Summary of different domains of outcome measures in spondyloarthritis

I. Disease Activity	*II. Physical Function*	*III. Structural Damage*	*IV. Disability/Quality of Life*
BASDAI ASDAS Enthesitis index	BASFI HAQ-S	BASMI	ASQoL
Peripheral joint count ESR/ CRP	ASPI (physical performance)	mSASSS	ASAS-HI

- Peripheral manifestations of arthritis, dactylitis, and enthesitis.
- Structural damage to the spine, root joints, peripheral joints, and other organs included.

Response and Remission Criteria

Response Criteria

The ASAS 20/40 response criteria are used in clinical trials to assess response to intervention. The domains included in these response measures include

1. Patient global assessment
2. Spinal pain
3. Function (assessed by BASFI)
4. Inflammation (mean of BASDAI questions 5 and 6)

To meet ASAS 20 response: 3 of 4 domains should improve by at least 20% with a minimum of 1 unit on a scale of 0–10 between two-time points and for ASAS 40 at least 40% and a minimum of 2 units on a scale of 0–10. In the remaining domain, there should be no worsening of 20% and a minimum of 1 unit, on a 0–10 scale.

The ASAS 5/6 improvement criteria include 6 domains: all of the above four criteria with CRP and spinal mobility (assessed by lateral spinal flexion). In order to meet this improvement criteria, there should be an improvement of at least 20% in at least 5 of these 6 domains.

CONCLUSION

To conclude the outcome measures in SpA (Table 5.4.7) can be grouped as those that assess activity, physical function, structural damage, and quality of life.

LEARNING POINTS

- Differentiation between disease activity and damage is crucial in planning treatment for a patient with spondyloarthritis.
- The BASDAI and ASDAS are valid and reliable measures of disease severity/activity and must be a routine part of practice
- BASFI and HAQ-S are useful to assess functional outcome to treatment.

- BASMI is a clinical measure of structural damage.
- mSASS are used to score radiographs to assess radiographic progression.
- The latest update to ASAS-OMERACT core domain includes extra-musculoskeletal domain, structural damage, and peripheral arthritis, enthesitis, and dactylitis.

FURTHER READING

1. Meghnathi B, Sood I, Patil A. Rheumatology Clinics Spondyloarthritis. 1st Edition. New Delhi. 2020. Evangel. Chapter 9, Disease assessment in spondyloarthritis: 119–46.
2. Molto A, Gossec L, Meghnathi B, et al. An Assessment in SpondyloArthritis International Society (ASAS)-endorsed definition of clinically important worsening in axial spondyloarthritis based on ASDAS. Ann Rheum Dis 2018; 77:124–7.
3. Navarro-Compán V, Boel A, Boonen A, et al. The ASAS-OMERACT core domain set for axial spondyloarthritis. Semin Arthritis Rheum. 2021;51:1342–9.
4. Rezvani A, Ergin O, Karacan I, Oncu M. Validity and reliability of the metric measurements in the assessment of lumbar spine motion in patients with ankylosing spondylitis. Spine (Phila. Pa. 1976) 2012;37.
5. Sieper J, Rudwaleit M, Baraliakos X, et al. The Assessment of SpondyloArthritis International Society (ASAS) handbook: a guide to assess spondyloarthritis. Ann Rheum Dis. 2009; 68(Suppl 2):ii1–44.
6. van Der Heijde D, Landewé R, Feldtkeller E. Proposal of a linear definition of the Bath Ankylosing Spondylitis Metrology Index (BASMI) and comparison with the 2-step and 10-step definitions. Ann. Rheum. Dis. 2008; 67:489–93.

Outcome Measures in Primary Sjögren's Syndrome

Ramya Janardana

INTRODUCTION

Sjögren's syndrome (SS) is characterized by exocrine glandular dysfunction. In about 20–40% of the patients, it may be associated with organ threatening systemic manifestations which may or may not be associated with subjective oral and/or ocular sicca at initial presentation.

OUTCOME MEASURES

There are two composite indices to assess the outcome of patients with primary Sjögren's syndrome. The first one assesses patient's symptoms and is called the EULAR Sjögren's syndrome patient reported index (ESSPRI). For systemic involvement, it is the EULAR Sjögren's syndrome disease activity index (ESSDAI). These indices were developed in 2009 and were subsequently validated. The ESSDAI and ESSPRI are employed as primary outcome measures in recent and ongoing clinical trials. To assess sicca, the sicca symptoms inventory (SSI) is used, whereas for fatigue the profile of fatigue and discomfort (PROFAD) is employed.

ESSDAI

The ESSDAI includes 12 domains. Each domain has 3–4 levels of activity (Table 5.5.1). A score between 1 to 6 has been assigned to each domain according to regression coefficient of the individual domain during the process of ESSDAI development. Each domain score is obtained by multiplying the activity level of the involved domain with the domain score. In each domain, features that are stable for at least 12 months get a score of 0. The total score of ESSDAI ranges from 0 to 123. It has been shown in a large cohort of SS that high activity in any of the domains, a score greater than or equal to 14 or the presence of more than one laboratory predictive markers were associated with mortality. High baseline ESSDAI score was also found to be associated development of hematological cancer at follow-up.

The minimal clinically significant improvement is a reduction in ESSDAI score of at least 3 points as compared to baseline. ClinESSDAI is a modification of ESSDAI where the biologic domain of ESSDAI is omitted. The sensitivity to change and reliability of ClinESSDAI is similar to ESSDAI.

ESSPRI

ESSPRI is patient-reported and measures subjective symptoms of primary SS namely pain, dryness, and fatigue. The total score of ESSPRI is the mean of the three Likert's numerical scale rating fatigue, pain and dryness with a range of 0–10. ESSPRI is easy to perform. An improvement of at least in 1 score or 15% from baseline is considered clinically significant. A web based ESSPRI and ESSDAI is available at *https://www.sanoia-fiche-sante.com/sjogren*.

The ESSDAI and ESSPRI have good correlation with physician and patient global assessment respectively. The ESSDAI and ESSPRI scores do not correlate with one another since they measure two different aspects of the disease.

Table 5.5.1: Salient features of ESSDAI and ESSPRI

Properties	*ESSDAI*	*ESSPRI*
Domains	• Constitutional • Glandular • Lymphadenopathy • Articular • Skin • Renal • Hematological • Muscular • Peripheral nervous system • Central nervous system • Respiratory • Biological	Fatigue Pain Dryness Each of these domains are scored on a scale of 0–10
Scoring	Sum of weighted scores of individual domains	Mean of 3 Likert scale
Administered by	Care provider	Self-administered
Range	Score range is 0–123	0–10
Severity	ESSDAI <5 is low, 5–13 is moderate, ≥14 is high disease activity	—
Duration	4 weeks	2 weeks
Minimal clinically significant improvement	3 points	Improvement in score by 1 or ≥15% from baseline
Psychometrics	feasible, valid, reliable, and sensitive to change	Feasible, valid, and reliable
Disadvantages	Large responses in placebo arm in clinical trials	Lesser sensitivity to change with treatment as compared to ESSDAI

ESSDAI: EULAR Sjögren's syndrome disease activity index; *ESSPRI:* EULAR Sjogren's syndrome patient reported index

Shortcomings

Although ESSDAI is found to be a useful measure to assess systemic activity and is sensitive to change in open label studies, it has failed to differentiate between treatment and placebo arms in several randomised controlled trials. This is mainly due to large decreases in ESSDAI score in placebo arms during study period, likely due to strong placebo effects on constitutional, glandular, and articular domains. Salient features of ESSDAI and ESSPRI are summarised in Table 5.5.1.

Fatigue and Sicca

The PROFAD and sicca symptom inventory questionnaires are PROs to measure fatigue and dryness, respectively. The brief forms of PROFAD and SSI were precursors of ESSPRI.

Other tools to assess fatigue, the FACIT-F scale and the fatigue severity scale which are uni-dimensional and scores only fatigue. Multidimensional fatigue inventory or the piper fatigue scale are multidimen-sional; however, they have not been specifically developed as measures of fatigue in SS but have been used as secondary outcome measures in some trials.

Although unstimulated whole salivary flow, Schimer's test, van Bijsterveld schema, and the ocular staining score (OSS) are used in primary SS diagnosis and were/are part of primary SS classification criteria; none have been validated for use as an outcome measure.

Quality of Life

Short form-36 and EuroQoL-5D are generic tools commonly used to study health-related quality of life (HRQoL) in primary SS. These are used to study QoL in other chronic diseases as well. These measures do not change over the trial period; however, they are used as secondary outcome measures and as markers of economic benefit of novel therapies.

LEARNING POINTS

- ESSDAI and ESSPRI are valid outcome measures in primary SS which assess systemic disease activity and patient perception of symptoms respectively. These are complementary to each other.
- ESSDAI, although useful in clinical practice and large cohort studies to assess organ involvement, has failed to show differential response between treatment and placebo arms in several randomised controlled trials (RCTs).
- Patient-reported outcomes are less sensitive to change with treatment, especially PROFAD and SSI.
- A combination of outcome measures including ESSDAI, PROs and glandular function may be preferable in RCTs.

FURTHER READING

1. Del Papa N, Vitali C. Management of primary Sjögren's syndrome: recent developments and new classification criteria. Ther Adv Musculoskelet Dis. 2018;10:39–54.
2. de Wolff L, Arends S, van Nimwegen JF, Bootsma H. Ten years of the ESSDAI: is it fit for purpose? Clin Exp Rheumatol. 2020;38 Suppl 126:283–90.
3. Seror R, Bowman S. Outcome measures in primary Sjögren's syndrome. Arthritis Care Res. 2020;72:134–49.
4. Seror R, Rauz S, Gosset M, Bowman SJ. Disease activity and patient reported outcome measures in Sjögren's-what are the best tools to evaluate? Rheumatology (Oxford). 2019:kez201.
5. Seror R, Theander E, Brun JG, et.al., EULAR Sjögren's Task Force. Validation of EULAR primary Sjögren's syndrome disease activity (ESSDAI) and patient indexes (ESSPRI). Ann Rheum Dis. 2015;74:859–66.

Chapter 5.6

Outcome Measures in Systemic Sclerosis

Anuj Shukla

INTRODUCTION

Systemic sclerosis (SSc) is characterized by microangiopathy, obliterative vasculopathy, immune dysregulation, and fibrosis. Its clinical manifestations have marked patient-to-patient variability in the organs involved, disease course, severity, and outcome. The skin is the primary organ involved with high morbidity leading to limitation of mouth opening, limitation of movements of hands, and other joints such as the elbows and knees. Raynaud's phenomenon and poor skin repair can result in frequent cutaneous ulcers. Interstitial lung disease (ILD), heart, gastrointestinal tract, and kidney involvement is directly associated with mortality.

In SSc outcome measures were primarily developed and validated for clinical trials but simpler short versions can be used for clinical practice. These outcome measures can be composite or organ-specific, and physician or patient-reported.

OUTCOME MEASURES

Raynaud's Phenomenon

Raynaud's phenomenon being the most common manifestation of SSc is easily assessed on a visual analog scale (VAS). Patients can also maintain a diary to document the number and severity of episodes (Table 5.6.1).

Skin Involvement

The modified-Rodnan skin score (mRSS) is the standard modality to date to measure skin involvement in scleroderma. The mRSS is a clinical method of assessing the thickness of the skin. The assessor uses the fingers to assess the thickness of the patient's skin and grades the skin as normal skin, mild thickness, moderate thickness, and severe thickness, based on which a score from 0 to 3 is assigned. Seventeen sites of the body are assessed, giving a possible final score of 51. The posterior chest is not scored.

The mRSS correlates with interstitial lung disease and a decline in forced vital capacity (FVC). The major limitations are that it is subjective and scores can vary from one assessor to another. Of the three changes that occur in the skin in scleroderma, mRSS can only measure skin thickness but not skin tightening or skin tethering.

Mouth opening in SSc can get hampered as a result of skin thickness and tightening. Therefore the distance between the maxillary and mandibular incisor is reduced in scleroderma. The physician can assess patients using a scale called the mouth handicap in systemic sclerosis scale (Table 5.6.1).

Hand Mobility and Function

Skin tightening and thickening lead to joint contractures affecting both large and small joints. There can be calcinosis. Additional problems are ischemic ulcers of the fingertips, all leading to impaired hand function. Hand function in SSc can be measured as follows:

- By assessing grip strength
- Finger to palm distance: measures flexion of the third finger up to the wrist. This test has been modified as delta finger to palm
- The hand mobility in scleroderma (HAMIS) score

The Cochin hand functional scale (CHFS) measures hand function (Table 5.6.1) based on

Table 5.6.1: Organ-specific (Raynaud's phenomenon. skin, hand, mouth opening, and digital ulcers) outcome measures in systemic sclerosis

Outcome measure domains	*Outcome measure*	*Year*	*Comment*
Raynaud's phenomenon Patient reported	Raynaud's condition score diary	2002	It is scored daily by the patient on a 11-point scale (0–10). The patient scores how much difficulty they experience as a result of Raynaud's.
Skin Physician assessed	Modified Rodnan skin score (mRSS)	–	Score ranges from 0 to 51. A good marker of disease severity and activity and severity. The mRSS contributes to CRISS score, 3–5-unit change in 12 months is significant, it may not be sufficient to document a change and patient-reported outcomes can be complementary to assess skin
Patient reported	Scleroderma skin patient-reported outcome (SSPRO)	2017	This scale has four domains assessed over 4-weeks. The domains are physical effects, physical limitations caused due to skin tightness, social effects, and emotional effects. Each item on each domain is scored on a Likert scale
Hand function Physician assessed	Hand mobility in systemic sclerosis (HAMIS). Four items modified mHAMIS test	2000	HAMIS has nine items viz finger extension, finger flexion, thumb abduction, finger abduction, pincer grip, dorsal extension of wrist, volar flexion of wrist, pronation, and supination. Each is graded from 0 to 3, which indicates normal to inability to perform.
Patient reported	Cochin hand functional scale (CHFS), and short form – CHFS-6	1996	This scale assesses the patient's ability to perform 18-tasks, in five areas namely kitchen (8 items), hygiene (2 items), dressing (2 items), office (2 items), and others (4 items). Each item is score from 0 to 5 i.e. without difficulty to impossible.
Oral Physician assessed	Mouth handicap in systemic sclerosis (MHISS) scale	2007	This scale consists of 12 items: 5 items are related to handicap caused by reduction in opening mouth, 5 items are handicap by sicca syndrome, and another 2 items due to aesthetic concerns
Digital ulcers* Physician assessed	Digital ulcers clinical assessment scores (DUCAS)	2019	There are seven items: number of ulcers, new ulcers, gangrene, need for surgical procedures, infection, hospitalization, and need analgesics due to ulcer related issues. Score ranges from 0 to 19.5
Patient reported	Hand disability in systemic sclerosis digital ulcers (HDISS-DU)	2020	A questionnaire adapted from CHFS has 24 items. Each item is scored from 1 to 6, i.e. without difficulty impossible. The final mean score ranges from 1 to 6
Physician assessed	Digital ulcer score (DUS)	2016	Individual ulcers arescored. One point is assigned if there is only hyperkeratosis, while 10 points is assigned for presence of an ulcer, this is multiplied by the diameter of the ulcer, where one point is assigned for diameter <0.5 cm and 2 points for 0.5 cm. The total is the sum of all ulcers. However, it is yet to be validated.

CRISS: Composite response index in systemic sclerosis

activities as reported by the patient. There are also scales to measure the number, and extent of digital ulcers and gangrene, etc. (Table 5.6.1)

Assessing Internal Organ Complications of SSc

SSc-ILD and Pulmonary Hypertension

ILD and pulmonary hypertension are major complications of SSc. The following tests are used to measure outcomes of lung involvement:

- The 6-minute walk test is easy to perform.
- Forced-vital-capacity (FVC) is a good measure of lung function even in clinical trials.
- Diffusing capacity of carbon monoxide (DLCO) a sensitive measure of ILD
- 2D-echocardiography to measure pulmonary artery hypertension (PAH)
- High-resolution CT chest to document fibrosis and ground-glass opacity.

The patient-reported outcome of ILD and cough questionnaires (Table 5.6.2) also help quantify the cardiopulmonary disease.

Gastrointestinal Tract (GIT)

GIT disease is a disabling manifestation of SSc. Objectively, we can assess with gastrointestinal endoscopy and esophageal manometry. Patient-reported outcomes are available that capture GI manifestations and complications (Table 5.6.2)

Mental Health

Of equal importance is mental health, given that SSc alters the patient's physical appearance due to skin involvement. Patients can report anxiety, depression, body appearance, and satisfaction using certain tools listed in Table 5.6.2.

Composite Measures

The EULAR and EUSTAR research groups have developed indices to assess overall disease activity (Table 5.6.3), while severity can be measured using the Medsger disease severity index. Physical function and quality of life can be measured using HAQ modified for scleroderma (Table 5.6.3).

Table 5.6.2: Organ-specific (lungs, cough, gastrointestinal, and mental health) outcome measures in systemic sclerosis

Outcome measure domains	*Outcome measure*	*Year*	*Comment*
Lungs Patient reported	UCSD-SOBQ	2013	This scale consists of 24-items which are different activities of daily living (21 items), one item each on fear of dyspnea, limitation due to dyspnea, and fear of harm from overexertion. Each item is scored on a scale of 0 = not at all to 5 = maximal or unable to do because of breathlessness. The total score possible is 120
Patient reported	Functional assessment of chronic illness therapy (FACIT)–dyspnea	2011	This scale is validated. It has 10 items related to dyspnea severity, and limitation of function due to dyspnea. Applied for symptoms over past 7 days in common day to day activities, scale ranges from 0 (no) to 3 (severe)
Patient reported	Dyspnea-12	2010	12-items in this scale: 6 items on breathing act, 6 on affective aspects of breathing. It helps the patient respond separately and differentiate systemic symptoms from breathing symptoms
Composite measure for lungs	Composite measure from scleroderma lung study-1 (SLS-1)	2015	composed of FVC (%) predicted, CT based quantitative lung fibrosis, total duration of illness and the HAQ-DI; needs further evaluation of psychometric properties

(*Contd.*)

Table 5.6.2: Organ-specific (lungs, cough, gastrointestinal, and mental health) outcome measures in systemic sclerosis *(Contd.)*

Outcome measure domains	*Outcome measure*	*Year*	*Comment*
Cough Patient reported	Leicester cough questionnaire (LCQ), The cough quality of life questionnaire (CQLQ), the modified cough index (MCI)	2003–2013	Not validated for systemic sclerosis, assesses cough frequency, severity, intensity and/or impact on quality of life
GIT measures Patient reported	Patient-reported outcomes measurement information system (PROMIS-29) GI scale	2014	Eight domains: Four items on bowel incontinence, belly pain, constipation, diarrhea, disrupted swallowing, gastroesophageal reflux, nausea and vomiting, and gas and bloating over last 7 days
Patient reported	UCLA scleroderma clinical trials consortium (SCTC)-GIT 2.0	2011	Assesses reflux, distention and/or bloating, constipation, diarrhea, fecal soilage, social functioning, and emotional well-being, and a total GIT score to assess quality of life and GI tract symptoms severity. Validated for systemic sclerosis
Pain measures	–	–	Assessed as part of a quality-of-life assessment using systemic sclerosis HAQ or the PROMIS-29. Also assessed along with its cause such as belly pain PROMIS GI scale or digital ulcer – DUCAS.
Mental health Patient reported	Social appearance anxiety scale (SAAS) short SAAS-5, Social interaction anxiety scale 6 (SIAS-6)	2018	SAAS assesses social anxiety and fear in situations where one's appearance is evaluated.
Depression Patient reported	Physical health questionnaire (PHQ-9), Center for epidemiological studies (CES-D)	2010	PHQ-9 is easy to use compared to 20-item CES-D. PHQ-8 is a shorter version removing 9th item of suicidal ideation
Appearance Patient reported	Body concealment scale for scleroderma (BCSS)	2016	This scale has 9-items, each is scored 0 (never) to 5 (always). The higher the total score the more it indicates concealment behaviors
Patient reported	Satisfaction with appearance (SWAP), adapted SWAP(ASWAP), brief SWAP	2015	SWAP has 14-items. Each is scored from 1 to 7, strongly disagree to strongly agree. ASWAP is 15-item adapted version for SSc, while brief is a 6-item version

UCSD-SOBQ: University of California–San Diego-shortness of breath questionnaire; *HAQ-DI:* Health assessment questionnaire–disability index; *FVC:* Forced vital capacity; *CT:* Computer tomography; *GIT:* Gastrointestinal tract; *HRQOL:* health related quality of life; *S-HAQ:* Scleroderma health assessment questionnaire

Table 5.6.3: Composite outcome measures in systemic sclerosis

Domains	*Outcome measure*	*Year*	*Comment*
Disease activity	European scleroderma study group activity index (EScSG-AI)	2003	Comprises 10 domains: total skin score, scleredema, arthritis, digital necrosis, ESR, decreased DLco, low serum complements. Also included are patient reported skin, cardiopulmonary, and vascular changes. Each variable ranges from 0.5 to 2 with a total score of 0–10.
	European scleroderma trials and research activity index (EUSTAR-AI)	2017	Revised version EScSC-AI; 6 variables-Changes in skin, mRSS >18, tendon friction rub, digital ulcers, C-reactive protein >1 mg/dL, DLCO<70%, >2.5 is active disease
Disease severity	Medsger disease severity scale	2003	Encompasses both damage and activity Nine domains—general health, peripheral vascular, skin, GI tract, lungs, joint/tendon, muscle, heart and kidneys. Total score is 36
Physical function	Scleroderma health assessment questionnaire (S-HAQ)	1997	Composed of the HAQ disability index (HAQ-DI) and additional six-VAS scales-pain, intestinal, breathing, Raynaud's and finger ulcers interference in past week and total disease severity today
Treatment response	Composite response index in systemic sclerosis	2016	First is to assess whether the disease is worsening or there is new end organ damage. Second step is to assess improvement of five variables determined over 1-year. There five variables include– skin scores (modified Rodnan), lung capacity (FVC), physician global, patient global assessment, and HAQ-DI
Organ damage Physician-assessed measure	Scleroderma clinical trials consortium damage index (SCTC-DI)	2019	23-weighted items covering domains: skin, gastrointestinal tract, vascular, musculoskeletal, respiratory, cardiovascular, and kidney. Maximum score is 55.
General health status (generic measure)	Patient-reported outcomes measurement information system PROMIS-29 (2.1)	2018	Seven domains assessed over last week, i.e. fatigue, depression, anxiety, pain interference, sleep, physical function, social functioning, and a pain intensity numeric rating scale.

mRSS: modified-Rodnan Skin score; *DLCO:* Diffusion capacity of the lungs for carbon monoxide; *GI:* Gastrointestinal; *VAS:* Visual analog scale; *FVC:* Forced vital capacity

CONCLUSION

With plenty of outcome measures emerging comparative studies are needed to test reliability, feasibility, validity, and sensitivity to change with newer therapies. In the process, many changes will be required to get the final tools that can represent such a heterogeneous disease while at the same time maintaining the feasibility for use both in clinical trials and daily practice.

LEARNING POINTS

- The mRSS is a standard tool to measure skin involvement in SSc.
- Hand function is measured using hand mobility in scleroderma (HAMIS) score (physician

assessed) and the Cochin hand functional scale (CHFS) (patient-reported)

- Digital ulcers can also be quantified using digital ulcers clinical assessment scores (DUCAS) and digital ulcer score (DUS). Both are physicians assessed.
- SSc-ILD is measured with 6-minute walk distance test, FVC, and CT chest
- SSc-PAH is measured with a 6-minute walk distance
- GIT involvement is measured using a patient reported measure the scleroderma clinical trial consortium GIT 2.0

FURTHER READING

1. Chang TYJ, Pope JE. An Update of Outcome Measures in Systemic Sclerosis. Arthritis Care Res (Hoboken). 2020;72 Suppl 10:110–33.
2. Lafyatis R, Valenzi E. Assessment of disease outcome measures in systemic sclerosis. Nat Rev Rheumatol. 2022;18:527–41.
3. Pellar RE, Tingey TM, Pope JE. Patient-Reported Outcome Measures in Systemic Sclerosis (Scleroderma). Rheum Dis Clin North Am. 2016;42:301–16.
4. Wells AU, Behr J, Silver R. Outcome measures in the lung. Rheumatology (Oxford). 2008;47 Suppl 5:v48–50.

Outcome Measures in Systemic Vasculitis

Saket Jha, Aadhar Dhooria

INTRODUCTION

Vasculitic syndromes are an exciting field of research and treatment, with most trials and clinical research being performed in the last two decades. With an explosion of knowledge also comes a question on how to assess outcomes in a given vasculitis patient and also whether the clinical tools used to measure outcome in published trials, are relevant in routine clinical practice. Similar to other rheumatic diseases outcome measures in vasculitis can be grouped as follows:

- To assess disease activity
- To assess damage
- Prognosis
- Patient-reported outcomes.

The outcome measures deployed depend on the vasculitis under purview. Whereas Birmingham vasculitis activity score version 3 (BVAS v3) is used most commonly in antineutrophil cytoplasmic antibodies (ANCA)-associated vasculitis (AAV), the Indian Takayasu activity score (ITAS2010) is employed in Takayasu arteritis.

DISEASE ACTIVITY ASSESSMENT

Birmingham Vasculitis Activity Score (BVAS)

The BVAS is the most common outcome measure used in clinical practice and vasculitis research. It was first described and validated in 1994 in patients with various types of vasculitis. The scoring includes nine organ-based systems with a maximum possible score of 63. The second version of modification BVAS (BVAS v2) has two components: BVAS1 shows the disease either to be new or to be worse. Similarly, BVAS2 shows disease to be persistent.

BVAS v3 in use since 2008, reduced the number of items scored from 66 to 56 and eliminated the need for two separate scores. The weightage of individual item varies from 1–9. The variability in weight of each item depends upon how severe the manifestation is, and whether it is new manifestation or worsening of previous manifestations (activity has recurred or worsened within the past 4 weeks) or continuing or persistent disease activity (activity present continuously without worsening for past 4 weeks). It is important that disease manifestations should be scored only when it is due to active vasculitis.

Advantage of BVAS is that it can be applied across various types of vasculitis except for giant cell arteritis, especially early in the clinical course where exact classification may not be possible. The major limitation of BVAS is an imperfect correlation with treatment decisions.

BVAS/WG: It is specifically used for activity assessment in patients with granulomatosis with polyangiitis (GPA).

Indian Takayasu Clinical Activity Score 2010 (ITAS 2010)

This is a tool developed specifically for activity assessment in patients with Takayasu arteritis (TA). Six organ-based systems with 44 items is used to score the activity. The cardiovascular system with 33 items, is the most dominant organ system in activity assessment. Other organ systems included are gastrointestinal, genitourinary, renal, and nervous systems. New manifestations or worsening manifestations in the past 3 months which have contributed to disease activity are scored. ITAS 2010 is a numerical tool and is sensitive to change and has clinical utility in following up on these patients. ITAS-A includes ITAS2010 along with inflammatory markers, namely ESR or CRP. A summary of these outcome assessment measures is outlined in Table 5.7.1.

Table 5.7.1: Summary of outcome measures in systemic vasculitis

Outcome measure	*Vasculitis*	*Domain*	*Salient features*	*Scoring*	*Limitations*
BVASv3	All systemic vasculitis	9 domain 56 manifestations	1. Ability to score persistent disease 2. Best tool to measure early/ unclassified vasculitis	Maximum persistent score = 33, Maximum new/ worse score = 63, Remission = 0	Not disease specific
BVAS/ WG	GPA/WG	9 domain, 36 manifestations, Section for physician global assessment	Disease specific	Maximum score = 68	Lacks grading of severity
VDI	All systemic vasculitis	10 domains 64 manifestations	Measures cumulative damage, The score never improves	Maximum score = 64	Measures cumulative damage, needs the previous score
ITAS 2010	Takayasu arteritis	6 domains 44 items (33 items from the cardiovascular system)	Disease-specific, Sensitive to treatment, Use both clinical and acute phase reactants.	Maximum score = 51	First assessment may falsely represent activity due to scoring of damage due to slow grumbling disease
DEI.Tak	Takayasu arteritis	11 domains, Special emphasis on cardiovascular domain	Measures disease extent includes both activity and damage	Maximum score = 75	Poor differentiation between activity and remission
SF 36	All systemic vasculitis	8 domains, 36 questions	Patient's perspective on the impact of the disease	Maximum score = 100 (score 0 max disability, score 100 min disability)	Not disease-specific
PETVAS	Large vessel vasculitis	4 segments of aorta and 11 branch arteries	PET scan (vascular uptake) based activity assessment	PETVAS ≥20 predicts active disease or relapse	Not applicable in all healthcare settings

BVAS v3: Birmingham vasculitis activity score (BVAS) version3; *WG:* Wegener's granulomatosis; *VDI:* Vasculitis damage index; *ITAS2010:* Indian Takayasu clinical activity score; *DEI.Tak:* Disease extent index Takayasu; *SF 36:* Short forms 36; *PETVAS:* PET vasculitis activity score

Disease Damage Assessment

Vasculitis damage index (VDI): It measures damage in vasculitis. It constitutes a total of 64 items. The items were selected by expert consensus. It reflects damage due to vasculitis, irrespective of the activity status of disease or adverse effects related to drugs. Manifestations which show irreversible damage and which has been present for a minimum of 3 months are scored. Thus, VDI score should not fall with time during longitudinal follow-up. VDI has also been found to be associated with poor survival in previous studies.

PROGNOSTIC ASSESSMENT

Five Factor Score (FFS)

The FFS is used as a prognostic tool. It is used to predict mortality in systemic necrotising vasculitis. It was devised in the year 1996 by the French Vasculitis Study Group. It was first validated in 342 patients with polyarteritis nodosa (n = 260) and Churg-Strauss syndrome (n = 82) now called eosinophilic granulomatosis with polyangiitis (EGPA).

The FFS includes items that, if present at baseline, predict mortality (Table 5.7.2). A score of 1 for each feature: proteinuria >1 g/24 hours, serum creatinine >1.58 mg/dL, gastrointestinal (GIT) involvement, cardiomyopathy, and central nervous system (CNS) signs was assigned. In 2009 it was revised to include age >65 years. Proteinuria was removed. Involvement of throat, nose, and ear received a negative score, as its presence carried a negative risk with mortality.

The 2009 FFS carried a score of +1 for each of age >65 years, cardiac symptoms, GI involvement, renal insufficiency, and -1 for ENT involvement. The revised score was validated in PAN, EGPA, microscopic polyangiitis, and GPA. The 5-year mortality of patients with 2009 FFS scores of 0, 1, and ≥2 were 9%, 21%, and 40%, respectively.

Patient-reported Outcomes

Till date no disease-specific, patient-reported measure has been materialized in vasculitis research. There are generic measuring tools like short form 36 (SF-36). It includes 26 items in 8 health dimensions, accessing health-related quality of life (HRQoL). Each dimension has a scale range from 0 to 100, with higher scores indicating better HRQoL. It has been shown that it captures morbidity burden which is not accessed by BVAS.

LEARNING POINTS

- Activity status of the disease and damage status due to previous insult is the core area of assessment by various outcome measures tools in vasculitis.
- BVASv3 and BVAS-WG for small vessel vasculitis and ITAS2010 for TA are the currently used outcome measures for disease activity assessment.
- VDI is used to assess damage
- FFS: Presence of at least one risk factor carries a higher risk of mortality at 5 years

Table 5.7.2: The five factor score (FFS)

1996 FFS	*2009 FFS*
Presence of any one of the following items increases the 5-year risk of mortality.	Presence of any of the first 4 items increases the 5-year mortality, but presence of ear nose throat (ENT) symptoms has a negative risk for mortality.
1. Renal insufficiency: Serum creatinine >140 µmol/L (1.58 mg/dL) 2. Proteinuria of >1g/day 3. Central nervous system involvement (encephalopathy) 4. Cardiac involvement 5. Gastrointestinal (GI) involvement	1. Age >65 years 2. Renal insufficiency: Peak serum creatinine ≥150 µmol/L (1.67 mg/dL) 3. Cardiac involvement 4. GI involvement 5. ENT involvement: negative risk of mortality

1996 FFS was validated in polyarteritis nodosa, microscopic polyangiitis, and eosinophilic granulomatosis with polyangiitis (EGPA), 2009 FFS was validated in granulomatosis with polyangiitis (GPA) also

FURTHER READING

1. Exley AR, Bacon PA, Luqmani RA, et al. Development and initial validation of the Vasculitis Damage Index for the standardized clinical assessment of damage in the systemic vasculitides. Arthritis Rheum. 1997;40: 371–80.
2. Guillevin L, Pagnoux C, Seror R, et al.; French Vasculitis Study Group (FVSG). The Five-Factor Score revisited: assessment of prognoses of systemic necrotizing vasculitides based on the French Vasculitis Study Group (FVSG) cohort. Medicine (Baltimore). 2011; 90:19–27.
3. Luqmani RA, Bacon PA, Moots RJ, et al. Birmingham Vasculitis Activity Score (BVAS) in systemic necrotizing vasculitis. QJM. 1994;87:671–8.
4. Misra R, Danda D, Rajappa SM, et al.; Indian Rheumatology Vasculitis (IRAVAS) group. Development and initial validation of the Indian Takayasu Clinical Activity Score (ITAS2010). Rheumatology (Oxford). 2013;52:1795–801.
5. Mukhtyar C, Lee R, Brown D, et al. Modification and validation of the Birmingham Vasculitis Activity Score (version 3). Ann Rheum Dis. 2009;68:1827–32.
6. Tomasson G. Quality of life and outcome measures in vasculitis. Best Practice Res Clin Rheumat. 2013;27: 69–77.

Outcome Measures in Osteoarthritis

Pooja Belani

INTRODUCTION

The dearth of advances in the treatment for osteoarthritis (OA) is multifactorial, one of which is the lack of a single specific tool for measuring the effectiveness of treatment.

OUTCOME MEASURES

Outcome measures in OA can be classified using the WHO-International classification of functioning, disability, and health (ICF) model of impairment, disability, and handicap (Tables 5.8.1 and 5.8.2).

Table 5.8.1: Classification of outcome measures in osteoarthritis according to International classification of functioning, disability and health (ICF)

Impairment		*Disability (Activity limitation)*		*Handicap/participation*
Pain	Visual analogue scale	Hip And/Or Knee OA WOMAC Timed chair stand test Timed up-and-go test Stair climb test 40-m fast paced walk test 6-min walk test		Jette Late-Life Function and Disability Instrument
	McGill Pain Questionnaire			
	PainDETECT			
	Numeric rating scale			
	S-LANSS			
	ICOAP			
Fatigue	Visual analogue scale			
	Numeric rating scale	Hip OA-HOOS Knee OA-KOOS		
	Functional Assessment of Chronic Illness Therapy–Fatigue scale	Hand OA Subjective-	Objective –	
	Profile of Mood States Fatigue Scale	DASH AUSCAN Cochin FIHOA SACRAH	Button test Dexterity JTHFT Grip strength Pinch strength	
	Multidimensional Fatigue Symptom Inventory			
Sleep	Visual analogue scale			
	Numeric rating scale			
	Chronic Pain Sleep Inventory			
	Sleep Disorders Questionnaire			
	Pittsburgh Sleep Quality Index			

(*Contd.*)

Table 5.8.1: Classification of outcome measures in osteoarthritis according to International classification of functioning, disability and health (ICF) *(Contd.)*

Impairment		*Disability (Activity Limitation)*	*Handicap/Participation*
Mood	CES-D	Work productivity	
	HADS		
	PHQ-8		
Clinical examination	Tender/ swollen joint	Need of walking aid	
	Joint deformity		
	Joint instability		
	Heberden's/Bouchard's nodes		
Imaging	Joint space narrowing		
	Bone marrow edema		
	Cartilage assessment on MRI		
	TOMS		
Biomarkers	MMP-1 , MMP 3		
	CTX-I, CTX- II		
	COMP		
	VCAM-1		
Treatment	Pill count (NSAIDs)		
	Need for joint replacement surgery		

OA: Osteoarthritis; *AUSCAN:* Australian-Canadian hand osteoarthritis index; *Cochin:* Cochin hand functional disability scale; *CES-D:* Center for epidemiologic studies depression scale; *DASH:* Disabilities of the arm, shoulder and hand questionnaire; *FIHOA:* Functional index for hand osteoarthritis; *HADS:* Hospital anxiety and depression scale; *HOOS:* Hip disability and osteoarthritis outcome score; *ICOAP:* Measure of intermittent and constant osteoarthritis pain; *KOOS:* Knee injury and osteoarthritis outcome score; *S-LANSS:* Self-report leeds assessment of neuropathic symptoms and signs pain scale; *VAS:* Visual analog scale; *WOMAC:* Western Ontario and McMaster universities osteoarthritis index; *ICOAP:* Intermittent and constant osteoarthritis pain; *MMP:* Matrix metalloproteinase, *SACRAH:* Score for the assessment and quantification of chronic rheumatoid affections of the hands, *JTHFT:* Jebsen-Taylor hand function test; *CTX-I:* C-telopeptide of type I collagen; *CTX-II:* C-telopeptide of type II collagen, *COMP:* Cartilage oligomeric matrix protein; *VCAM-1:* Vascular cell adhesion molecule

Table 5.8.2: International classification of functioning, disability, and health (ICF) domains measured by different composite outcome measures

Questionnaire (Patient reported)	*OA*	*Impairment*	*Disability*	*Handicap*
WOMAC	Hip/knee OA	+	+	–
Lequesne's index	Hip/knee OA	+	+	–
SACRAH	Hand OA	+	+	–
AUSCAN	Hand OA	+	+	–
ASES	Any OA	+	+	–
DASH	Hand OA	+	+	+
PROMIS 29	Any OA	+	+	+
ODI	Spine OA	+	+	+
RDQ	Spine OA	+	+	–

WOMAC: Western Ontario and McMaster universities osteoarthritis index; *SACRAH:* Score for assessment and quantification of chronic rheumatoid affection of the hand; *DASH:* Disabilities of arm, shoulder and hand; *PROMIS 29:* Patient reported outcome measurement information system 29; *ASES:* Arthritis self efficacy scale; *AUSCAN:* Australian/Canadian hand OA index; *ODI:* Oswestry disability index; *RDQ:* Roland-Morris disability questionnaire

Some outcome measures are OA specific, whereas others are generic that are used in other rheumatic diseases as well, some are joint-specific and some are for generalized OA.

Outcome measures in OA can further be classified as subjective or patient-based measures, for example, the Western Ontario and McMaster Universities osteoarthritis index (WOMAC), and objective or performance-based measures. Subjective measures may evaluate all three aspects of ICF categories (namely impairment, disability, and handicap) whereas objective measures evaluate mainly the disability and functional aspect of the disease.

Psychometric Properties of an Ideal Outcome Measure

The desired outcome measure should be reliable (able to discriminate), valid (measures what it is intended to measure), and responsive to change (Figure 5.8.1). The psychometric properties of the outcome measures in OA are described in Table 5.8.3.

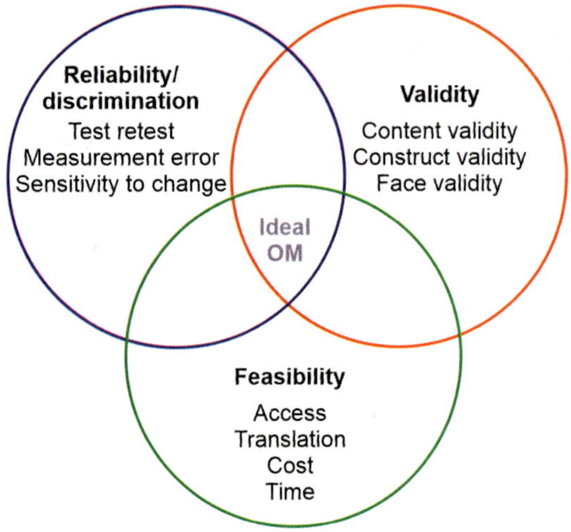

Fig. 5.8.1: Psychometric properties of outcome measure

ASSESSMENT OF IMPAIRMENTS IN OSTEOARTHRITIS

The ICF core set measures in OA includes the following under impairment of body function—pain, fatigue, sleep, and mood: body structure deformities, crepitus, radiographic changes,

Table 5.8.3: Psychometric properties of various outcome measures for osteoarthritis

	Validity	*Discrimination*	*Feasibility*	*Responsiveness*	*Generic/specific*
PainDETECT	++	++	++	++	Any
ICOAP	++	++	++	++	Hip/knee
PSQI	++	++	++	++	Any
WOMAC	++	++	++	++	Hip/knee
Lequesne's index	++	++	++	—	Hip/knee
AUSCAN	++	++	—	++	Hand
FIHOA	++	++	+	++	Hand
Grip strength	++	+	—	++	Hand
DASH	++	++	++	++	Hand/shoulder
30s chair stand test, 40 m fast-paced walk test, stair climb test	+	++	++	—	Hip/knee
HADS	++	++	++	++	Any
HAMIS, FPD, MKI	++	++	++	NA	Hand
ODI	++	++	++	++	Spine
RDQ	++	++	++	++	Spine
Radiography JSN	+	++	++	+	Any

(Contd.)

Table 5.8.3: Psychometric properties of various outcome measures for osteoarthritis *(Contd.)*

	Validity	*Discrimination*	*Feasibility*	*Responsiveness*	*Generic/specific*
Kellgren and Lawrence scoring	++	++	++	++	Any
OARSI Atlas	++	++	++	++	Any
SQ MRI (WORMS, BLOKS, MOCKS, KOSS)	++	++	+	++	Knee
SQ MRI (HOAMS)	++	++	+	++	Hip
Quantitative MRI	++	++	—	++	Knee/hip
Compositional MRI	++	++	—	++	Hip/knee
TOMS	++	NA	—	NA	Hand
HOAMRIS	++	++	—	++	Hand

ICOAP: Intermittent and constant osteoarthritis pain; *PSQI:* Pittsburgh sleep quality index; *HADS:* Hospital anxiety and depression scale; *HAMIS:* Hand mobility in scleroderma; *FPD:* Finger palm distance; *MKI:* Modified Kapandji test; *ODI:* Oswestry disability index; *RDQ:* Roland-Morris disability questionnaire; *SQ:* Semi-quantitative, *WORMS:* Whole organ magnetic resonance imaging score; *KOSS:* The knee osteoarthritis scoring system; *BLOKS:* The Boston Leeds osteoarthritis knee score; *TOMS:* Thumb base osteoarthritis magnetic resonance imaging scoring system; *HOAMRIS:* Hand osteoarthritis MRI score.

and biomarkers indicating cartilage damage (Table 5.8.1).

Assessment of Pain

The most often utilized general measures for pain are the 10 cm visual analog scale (VAS) or numerical rating scale. OA-specific measures for pain include WOMAC, Hip disability and osteoarthritis outcome score (HOOS), and specific to hand osteoarthritis is the AUSCAN (Australian–Canadian hand osteoarthritis index).

WOMAC is self-administered and has 24 items (questions). It includes 3 subscales (pain, stiffness, and physical function). Pain due to central sensitization in OA can be evaluated by either pain DETECT, or the McGill pain questionnaire, or the Self-report Leeds assessment of neuropathic symptoms and signs (S-LANSS) pain scale.

Assessment of Fatigue, Sleep, and Mood

No specific measures to assess fatigue, sleep, and mood for OA exist. The generic measures used in OA clinical trials are shown in Table 5.8.1.

Outcome Measures for Structural Damage

Disease modification is defined as an improvement in OA-related symptoms with arrest/reversal of structural changes of the disease. The current FDA guidelines require the demonstration of slowing of the loss of joint space on radiographs, for any drug to classify as disease-modifying therapies for osteoarthritis (DMOAD).

Structure damage can be assessed clinically (deformities, joint instability) or by imaging.

Radiographs as an Outcome Measure in Osteoarthritis

Radiographic assessment can be quantitative–joint space width (JSW) or semiquantitative using the Kellgren and Lawrence (KL) grading and/or OARSI atlas. Joint space narrowing (JSN) on radiographs are valid and reliable markers of structural progression in OA in clinical trials. The drawbacks include lack of reproducibility, inability to directly visualize cartilage, low sensitivity and specificity, and inability to capture other aspects of this multi-dimensional disease like bone marrow lesions, and effusion.

MRI in Osteoarthritis

MRI is now increasingly used as the primary endpoint in clinical trials for assessing cartilage morphology and OA progression. Three types of MRI techniques are used as an outcome measure in OA

- **Semiquantitative MRI:** The MRI pathology in OA is graded according to the severity on an ordinal scale (e.g. severity 1, 2, 3). Examples of these are given in Table 5.8.3.

- **Quantitative MRI:** Quantitative MRI involves specialized MRI techniques (labor intensive, expert analyst, specialized computer software, special training for segmentation technique) for accurate quantification of tissue characteristics.
- **Compositional MRI:** In this collagen and proteoglycan-associated glycosaminoglycans content is evaluated. Techniques of compositional MRI to evaluate cartilage changes includes T2 mapping, T1rho, diffusion tensor imaging, dGEMRIC (delayed gadolinium-enhanced MRI of cartilage) amongst other techniques.

Biomarker

Currently, no biomarker is approved as valid outcome measure in OA.

Assessment of Activity Limitations in Osteoarthritis

Tools for measuring activity limitation (disability) is joint-specific. Subjective (questionnaire-based) and objective (patient-based measures) are complementary to each other.

Measurement of Activity Limitations (Hip and Knee OA)

Standardized questionnaires to evaluate activity limitations include the WOMAC and HOOS for hip OA, and WOMAC and KOOS for knee OA. The Timed up and Go test, the 30-second chair stand test, 40-meter fast-paced walk test, the stair climb test, 6-minute walk test is used to assess functional activity.

Measurement of Activity Limitations (Hand OA)

Generic measures: The disabilities of the arm, shoulder, and hand questionnaire, and OA-specific AUSCAN is reliable, valid, and responsive. However, AUSCAN is not freely available, making it less feasible. Objectively, hand OA can be assessed by evaluating grip strength, pinch strength, and hand mobility.

No disease-specific instruments exist. The hand mobility in the scleroderma test, the fingertip-to-palm distance, and the modified Kapandji index have been validated and are reliable and feasible in OA.

Assessment of Participation Restrictions (Handicap)

Generic instruments may be used to assess handicaps in occupations, leisure, relationships with others, and community involvement due to the lack of any specific OA measure to assess the handicap in OA.

LEARNING POINTS

- Outcome measures in osteoarthritis can be classified based on 3 domains of the International classification of functioning, disability, and Health (ICF)
- Ideal outcome measures should encompass all aspects of ICF domains
- The outcome measures should be valid, reliable, and responsive to change.

FURTHER READING

1. Lundgren-Nilsson Å, Dencker A, Palstam A, et al. Patient-reported outcome measures in osteoarthritis: a systematic search and review of their use and psychometric properties. RMD Open. 2018;4:e000715.
2. Nilsdotter A, Bremander A. Measures of hip function and symptoms: Harris Hip Score (HHS), Hip Disability and Osteoarthritis Outcome Score (HOOS), Oxford Hip Score (OHS), Lequesne Index of Severity for Osteoarthritis of the Hip (LISOH), and American Academy of Orthopedic Surgeons (AAOS) Hip and Knee Questionnaire. Arthritis Care Res (Hoboken). 2011;63 Suppl 11:S200–7.
3. Osteoarthritis Research Society International. Outcome measures. https://oarsi.org/research/outcome-measures (accessed on 25/08/2022).
4. Strand V, Kelman A. Outcome measures in osteoarthritis: randomized controlled trials. Curr Rheumatol Rep. 2004;6:20–30.
5. Veenhof C, Bijlsma JW, van den Ende CH, et al. Psychometric evaluation of osteoarthritis questionnaires: a systematic review of the literature. Arthritis Rheum. 2006;55:480–92.

Chapter 5.9

Outcome Measures in Juvenile Idiopathic Arthritis

Manjari Agarwal

INTRODUCTION

Pain was the most common outcome measure in juvenile idiopathic arthritis (JIA) as it is easily comprehended by the child and caregiver. However, only measuring pain ignores various other components that affect the life of the child with JIA. Therefore, over the years with better patient participation, outcome measures in JIA have included functional status, and quality of life also.

A good set of outcome measures helps a clinician objectively decide on drug therapy (especially biological agents), psychological counseling, and physical therapy to improve the functional status.

The majority of JIA outcome measures are employed in clinical trials and less frequently in everyday practice since they are time-consuming and difficult to fit into a busy clinical practice. Moreover, several of the outcome measures may not be suitable for use in different socioeconomic and cultural situations. It is however felt that the outcome measures are required to be integrated with health care to improve the care provided to these children.

Outcome measures in JIA include the following domains:

1. Disease activity
2. Damage
3. Function
4. Quality of life

DISEASE ACTIVITY

Several tools are available to assess disease activity.

a. **Physician global assessment:** This is also called MD global. This is a simple analog scale that measures the overall impact of JIA on the child at the time of visit. There is no subscale, takes less than 20 seconds to complete, and answers the question of "how is the patient doing overall"

b. **Patient and parent assessment of disease activity:** This is a simple visual analog scale (VAS) completed by a parent or the patient. This is based on a recall of disease activity of the last one week.

c. **Juvenile arthritis disease activity score (JADAS):** This is a single measure that include the following components: Physician global assessment on a VAS, Parent/patient Global assessment (VAS 10 cm), ESR (0–10), and active joint count. There are three versions based on joint count:

   JADAS 10 has a selected joint count, total score: 0–40

   JADAS 27 has a selected joint count, total score: 0–57

   JADAS 71 has unrestricted joint count, total score: 0–101

   Inactive disease according to JADAS is summarized in Table 5.9.1.

   JADAS with CRP has a higher correlation with disease activity as compared to ESR. The disadvantages of the JADAS are that it does not capture extra-articular disease namely ocular symptoms and systemic features of JIA

d. **Clinical juvenile arthritis disease activity score (cJADAS):** This is easy to use in practice and does not require any laboratory values. It includes active joint count, parent/patient global assessment, and MD global assessment. This has

Table 5.9.1: Disease activity assessments as per the original JADAS and clinical JADAS (cJADAS)

Activity	*cJADAS10*	*JADAS 10/71*	*JADAS 27*
Polyarthritis			
Inactive disease	≤1	≤1	≤1
Low	1.1–2.5	1.1–3.8	1.1–3.8
Moderate	2.51–8.5	3.9–10.5	3.9–8.5
High	>8.5	>10.5	>8.5
Oligoarthritis			
Inactive disease	≤1	≤1	≤1
Low	1.1–1.5	1.1–2	1.1–2
Moderate	1.51–4	2.1–4.2	2.1–4.2
High	>4	>4.2	>4.2

Adapted from: Consolaro A et al., Clinical outcome measures in juvenile idiopathic arthritis. Pediatric Rheumatology. 2016;14:1–8.

three versions based on the active joint count of 10, 27, and 71 joints. The cJADAS has a good correlation with the original JADAS.

e. **Juvenile spondyloarthropathy disease activity (JSpADA) index:** This a disease activity tool for assessment of JIA enthesitis-related arthritis (Table 5.9.2).

The definition of remission in JIA are (A) clinical remission on medication, when on medication there is 6 months of continuous inactive disease. (B) Clinical remission off medication, when there is 1 year inactive disease and the child is off all medications for uveitis and arthritis.

DAMAGE INDICES

Damage is defined as persistent manifestations due to disease or its treatment that are present for at least 6 months. The juvenile arthritis damage index (JADI) has two versions these include:

- **JADI-A:** Articular domain
- **JADI-E:** Extra-articular domain

Various radiographic scores are available that assess joint damage radiologically. A few of them are: the Poznanski score (for wrist damage assessment), Dijkstra score, Sharp and Larsen score, and childhood arthritis radiographic score of the hip (CARSH).

Table 5.9.2: Juvenile spondyloarthritis disease activity (JSpADA) index

JSpADA Index includes 8 items:

1. Active joint count
2. Active enthesitis
3. Clinically active sacroiliitis
4. Presence of uveitis
5. Presence of morning stiffness for >15 minutes
6. Lumbar spine mobility
7. Presence of inflammatory markers
8. Parent/patient assessment of pain and morning stiffness

FUNCTIONAL ASSESSMENT

Functional assessment of JIA is focused on the activities affecting daily routine with an aim of evaluating the impairment in these functional aspects. Various instruments have been derived from adult counterparts. The clinician must be aware of the various domains assessed by the tool that they wish to use.

a. **Childhood health assessment questionnaire (CHAQ):** Published in 1994, it is the most widely used. It is a valid and reliable to measure the functional status in childhood arthritis. It does not measure the quality of life.

b. **Juvenile arthritis functional assessment scale and report (JAFAR):** Developed in the early 90s', it is a questionnaire to measure functional ability and is both valid and reliable. It has a child self-report and parent report form.

c. **Juvenile arthritis self report index (JASI):** Is designed for children more than 8 years of age. It measures various aspects of function such as school, self care. It does not measure the quality of life.
d. **Juvenile arthritis quality of life questionnaire JAQQ:** This measures both physical functional status and psychosocial function.
e. **The childhood arthritis health profile (CAHP):** It Measures physical functional status, pain, mental health, self impact, psychosocial functioning impact of the disease. It is a specific JIA module that focuses on function both gross and fine motor, disability, pain, and activities of daily living. It has a parent report form and children >13 years can also report.

CHAQ and JAFAR are easier to use and are less time consuming. A parent/child may complete it prior to clinic appointment as well and these can be replicated with reliability.

QUALITY OF LIFE (QoL)

This domain of outcome (oft neglected) is important. It is the gap between the achievements and the expectations that an individual has. Mental health and physical functioning are two important determinants of QoL. The QoL instruments incorporate health status, nonmedical aspects of life such as emotional function, relationships with peer and family, and social functioning, as these are indirectly related to ones' health status.

a. **Child health questionnaire:** This is designed for children and the primary domains are self esteem and family functioning. It measures pain, physical function, emotional and mental health, self-esteem, and family cohesion among others.
b. **Pediatric quality of life (PedQL) inventory:** It measures health related QoL in children between 2–18 years of age. It consists of a generic measure combined with a disease specific module. The PedsQL rheumatology module includes daily activities, pain, medications, worry, and communication.

CONCLUSION

There are several outcome measures available for various aspects of health in childhood arthritis. There is, however, a gap between the availability of an appropriate tool and its implementation for routine clinical use. There are areas of research like instruments for young children and the appropriate selection of children for parent proxy reporting. Also, just the availability and the completion of the tool is not enough. The appropriate clinical implementation and action is also necessary.

LEARNING POINTS

- An outcome measure must be simple, easy to use, and reproducible.
- Disease activity, damage, functional status, and quality of life can be assessed using outcome measures in juvenile arthritis
- Outcome measures enable a treat-to-target approach towards patient management.

FURTHER READING

1. Duffy CM. Health outcomes in pediatric rheumatic diseases. Curr Opin Rheumatol. 2004;16:102–8.
2. Consolaro A, Giancane G, Schiappapietra B, et al. Clinical outcome measures in juvenile idiopathic arthritis. Pediatric Rheumatology. 2016;14:1–8.
3. Ringold S, Wallace CA. Measuring clinical response and remission in juvenile idiopathic arthritis. Curr Opin Rheumatol. 2007;19:471–6.
4. Zulian F. Outcome measures and medical progress: why outcome measures are needed in childhood arthritis. Curr Rheumatol Rep. 2003;5:463–70.

Section

VI

IMAGING INVESTIGATIONS AND JOINT INJECTIONS

Chapter 6.1

Conventional Radiology in Rheumatological Disorders

Ramakrishna Rao Uppuluri, U Ravi Theja

INTRODUCTION

Conventional radiographs are inexpensive, widely available and can be easily obtained. Radiographs depict bone erosions, joint space narrowing, subluxation, misalignment and ankylosis of the joints (Table 6.1.1).

Table 6.1.1: Commonly requested radiographic projections

Hand and wrist	Ball-catcher view or Nørgaard projection Anteroposterior (AP)
Elbow	Oblique AP, lateral
Shoulder	AP (with internal and/or external rotation of humerus)
Hip	Pelvis AP [internal rotation and/or external rotation of leg (frog leg)]
Knee	AP (standing), lateral (AP in semi-flexion-tunnel view and sunrise); Skyline view
Ankle	AP, lateral/oblique
Foot	AP (lateral/oblique)
Sacroiliac joints	Pelvis AP (SI oblique)
Lumbar spine	AP, lateral (oblique, coned views)
Thoracic spine	AP, lateral
Cervical spine	AP, lateral (flexion, extension and open mouth view)
Chest	PA, lateral

Note: Projections mentioned in brackets are for special circumstances

Disadvantages: Insensitivity in detecting early bone disease or soft tissue manifestations.

Mnemonic for evaluation of a plain radiograph:

A: Alignment
B: Bone density
C: Cartilage
D: Distribution of lesions
E: Erosions/enthesopathy/eburnation
S: Soft tissue evaluation

CHEST RADIOGRAPH IN RHEUMATOLOGY

I. Pleural/pericardial effusions.
II. Interstitial lung disease (reticulonodular).
III. Pulmonary infiltrates/nodules/mediastinal nodes (Fig. 6.1.1).
IV. Pulmonary hemorrhage (ground glass).

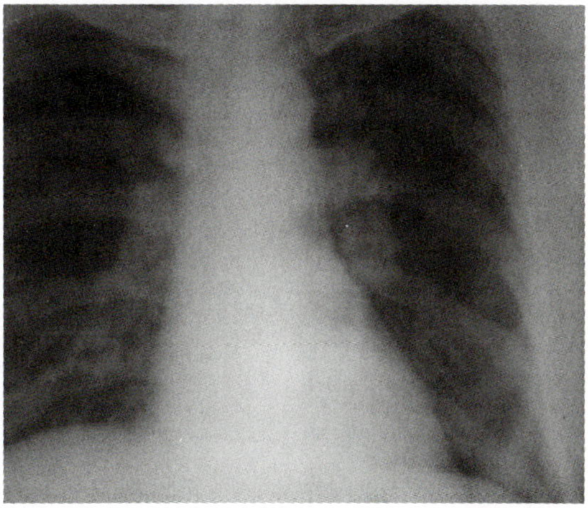

Fig. 6.1.1: Chest (PA view): Bilateral hilar lymph nodes—sarcoidosis

V. Drug complications: Methotrexate pneumonitis shows infiltrates mostly at bases and out of proportion to chest signs.

VI. Calcification.

VII. Cardiac status (size, position, etc.)

RADIOGRAPHS IN RHEUMATOID ARTHRITIS

The most commonly involved joints are metacarpophalangeal (MCP) and proximal interphalangeal (PIP) joints of hands, metatarsophalangeal (MTP) and interphalangeal joints of feet, wrists, elbows, knees, and hips (Figs. 6.1.2 to 6.1.8). Soft tissue swelling around the joints and periarticular osteopenia are early manifestations of RA (Figs. 6.1.2 and 6.1.3) (Table 6.1.2).

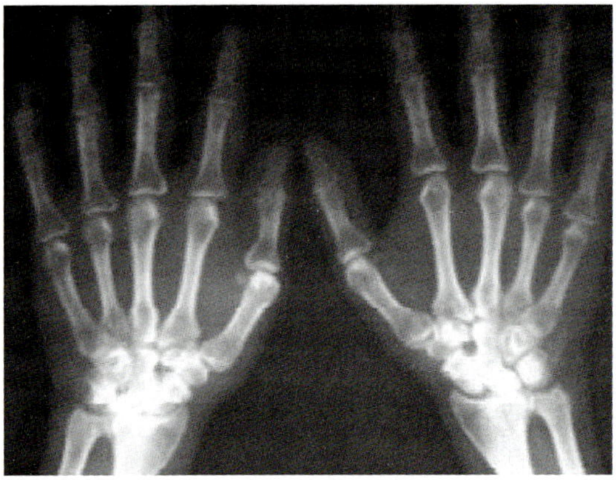

Fig. 6.1.2: Hands (AP view): Early RA with bilateral symmetrical soft tissue swelling at PIP joints

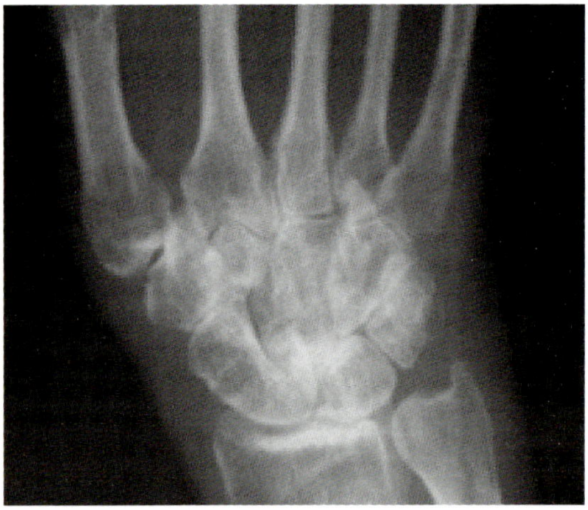

Fig. 6.1.3: Wrist (AP view): Early RA with subarticular osteopenia and joint space narrowing at carpometacarpal, intercarpal, and radiocarpal joints

Table 6.1.2: Features of rheumatoid arthritis

Early	*Delayed*
Soft tissue prominence around the joint	Periarticular erosions
Joint space narrowing (Fig. 6.1.8)	Cystic spaces
Periarticular osteopenia	Subluxations and deformities Ankylosis

The swelling of the PIP joint is usually fusiform. Bilateral and symmetrical swelling of MCP joints, especially 2nd and 3rd are very common. The distal interphalangeal (DIP) joints are spared in RA. As the disease progresses, the erosions appear at synovial attachment sites (Fig. 6.1.4). Subarticular cystic lesions, bony ankylosis or subluxation of MCP joints and ulnar deviation of fingers are noted in the more advanced disease (Fig. 6.1.5).

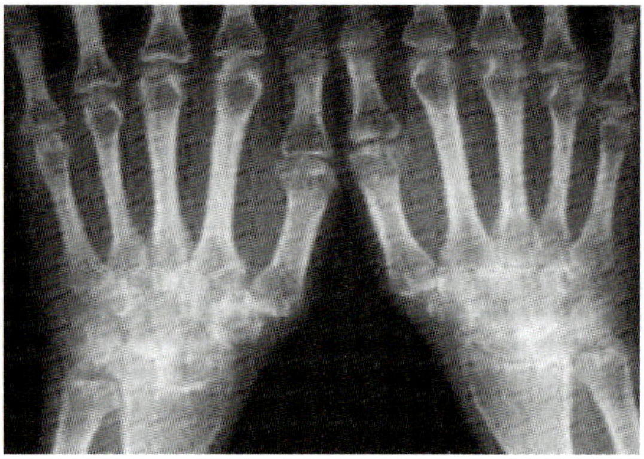

Fig. 6.1.4: Hands (AP view): RA with erosions and narrow joint space in bilateral 2nd, 3rd MCP joints and wrist joints

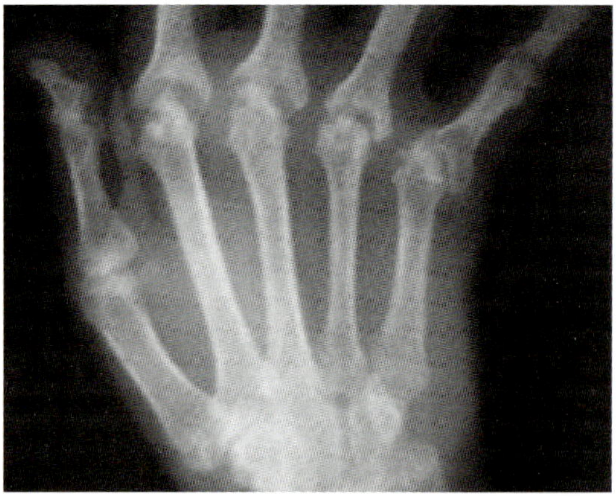

Fig. 6.1.5: Hand (AP view): Advanced RA with erosions, subluxation, and ulnar deviation at MCP joints

Secondary osteoarthritis of the knee is characterized by symmetrical loss of joint space (Fig. 6.1.6). In the feet, the earliest erosive change is seen on the lateral aspect of 5th metatarsal head (Fig. 6.1.7).

Except for the upper cervical spine, the axial skeleton is seldom involved in RA. Subluxation at atlantoaxial (C1–C2) joint due to progressive erosive RA affecting the odontoid process is seen in some of the patients with advanced RA (Table 6.1.3) (Fig. 6.1.9).

Juvenile Idiopathic Arthritis

Radiologically, soft tissue swelling around an affected joint is typical with periarticular osteoporosis. Erosions are late finding in JIA (Fig. 6.1.10), since erosions in the cartilaginous epiphysis will not be visible until ossification is complete. In systemic JIA, there may be fusion of segments of 2–4 cervical vertebrae. Altantoaxial subluxation is found in seropositive, polyarticular RA.

Seronegative Spondyloarthropathy

In these disorders, spinal predilection is common resulting in sacroiliitis and spondylitis (Fig. 6.1.11). Inflammation at the bony insertions of ligaments and tendons (enthesopathy) is radiologically characterized by bony erosions followed by bony proliferation and eventually ankylosis of the adjacent bones.

Ankylosing Spondylitis

The disease starts in the sacroiliac (SI) joints with subchondral bony erosions on the iliac side of the joint with "saw-teeth" appearance. The erosions are followed by bony proliferation and sclerosis. The changes start appearing in the lower third of the SI joint which is synovial. Initially, the joint may look widened due to erosions. The changes gradually affect whole of the SI joint and the joint eventually fuses. Once the fusion is complete, sclerosis

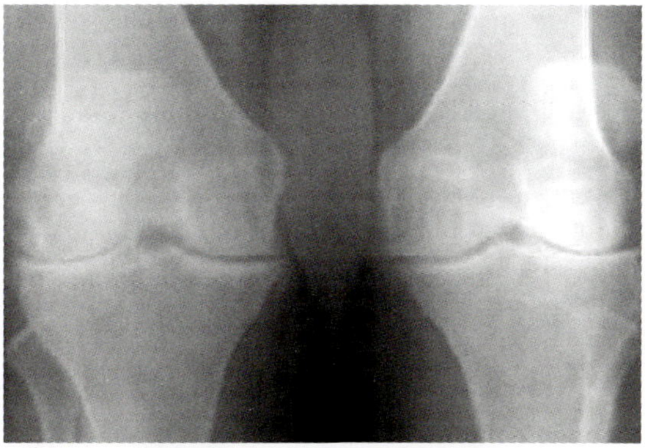

Fig. 6.1.6: Knees (AP view): RA with both compartments narrow, lateral more than medial

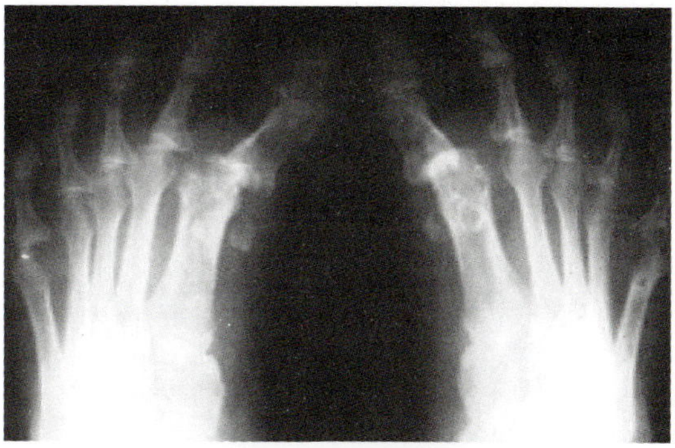

Fig. 6.1.7: Feet (AP view): RA-Dorsi flexion deformities of IP joints and hallux varus deformities of big toe with erosions noted at 1st and 5th MTP joints

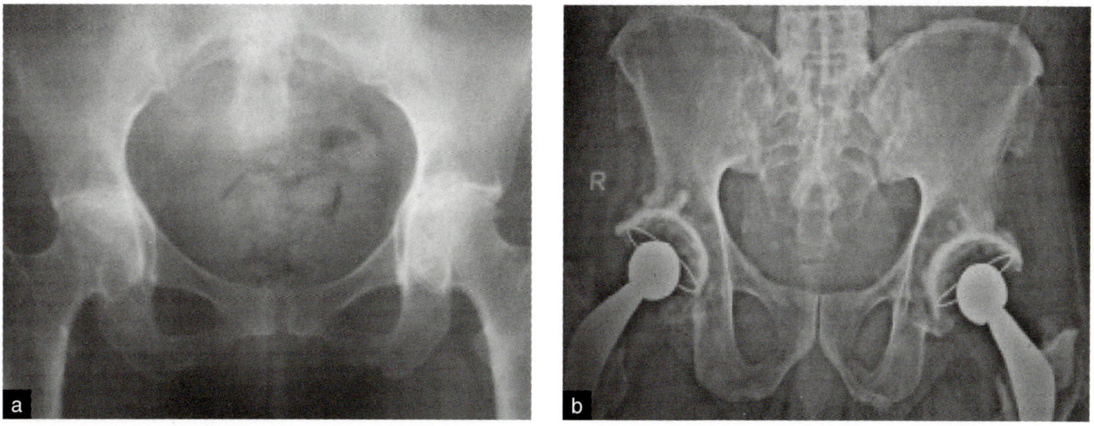

Fig. 6.1.8: (a) Pelvis (AP view): RA-bilateral uniform hip space narrowing with erosions. (b) Pelvis (AP view): RA-bilateral hip replacement

Table 6.1.3: Deformities in rheumatoid arthritis		
Site	*Abnormality*	*Name*
Hand		
• PIP and DIP joints	Flexion PIP, extension DIP	Boutonniere deformity
	Extension PIP, flexion DIP	Swan-neck deformity
• MCP joints	Ulnar deviation, volar subluxation	
Wrist		
• Radiocarpal joint	Radial deviation	
Hip	Acetabular wall medial to Ilioischial line	Protrusio acetabuli
Knee	Outward deviation of knee	Genu varus
	Inward deviation of knee	Genu valgum
Feet		
• First MTP joint	Lateral deviation	Hallux valgus
	Deviation away from 2nd toe	Hallux varus
• PIP and DIP	Hyperextension and dorsal	
	Subluxation of MTP	Cock-up toe
	Hyperflexion PIP or DIP	Hammer toe
Cervical spine		
• Atlantoaxial joint	Atlanto-odontoid space >3 mm	Atlantoaxial subluxation
• All levels	Subluxation of apophyseal joints	Stair-step deformity

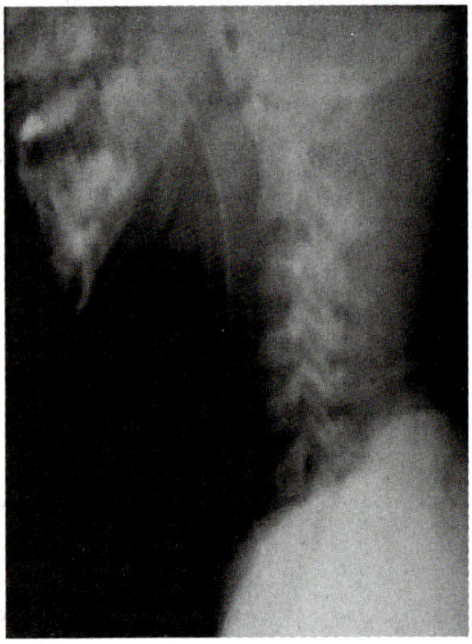

Fig. 6.1.9: Cervical spine (Lateral view): Subluxation at atlantoaxial joint

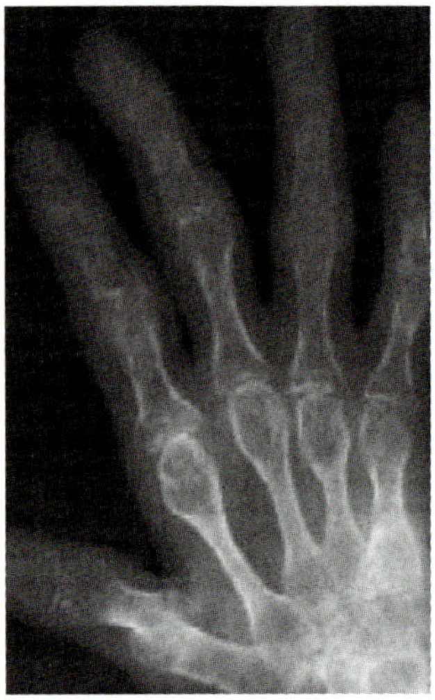

Fig. 6.1.10: Hand (AP view): JIA-diffuse osteoporosis. Erosions noted 2nd and 3rd PIP joints

disappears (Fig. 6.1.12). In psoriatic arthritis and reactive arthritis, no such orderly spread is seen and paravertebral ossifications tend to appear in a random fashion.

The enthesopathy in the spine manifests as small erosions surrounded by bony sclerosis at the vertebral corners seen as "shiny corners". This is followed by ossification of the outer annular fibers to form marginal and symmetric syndesmophytes (Fig. 6.1.13). They are different from osteophytes seen with degenerative disc disease in that syndesmophytes are parallel to the spinal axis whereas osteophytes are perpendicular (grow outwards). Squaring of the vertebral bodies is characteristic of early AS caused by the corner erosions and anterior apposition of

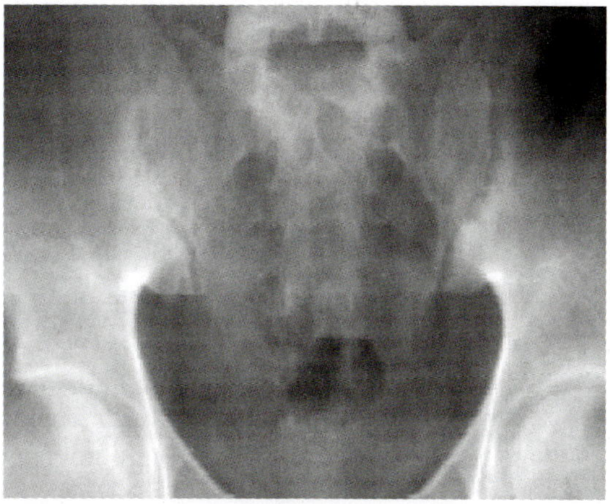

Fig. 6.1.11: Pelvis (AP view): Sacroiliitis—early sclerosis and erosions of both SI joints

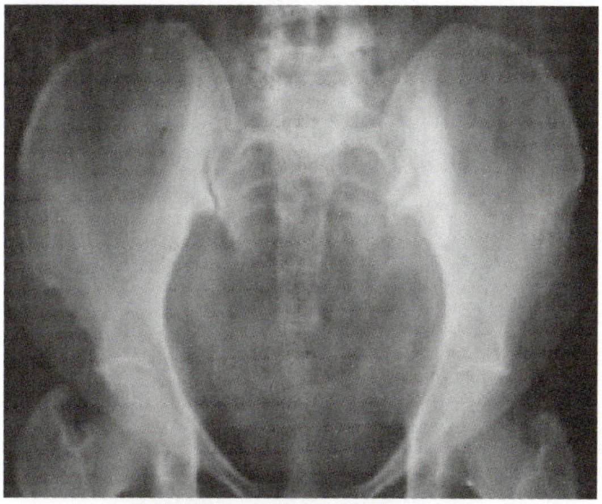

Fig. 6.1.12: Pelvis (AP view): Plain radiograph demonstrating sclerosis of iliac side of the SI joint, left > right

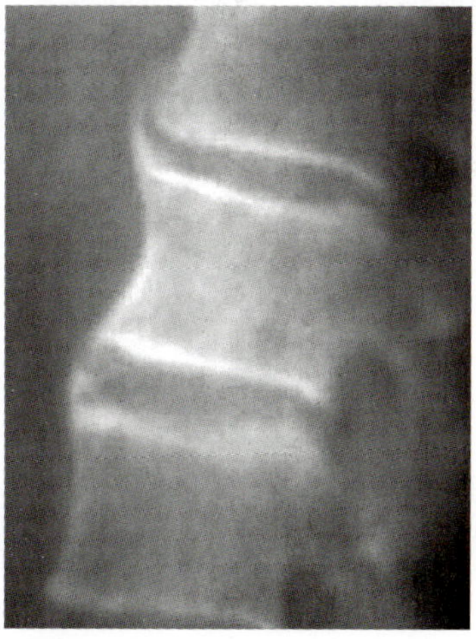

Fig. 6.1.13: Lumbar spine (Lateral view): AS—early syndesmophytes noted

periosteal new bone formation. Squaring is easier to appreciate in the lumbar spine. The complete fusion of syndesmophytes leads to the appearance of "bamboo-spine" which is a late feature (Fig. 6.1.14 and 6.1.15). Erosions are seen in the apophyseal and costovertebral joints followed by ankylosis of these joints. Following spinal fusion, the spine becomes osteoporotic and is vulnerable to stress. Fractures in AS occur most commonly at the thoracolumbar and cervicothoracic junctions. It may proceed to non-union with pseudoarthrosis, an appearance resembling disc space infection (Andersson lesion) (Fig. 6.1.16). Enthesopathy of ischial tuberosities is described as "Whiskering".

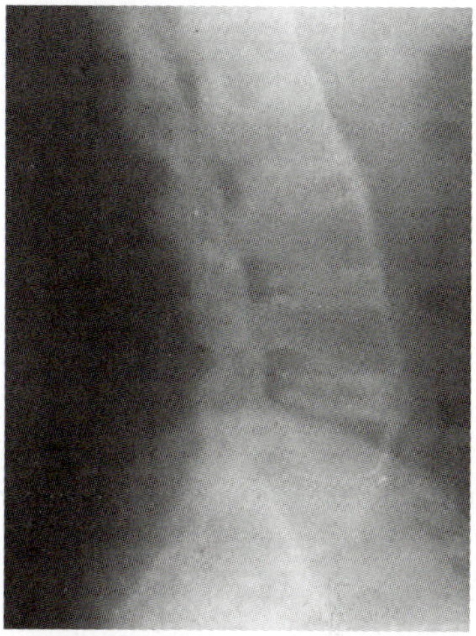

Fig. 6.1.14: Lumbar spine (Lateral view): AS—syndesmophytes joining anterior vertebral margins

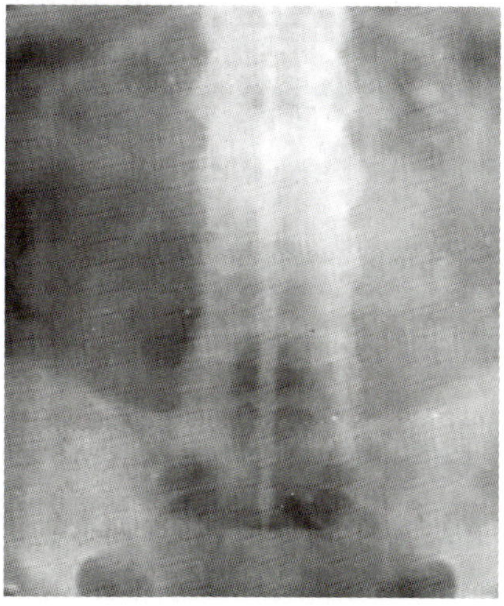

Fig. 6.1.15: Lumbar spine (AP view): AS—with bamboo spine

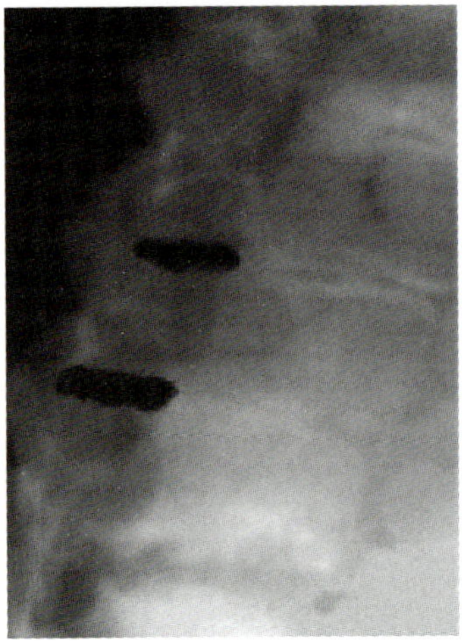

Fig. 6.1.16: Dorso lumbar spine (Lateral view): AS with pseudoarthrosis

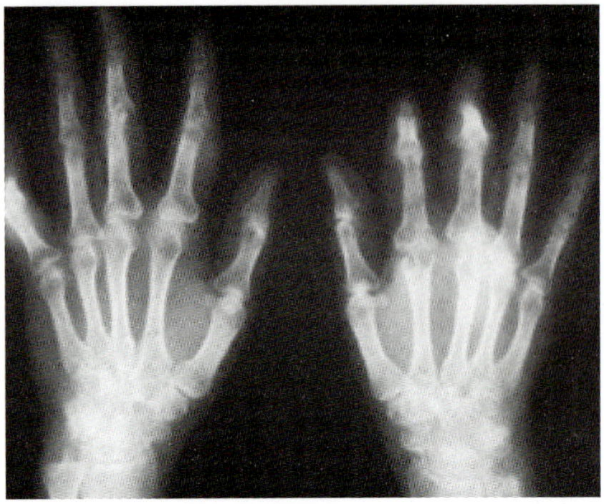

Fig. 6.1.17: Hands (AP view): Left 2nd, 3rd and right 5th DIP joint involvement in PsA

Psoriatic Arthritis (PsA) and Reactive Arthritis (ReA)

SI joint and spine involvement occur in 20–40% of patients with PsA. The sacroiliitis in PsA and ReA may or may not be symmetrical and spondylitis occurs in a more random fashion. It is associated with presence of coarse, symmetric paravertebral ossification (non-marginal syndesmophytes). The joint involvement in psoriasis can be variable (Table 6.1.4).

Erosions in the phalanges are seen in the bare areas with associated fluffy bone formation (mouse ears) and sometimes followed by fusion (Fig. 6.1.17 and 6.1.18). The distal erosions can evolve into the so called 'pencil and cup' appearance (Fig. 6.1.18). In the feet, Tuftal proliferation of the digit results in a shaggy dense distal phalanx (ivory phalanx). Periosteal reaction can be seen early in the disease along with shafts of the phalanges and metatarsals and is associated in the feet with sausage digits. Radiographic features of reactive arthritis are similar to that of psoriatic arthritis, (Fig. 6.1.17 and 6.1.18).

Table 6.1.4: Modes of presentation in psoriatic arthritis
Distal interphalangeal joint involvement.
Proximal interphalangeal and metacarpophalangeal joint involvement that resemble seronegative RA.
Asymmetric oligoarthritis affecting large joints Destructive form of arthropathy (arthritis mutilans) Seronegative spondyloarthropathy.

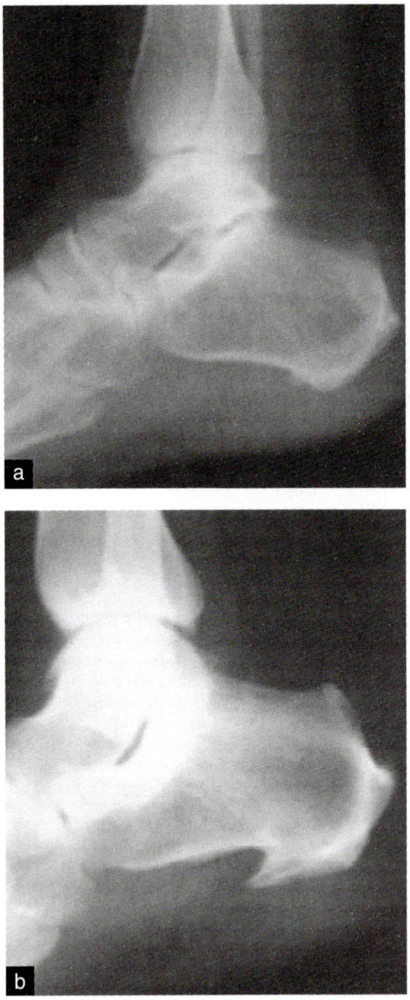

Fig. 6.1.18: (a) Ankle (Lateral view); Reiter's disease: Fluffy appearance of calcaneal spur. (b) Ankle (Lateral): Degenerative calcaneal spur

Osteoarthritis

The common joints involved in osteoarthritis (OA) are knees, hips, DIP, first carpometacarpal (CMC) joints, first MTP joint and spine (cervical, lumbar and lumbosacral). The radiographic appearance of OA in different joints varies, being dependent on anatomic relationships and on the stress to which each joint is subjected. The most typical pattern is the presence of reparative changes in both the "stressed and non-stressed" segments of the joints. In the stressed segment, there is narrowing of joint space due to thinning of cartilage with the development of erosions and eburnation. Subchondral bone sclerosis with formation of cystic lesions follows. In nonstressed segment, reparative changes lead to osteophytosis. Osteophytes are classified as marginal, central, periosteal and capsular. Degeneration of surrounding tissues such as ligaments and capsule may lead to malalignment and subluxation of the joint. In advanced OA, fragmentation of the cartilaginous or osseous surface can lead to the formation of intra-articular "loose bodies" (Table 6.1.5).

Hip: Asymmetric joint space narrowing is the most reliable sign of OA in the hip joint. The femoral head displacement can be categorized into three different migration patterns—superior migration, medial migration, and axial migration. The superior migration pattern in turn is of two types—superolateral and superomedial.

Knee: Weight bearing AP view of the knee is better for accurate assessment. This view shows the extent of joint space loss and the degree of angulation (varus or valgus) and subluxation. The knee joint is divided into three compartments-the medial femorotibial, lateral femorotibial and patellofemoral. Most frequently, the medial compartment is involved in primary OA of knees (Fig. 6.1.19). Both or only lateral compartment are/is involved in secondary OA knees due to inflammatory arthropathies such as RA. The patellofemoral compartment (Fig. 6.1.20) is affected usually in association with medial compartment disease.

Table 6.1.5: Features of OA
Narrowing of joint space
Osteophytosis
Subarticular sclerosis

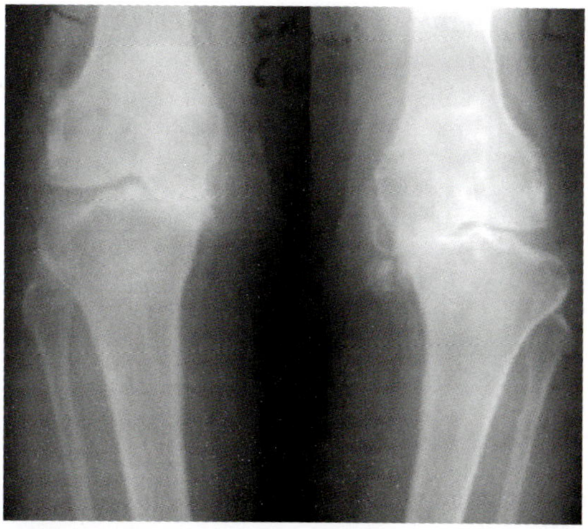

Fig. 6.1.19: Knees (AP view): Gross osteoarthritis knees with obliteration of medial compartments (OA)

Conventional radiography is one of the parameters useful in the assessment of outcome measurements in RA, PsA, OA and SpA and other autoimmune diseases.

Additional signs of OA are angulation and subluxation with varus (primary OA) or valgus (secondary OA) deformities, small joint effusions and presence of intraarticular bodies (loose bodies), called secondary osteocondromatosis.

Spine: In the spine, cervical (C5–6, C6–7) (Fig. 6.1.21) and lumbosacral (L4–5, L5–S1) (Fig. 6.1.22) areas are most commonly affected.

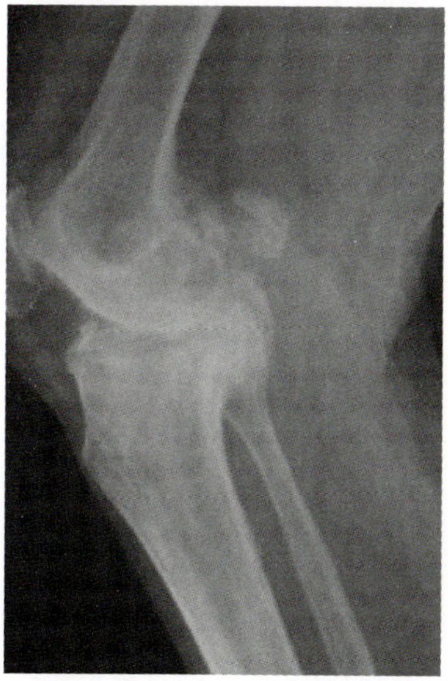

Fig. 6.1.20: Knees (Lateral view): Patellofemoral joint space narrowing with loose bodies (OA)

In intervertebral (disc) spaces, marginal osteophytes are observed early. As the disease advances, thinning of the disc space with sclerosis of subchondral bone takes place with subluxation of various degrees leading to instability and pain. The hyaline cartilage of the facet joints may also be involved by the degenerative process.

Hands and feet: The degenerative joint disease can occur primarily in nonweight bearing joints such as DIP joints (Fig. 6.1.23), first CMC joint (Fig. 6.1.24) and first metatarsal joints (Fig. 6.1.25). The erosive and nodal osteoarthritis may mimic RA or PsA. However, subarticular osteoporosis is not encountered in OA.

Crystal Arthropathies

Gout: Classical findings are summarized in (Table 6.1.6). Though lesion is more common in first metatarsophalangeal joint, similar lesions are also seen in ankles, elbows, wrists and hands (Fig. 6.1.26). Intra-articular erosions tend to involve the joint margins before extending centrally. An elevated margin of the bone may extend outside the erosions as "overhanging edge" which is very suggestive

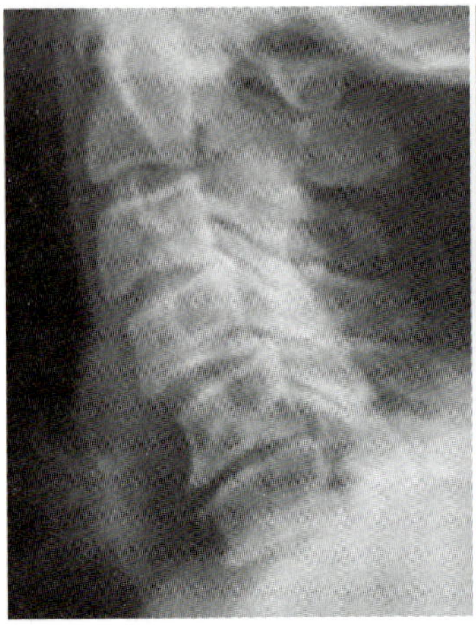

Fig. 6.1.21: Cervical spine (Lateral view): cervical spondylosis with narrow C5–6 intervertebral space and osteophytosis

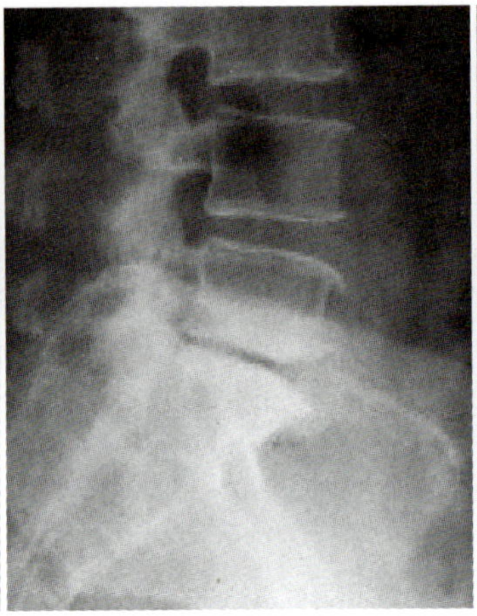

Fig. 6.1.22: Lumbosacral spine (Lateral view): Lumbar spondylosis with narrow L5–S1 and anterior osteophytes noted at L5 with vacuum sign L5–S1

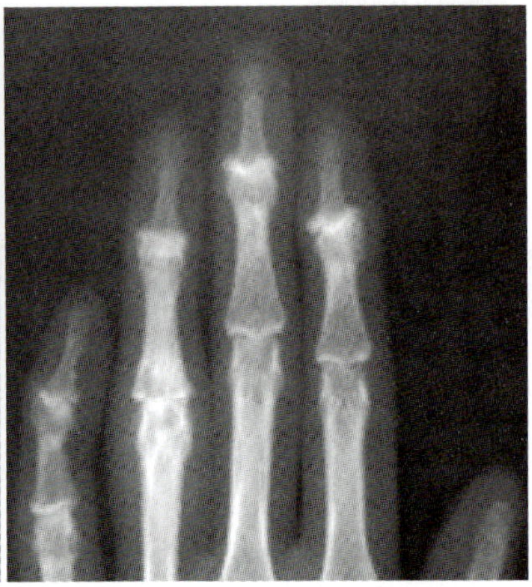

Fig. 6.1.23: Hand (AP view): OA DIP joints with narrow joint space, subarticular sclerosis and erosions

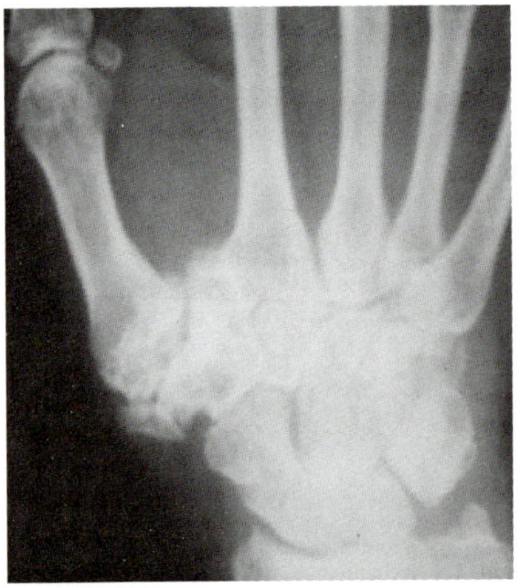

Fig. 6.1.24: Wrist (AP view): OA first CMC joint with narrow joint space, subarticular sclerosis, and osteophytes

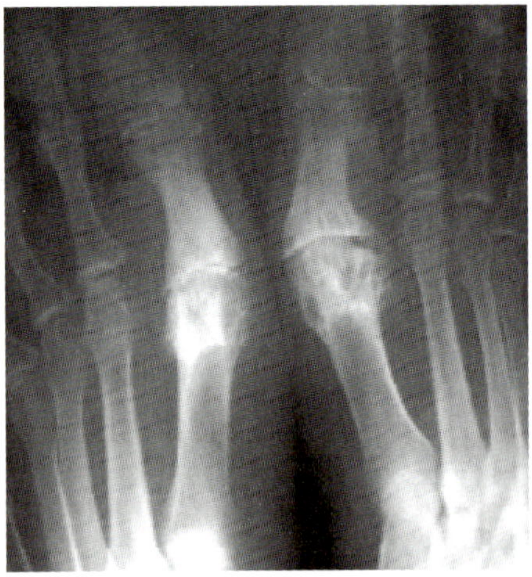

Fig. 6.1.25: Feet (AP view): First MTP joints with narrow joint space, subarticular sclerosis, and osteophytes (OA)

Table 6.1.6: Characteristic radiographic features of gouty arthritis

Asymmetrical involvement	Relative preservation of joint space
Eccentric soft tissue prominence	Relative preservation of bone density
Punched out erosions	Intraosseous calcification/ lytic lesions
Overhanging margins	

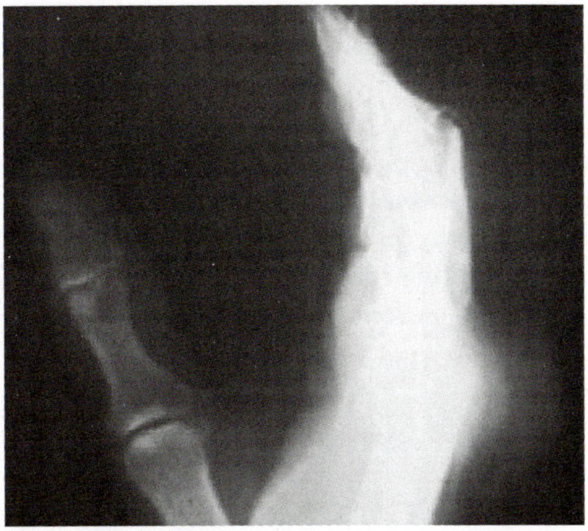

Fig. 6.1.26: Hand (Oblique view): Gouty tophus at 2nd MCP joint with mouse ears (overhanging margins) at 2nd PIP

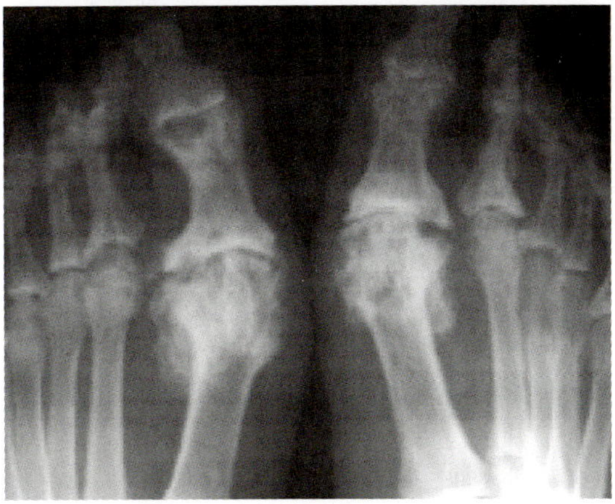

Fig. 6.1.27: Feet (AP view): Interosseous osteolysis at both 1st MTP joints with overhanging margins. Punched out erosions are also noted near IP joints

of gout (Fig. 6.1.27). Intraosseous MSU crystals deposition and tophus formation may give rise to osteolytic lesions that simulate neoplastic disease.

CPPD Disease

Articular calcification related to calcium pyrophosphate crystals deposition (CPPD) is most frequent in the knee followed by symphysis pubis, wrist, elbow, shoulder and hip. Calcification in the hyaline cartilage and/or fibrocartilage (chondrocalcinosis) is present (Fig. 6.1.28a and 6.1.28b). Fibrocartilage calcification is coarse and irregular, commonly occurring within the meniscus of the wrist and the pubic symphysis. Hyaline cartilage calcification is fine and linear following the contour of underlying subchondral bone. Apart from the cartilage, CPPD deposition may also occur in the capsule, synovium, ligaments, and soft tissue mostly appearing as curvy linear calcifications.

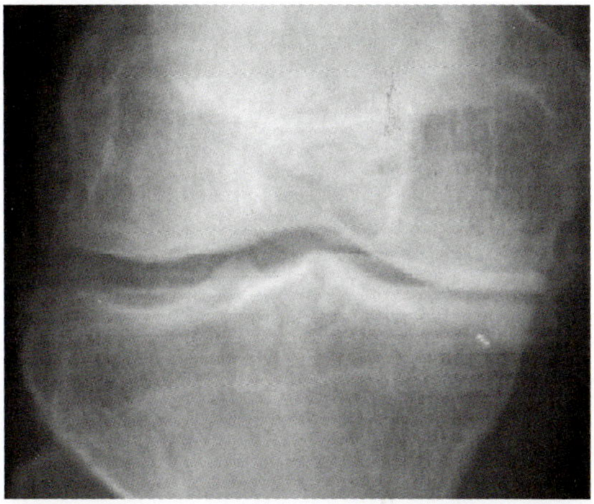

Fig. 6.1.28a: Knee (AP view): Linear calcification seen in hyaline cartilage at lateral compartment (CPPD)

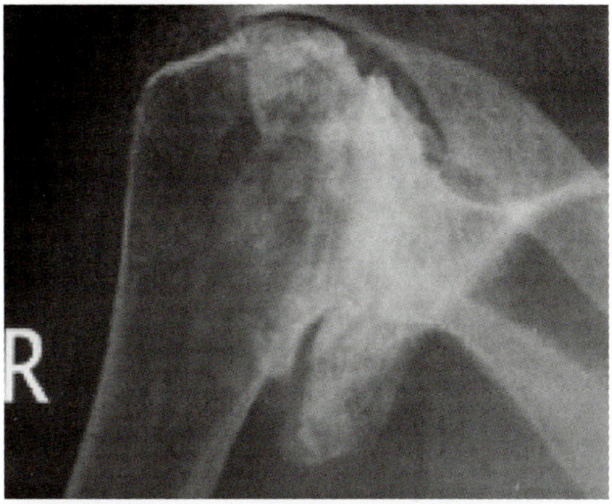

Fig. 6.1.28b: Shoulder (AP view): Shoulder with CPPD arthropathy. There is loss of the glenohumeral joint space with osteophyte formation, subchondral sclerosis and cyst formation

Calcium hydroxyapatite (CHA) crystal depositon commonly occurs in shoulder and is called peritendinitis calcarea. But it may also be seen in hip, elbow and wrist joints. Radiographically amorphous calcific deposits are noted (Fig. 6.1.28c).

Other Collagen Vascular Diseases

Systemic lupus erythematosus (SLE): The radiological features of SLE may mimic early RA, but erosions are uncommon in SLE. However, deforming arthropathy can occur due to soft tissue involvement. Osteonecrosis may occur in patients with SLE especially on glucocorticosteroids (GCs) (Fig. 6.1.29).

Systemic sclerosis (SSc) or scleroderma: Articular or non-articular features are commonly seen in scleroderma especially with Raynaud's phenomena (Fig. 6.1.30) (Table 6.1.7). CREST syndrome in localized scleroderma includes calcinosis, Raynaud's phenomenon, esophageal hypomotility, sclerodactyly and telangiectasia.

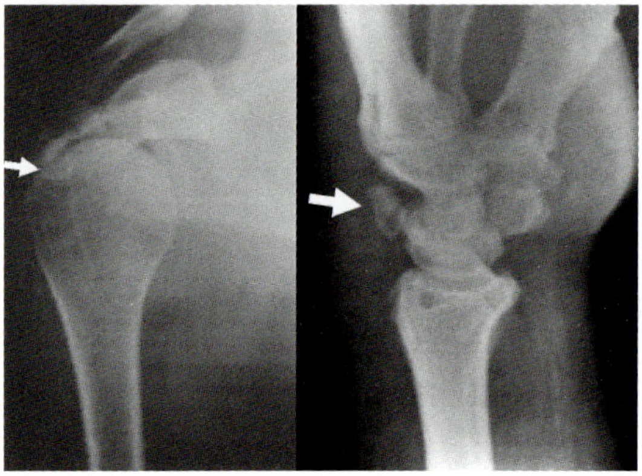

Fig. 6.1.28c: Shoulder (AP view) and wrist (oblique view): Calcium hydroxyapatite crystal depositions

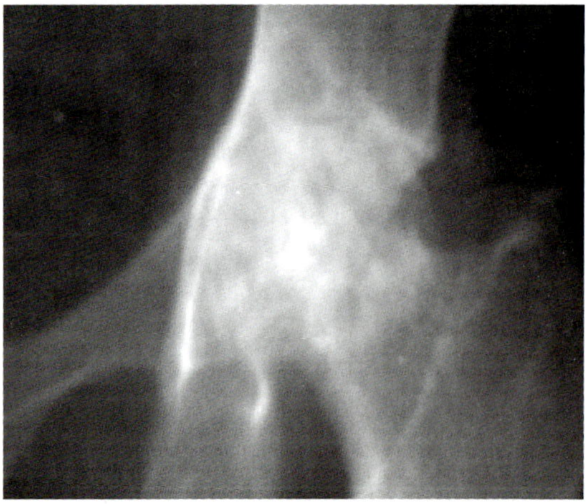

Fig. 6.1.29: Hip (AP view): SLE on GCs-osteonecrosis with secondary OA

Inflammatory myositis: The most characteristic soft tissue abnormality in dermato/polymyositis is calcification in subcutaneous tissue and intermuscular fascia.

Miscellaneous Disorders

Osteonecrosis: The most common sites of osteonecrosis (avasular necrosis) are the femoral heads, femoral condyles, humeral head (Fig. 6.1.31), talus, scaphoid and lunate. In children, the idiopathic form of osteonecrosis of the femoral head is called Legg–Calve–Perthes disease.

Secondary osteonecrosis is commonly seen in adults. Radiographic changes are not evident in early epiphyseal osteonecrosis. As the disease progresses, arc like radiolucent subchondral band (crescent sign) and the formation of patchy subchondral lucent and sclerotic foci are seen. Fragmentation and collapse of

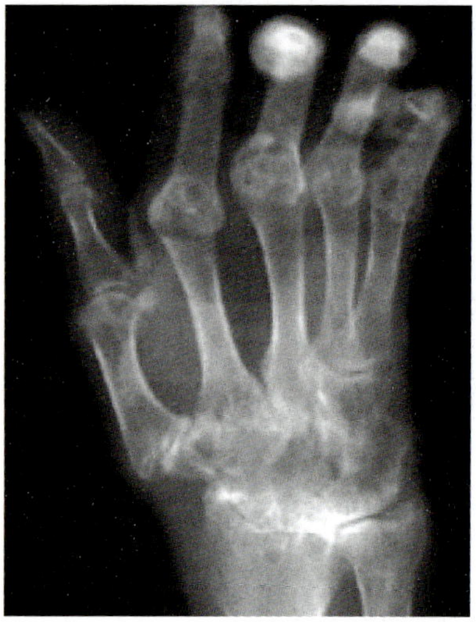

Fig. 6.1.30: Hand (AP view): Scleroderma–acroosteolysis, subcutaneous calcification finger tufts with erosive articular disease of wrist

Table 6.1.7: Radiographic features in systemic sclerosis
Soft tissue resorption—most commonly at finger tips
Soft tissue calcification—subcutaneous tissue, joint capsule, tendons or ligaments
Osteolysis—resorption of terminal phalanges (acroosteolysis)
Erosive articular disease

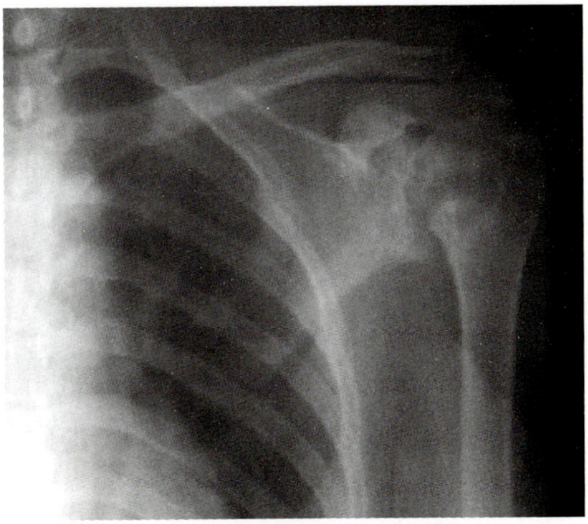

Fig. 6.1.31: Shoulder (AP view): Osteonecrosis of humeral head in a patient with SLE on GCs

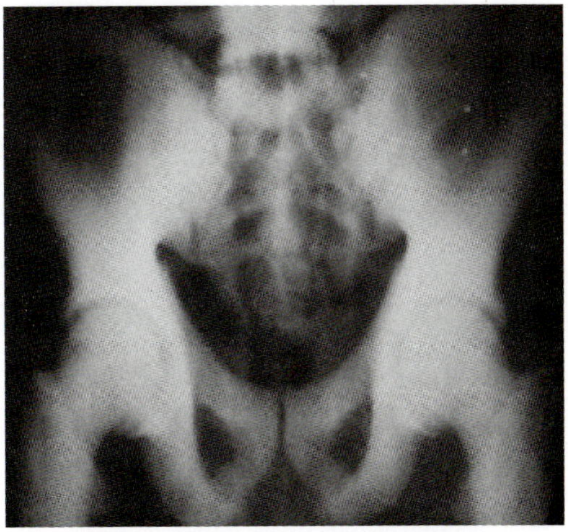

Fig. 6.1.32: Pelvis (AP view): Dense bones in fluorosis

the articular surface follows. The joint space is usually preserved until late in the course of the disease when secondary osteoarthritis may develop (Fig. 6.1.29).

Fluorosis: Excessive ingestion of fluoride through water or food causes toxicity or a debilitating disease called 'fluorosis'. Excessive intake during pre-eruptive stage of teeth leads to dental fluorosis and further continued ingestion over years and decades causes bony or skeletal fluorosis. Patient complains of pains in the small joints of the limbs and back, which are often mistaken for RA or AS. Radiological findings show calcification and ossification of various bones (Fig. 6.1.32), joints, spine (Fig. 6.1.33), related ligaments and tendinous attachments to the bones and interosseous membranes (Fig. 6.1.34).

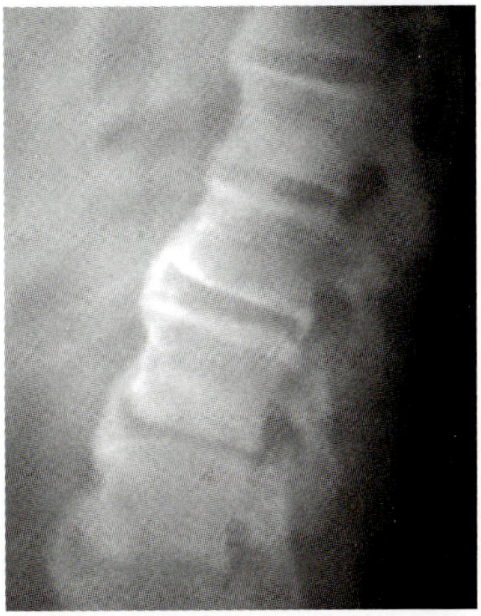

Fig. 6.1.33: Lumbar spine (Lateral view): Dense vertebrae with bridging osteophytes (Fluorosis)

Diffuse idiopathic skeletal hyperostosis (DISH): DISH radiologically resembles fluorosis. Since it is seen in older people, density of the bones is not that of fluorosis, flowing hyperostosis is added feature (Fig. 6.1.35).

Osteoporosis and osteomalacia: Radiologically reduced bone density is observed in vertebrae, wrist, hips, humerus and tibial bones. The bones have prominent vertical striations resulting from a relatively greater loss of the horizontally oriented trabeculae (Fig. 6.1.36). In severe osteoporosis vertebral fractures (wedge compression) can be seen (Fig. 6.1.37).

The characteristic feature of osteomalacia is ground glass appearance without differentiation between cortex and spongiosa the detection of Looser's zone or pseudofractures commonly seen in upper femur, pelvis and scapula (Fig. 6.1.38)

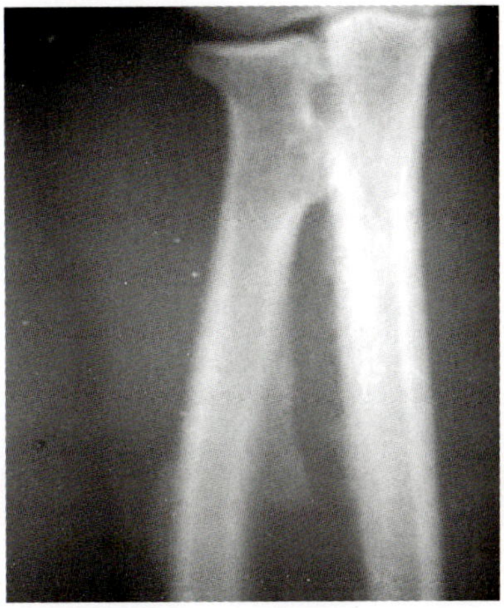

Fig. 6.1.34: Forearm (AP veiw): Calcification of interosseous membrane (Fluorosis)

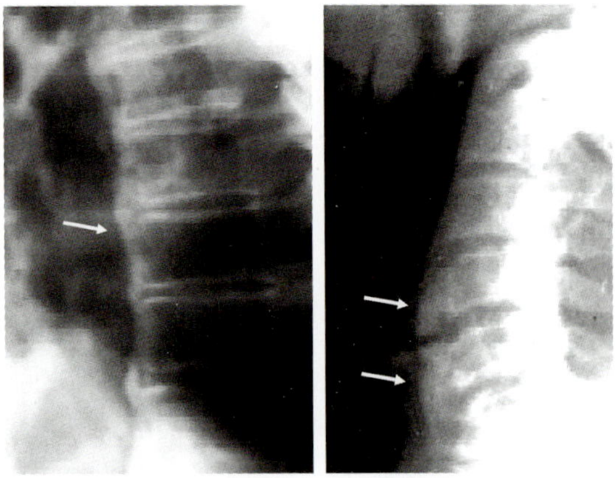

Fig. 6.1.35: Lumbar spine and cervical spine (Lateral view): DISH with flowing hyperostosis

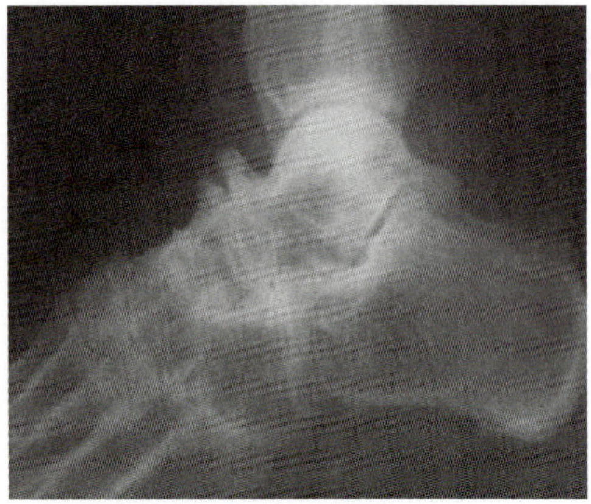

Fig. 6.1.36: Ankle (Lateral view): Osteoporosis with vertical striations at calcaneal bone

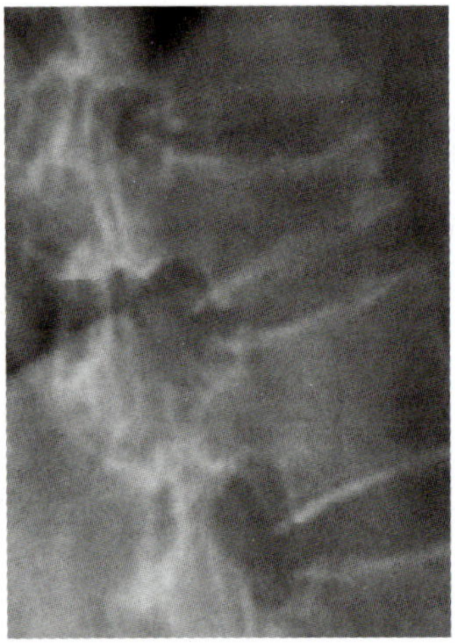

Fig. 6.1.37: Dorsal spine (Lateral view): Wedge compression at D10 due to osteoporosis

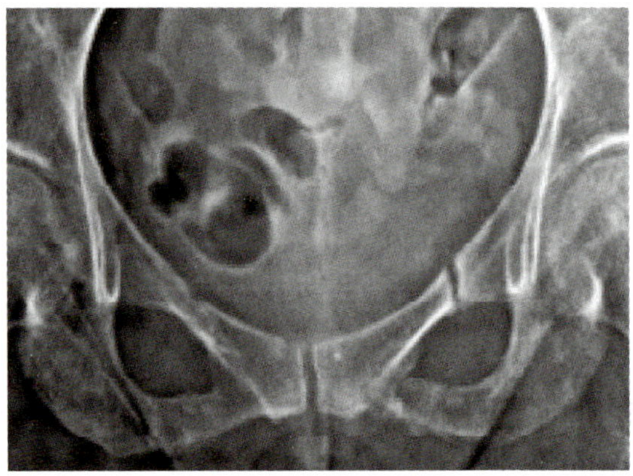

Fig. 6.1.38: Pelvis (AP view): Osteomalacia with pseudofractures at superior ramus of pubic bone on both sides

LEARNING POINTS

- Radiographs are requested after obtaining the patient's complete history and physical examination.
- Conventional radiography is one of the parameters useful in the assessment of damage of RA, PsA, OA and SpA and other autoimmune diseases.
- Classical features of arthritis include erosions, peri-articular osteopenia and soft tissue swelling.

FURTHER READING

1. Hellio Le Graverand MP, Mazzuca S, Duryea J, Brett A. Radiographic grading and measurement of joint space width in osteoarthritis. Rheum Dis Clin North Am. 2009;35:485–502.
2. Østergaard M, Jen H, Jaremko JL, Lambert GW. Imaging in rheumatic diseases. In: Firestein G, Budd RC, Gabriel SE, Koretsky GA, McInnes IB, O'Dell JR, editors, Kelley's Textbook of Rheumatology. 11th edition. Elsevier: Philadelphia; 2021. p.920–64.
3. Østergaard M, Ejbjerg B, Szkudlarek M. Imaging in early rheumatoid arthritis: roles of magnetic resonance imaging, ultrasonography, conventional radiography and computed tomography. Best Pract Res Clin Rheumatol. 2005;19:91–116.
4. Subbarao K. Arthritides (disorder of joints). In Subbarao K, Banerjee S, Aggarwal S, Bhargava S, editors. Diagnostic Radiology and Imaging. Jaypee Brothers: New Delhi; 1997. p. 269–71.
5. van der Heijde D. Quantification of radiological damage in inflammatory arthritis: rheumatoid arthritis, psoriatic arthritis and ankylosing spondylitis. Best Pract Res Clin Rheumatol. 2004;18: 847–60.

CT Interpretation of ILD

Sachin Kumar, Sanket Shah

INTRODUCTION

Computed tomography (CT) scan is an important tool to identify interstitial lung disease (ILD) in autoimmune rheumatic diseases (AIRD). Occasionally, a CT scan shows changes in a patient who does not have respiratory symptoms, and these findings may impact the classification of the disease and the management plan. In this chapter, we will discuss the basic patterns of CT findings that are observed in patients with AIRDs.

BASICS BEFORE WE START

The most cost-effective method to diagnose ILD in current use is a high-resolution CT scan (HRCT) of the thorax. HRCT images are extremely thin slices of the lungs (usually <1.5 mm) and post-processing those images using a high spatial frequency algorithm which yields outstanding spatial resolution and anatomical detail. It is essential to be familiar with various terms that are used during reporting of HRCT of lungs (Fig. 6.2.1). A knowledge of these

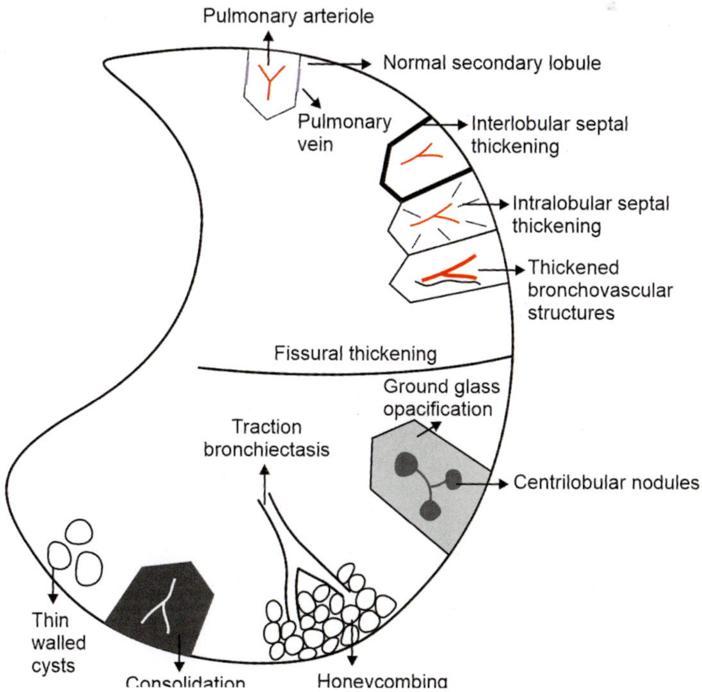

Fig. 6.2.1: Terminology of findings on CT scan

terms help us know the pattern and narrow down the differential diagnosis.

APPROACH TO INTERPRETATION

In most cases in practice, a clinical diagnosis of ILD is assumed, and then a CT scan helps confirm the clinical suspicion. Moreover, a CT scan helps identify the pattern of ILD and points us toward the presence or absence of pulmonary artery hypertension in a given case. An algorithmic approach to ILD in connective tissue disease (CTD) is illustrated in Figure 6.2.2, while Figure 6.2.3 shows the four major patterns of ILD seen with AIRDs. In addition to this typical pattern,

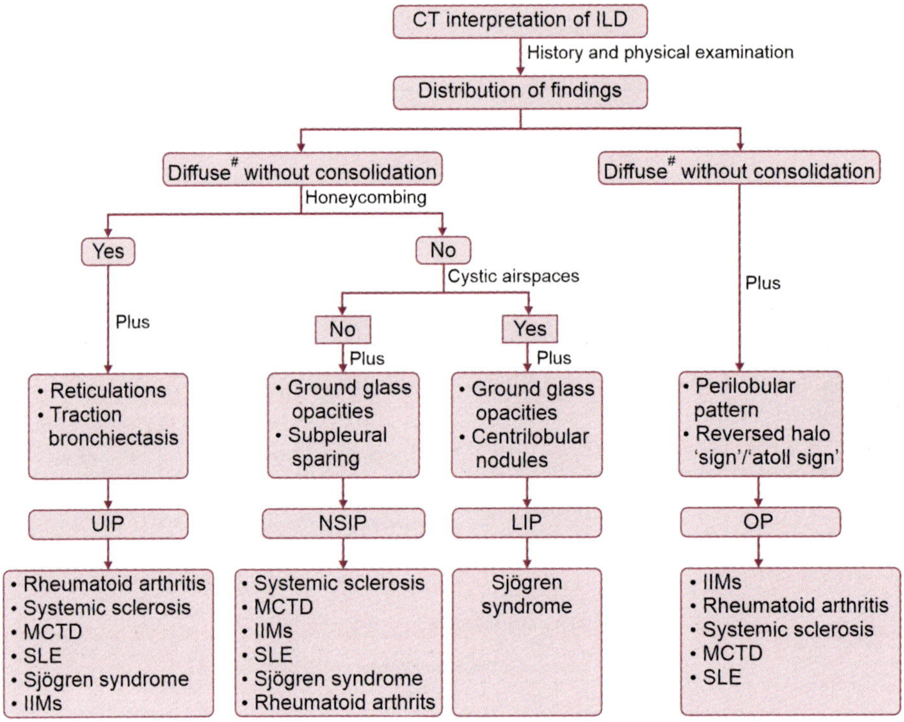

Fig. 6.2.2: Algorithmic approach to interpretation of CT scan in ILD

IIMs: Idiopathic inflammatory myositis; *LIP:* Lymphoid interstitial pneumonia; *MCTD:* Mixed connective tissue disorder; *NSIP:* Nonspecific interstitial pneumonia; *OP:* Organizing pneumonia; *SLE:* Systemic lupus erythematosus; *UIP:* Usual interstitial pneumonia

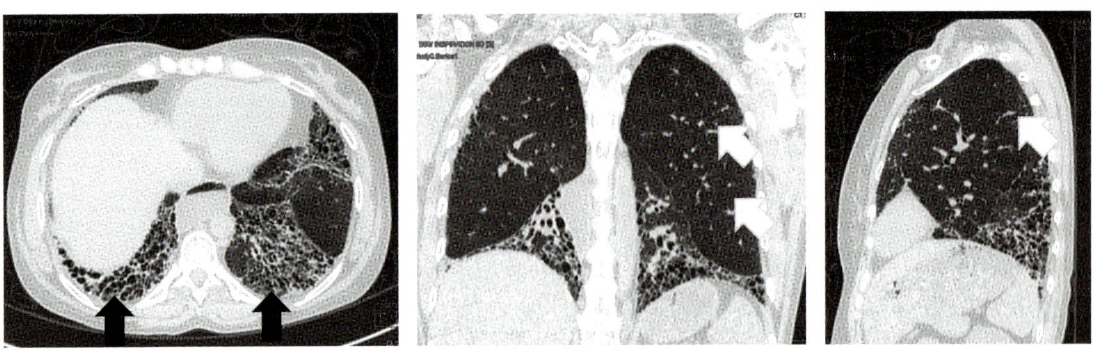

Fig. 6.2.3a: UIP pattern on HRCT: From left to right: axial, coronal, and sagittal sections depicting UIP pattern. Note the lower lobe predominance of the honeycombing (black arrows) along with the presence of subpleural reticulations (white arrows)

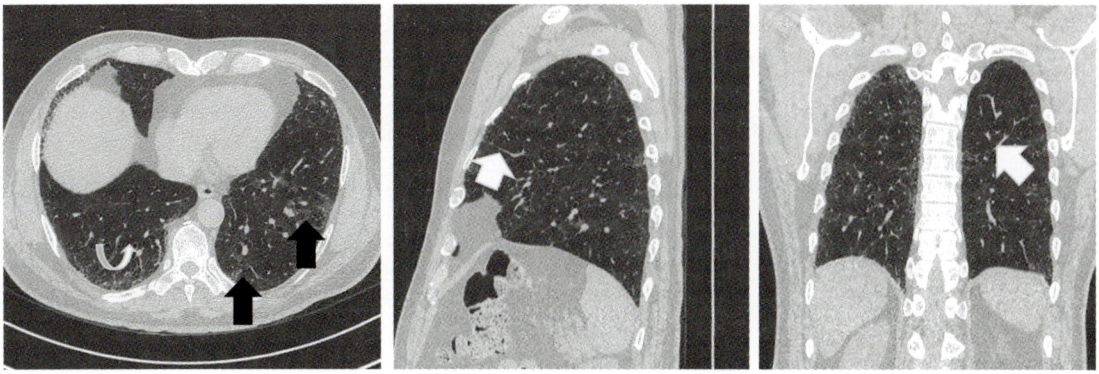

Fig. 6.2.3b: NSIP pattern on HRCT: From left to right: axial, sagittal, and coronal sections depicting the NSIP pattern with ground glass opacifications (black solid arrows), reticulations (white arrows), and traction bronchiectasis (curved arrows)

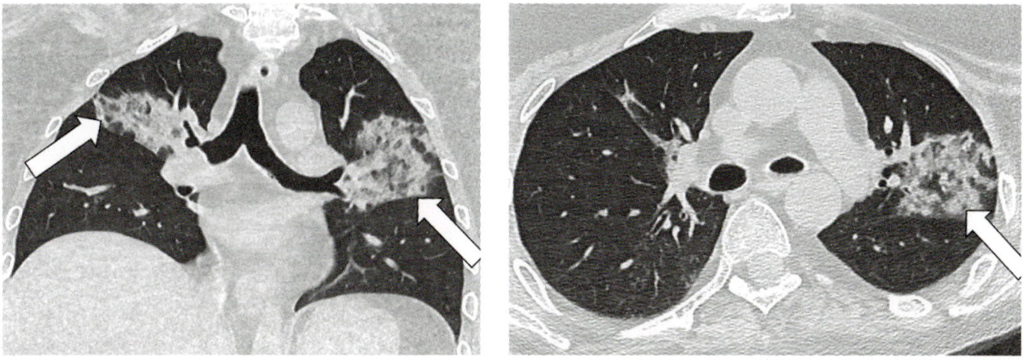

Fig. 6.2.3c: Cryptogenic organizing pneumonia (COP) pattern on HRCT: Coronal and axial images showing organizing pneumonia pattern with multifocal, bilateral areas of subpleural and peribronchovascular consolidations (arrows)

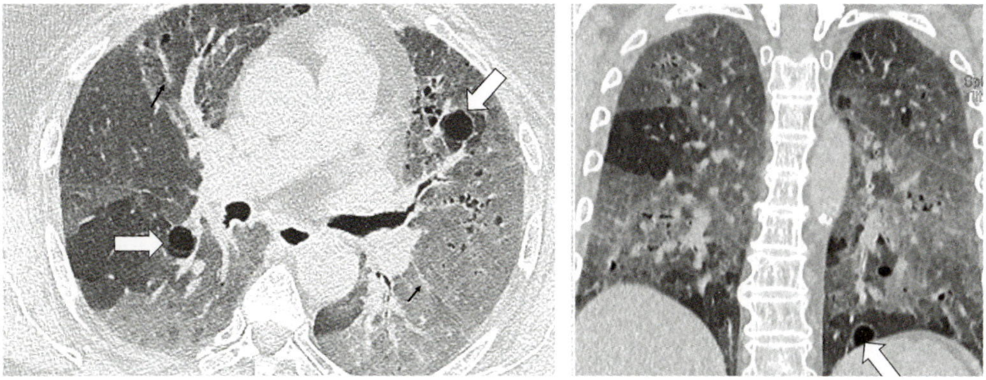

Fig. 6.2.3d: Axial and coronal HRCT images of a patient with Sjögren's syndrome depicting lymphocytic interstitial pattern (LIP) pattern. Note the diffuse bilateral ground-glass opacifications, multiple scattered thin-walled cysts (white arrows), and thickened bronchovascular bundles (black arrows). CT images *Courtsey:* Dr. Abhijit A Rout, Consultant Radiologist, Kokilaben Dhirubhai Ambani Hospital, Mumbai.

LIP: Lymphoid interstitial pneumonia; *NSIP:* Nonspecific interstitial pneumonia; *OP:* Organizing pneumonia; *UIP:* Usual interstitial pneumonia.

Table 6.2.1: Pattern of ILD and other clues on CT scan in AIRDs

Autoimmune rheumatic disease	*Most common ILD pattern*	*Additional findings on CT scan*
Rheumatoid arthritis	UIP > NSIP > OP	• Pleural thickening and effusion • Follicular bronchiolitis • Obliterative bronchiolitis • Rheumatoid nodules
Systemic sclerosis	NSIP> UIP > OP	• Evidence of PAH: enlarged pulmonary trunk (>2.9 cm in diameter), main pulmonary artery and their segments • Esophageal dilatation • Pleural thickening
Inflammatory myositis	NSIP with OP > OP > UIP	• Rapidly progressive ILD with Anti MDA-5 antibody seropositivity
Mixed connective tissue disorder	NSIP > UIP > OP	• Evidence of PAH: As mentioned above
Systemic lupus erythematosus	NSIP > UIP > OP	• Pleural effusion and pleural thickening • Diffuse alveolar haemorrhage (rare but severe complication)
Sjögren's syndrome	NSIP > LIP> UIP and OP	• Lymphoma—may result in patchy consolidations, ground glass opacities and multiple nodules

LIP: Lymphoid interstial pneumonia; *NSIP:* Non specific interstitial pneumonia; *OP:* Organising pneumonia; *UIP:* Usual interstitial pneumonia

individual AIRD shows additional findings that help narrow down diagnosis further with the CT scan as described in Table 6.2.1.

In addition to above mentioned rheumatic disease, sarcoidosis related ILD needs a special mention which can have findings in the form of upper lobe predominant fibrosis and traction bronchiectasis in the advanced disease. Overall pulmonary fibrosis has been reported in 20–40% cases of ANCA associated vasculitis especially with the Anti-MPO ANCA vasculitis. The pattern of UIP was observed more commonly compared to NSIP in the French vasculitis cohort.

LEARNING POINTS

- CT scan serves as the most sensitive tool to identify interstitial lung disease in clinical practice.
- The most common pattern observed in patient with rheumatic disease is NSIP except in case of RA where the UIP is the most common pattern.
- Presence of NSIP with OP is a peculiar pattern observed in case of Inflammatory myositis and LIP pattern in specific to Sjogren syndrome among the rheumatic diseases.

FURTHER READING

1. Kim EA, Lee KS, Johkoh T, et al. Interstitial lung diseases associated with collagen vascular diseases: radiologic and histopathologic findings [published correction appears in Radiographics. 2003 Sep-Oct;23(5):1340]. Radiographics. 2002;22 Spec No:S151–65.
2. Marten K, Schnyder P, Schirg E, et al. Pattern-based differential diagnosis in pulmonary vasculitis using volumetric CT. AJR Am J Roentgenol. 2005;184(3):720–33.

Probe Positioning and Normal Sonoanatomy of Joints

Ankit B Shah, Bipin R Shah

INTRODUCTION

Musculoskeletal ultrasound is generally performed with linear probes which operate at a higher frequency compared to the convex probes. Standard linear probes operate between frequencies of 9 and 16 MHz. Convex probes operate at lower frequencies ranging from 1 to 7 MHz. Convex probes can be used to scan deeper structures like hip, gluteal region and sacroiliac joints. Hockey-stick probes operate at higher frequencies (8–24 MHz) and have better spatial resolution than standard linear probes. Their smaller footprint allows easier scanning of difficult anatomical areas like the web spaces of hands and feet. Hence, the selection of the probe must be made depending on the area that needs to be scanned.

A SIMPLE RULE OF THUMB

- **Higher the probe frequency:** Better visualization of the superficial structures (e.g. dermis, subcutaneous fat, peripheral nerves, tendons of fingers and feet, joints of hands and feet).
- **Lower probe frequency:** Better visualization of deeper structures (e.g. hip joint, sacroiliac joint, the posterior recess of glenohumeral joint).

The image quality of superficial structures like subcutaneous fat, cutaneous nodules and nail bed can be greatly improved by using a water-bath technique or copious quantities of gel.

It is absolutely essential to have appropriate power Doppler settings. The pulse repetition frequency (PRF) and Doppler gain need to be adjusted so as to detect low-velocity flows in the pannus. Care should be taken that the PRF is neither too high (which would not detect low-flow) nor too low (Which would result in the detection of a false-positive power Doppler signal). Figures 6.3.1 to 6.3.60 illustrate probe positioning in various joints.

SHOULDER

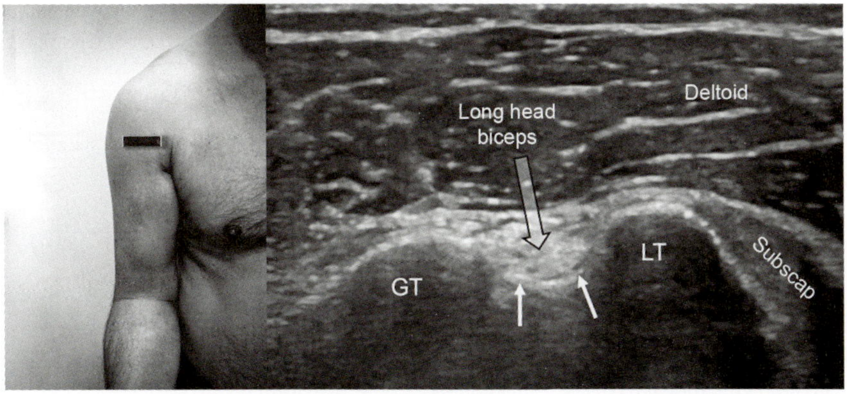

Fig. 6.3.1: On short-axis imaging, the long head of biceps is identified as an oval echogenic structure in the bicipital groove (arrows) which is located between the greater tuberosity (GT) laterally and the lesser tuberosity (LT) medially

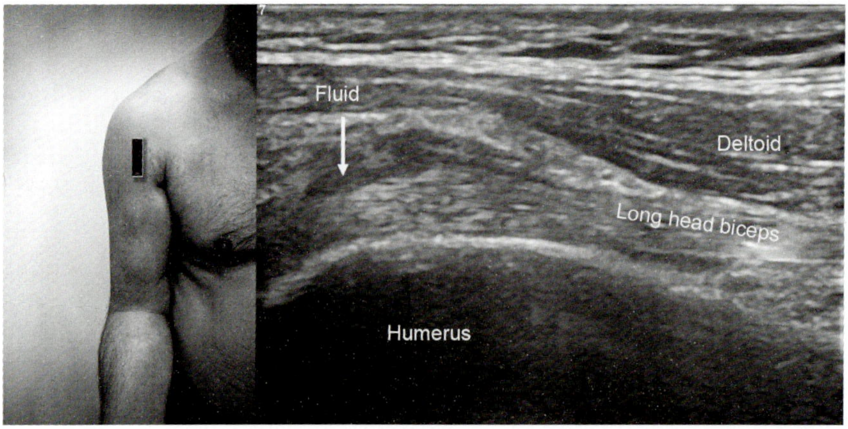

Fig. 6.3.2: Long head of biceps is seen as an echogenic structure with fibrillary pattern. Small volume of fluid in the biceps tendon sheath, partially encircling the biceps tendon, is seen in normal subjects

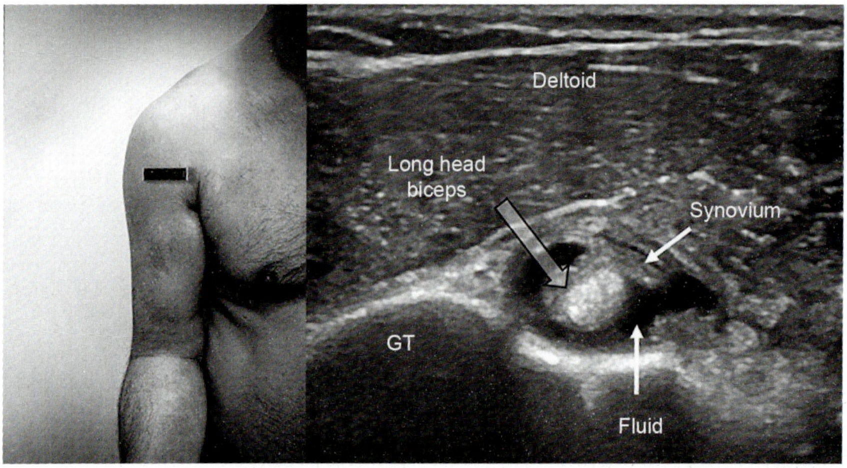

Fig. 6.3.3: Tenosynovitis involving the biceps tendon sheath. The short-axis image shows nodular synovial hypertrophy with anechoic effusion surrounding the biceps tendon. GT: Greater tuberosity

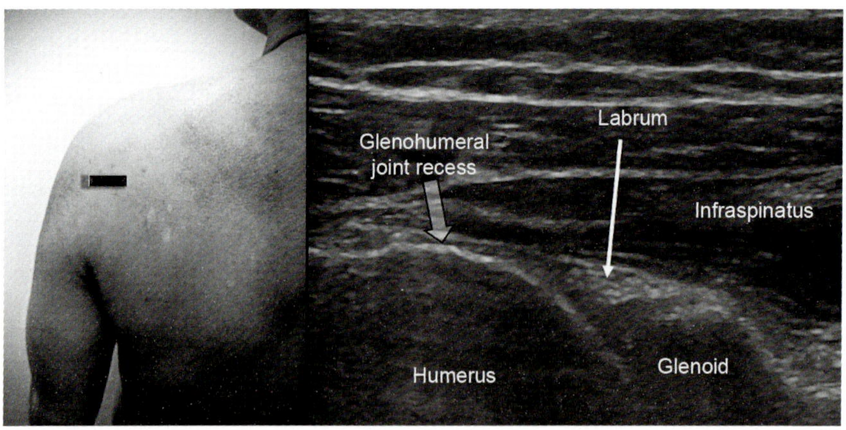

Fig. 6.3.4: Effusion in the glenohumeral joint can be easily visualized in the posterior glenohumeral joint recess. The probe is placed along the long axis of the infraspinatus muscle. The joint recess is identified between the humeral head and glenoid. Posterosuperior glenoid labrum is identified as an echogenic triangular structure flush with the glenoid cortex. Slow external and internal rotation of the arm can help in better visualization of the joint fluid

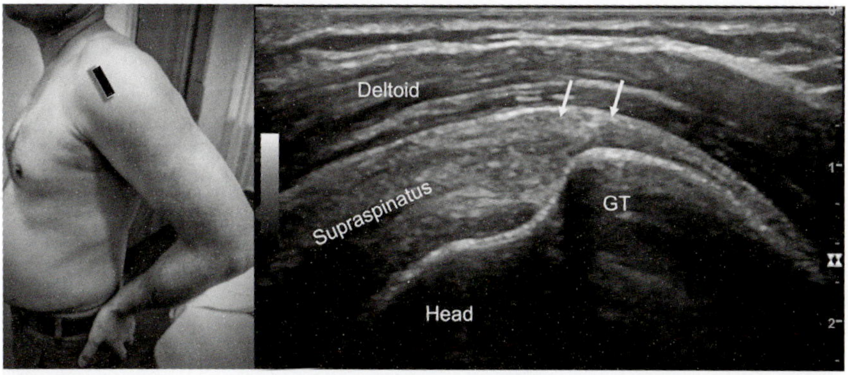

Fig. 6.3.5: The rotator cuff tendons and the subacromial subdeltoid bursa are evaluated in the modified Crass position. Beginning from the deltopectoral groove, the probe is positioned parallel to the long head of biceps and swept posteriorly to identify Supraspinatus and infraspinatus tendons. The tendons are seen as an echogenic beak-shaped structure inserting on the greater tuberosity (GT). The collapsed subacromial subdeltoid bursa (white arrows) is seen as a thin echogenic structure between the rotator cuff tendons and the deltoid muscle belly

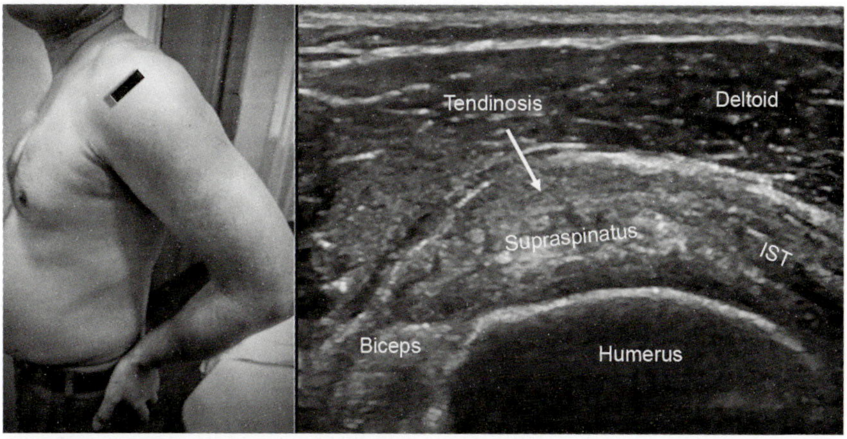

Fig. 6.3.6: The supraspinatus and infraspinatus tendons are evaluated in the short-axis by turning the probe perpendicular to the position that was used to evaluate supraspinatus tendon in the long axis. In a case of tendinosis, the supraspinatus tendon appears mildly thickened and heterogeneously hypoechoic (arrow). IST: Infraspinatus

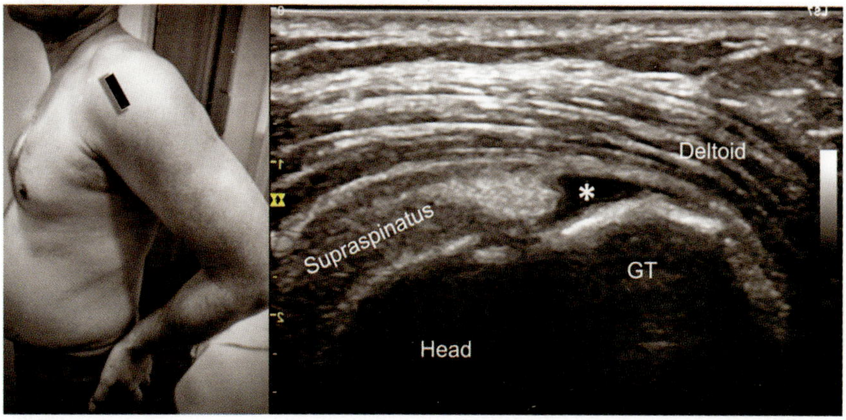

Fig. 6.3.7: Full thickness tear (asterisk) of supraspinatus tendon along its footprint. GT: Greater tuberosity

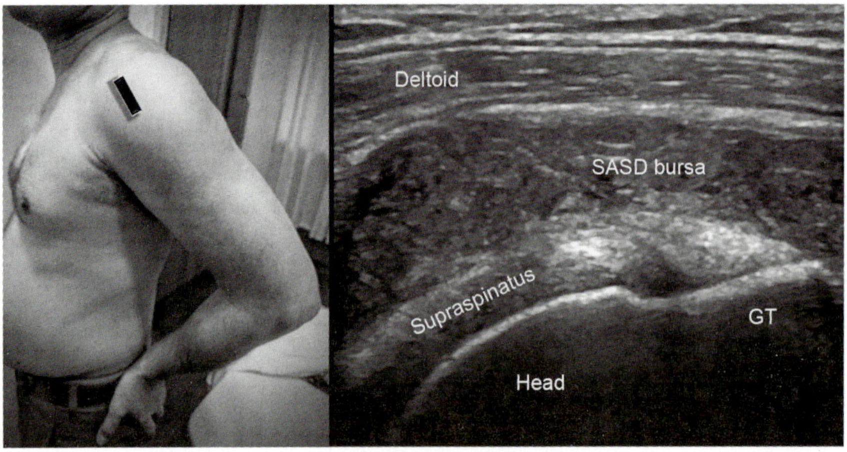

Fig. 6.3.8: Subacromial subdeltoid bursitis is seen as a thickened hypoechoic structure between the rotator cuff tendons and the deltoid muscle. GT: Greater tuberosity

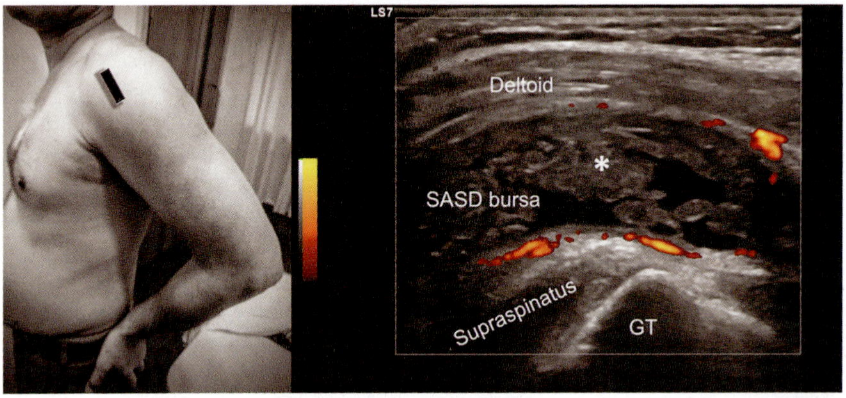

Fig. 6.3.9: Marked synovial hypertrophy (asterisk) along with anechoic fluid are seen to distend the subacromial subdeltoid bursa in a patient having rheumatoid arthritis. Power Doppler shows hyperemia along the walls of the thickened bursa. GT: Greater tuberosity

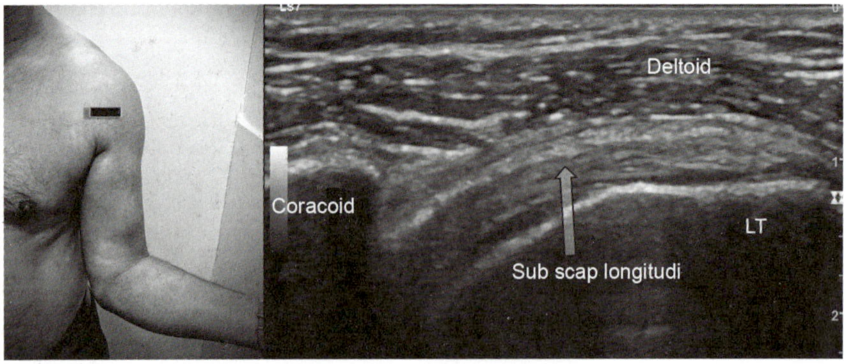

Fig. 6.3.10: The subscapularis tendon is scanned from the anterior aspect while asking the patient to externally rotate the arm as much as possible. Coracoid process (medially) and the lesser tuberosity (LT) are the two osseous landmarks that are used to identify the subscapularis tendon (arrow) in the long-axis

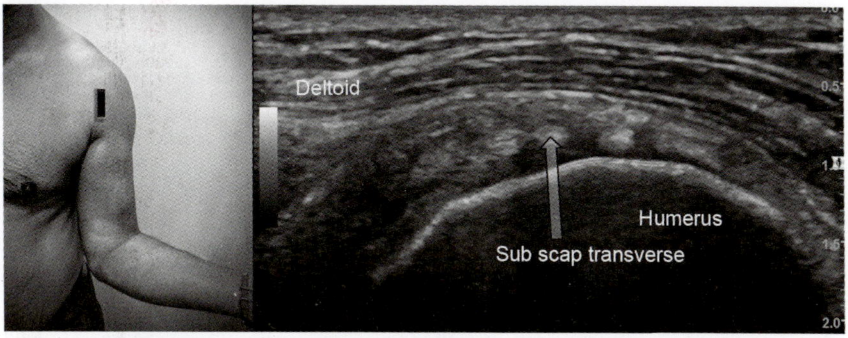

Fig. 6.3.11: On short-axis, multipennate morphology of the subscapularis tendon results in appearance of alternate hypoechoic bands between the echogenic tendon slips. The hypoechoic bands representing muscle tissue may be mistaken as tendinosis or a partial thickness tear

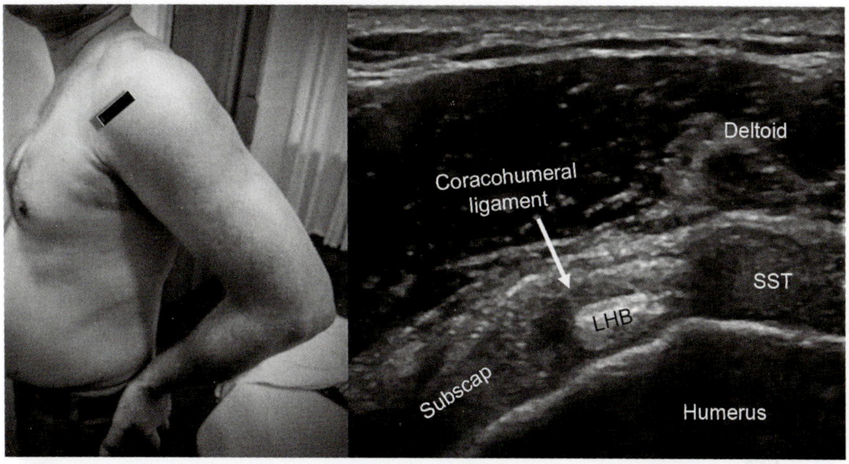

Fig. 6.3.12: . On short-axis imaging, the rotator interval is visualized between the subscapularis tendon anteriorly and the supraspinatus tendon (SST) posteriorly. The rotator interval contains the coracohumeral ligament (arrow), long head of biceps (LHB) and the superior glenohumeral ligament. In patients with frozen shoulder, the rotator cuff interval is scanned to evaluate the thickness of the coracohumeral ligament

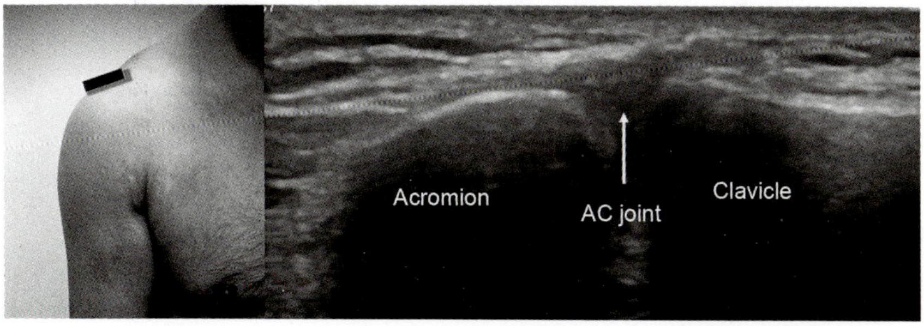

Fig. 6.3.13: Acromioclavicular joint is evaluated along the its short-axis. The probe is gently swept from the anterior to posterior direction. The superior acromioclavicular ligament is a capsular ligament. The intra-articular disc (fibrocartilaginous structure) is seen as an echogenic inverted triangle

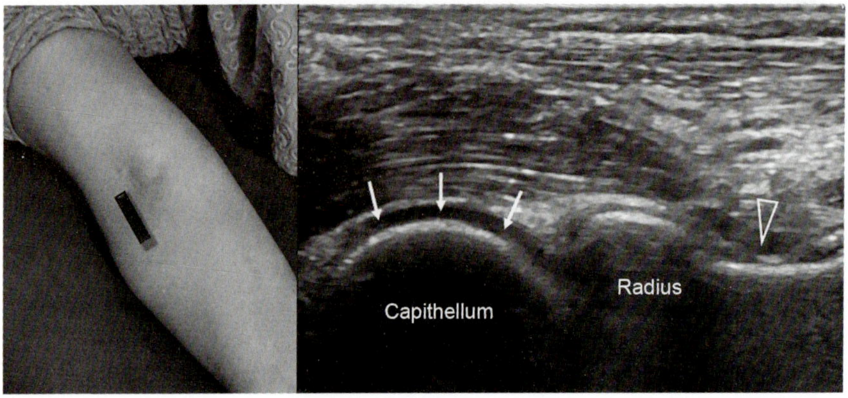

Fig. 6.3.14: Anterior recess (radiocapitellar recess) of the elbow is located in the long-axis by identifying the round capitellum of the humerus and the box-like appearance of the radial head. The articular cartilage over the capitellum is seen as a hypoechoic strip (white arrows) covering the smooth echogenic bone of capitellum. The annular recess communicates with rest of the anterior joint recess (white arrow-head) and is located at the level of radial neck

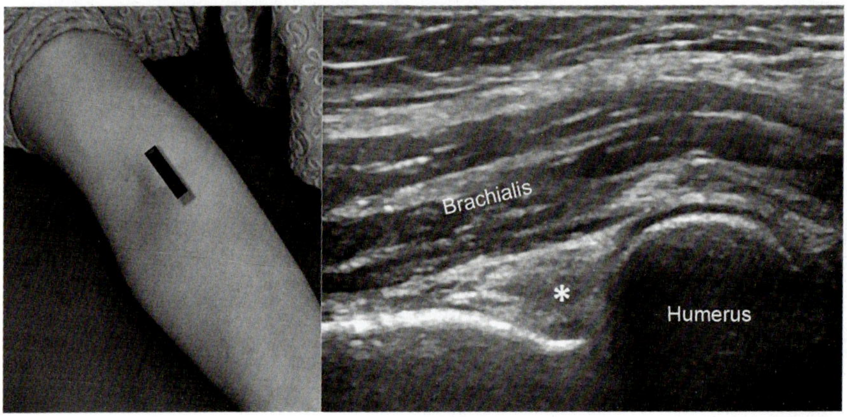

Fig. 6.3.15: The anterior fat pad (asterisk) is seen along the coronoid fossa. The intra-articular fat pad is extra-synovial in location. In presence of joint effusion, the fat pad is displaced anteriorly

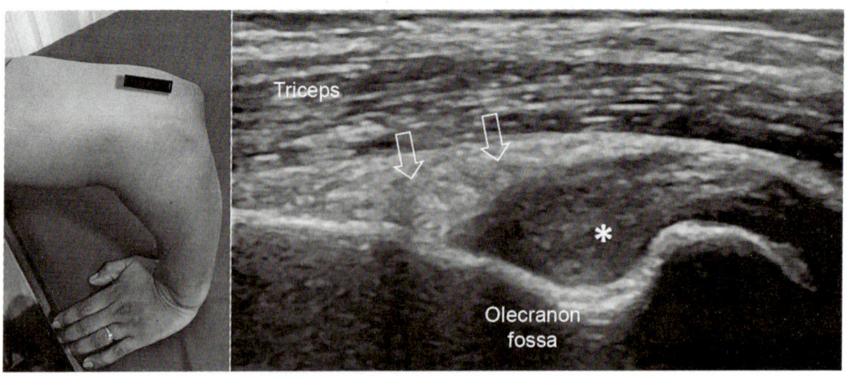

Fig. 6.3.16: Posterior joint recess or the olecranon recess is the largest recess of the elbow joint. The recess is evaluated with the elbow flexed at 90° so that the olecranon process disengages from the olecranon fossa. Synovial hypertrophy (asterisk) results in posterior displacement of the intra-articular extra-synovial fat pad (clear arrows)

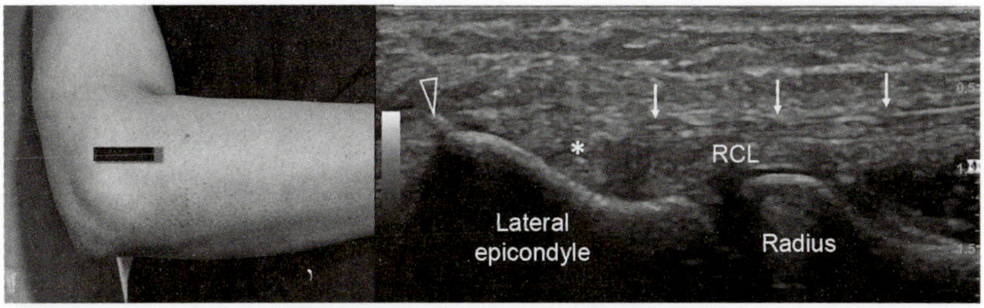

Fig. 6.3.17: Common extensor tendon (CET) is evaluated by aligning the lateral epicondyle, the radial head and radial neck in one plane. The CET (white arrows) is seen as an echogenic fibrillar structure. Tendinosis of the CET is seen as an intratendinous focal hypoechoic area (asterisk) and formation of an enthesophyte (clear triangle). The radial collateral ligament (RCL) is an echogenic structure flush with the CET. Often it might be difficult to differentiate the RCL from the deep fibers of CET

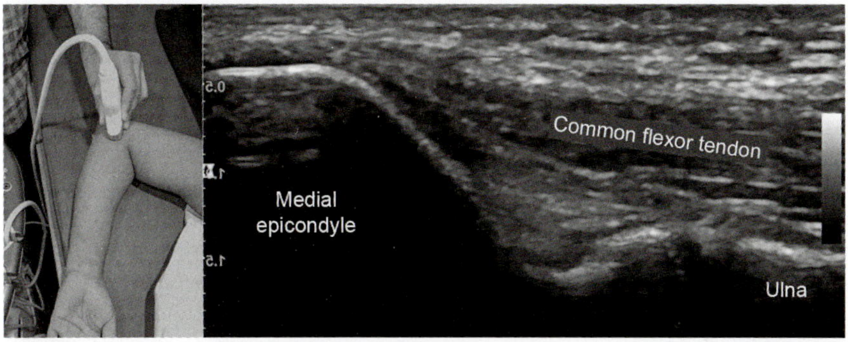

Fig. 6.3.18: Common flexor tendon is visualized by placing the proximal end of the probe over the medial epicondyle and distal end of the probe pointing to wards the base of thumb

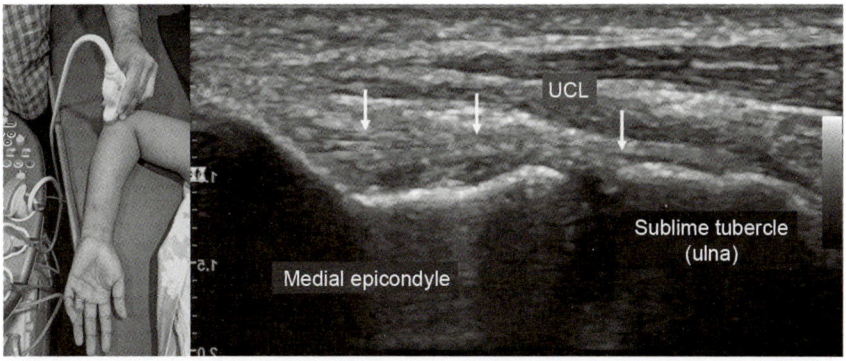

Fig. 6.3.19: Anterior band of the ulnar collateral ligament (UCL) is an important medial stabilizer of the elbow. The UCL is located deep to the common flexor tendon. The UCL is identified by placing the proximal end of the probe over the medial epicondyle and distal end of the probe pointing to wards the hypothenar eminence. The UCL is seen as a cone-shaped echogenic structure with its base at the medial epicondyle

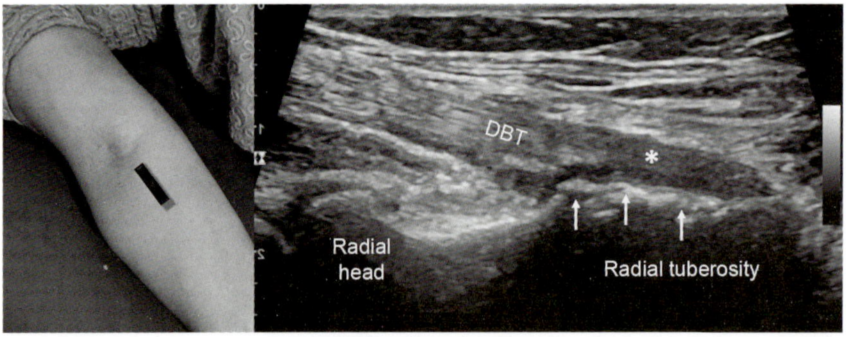

Fig. 6.3.20: Distal biceps tendon (DBT) is imaged in the longitudinal plane with forceful supination for better visualization of the DBT footprint over the radial tuberosity. A heel-toe maneuver would be helpful in removing anisotropy in the DBT. Chronic insertional tendinosis is visualized as an ill-defined hypoechoic area (asterisk) in the peri-insertional fibers of DBT along with presence of cortical irregularity (white arrows) in the radial tuberosity

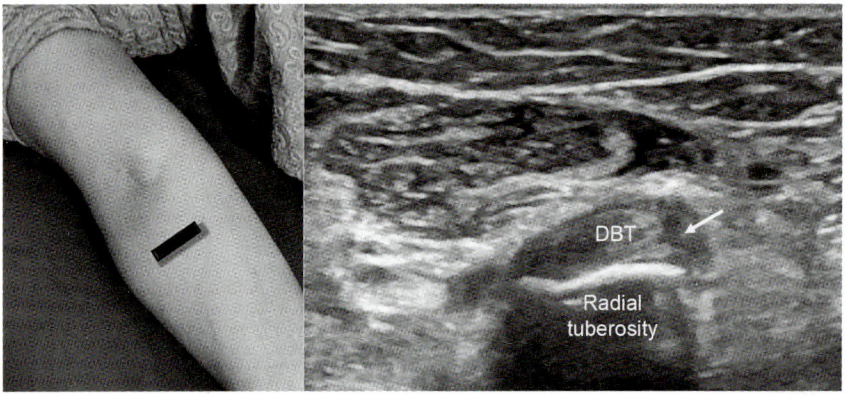

Fig. 6.3.21: Short-axis image of distal biceps tendon (DBT) at its insertion over the radial tuberosity. Chronic insertional tendinosis is visualized as an ill-defined hypoechoic area in the peri-insertional fibers of DBT. Mild peritendinous fluid is seen at the expected location of bicipitoradial bursa (white arrow)

WRIST AND HAND

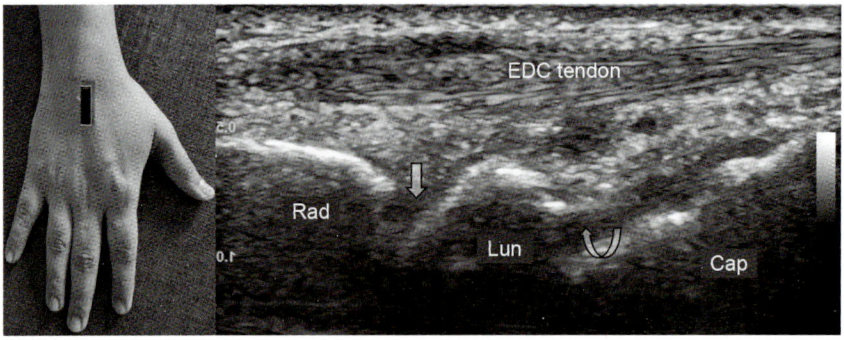

Fig. 6.3.22: Radiocarpal (white arrow) and intercarpal (curved arrow) joints are two separate joint recesses. Dorsal recesses of the wrist are evaluated in the log-axis by placing the probe over the radius (Rad), lunate (Lun) and capitate (Cap) bones. The entire width of the wrist joint should be scanned by gently sweeping the probe from medial to lateral direction

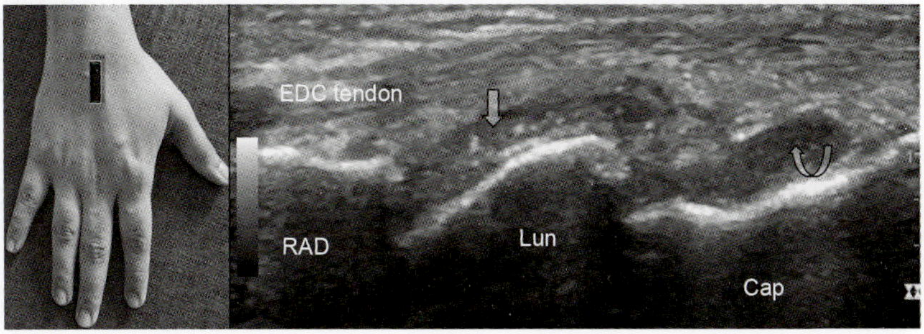

Fig. 6.3.23: Synovial hypertrophy is seen to cause distention of the dorsal radiocarpal (white arrow) and intercarpal (curved arrow) joint recesses. Observe the smooth cortex of lunate (Lun) and capitate (Cap). The patient is known to have rheumatoid arthritis. Rad: Radius

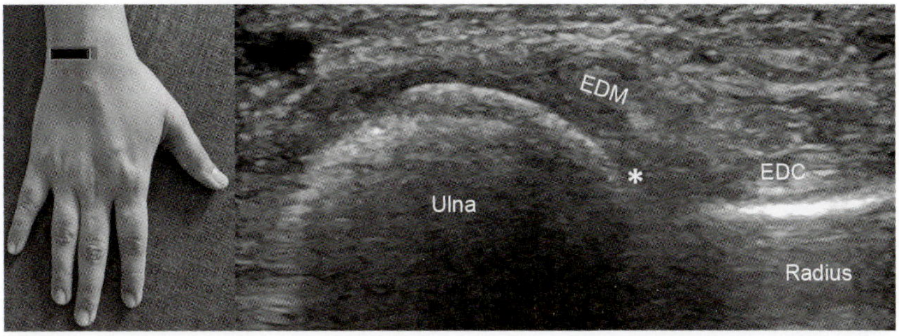

Fig. 6.3.24: Dorsal recess of the distal radioulnar joint is evaluated in the short-axis by identifying the distal radius and the rounded ulnar head. The asterisk represents dorsal recess of the distal radioulnar joint. The extensor digiti minimi (EDM) tendon lies passes over the distal radioulnar joint. EDC: Extensor digitorum communis tendon

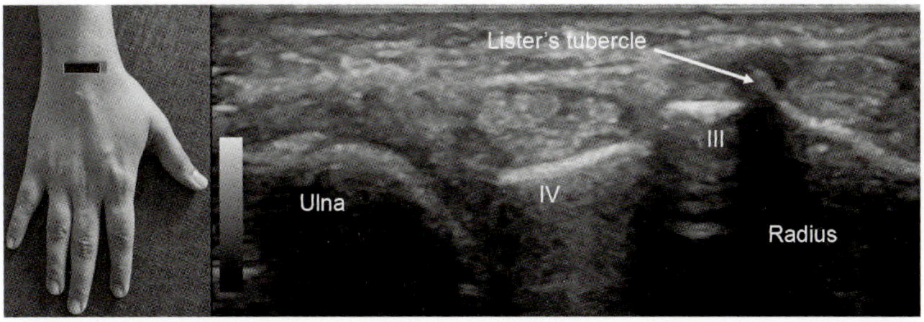

Fig. 6.3.25: On the short-axis, extensor tendons are visualized as echogenic rounded structures over the distal radius. Lister's tubercle is a pyramid shaped osseous projection along the dorsum of radius. The Lister's tubercle is used as a landmark to differentiate extensor compartment II and III tendons. III: Extensor pollicis longus tendon. IV: Extensor digitorum communis tendon

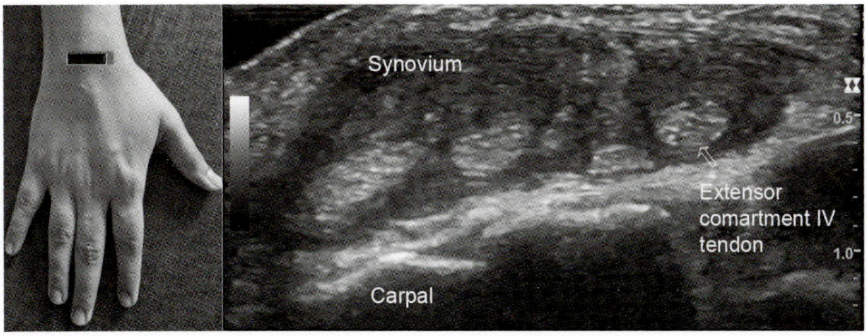

Fig. 6.3.26: Tenosynovitis of the extensor compartment IV tendon sheath. Hypoechoic synovial tissue is seen surrounding the echogenic tendon

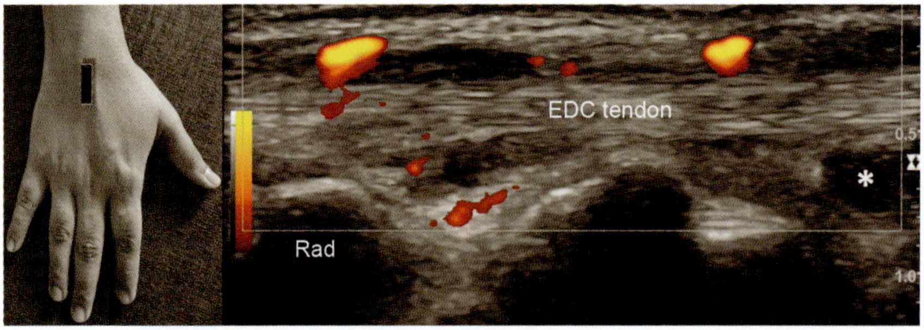

Fig. 6.3.27: Long-axis image shows tenosynovitis of the extensor compartment IV tendon sheath. Hypoechoic synovial tissue along with fluid (asterisk) is seen surrounding the echogenic tendon. Power Doppler shows mild vascularity within the thickened synovium. EDC: Extensor digitorum communis; Rad: Radius

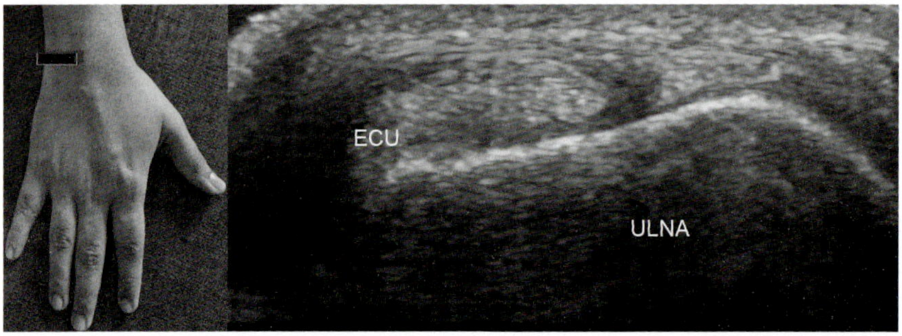

Fig. 6.3.28: On the short-axis, extensor carpi ulnaris (ECU) tendon is visualized as an echogenic round structure situated in the ECU groove located along the dorsolateral surface of ulnar head. The ECU tendon is located in the 6th extensor compartment along the dorsum of wrist

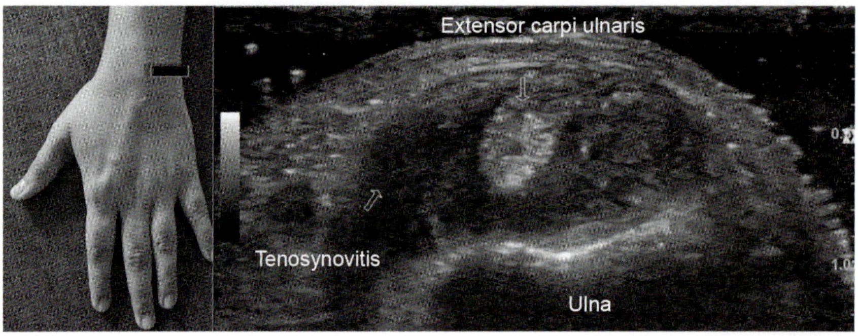

Fig. 6.3.29: Tenosynovitis involving the extensor carpi ulnaris (ECU) tendon sheath. Hypoechoic synovial tissue is seen surrounding the ECU tendon

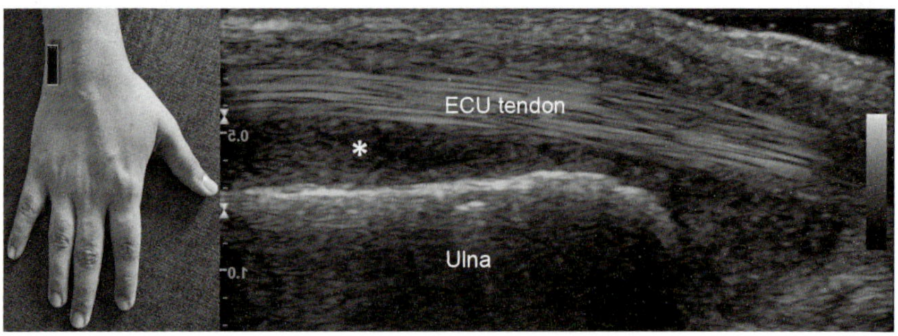

Fig. 6.3.30: Long-axis image shows tenosynovitis involving the extensor carpi ulnaris (ECU) tendon sheath. Hypoechoic synovial tissue (asterisk) is seen surrounding the echogenic tendon

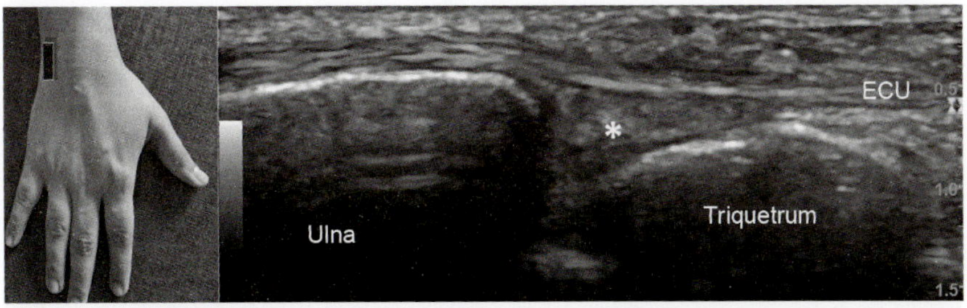

Fig. 6.3.31: Long-axis image echogenic appearance of the normal triangular fibrocartilage complex (asterisk) immediately distal to the ulnar styloid. Note the close relationship of the triangular fibrocartilage complex with the extensor carpi ulnaris (ECU) tendon

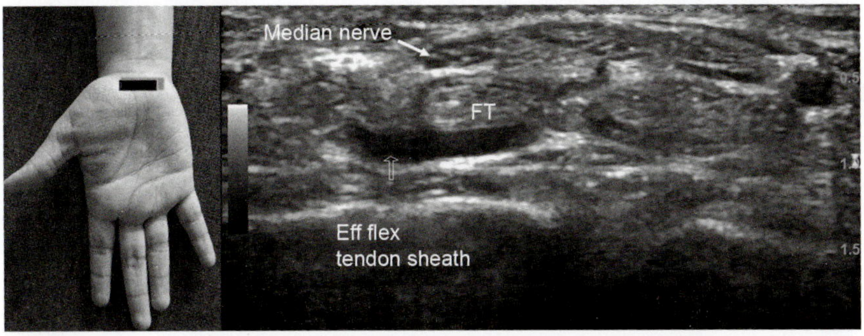

Fig. 6.3.32: Tenosynovitis involving the extensor flexor tendon (FT) sheath at the level of proximal carpal tunnel. Anechoic fluid (clear arrow) is seen partially encircling the common flexor tendon sheath in the carpal tunnel. Note the "honey-comb" appearance of median nerve in the short-axis

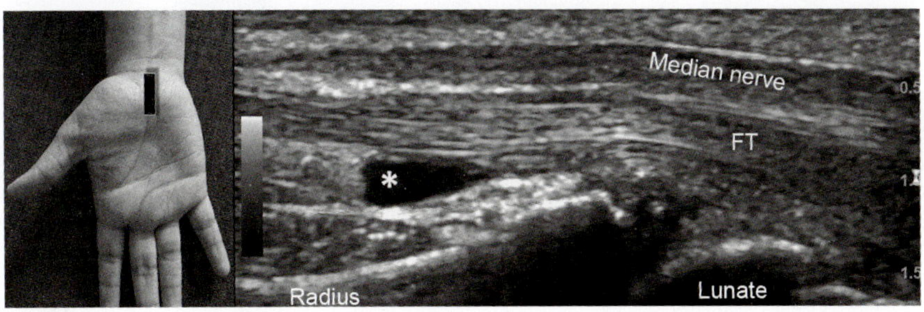

Fig. 6.3.33: Tenosynovitis involving the extensor flexor tendon (FT) sheath proximal to the carpal tunnel. Anechoic fluid (asterisk) is seen in the dependent region of the common flexor tendon sheath. Note the appearance of median nerve—differentiating the Median nerve from the adjacent flexor tendons can be challenging on long-axis images alone

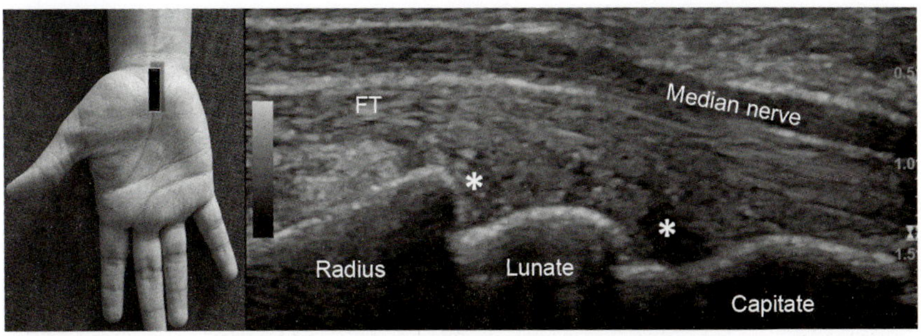

Fig. 6.3.34: Normal appearance of the volar recesses (asterisks) of radiocarpal and intercarpal joints. The volar recesses may be difficult to visualize on very high frequency probes. It would be worthwhile to lower the frequency of the ultrasound probe during evaluation of the volar recesses of the wrist joint. FT: Flexor tendon

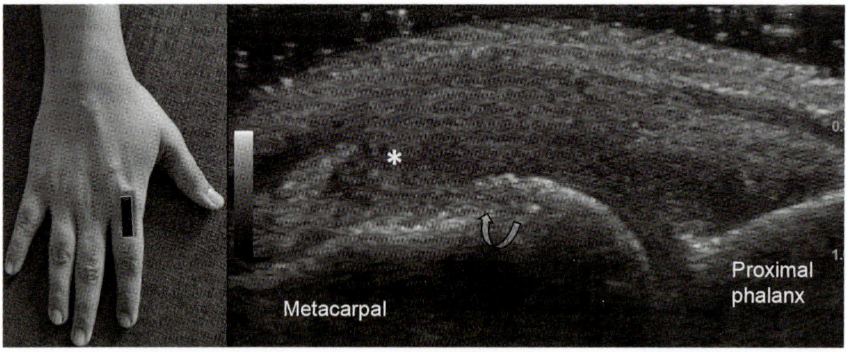

Fig. 6.3.35: Dorsal recesses of the metacarpophalangeal (MCP) joints should be evaluated with mild palmar flexion of the MCP joints. The dorsal recess of the MCP joint extends till the distal metaphysis of the metacarpal. In a patient with psoriatic arthropathy, we can see the thickened and mildly hypoechoic synovium (asterisk) in the dorsal recess along with multiple cortical erosions (curved arrow) in the head and neck of the metacarpal

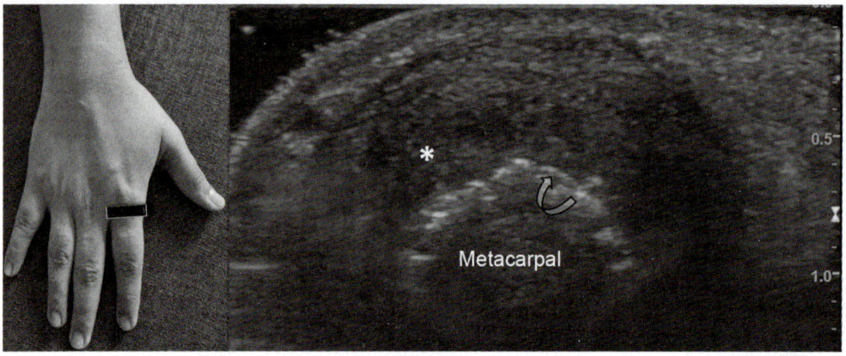

Fig. 6.3.36: Transverse section of the involved metacarpophalangeal joint (from Fig. 6.3.33). Thickened and mildly hypoechoic synovium (asterisk) in the dorsal, ulnar and radial recesses along with multiple cortical erosions (curved arrow) in the neck of the metacarpal

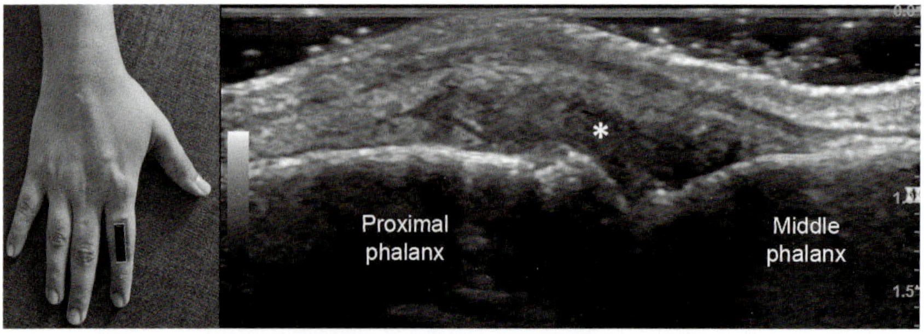

Fig. 6.3.37: Morphology of dorsal recess of the proximal interphalangeal (PIP) joint is similar to the metacarpophalangeal joint, i.e. the joint extends till the distal metaphysis of the proximal phalanx. In a patient with unknown inflammatory arthropathy, we can see the thickened and hypoechoic synovium (asterisk) in the dorsal recess of the PIP joint

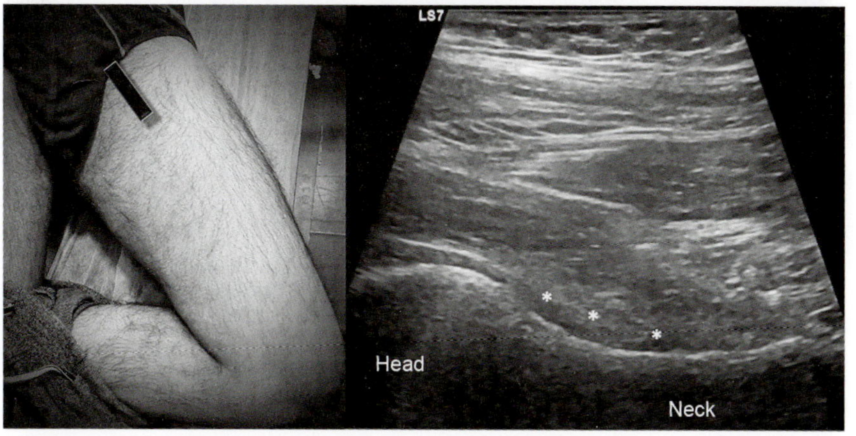

Fig. 6.3.38: Anterior recess of hip is evaluated with the hip in external rotation. The femoral head and neck are identified and the probe is placed parallel to the femoral neck. The anterior joint recess is located deep to the iliopsoas tendon and the anterior joint capsule (asterisks)

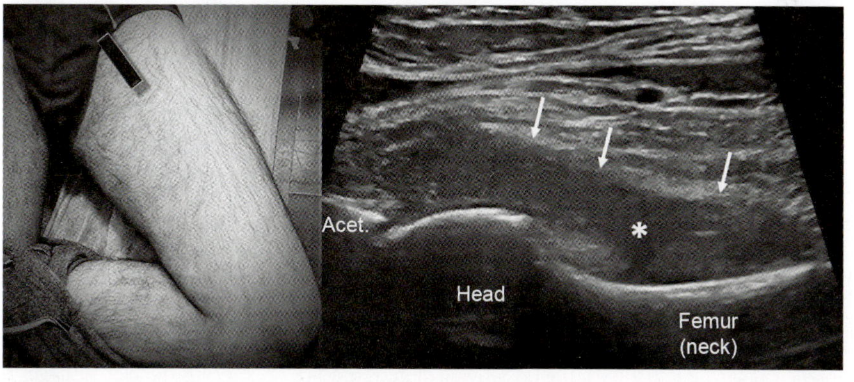

Fig. 6.3.39: Diffuse synovial hypertrophy along with joint effusion is seen to cause distension of joint capsule anterior joint capsule (asterisks). The patient is known to have juvenile idiopathic arthritis. Acet.: Acetabulum.

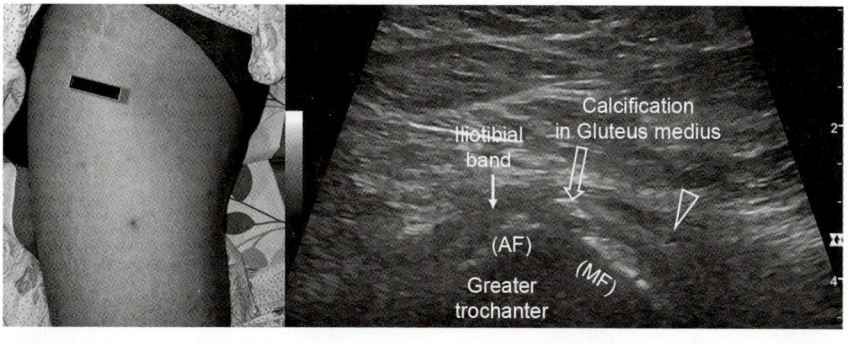

Fig. 6.3.40: The key to successful evaluation of greater trochanteric pain is identification of the anterior and middle facets of the greater trochanter on the short-axis. The gluteus minimus tendon inserts on the anterior facet (AF) whereas the Gluteus Medius tendon (clear arrow) inserts on the middle facet (MF). The iliotibial band (white arrow) is an isoechoic to hypoechoic band overlying the greater trochanter. The greater trochanteric bursa (clear triangle) is situated between the greater trochanter and the iliotibial band (white arrow). Note the focal intratendinous calcification in the gluteus medius tendon (clear arrow)

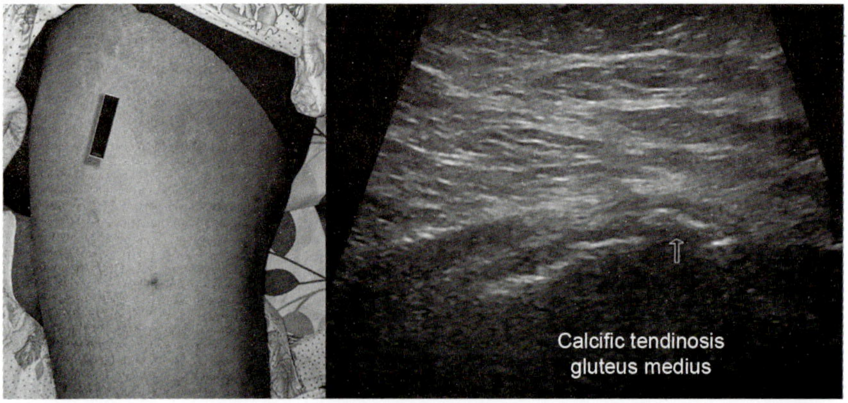

Fig. 6.3.41: Long-axis image obtained at the level of middle facet in the greater trochanter shows intratendinous calcification (clear arrow) in the peri-insertional fibers of gluteus medius tendon

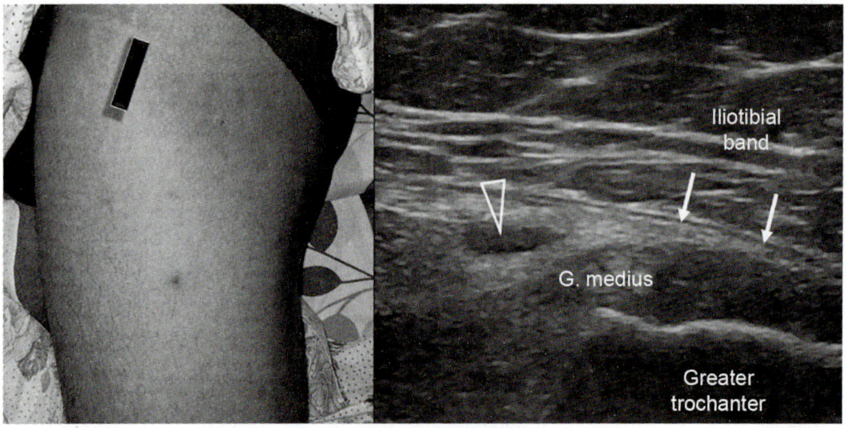

Fig. 6.3.42: Long-axis image obtained at the level of middle facet in the greater trochanter shows mild effusion in the greater trochanteric bursa (clear triangle). The underlying gluteus medius (G. medius) tendon appears hypoechoic—suggestive of tendinosis

KNEE

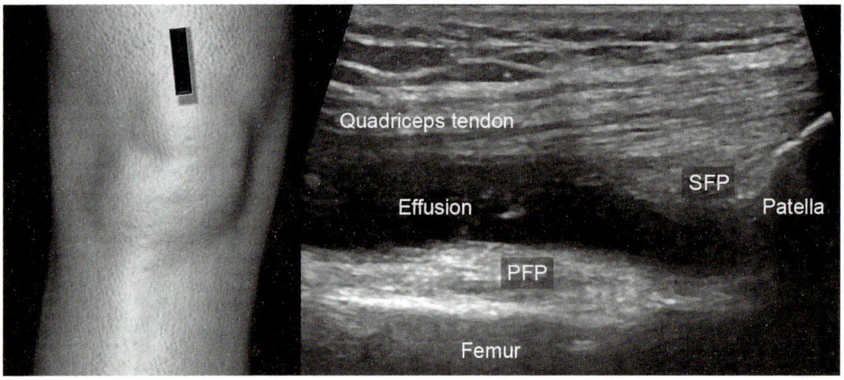

Fig. 6.3.43: On long-axis, the suprapatellar recess is located deep to the quadriceps tendon, between the suprapatellar fat pad (SFP) and prefemoral fat pad (PFP). Suprapatellar recess is commonly assessed to look for joint effusion, synovial hypertrophy and intra-articular loose bodies

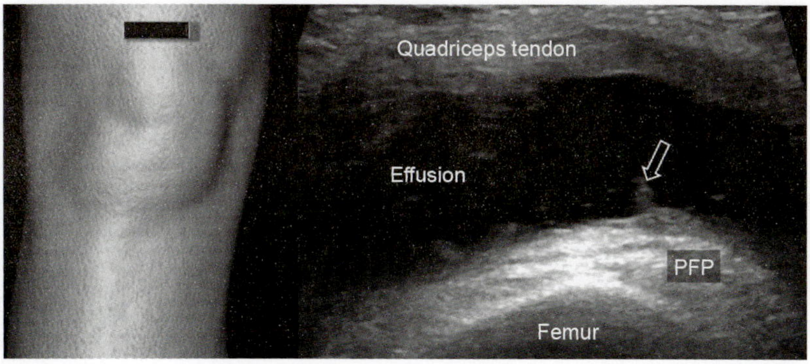

Fig. 6.3.44: Transverse section obtained at the level of suprapatellar recess shows mild to moderate effusion along with synovial hypertrophy (clear arrow). PFP: Prefemoral fat pad

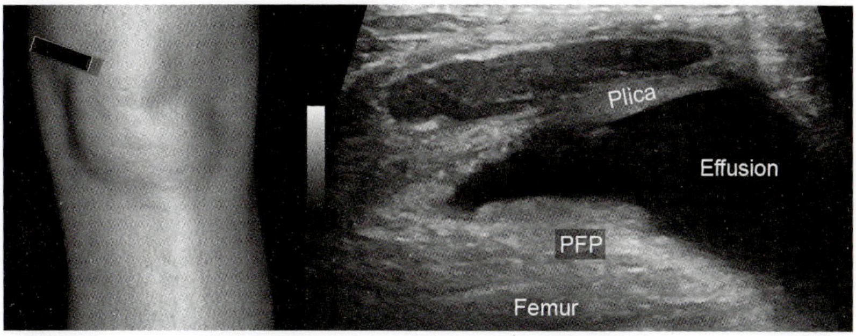

Fig. 6.3.45: Oblique section obtained at the level of medial parapatellar recess shows mild-to-moderate effusion along with a synovial plica. PFP: Prefemoral fat pad

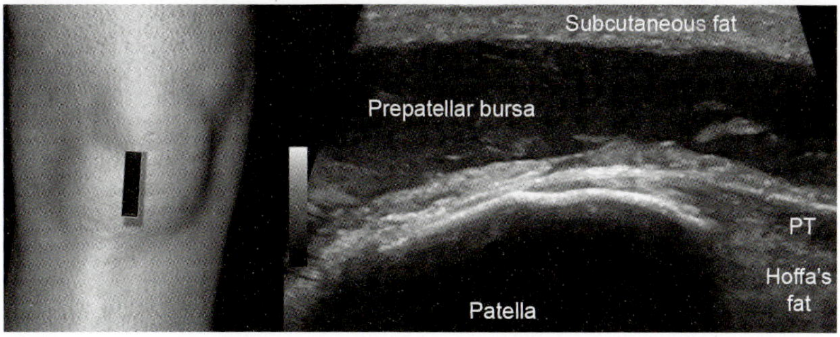

Fig. 6.3.46: Long-axis view over the patella shows a cystic lesion between the subcutaneous fat and the patella at the expected location of prepatellar bursa. PT: Patellar tendon

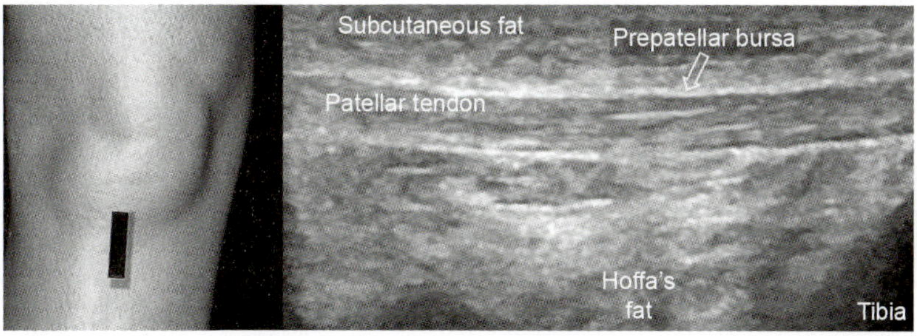

Fig. 6.3.47: Superficial infrapatellar bursa is located between the subcutaneous fat and the patellar tendon. Normally, the bursa would not be visualized in the collapsed state

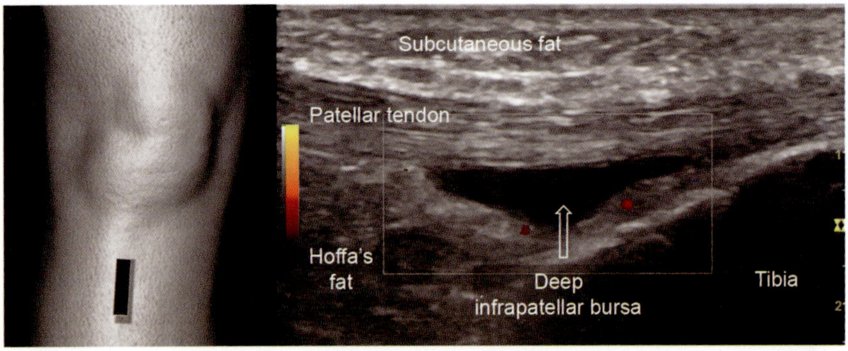

Fig. 6.3.48: Deep infrapatellar bursa is located between the patellar tendon (anteriorly) and the tibia and Hoffa's fat (posteriorly). Mild effusion with synovial hypertrophy is seen in the deep infrapatellar bursa (clear arrow)

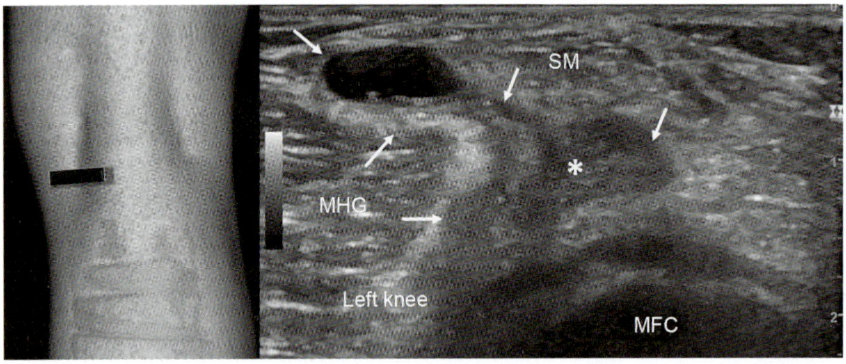

Fig. 6.3.49: Gastrocnemius-semimembranosus bursa (white arrows) is located between the medial head of gastrocnemius (MHG) and the semimembranosus (SM) tendon. The bursa is located on the transverse images by identifying the medial femoral condyle (MFC), MHG and SM tendons. Most of the times, the bursa communicates with the knee joint. Effusion, synovial hypertrophy (asterisk) and loose bodies can be identified in the distended bursa. An enlarged gastrocnemius semimembranosus bursa is also known as Baker's cyst

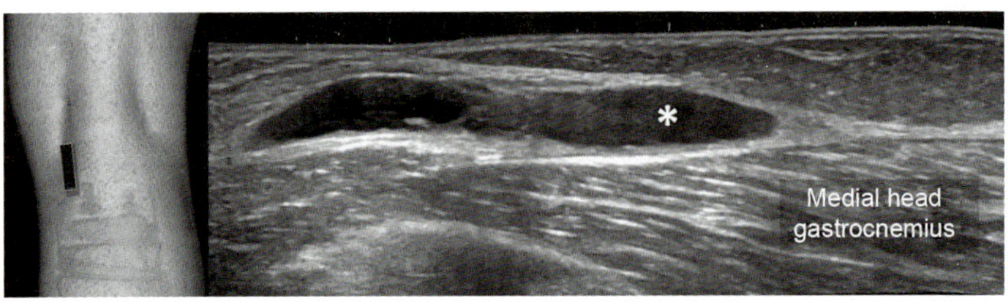

Fig. 6.3.50: As the gastrocnemius-semimembranosus bursa (asterisk) enlarges it grows in the craniocaudal direction. Pointing inferior edge of the Baker's cyst or disproportionate edema in the adjacent intermuscular planes suggests the possibility of rupture of the Baker's cyst

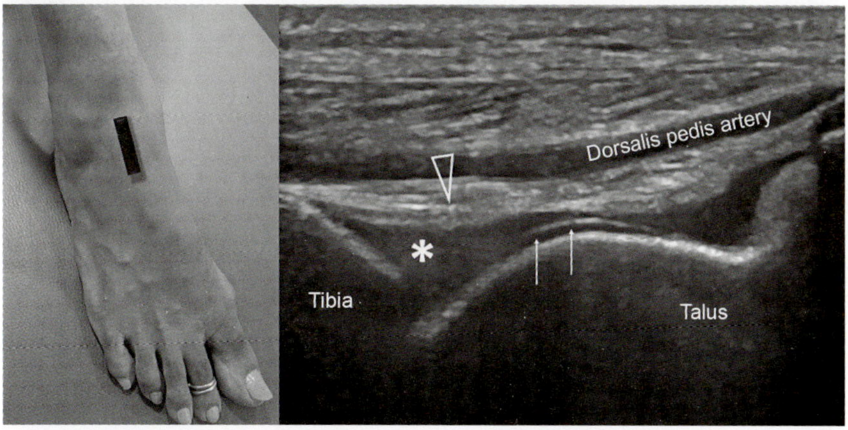

Fig. 6.3.51: Anterior recess of the tibiotalar joint is located by identifying the distal end of tibia and the talus. Articular cartilage over the talar head is seen as a hypoechoic stripe (white arrows) covering the talar dome. Joint effusion (asterisk) results in anterior displacement of the intra-articular extrasynovial fat pad (clear triangle)

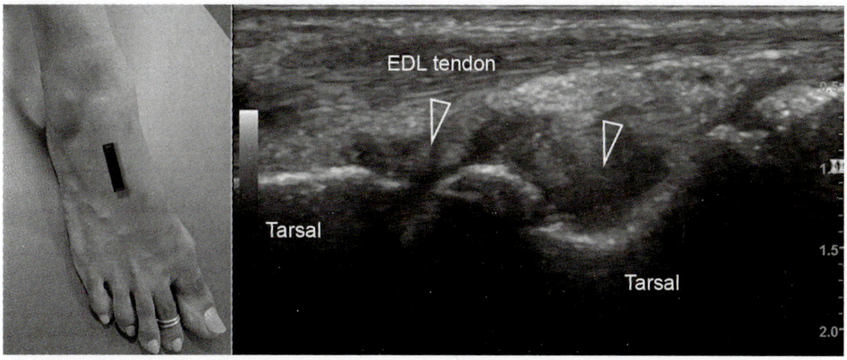

Fig. 6.3.52: Fluid and synovial hypertrophy (white triangles) can be identified in the dorsal recesses of the midfoot joints. This patient was known to have rheumatoid arthritis and had midfoot synovitis

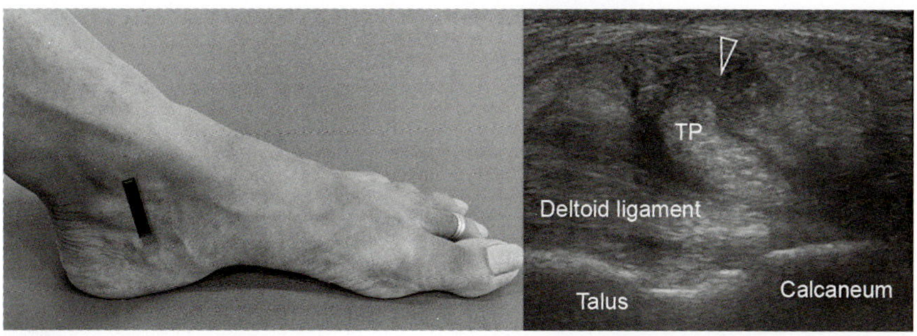

Fig. 6.3.53: Tibialis posterior (TP) tendon is located just posterior to the medial malleolus. The TP tendon is imaged in the short-axis after identifying the medial malleolus. The TP tendon is traced in the short-axis in the supramalleolar, retromalleolar and inframalleolar regions. Marked tenosynovitis (clear triangle) is seen in the TP tendon sheath along the inframalleolar segment. The TP tendon is closely related to the deltoid and spring ligaments in the inframalleolar segment

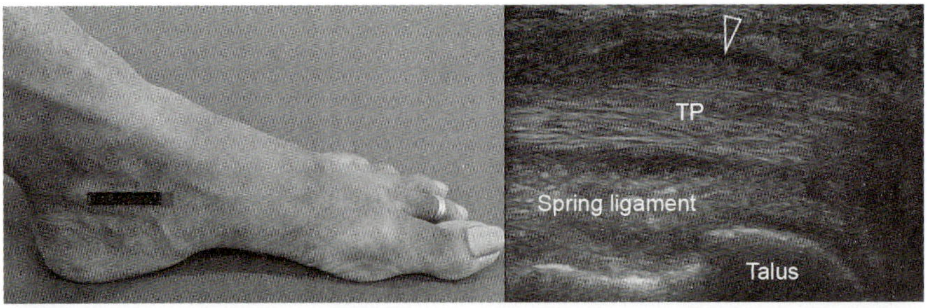

Fig. 6.3.54: Tibialis posterior (TP) tendon is evaluated in the long-axis at supramalleolar, retromalleolar and inframalleolar segments. Fluid (clear triangle) is seen along the inframalleolar segment of TP tendon—suggestive of tenosynovitis

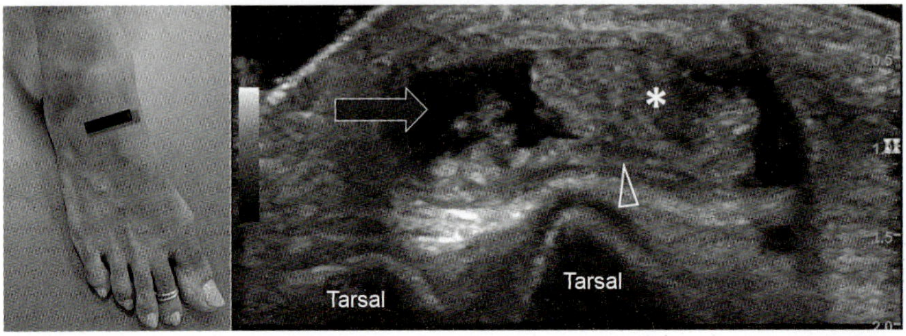

Fig. 6.3.55: Extensor tendons along the anterior aspect of ankle foot are evaluated in the short-axis. Nodular synovial hypertrophy (asterisk) along with effusion (black arrow) are seen along the extensor digitorum longus tendon (clear triangle)–suggestive of marked tenosynovitis. The patient is known to have juvenile HLA B27 positive spondyloarthropathy

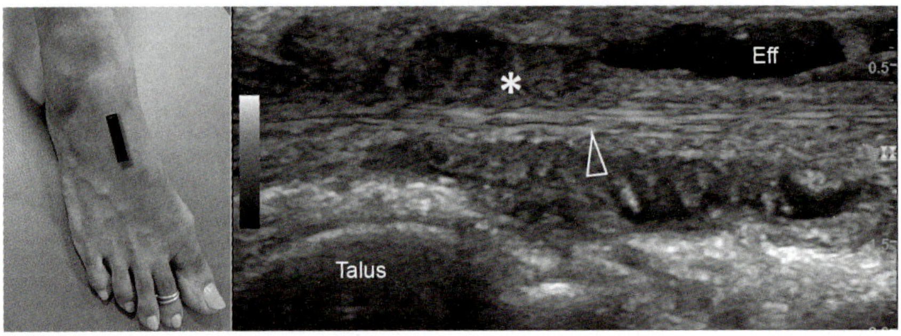

Fig. 6.3.56: Long-axis image shows nodular synovial hypertrophy (asterisk) along with effusion (Eff) along the extensor digitorum longus tendon (clear triangle) sheath—suggestive of marked tenosynovitis

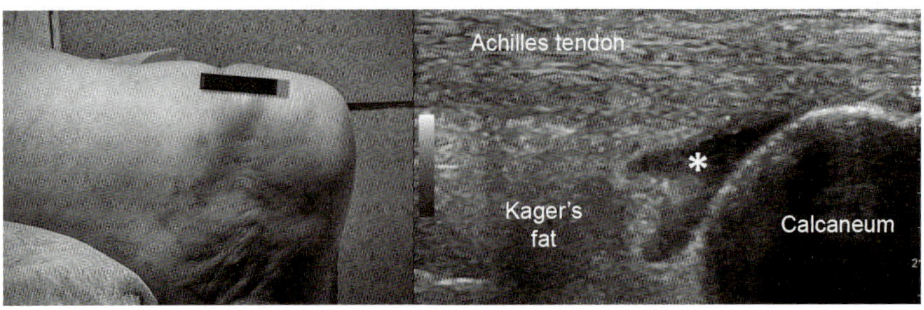

Fig. 6.3.57: Long-axis image shows the retrocalcanel bursa (asterisk) located between distal Achilles tendon and calcaneum

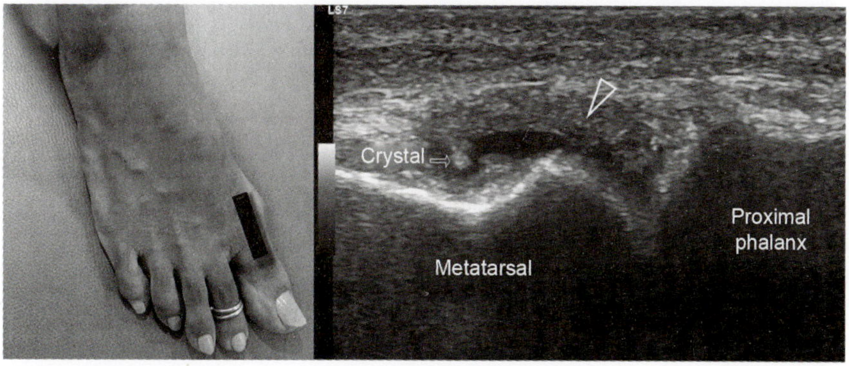

Fig. 6.3.58: Long-axis image shows the dorsal recess of metatarsophalangeal joint of the great toe. In a known case of gout, the long axis image shows thickening of the dorsal capsule (clear triangle) of 1st metatarsophalangeal joint along with echogenic crystal deposit (clear arrow) in the synovium

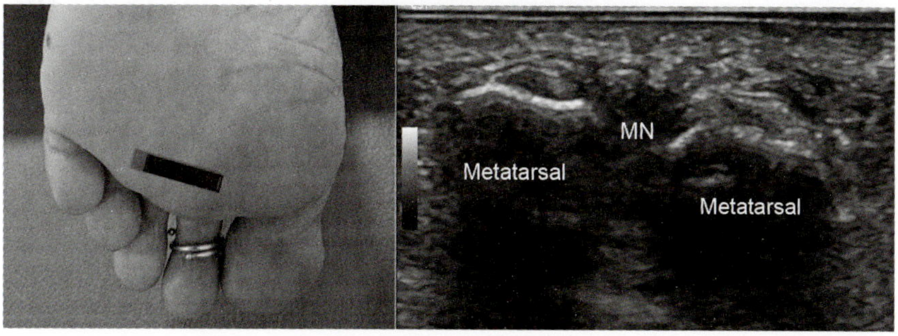

Fig. 6.3.59: Morton's neuroma represents focal perineural fibrosis along the digital nerve at the level of metatarsal heads. Typically, transverse scan at the level of the 2nd web space shows an ill-defined hypoechoic soft (MN) tissue between the metatarsal heads. Squeezing of the metatarsal heads results in better visualization of the protruding soft tissue. Imaging findings are consistent with a Morton's neuroma

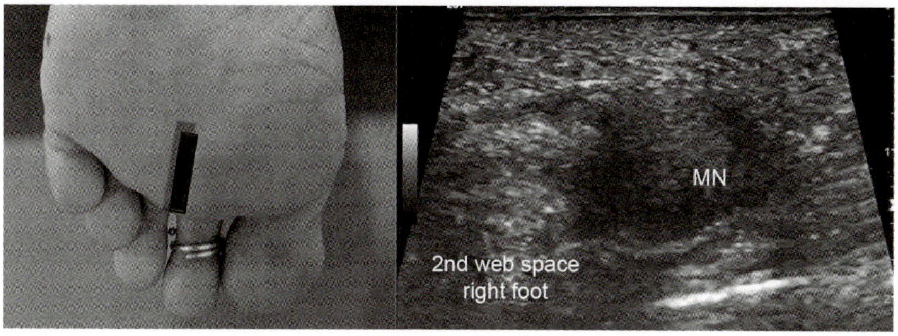

Fig. 6.3.60: On longitudinal images, Morton's neuroma is visualized as a hypoechoic soft tissue (MN) at the level of metatarsal heads. Sometimes, the digital nerve may be seen entering the lesion

MAIN LIMITATIONS OF MUSCULOSKELETAL ULTRASOUND

- Inability to detect bone inflammation (marrow edema).
- Inadequate visualization of deeper anatomical structures (hip, knee) and structures covered by bone (spine, femoral head, talar dome).
- Interobserver variability.

LEARNING POINTS

- Knowledge of appropriate musculoskeletal ultrasound scanning techniques is essential to obtain standardised high quality diagnostic images.
- Appropriate Power Doppler settings allow detection of early inflammation and avoid diagnostic pitfalls.
- Ultrasound can easily identify effusion, synovial hypertrophy and cortical erosions - the hallmarks of inflammation in superficial areas like wrist, hand, elbow, knee, ankle and foot.

FURTHER READING

1. Czyrny Z. Standards for musculoskeletal ultrasound. J Ultrason. 2017;17(70):182–7.
2. Martinoli, C. Musculoskeletal ultrasound: technical guidelines. Insights Imaging. 2010;1:99–141.

Chapter 6.4

Diagnostic Ultrasound in Arthritis (Upper Limb)

PD Rath, Amit Kumar Sahu, Jani Ami Kaushik

INTRODUCTION

Upper limb joints can be affected by inflammatory or non-inflammatory pathologies. The ultrasound (US) definitions for findings such as erosions, joint effusion, synovitis, and grading of synovitis include:

- **An articular erosions** is a discontinuity of >5 mm of the bone surface (intra-articular) that must be visualized in two perpendicular planes.
- **A joint effusion** is usually a hypoechoic or anechoic (though sometimes iso or hyperechoic) intra-articular material (as compared to subdermal fat) that is compressible and displaceable. An effusion generally will not show Doppler signal.
- **Synovitis [Gray scale ultrasound (GSUS) and Power doppler ultrasound (PDUS)]:** The definition of synovitis on ultrasound is similar to effusion only that the intra-articualr material is not displaceable, poorly compressible, and may exhibit Doppler signal.
- **GSUS grades of synovitis:** Grade 0: No synovial thickening; Grade 1 – minimal synovial thickening; Grade 2 – synovial thickening that exceeds the line connecting periarticular bones, without extension to the bone diaphysis; Grade 3 – synovial thickening that exceeds the line which connects periarticular bones and also extends on diaphysis.
- PDUS grades of synovitis: Grade 0—no Doppler signal; Grade 1—single vessel signal (up to 3); Grade 2—confluent vessel signal in less than half of the area of synovium; Grade 3— vessel signal in more than half of the synovium.

RHEUMATOID ARTHRITIS

Findings at the wrist and hands: Synovitis (with PDUS signal), joint effusion, flexor tenosynovitis and marginal bone erosions (Fig. 6.4.1). The common sites of marginal erosions are the 2nd metacarpal head (radial aspect), the 5th metacarpal head (ulnar aspect), the lunate and pisiform. *PDUS synovitis is more sensitive than GSUS.*

Glenohumeral synovitis with PDUS signal, subacromial bursitis with synovial thickening

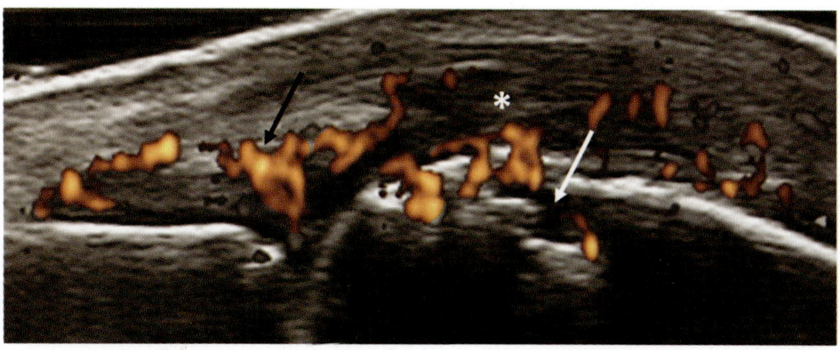

Fig. 6.4.1: Rheumatoid arthritis: Erosions in metacarpal head (white arrow); synovial thickening (asterisk) and power doppler signal in the thickened synovium (black arrow)

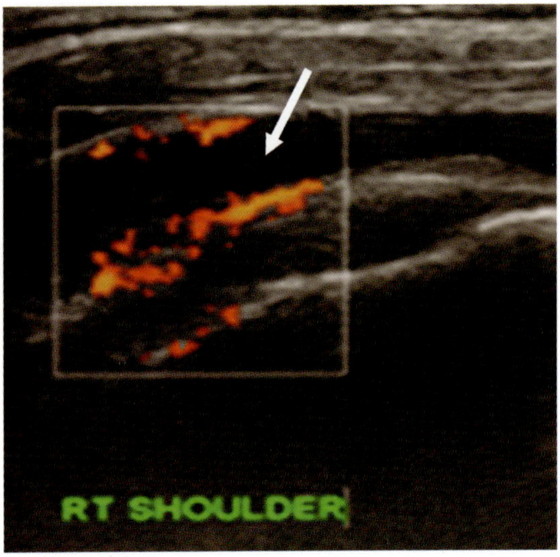

Fig. 6.4.2: Subacromial bursitis: Fluid in the subacromial bursa (arrow) with power doppler signal, suggesting inflammatory etiology

(Fig. 6.4.2) and bicipital tenosynovitis are common. In the elbow, marginal erosions and synovitis in anterior humeroradial fossa and humeroulnar fossa and posterior fossa along with joint effusion are also common findings.

PSORIATIC ARTHRITIS

The common findings are extensor paratenonitis, PDUS signal within the soft tissue, microenthesitis, periosteitis, synovitis, tenosynovitis/peritendinitis (Figs. 6.4.3 and 6.4.4), *pseudo-tenosynovitis* and erosions in wrist and small joints of hand. Pseudotenosynovitis represents hypoechoic soft tissue surrounding flexor tendon showing extensive power doppler signal. Peritendinitis is hypoechoic soft tissue with/without fluid within the flexor tendon sheaths or surrounding the extensor tendon.

Microenthesitis is PDUS signal at the attachment site of extensor tendons in fingers without any obvious enthesophytes detected on ultrasound. *Periosteitis* is inflammation of the periosteum which can be detected on ultrasound as hypoechoic thickening of periosteum with sub periosteal fluid and PDUS. It is indistinguishable from periosteal reaction in infective/neoplastic disease.

In the shoulder, acromioclavicular joint is more commonly involved than glenohumeral joint.

In the elbow enthesitis of common extensor (Fig. 6.4.5) and common flexor tendon is seen along with periosteitis.

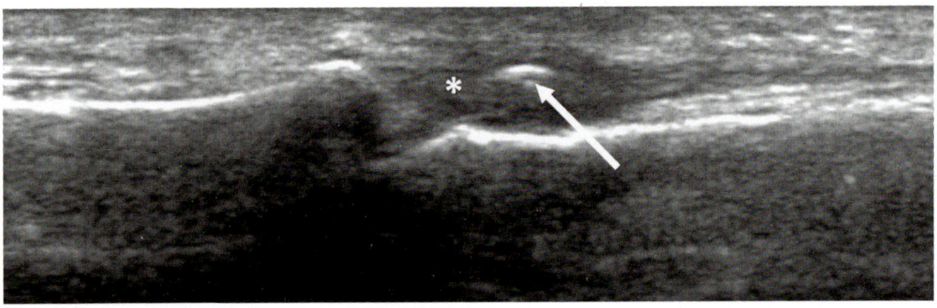

Fig. 6.4.3: Psoriatic arthritis: Diffuse thickening of the extensor tendon (asterisk) of finger at terminal phalangeal attachment with calcification (arrow), suggesting enthesitis

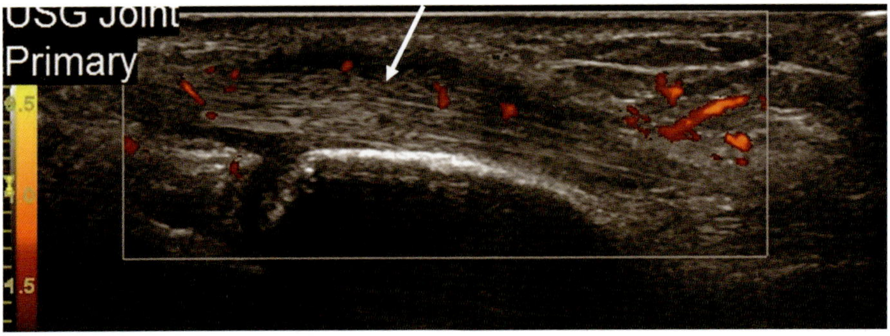

Fig. 6.4.4: Psoriatic arthritis: Diffuse thickening of the flexor tendon of finger with synovial hypoechogenicity (arrow) showing power Doppler signal, suggesting tenosynovitis

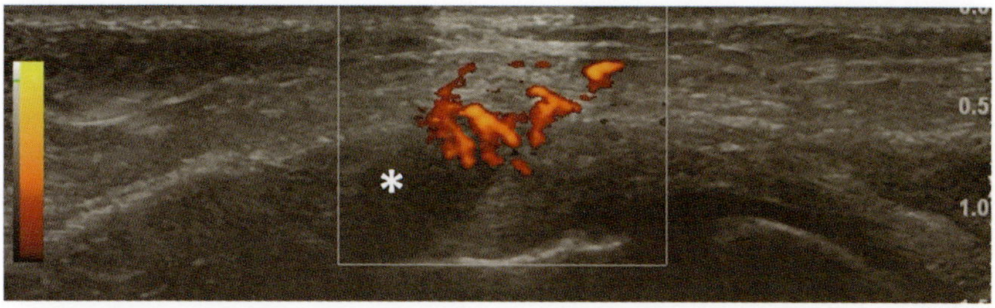

Fig. 6.4.5: Psoriatic arthritis: Diffusely thickened common extensor tendon (asterisk) at elbow joint with power Doppler signal, suggesting enthesitis

GOUT

Ultrasound findings are hyperechoic synovitis due to deposition of monosodium urate crystals[5] with PDUS signal. Visualization of tophus which appears as hyperechoic/hypoechoic aggregates with anechoic rim floating in synovial fluid. Intra-tendinous tophus appear hypoechoic with few hyperechoic foci and loss of normal fibrillar pattern of tendon. The most common site is in triceps tendon at attachment in elbow. Erosions can be intra-articular or extra-articular. Various stages of tophus from soft to hard with post acoustic shadowing. Double contour sign has very high sensitivity to diagnose gout. It is manifested as a hyperechoic line in the outer margin of the cartilage, its thickness is almost same as the subchondral bone (Fig. 6.4.6).

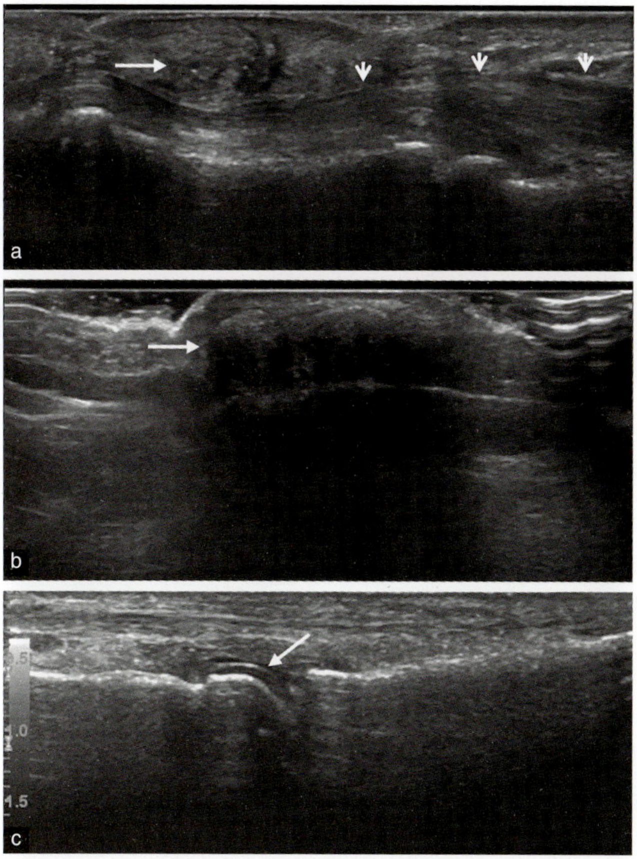

Fig. 6.4.6: Gout: (a) Soft tophus (large arrow) without posterior acoustic shadowing in the soft tissue over the flexor tendon (small arrows) of finger; (b) Hard tophus (arrow) with posterior acoustic shadowing in soft tissue of finger; (c) Double contour sign (arrow)

CALCIUM PYROPHOSPATE DEPOSITION (CPPD) DISEASE

The findings are hyperechoic foci within the hyaline cartilage without posterior acoustic shadowing in hand and wrist joints. Chondrocalcinosis: Lunotriquetral and scapholunate ligaments; predilection for 2nd and 3rd MCP joints (usually presents as advanced degenerative changes). Other findings of CPPD disease on US in the upper limbs are triangular fibrocartilage complex (TFCC) calcification in wrist (Fig. 6.4.7) and acromioclavicular joint calcification. There can also be entheseal thickening and intra-tendinuous hyperechoic linear bands with or without acoustic shadowing. CPPD crystals are usually uniformly round with well defined outer margins. They can also be seen in subacromial subdeltoid bursa.

POLYMYALGIA RHEUMATICA

US definitions according to the classification criteria is presence of any two of bursitis, synovitis and tenosynovitis in a proximal joint. These US findings when present bilaterally has increased diagnostic value.

US FINDINGS IN OTHER CONDITIONS

Beyond arthritis conditions, pathologies commonly encountered on US in other conditions are as follows.

SHOULDER

- **Bursitis:** fluid distension of the subdeltoid and subacromial bursa along with synovial thickening.
- **Rotator cuff:** In tendinosis, there is diffuse thickening of the tendon with decreased echogenicity and loss of normal fibrillar pattern. The tendon tear can be complete/partial tear; partial thickness/ full thickness tear. Partial tear can be articular/ bursal/intrasubstance/insertional. There is hypoechoic fluid like area within the tendon with discontinuity of fibres (Figs. 6.4.8 and 6.4.9).

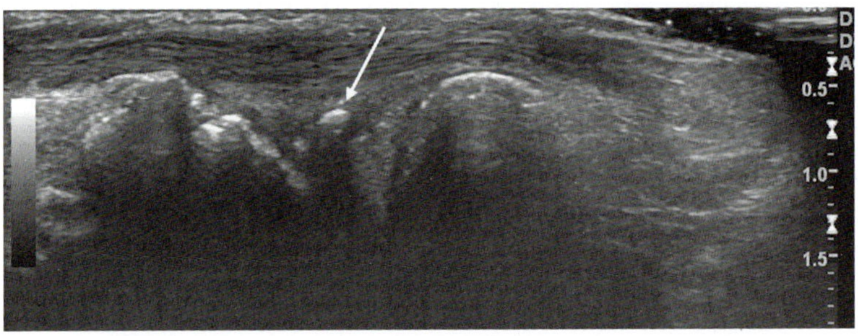

Fig. 6.4.7: CPPD: Calcification seen in the triangular fibrocartilage complex (arrow)

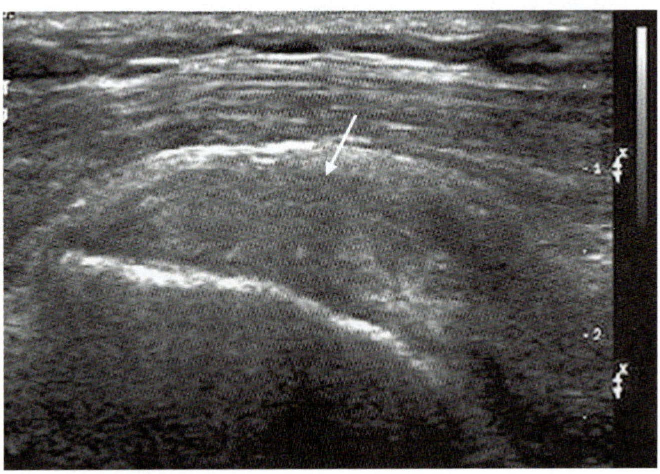

Fig. 6.4.8: Supraspinatus tendinosis: Diffuse thickening of the tendon with decreased echogenicity (arrow)

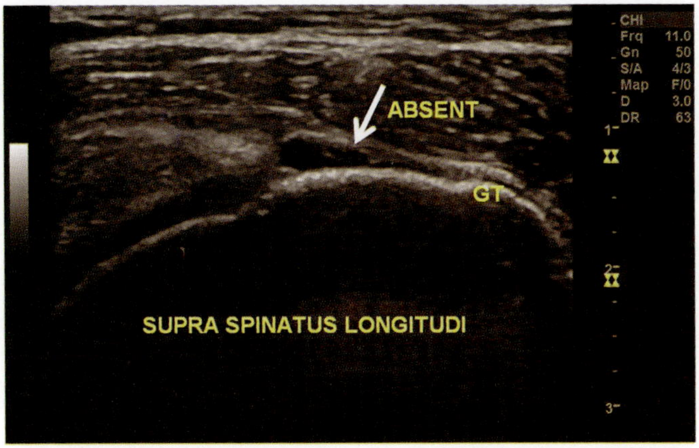

Fig. 6.4.9: Complete tear of supraspinatus tendon. There is absence of the tendon in the region of foot print (arrow). *GT:* Greater tuberosity

- **Adhesive capsulitis:** Presents with mainly normal ultrasound. US has a very low sensitivity and specificity for thickening of the axillary capsule and coracohumeral ligament. External rotation is markedly restricted which can be noted while doing dynamic US.
- **Subacromial impingement syndrome:** Although a clinical diagnosis, there is restricted movement and clumping of fibres of the supraspinatus tendon beneath the acromion on dynamic study .

ELBOW

- Tendinosis of common extensor tendon, common flexor tendon and triceps tendon.
- Degenerative enthesopathy—enthesophytes without any evidence of inflammation.
- Olecranon bursitis (Fig. 6.4.10).
- Ulnar nerve entrapment at cubital fossa: thickening of the ulnar nerve within the cubital fossa with or without retinaculum thickening. If the thickness ratio of the ulnar nerve at the cubital tunnel compared to that proximal to the tunnel is 1.5:1, it is diagnostic of cubital tunnel syndrome.

WRIST

- Ganglion cyst: fluid containing sac in the wrist (commonly in dorsal aspect) with/without articular communication (Fig. 6.4.11).

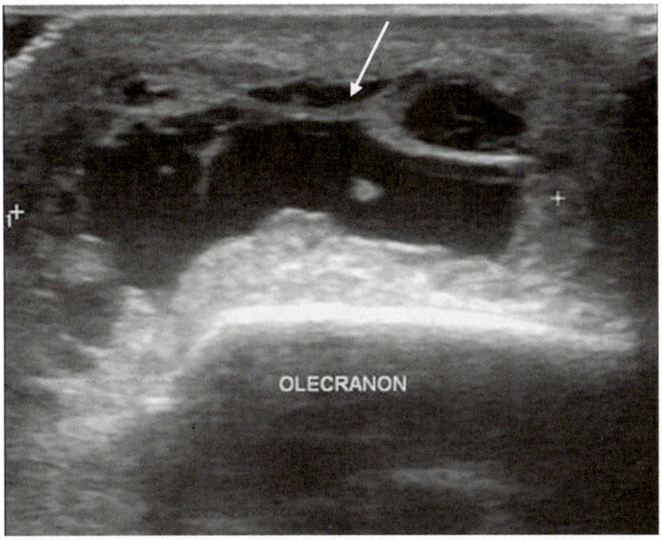

Fig. 6.4.10: Olecranon bursitis: Fluid in the olecranon bursa with thick internal septae

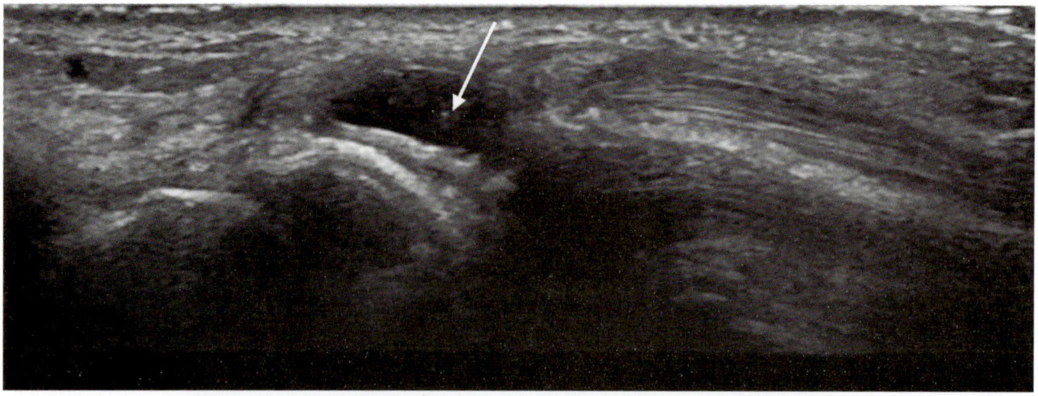

Fig. 6.4.11: Ganglion cyst: Anechoeic cyst (arrow) seen in the wrist joint dorsal aspect

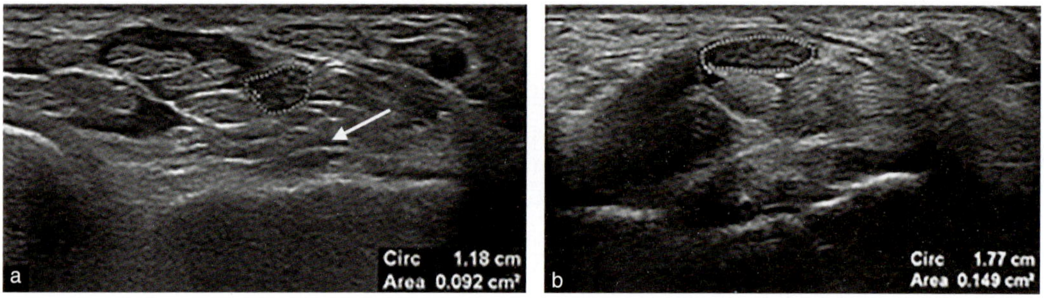

Fig. 6.4.12: Carpal tunnel syndrome: There is >2 mm^2 difference in cross sectional area in median nerve between the level of pronator quadratus (arrow in A) and carpal tunnel (B).

- Giant cell tumour of tendon sheath: nodular soft tissue thickening around the flexor tendon which is immobile in relation to the tendon on dynamic study.
- Carpal tunnel syndrome: Flattening, thickening and decreased echogenicity of the median nerve within the carpal tunnel with/without retinaculum thickening (Fig. 6.4.12). Diagnostic criteria of carpal tunnel syndrome are well described.
- Ulnar nerve entrapment at Guyon's canal: thickening and decreased echogenicity of the ulnar nerve in the Guyon's canal.
- Tendinosis can also be a finding in wrist ultrasound.

LEARNING POINTS

- The US findings at the wrist and hands in RA include synovitis (with PDUS signal), joint effusion, flexor tenosynovitis and marginal bone erosions.
- Findings in PsA on upper limb US are extensor paratenonitis, PDUS signal within the soft tissue, microenthesitis, periosteitis, synovitis, tenosynovitis, and peritendinitis.
- US detected bursitis, synovitis and tenosynovitis are included in the classification criteria for polymayalgia rheumatica.
- Other conditions where US is useful to confirm a clinical diagnosis is gout.
- US is a promising tool to diagnose CPPD disease.
- US is a good tool to diagnose carpal tunnel syndrome.

FURTHER READING

1. Filippou G, Sirotti S. How can ultrasonography help in the management of CPPD? From diagnosis to clinical subset identification. Curr Opin Rheumatol. 2023;35:185–93.
2. Kim MK, Jeon HJ, Park SH, et al. Value of ultrasonography in the diagnosis of carpal tunnel syndrome: correlation with electrophysiological abnormalities and clinical severity. J Korean Neurosurg Soc. 2014; 55:78–82.

3. Østergaard M, Lambert R, Ho J, et al. Imaging in Rheumatic Diseases. In: Firestein GS, Budd RC, Gabriel SE, McInnes IB, O'Dell JR, editors. Kelley and Firestein's Textbook of Rheumatology. Philadelphia: Elsevier; 2017.p.858-907.e8.
4. Suzuki T. Power Doppler ultrasonographic assessment of the ankle in patients with inflammatory rheumatic diseases. World J Orthop. 2014;5:574–84.
5. Terslev L, Naredo E, Aegerter P, et al. Scoring ultrasound synovitis in rheumatoid arthritis: a EULAR-OMERACT ultrasound taskforce-Part 2: reliability and application to multiple joints of a standardised consensus-based scoring system. RMD Open. 2017;3:e000427.
6. Thiele RG, Schlesinger N. Diagnosis of gout by ultrasound. Rheumatology (Oxford). 2007; 46: 1116–21.

Diagnostic Ultrasound in Arthritis (Lower Limb)

Jyoti Ranjan Parida, Ankit B Shah

INTRODUCTION

The key articular ultrasound (US) imaging findings are effusion, synovial hypertrophy and cortical erosions. Power Doppler aids in assessment of active inflammation in the thickened synovium. Extra-articular imaging findings include tenosynovitis, enthesitis, tendinosis, tendon tears and bursitis. Further, US can help in identification of intra-articular and peri-articular echogenic crystal deposits, which may be difficult to detect on plain radiographs.

Convex transducers with lower frequencies ranging from 2 to 5 MHz may sometimes be required to evaluate deep seated structures like anterior recess of the hip, greater trochanter, sacroiliac joint, ischiogluteal bursa and the hamstring tendons, particularly in patients with a large body habitus. High frequency (14–20 MHz) "hockey-stick" transducers with an extremely small footprint are widely used for assessment for extremely superficial structures including metatarsophalangeal (MTP) joints, interphalangeal (IP) joints, midfoot joints and subcutaneous tissues.

HIP

Focal US imaging of the hip (anterior joint recess) is done to detect joint effusion and synovial hypertrophy. The anterior joint recess is assessed in the longitudinal plane by placing the probe parallel to the neck of the femur. Characterization of the hip joint effusion (Fig. 6.5.1) is done as simple (anechoic) or complex (presence of internal echoes). Additional imaging findings may include synovial hypertrophy (focal or diffuse), cortical erosions and marginal osteophytes. Diagnostic aspiration of the joint fluid or biopsy of the thickened synovium can be easily done under ultrasound guidance as an outpatient procedure.

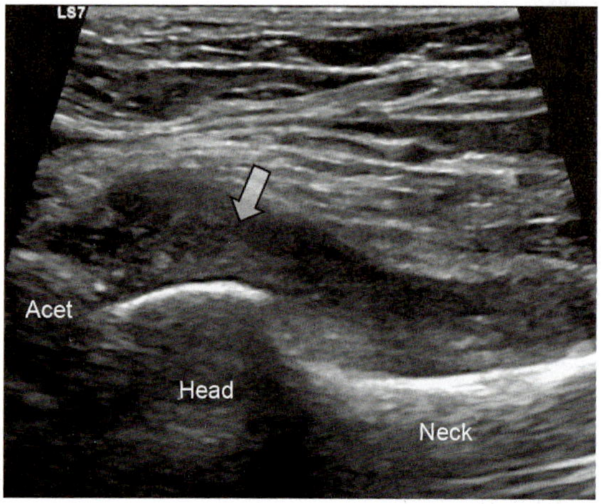

Fig. 6.5.1: Fluid in anterior joint recess (Hip joint effusion)

Greater trochanteric pain syndrome (GTPS): inflammation of the greater trochanteric bursa, gluteus medius tendinosis (including calcific tendinosis) (Fig. 6.5.2), gluteus medius tear, gluteus minimus tendinosis, subgluteus medius bursitis and snapping iliotibial band are some of the common causes resulting in lateral hip pain. US can be of great help in identifying these pathologies. Greater trochanteric bursitis (Fig. 6.5.3) is characterized on US imaging by identification of anechoic fluid or thickening of the greater trochanteric bursa.

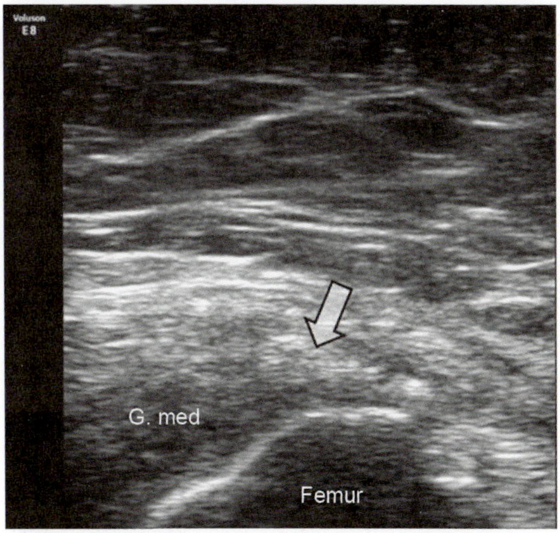

Fig. 6.5.2: Intratendinous calcification within the gluteal medius tendon

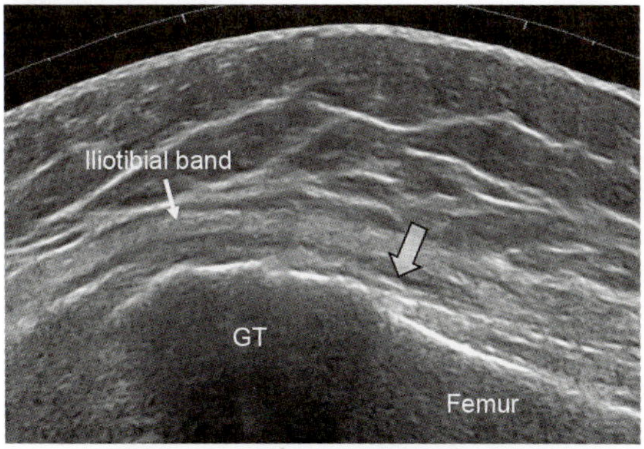

Fig. 6.5.3: Greater trochanteric bursitis

KNEE

Evaluation of the knee joint (anterior part) is done in mild (approximately 30°) knee flexion. Effusion in the suprapatellar recess is seen as an anechoic or hypoechoic area deep to the quadriceps tendon (Fig. 6.5.4). During US imaging, it is important to differentiate thickened synovium from underlying prefemoral fat pad.

Quadriceps and patellar tendinopathies can often result in anterior knee pain. On US imaging, the involved tendon appears enlarged and hypoechoic along with loss of fibrillary pattern (Fig. 6.5.5). Active inflammation is determined by increased vascularity on power Doppler images. Intratendinous calcification or clefts can be seen in chronic tendinopathies.

Baker's cyst: The gastrocnemius-semimembranosus (GSM) bursa is located along the posteromedial aspect of knee joint–between the medial head of gastrocnemius and semimembranosus tendon and immediately posterior to the medial femoral condyle. The bursa is most often connected with the knee joint. Enlargement of this bursa is a Baker cyst. (Fig. 6.5.6) A pointing inferior edge of the Baker cyst indicates a rupture.

ANKLE AND FOOT

US can image Achilles tendon pathologies, plantar fasciopathy, detection of joint effusion (Fig. 6.5.7), synovial hypertrophy, tenosynovitis (Fig. 6.5.8) and gout.

Common disorders of Achilles tendon that can be identified on US imaging are tendinosis and tears in the critical zone, insertional tendinosis (Fig. 6.5.9), paratenonitis, retrocalcaneal bursitis and Haglund's syndrome (insertional tendinosis of Achilles tendon, retrocalcaneal bursitis and pre-Achilles bursitis).

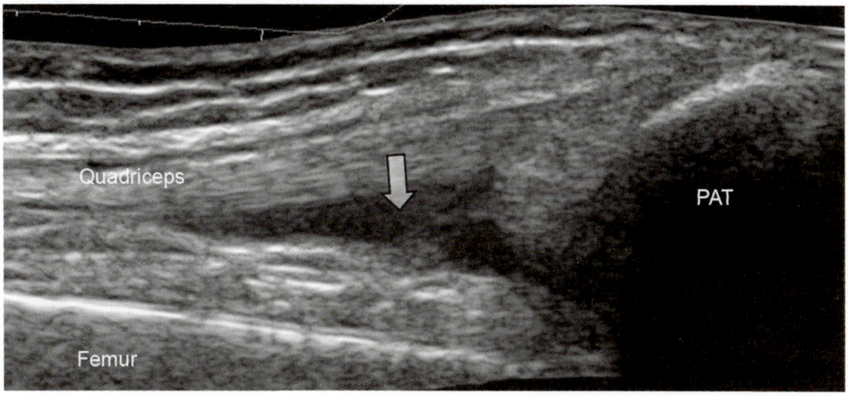

Fig. 6.5.4: Effusion in the suprapatellar recess (Knee effusion)

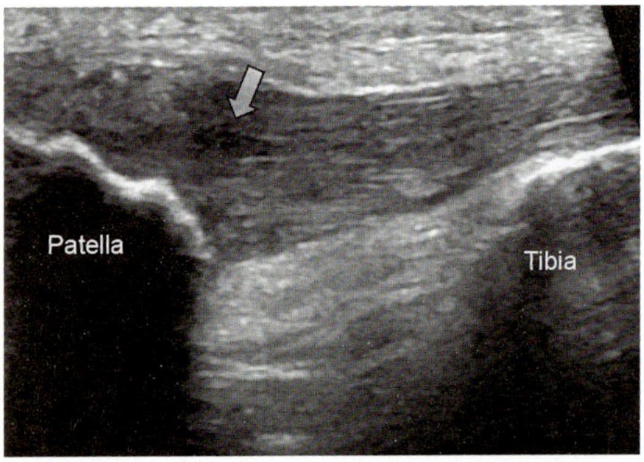

Fig. 6.5.5: Hypoechoic area with loss of fibrillary pattern and increased thickness at insertion of patellar tendon (Patellar tendinosis with an interstitial tear)

Plantar fasciopathy: The Plantar fascia appears thickened and hypoechoic on US imaging (Fig. 6.5.10). In presence of appropriate symptoms– plantar fascia thickness of more than 5 mm is considered diagnostic. US imaging can help in ruling out partial thickness tears of the plantar fascia, which can be a relative contraindication to steroid injection.

US is extremely helpful in identification of peri-articular and intra-articular crystal deposits at the first MTP joint in gout. Effusion with synovial hypertrophy is seen in acute gout along with hyperemia in the thickened synovium on Power Doppler images. Uric acid crystals get deposited over the most superficial layer of hyaline cartilage as an irregular echogenic line producing "double contour sign" (Fig. 6.5.11). US guided diagnostic aspiration of the joint fluid may be done in clinically suspected cases of gout (Fig. 6.5.12).

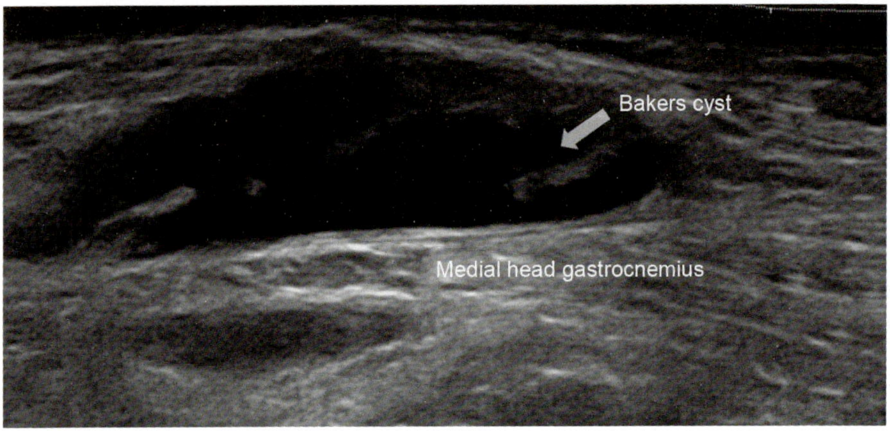

Fig. 6.5.6: Baker's cyst (Longitudinal view)

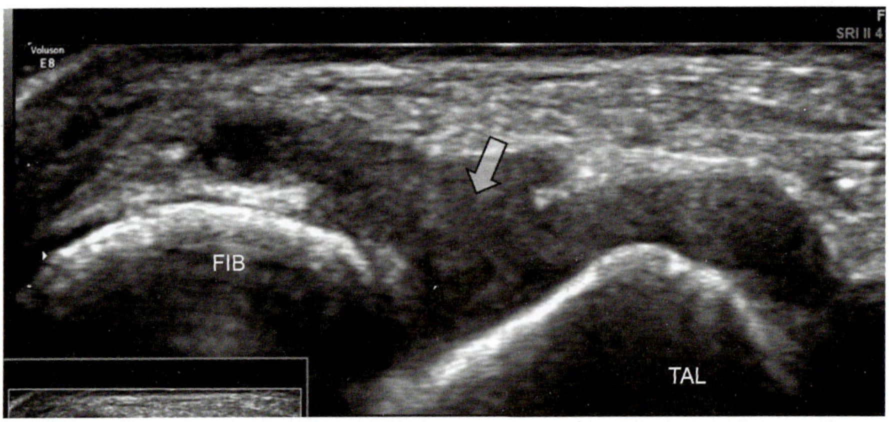

Fig. 6.5.7: Hypoechoic area indicating synovial hypertrophy in ankle joints

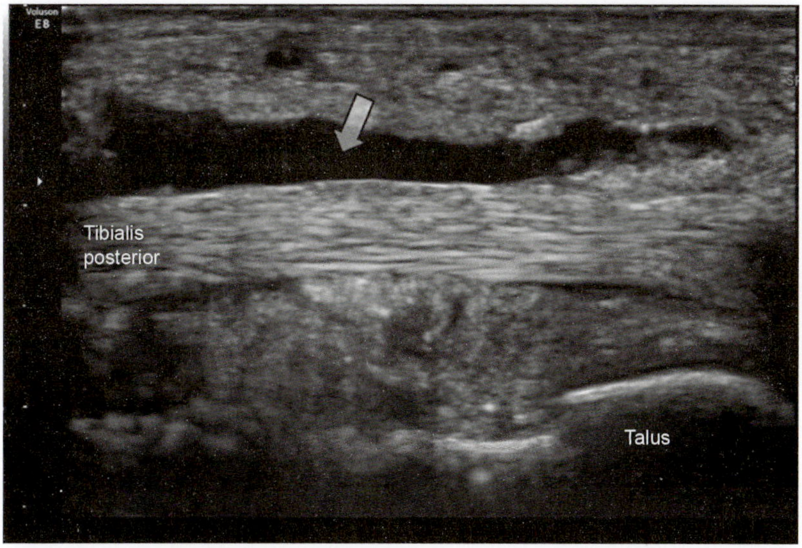

Fig. 6.5.8: Tenosynovitis of tibialis posterior tendon

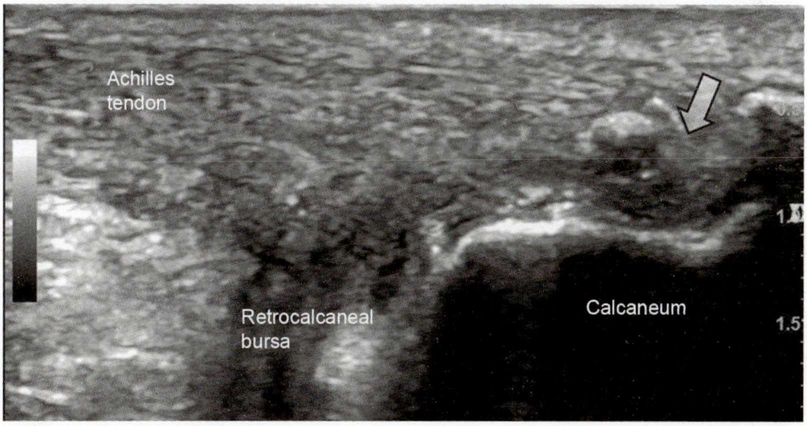

Fig. 6.5.9: Insertional tendinosis of Achilles tendon with calcification and partial thickness interstitial tear

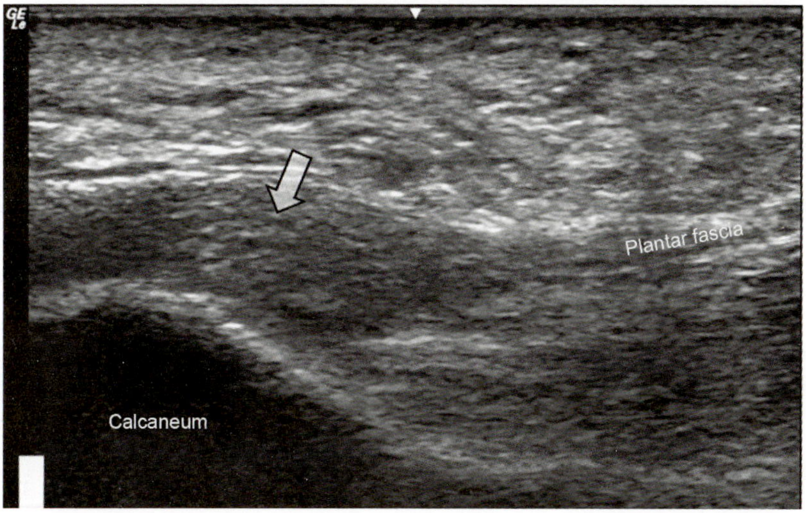

Fig. 6.5.10: Hypoechoic thickening of the peri-insertional fibers of plantar fascia (Plantar fascitis)

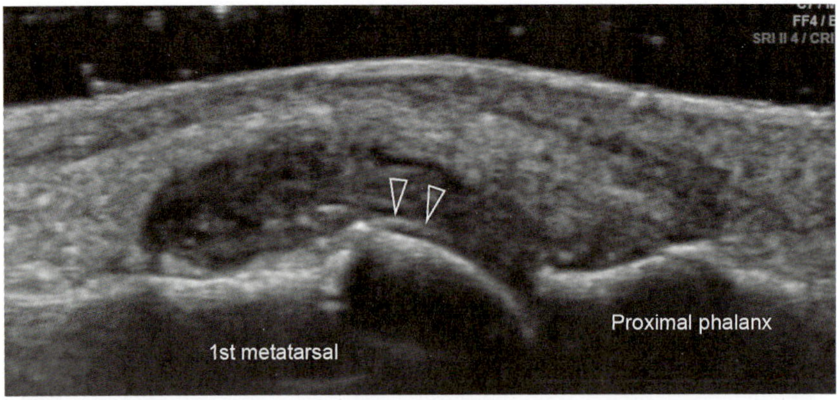

Fig. 6.5.11: 1st MTP joint synovitis with double countour sign (Open arrows) in a case of gout

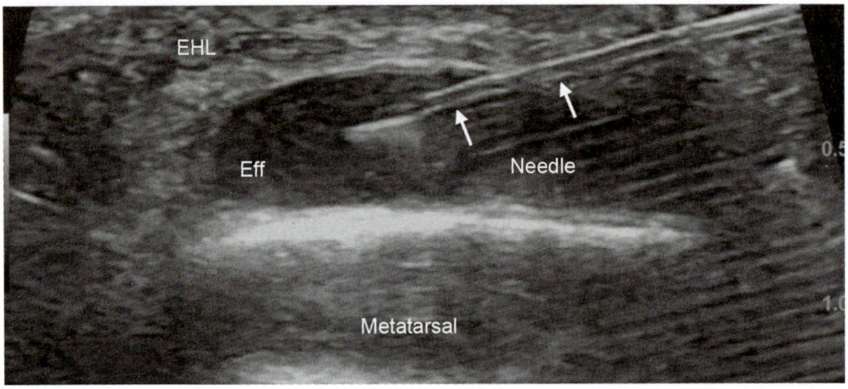

Fig. 6.5.12: Aspiration of 1st MTP joint effusion under US guidance

LEARNING POINTS (USEFULNESS OF US IN LOWER LIMB)

- **Hip:** Hip synovitis, joint aspiration, greater trochanter pain syndrome (GTPS).
- **Knee:** Suprapatellar bursitis, double contour sign (gout), quadriceps and patellar tendinopathies, Baker's cyst and its rupture.
- **Ankle:** Synovitis, Achilles tendinopathy, plantar fasciitis.
- **Foot:** 1st MTP synovitis, double contour sign (gout).

FURTHER READING

1. Malanga GA, Dentico R, Halperin JS. Ultrasonography of the hip and lower extremity. Phys Med Rehabil Clin N Am. 2010;21:533–47.
2. Micu MC, Nestorova R, Petranova T, et al. Ultrasound of the ankle and foot in Rheumatology. Med Ultrason. 2012;14:34–41.
3. Zhou H, Qiu L, Sun P, Let al. Clinical joints manifestations in patients with psoriatic arthritis on musculoskeletal ultrasound. Clin Rheumatol. 2022; 41:1211–18.

Chapter 6.6

Ultrasound in Pediatric Rheumatology

Abhra Chandra Chowdhury

INTRODUCTION

Why should we use musculoskeletal ultrasonography in pediatric rheumatology?

- History taking and physical examination in young patients is often difficult.
- Compared to other imaging modalities Musculoskeletal ultrasonography (MSUS) is non-invasive, mobile, instantly accessible and is suitable for use in children of all ages
- MSUS allows multiple joint assessment in one sitting and provides an opportunity to do ultrasonography-guide injections
- With the use of MSUS, it is easy to explain the abnormalities in joints to parents
- MSUS is well tolerated and does not need sedation in comparison to other imaging modalities.

CHALLENGES IN MSUS IN PEDIATRIC PATIENTS

- The growing bones and joints undergo a lot of changes with age. At birth, the bones are cartilaginous, and then ossify to form the bony skeleton.
- The joint space decreases with growth. It often becomes difficult to interpret whether the decrease is part of the growing process or due to erosion related to inflammation.
- The physiologic bony irregularities along with ossification centres are often confused with bony erosions.
- The cartilage vascularisation pattern in children is different from that in adults. Physiologic increased blood flow in the growing epiphyseal cartilage needs to be differentiated from increased vascularity caused by inflammation. Thus, a comprehensive knowledge of the vascularisation pattern of the growing skeleton is needed for proper interpretation of the juxta articular doppler signals.
- The epiphyseal cartilage is anechoic in children which can sometimes be confused with synovial effusion.

Mild joint effusion can be physiologic in children. Windscall et al. has shown 64% of healthy children had fluid accumulation in the suprapatellar recess. This needs to be distinguished from pathologic joint effusion. The indications of MSUS in children is summarised in Table 6.6.1.

Table 6.6.1: Indication for performing MSUS in pediatric rheumatology practice

1. Evaluation of a child presenting with painful or swollen joint
2. Diagnosis of suspected case of JIA
3. Follow up of a case of JIA
4. Apophysitis and Osteochondrosis in Pediatric age group e.g.
   i. Osgood Schlatter disease
   ii. Sinding Larsen Johansson disease
   iii. Osteochondritis dissecans of the knee
   iv. Sever's disease
5. Evaluation of a swollen joint in patient with hemophilia
6. For arthrocentesis in a patient with suspected septic arthritis
7. For therapeutic interventions-intra-articular and tendon sheath injections

MSUS IN JUVENILE IDIOPATHIC ARTHRITIS (JIA)

With the availability of advanced treatment options in JIA, the need for tools for early diagnosis and prognosis is high. MRI is a very sensitive technique, but its use is limited by high cost, limited availability and the need for sedation in young children. In comparison musculoskeletal ultrasound (MSUS) is much cheaper, easily available and does not need any sedation, thus is a popular tool with pediatric rheumatologists. Multiple joints can be scanned in a single setting with limited time whereas in MRI only a single joint can be imaged. MSUS is a very sensitive tool to detect joint effusion, synovial hypertrophy and signs of inflammation like increased vascularity in the form of positive power doppler signals.

MSUS helps in the differentiation between the articular and extra-articular origin of joint swelling. In a study by Rooney et al. involving 49 clinically swollen ankles, only 29% had tibiotalar effusion alone and 39% of cases did not have tibiotalar joint involvement. In the classification of the type of JIA, the number of joints involved in the first six months is of utmost importance. In some cases where patients had been clinically classified as having oligoarticular JIA, the use of MSUS has led to the reclassification of some of them as having polyarticular JIA.

MSUS can also help in the diagnosis of enthesitis-related arthritis (ERA). The superficial tendinous attachment of muscles can be easily seen by high-frequency probes. In a patient with recent onset inflammatory arthritis, the detection of enthesitis gives a clue to the type of disease. Jousse-Joulin has shown that out of all MSUS confirmed enthesitis, 50% were missed clinically.

Children affected with JIA often need intra-articular corticosteroid injection. However, unlike adults, in children, it is mostly carried out under general anaesthesia, hence the effect needs to be optimal and long-lasting. MSUS helps in correct needle placement inside the joint.

ASSESSMENT OF TREATMENT EFFICACY

Studies have shown that MSUS is able to assess treatment response in JIA. Lanni et al. have shown that both grey scale and power doppler MSUS scores improved in response to treatment in a cohort of new-onset JIA patients. De Lucia et al. have also shown that baseline ultrasound abnormalities can predict future relapse in JIA. However further studies are needed to establish the impact of MSUS in therapeutic decision-making in JIA.

MSUS is hugely operator dependent. There have not been many studies on the reproducibility of MSUS in the pediatric population. In order to overcome this problem, the OMERACT Ultrasound Task Force for JIA has recently proposed standardised scanning procedures and definitions of sonographic features of synovitis in children. The fallacies of MSUS in children that one should be aware of is summarised in Table 6.6.2.

Table 6.6.2: Common fallacies in interpretation of pediatric MSUS

1. Physiologic abnormalities around ossification centre mistaken as erosions
2. Epiphyseal cartilage is often mistaken as joint effusion
3. Mild joint effusion can be physiologic in children
4. Increased vascularity in epiphyseal cartilage can be physiologic

Although MSUS can scan many joints, scanning all joints is not possible on a daily clinical practice. The minimum number and optimal set of joints to be scanned is still a matter of debate. Collado et al. has shown that 10 joint ultrasound assessment including bilateral knees, ankles, wrists, elbows, and 2nd MCP joints was sensitive to detect synovitis in children with JIA in comparison to 44 joint assessments.

LEARNING POINTS

- MSUS is an useful tool both in diagnosis and management of JIA.
- A thorough knowledge of anatomy of the growing skeleton and vascularisation pattern is needed to correctly interpret images
- MSUS is much more sensitive than clinical examination in detecting joint inflammation and therefore improves diagnostic accuracy and classification of JIA.
- MSUS can be a useful tool to assess treatment response and stratify the risk of flare in JIA patients.
- MSUS is also useful for intra- articular and tendon sheath injections.

FURTHER READING

1. Colebatch-Bourn AN, Edwards CJ, Collado P, et al. EULAR-PReS points to consider for the use of imaging in the diagnosis and management of juvenile idiopathic arthritis in clinical practice. Ann Rheum Dis. 2015;74:1946–57.
2. De Lucia O, Ravagnani V, Pregnolato F, et al. Baseline ultrasound examination as possible predictor of relapse in patients affected by juvenile idiopathic arthritis (JIA). Ann Rheum Dis. 2018;77:1426–43.
3. Lanni S, van Dijkhuizen EHP, Vanoni F, et al. Ultrasound changes in synovial abnormalities induced by treatment in juvenile idiopathic arthritis. Clin Exp Rheumatol. 2018;36:329–34.
4. Rooney ME, McAllister C, Burns JF. Ankle disease in juvenile idiopathic arthritis: ultrasound findings in clinically swollen ankles. J Rheumatol. 2009; 36: 1725–9.
5. Roth J, Jousse-Joulin S, Magni-Manzoni S, et al. Definitions for the sonographic features of joints in healthy children. Arthritis Care Res. 2015;67:136–42.
6. Roth J, Ravagnani V, Backhaus M, et al. Preliminary definitions for the sonographic features of synovitis in children. Arthritis Care Res (Hoboken). 2017;69: 1217–23.

Magnetic Resonance Imaging in Rheumatology

Ashish J Mathew, Madhavi Kandagaddala

INTRODUCTION

Magnetic resonance imaging (MRI) enables non-ionizing, multiplanar assessment of all the structures involved in musculoskeletal diseases with remarkable soft-tissue resolution. This chapter discusses the potential utility of MRI in various inflammatory arthritides.

TECHNICAL CONSIDERATIONS

T1-weighted (T1w), T2-weighted (T2w) with fat-saturation (FS), short-tau inversion recovery (STIR) and proton density (PD) sequences are detailed in Table 6.7.1.

Table 6.7.1: MRI sequences—strengths and weaknesses

Sequence	*Visualization of pathologies*	*Strengths*	*Drawbacks*
T1w	Structural changes Meniscal pathology	High resolution Good detection of anatomic details Relatively short imaging times	Poor detection of inflammatory changes Not sensitive for marrow pathology
T1w post gadolinium (Gd) with fat saturation (FS)	Inflamed synovium	Best contrast for paramagnetic contrast agents Increases contrast between inflamed synovium and adjacent structures	Gadolinium-related complications
T2w	Fat Fluid/ edematous tissue	High signal intensity	Long imaging times
T2wFS	Inflammatory changes Bone marrow edema	No need for Gd Increases detection of edematous tissue/fluid located in areas with fatty tissue	Could increase imaging times
Short-tau inversion recovery (STIR)	Bone marrow edema Soft tissue pathology	Fat suppressed sequence Can be performed on machines with any magnetic field strength Can be used with fast (turbo) spin echo sequences reducing imaging times	Increase in flow-related artifacts Should not be used after gadolinium injection Potential decrease in signal to noise ratio
Proton density (PD)	Cartilage degeneration Meniscal pathology	Good anatomic details	Poor detection of fluid and marrow pathology

MRI in Rheumatoid Arthritis

MRI allows visualization of articular (synovium, cartilage), extra-articular (ligaments, tendons, tendon sheath) and intra-osseous pathologies. Bone marrow edema (BME) represents inflammatory infiltrates, i.e. osteitis.

Role of MRI in Early Diagnosis, Monitoring and Prognostication of Rheumatoid Arthritis

MRI aids in defining the extent of peripheral joint involvement in rheumatoid arthritis. The outcome measures in rheumatology (OMERACT) RA MRI scoring system (RAMRIS) has been used in many clinical trials. Table 6.7.2 describes the RAMRIS sequences and description of inflammatory and structural damage pathologies observed in patients with RA. BME is acclaimed to be an independent predictor of future radiographic progression in early RA. MRI can be a valuable supplement to radiography in diagnosing cervical spine involvement and secondary medullary compression in patients with RA.

Table 6.7.2: MRI sequences and definitions of pathologies in RAMRIS, PsAMRIS and MRI peripheral enthesitis scoring system

"Core set" of basic MRI sequences for RAMRIS and PsAMRIS T1w images before and after IV gadolinium-contrast injection-visualization in two planes T2wFS or STIR images	
Definitions of important MRI RA and peripheral PsA joint pathologies	
Synovitis (Fig. 6.7.1) (RAMRIS, PsAMRIS)	An area of thickness greater than the width of normal synovium, showing increased signal intensity following gadolinium enhancement.
Bone erosion (RAMRIS, PsAMRIS)	A sharply marginated bone lesion on T1w image with discontinuity of signal void of cortical bone and loss of normal high signal intensity of bone marrow fat, in the correct juxta-articular location, that is visible in 2 planes with a cortical break seen in at least 1 plane.
Osteitis/BME (RAMRIS, PsAMRIS)	A lesion with ill-defined margins, within the trabecular bone, with high signal intensity on T2wFS or STIR images, and low signal intensity on T1w images.
Joint-space narrowing (RAMRIS)	Decrease in the width of joint space compared to normal, when assessed in a slice perpendicular to the joint surface.
Tenosynovitis (Fig. 6.7.2) (RAMRIS, PsAMRIS)	High signal intensity on T2wFS/STIR around the tendon and/or tenosynovial postcontrast enhancement determined in comparison to T1w images obtained before and after IV-gadolivnium contrast, assessed on axial sequences over ≥3 consecutive slices.
Periarticular inflammation (PsAMRIS)	High signal intensity on STIR/T2wFS images and/or above normal post-Gd enhancement on T1w images, at extra-articular areas, including the periosteum (periostitis) and entheses (enthesitis), but not in the tendon sheaths.
Peritendonitis (PsAMRIS)	High signal intensity on STIR/T2wFS images and/or above normal post-Gd enhancement on T1w images, adjacent to a tendon in an area without a tendon sheath.
Tendonitis (PsAMRIS)	Abnormal thickness and high signal intensity on STIR/T2wFS images and/or above normal post-Gd enhancement on T1w images, inside a tendon.
Tendinopathy (PsAMRIS)	Morphological abnormality (abnormal thickening, attenuation or complete disruption) and/or high signal intensity on STIR/T2wFS images and/or above normal post-Gd enhancement on T1w images, inside a tendon.

(Contd.)

Table 6.7.2: MRI sequences and definitions of pathologies in RAMRIS, PsAMRIS and MRI peripheral enthesitis scoring system *(Contd.)*

Bone proliferation (PsAMRIS)	Abnormal bone formation in the periarticular region, including entheses (enthesophytes) and across the jont (ankylosis).
Key MRI entheseal pathologies associated with inflammation	
Intra-tendon hypersignal (entheseal tendonitis)	High signal intensity within the tendon/ligament/fascia on STIR/T2wFS images and/or above normal post-Gd enhancement on T1w images close to its insertion.
Peri-tendon hypersignal (entheseal peri-tendonitis)	High signal intensity in the soft tissues surrounding the tendon/ligament/fascia, on STIR/T2wFS images and/or above normal post-Gd enhancement on T1w images, close to its insertion.
Bone marrow edema (Fig. 6.7.3)	Bone lesion with ill-defined margins on STIR/T2wFS images, close to the tendon/fascia insertion.
Bursitis (in the presence of a relevant bursa) (Fig. 6.7.4)	High signal intensity on STIR/T2wFS images and/or above normal post-Gd enhancement on T1w images, in an above normal-sized bursa.
Key MRI entheseal pathologies associated with structural damage	
Tendon/aponeurosis thickening	Abnormal thickening of tendon/fascia close to its insertion.
Enthesophyte	Abnormal bone formation at the insertion of tendon/ligament/fascia into the bone.
Bone erosion (entheseal bone erosion)	Sharply marginated bone lesion with loss of normal low signal intensity of cortical bone and loss of normal high signal intensity of fat, on T1w images without Gd injection, and a visible cortical break located close to the tendon/fascia insertion.
Intra-tendon hypersignal on T1w	Increased signal in T1w sequence within the tendon/fascia close to its insertion.

Adapted from: Østergaard M, et al. J Rheumatol 2017;44:1706-12; Østergaard M, et al. J Rheumatol 2009;36:1816–24; Mathew AJ, et al. J Rheumatol 2019;46:1232–8

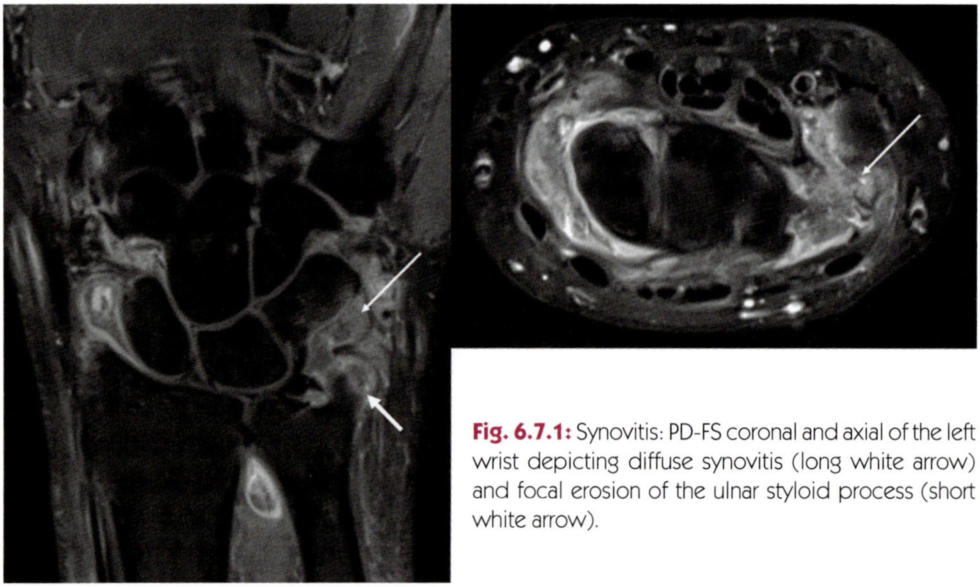

Fig. 6.7.1: Synovitis: PD-FS coronal and axial of the left wrist depicting diffuse synovitis (long white arrow) and focal erosion of the ulnar styloid process (short white arrow).

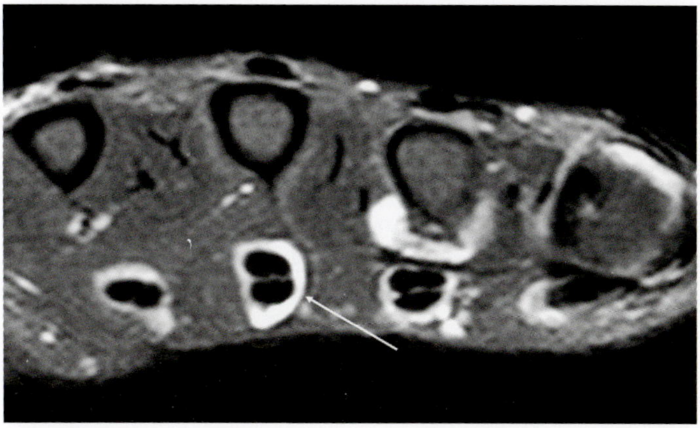

Fig. 6.7.2: Tenosynovitis: STIR axial of the right-hand showing tenosynovitis of flexor tendons

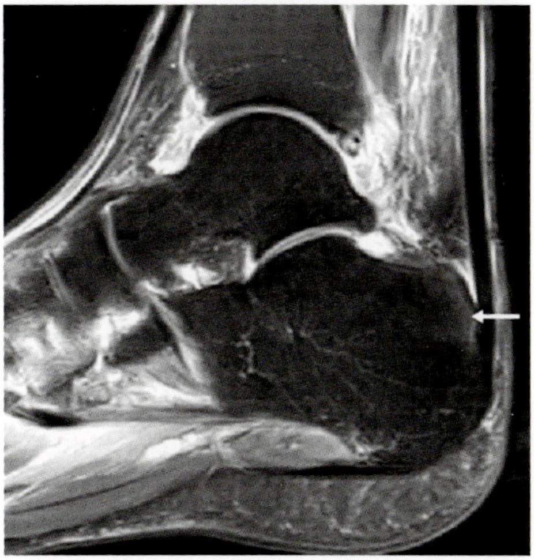

Fig. 6.7.3: Bone marrow edema at and immediately near the attachment of Achilles tendon to the postero-superior part of calcaneum: T2W-FS sagittal MR image of the heel region demonstrating BME (arrow)

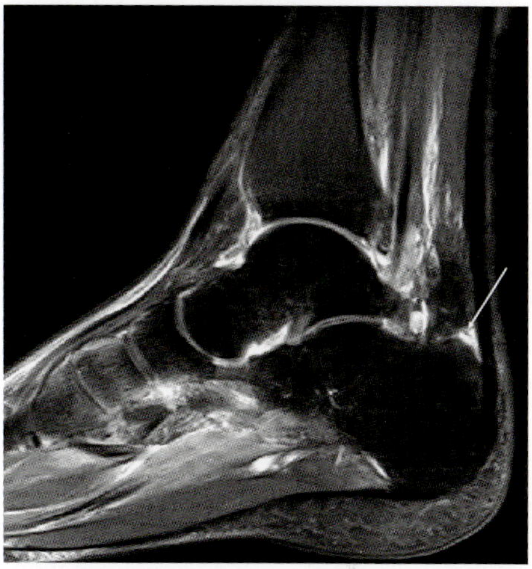

Fig. 6.7.4: Bursitis: T2W-FS sagittal MR image of the heel region with the white arrow pointing at retrocalcaneal bursitis

MRI in Psoriatic Arthritis (PsA)

MRI features of PsA include peripheral joints and/or entheses, sacroiliac joints and the spine. MRI synovitis and erosions in the peripheral joints share the same characteristics as in RA. Whole-body MRI (WBMRI) allows visualization of both peripheral and axial joints, along with entheses throughout the body in one examination, and may evolve as the preferred imaging modality in patients with PsA. The OMERACT MRI in arthritis working group has developed consensus-based definitions for MRI features of enthesitis, along with a scoring system focused around the heel region (HEMRIS). Table 6.7.2 MRI features of dactylitis include tenosynovitis with effusion, diffuse soft tissue edema, BME and/or synovitis in the nearby finger or toe joint.

Role of MRI in Early Diagnosis, Prognostication and Monitoring of PsA

BME in PsA has been shown to be closer to the entheses, as opposed to synovial attachments in RA and subchondral location in osteoarthritis (OA). Diaphyseal BME with extracapsular inflammation and increased frequency of flexor tenosynovitis has been reported in patients with PsA. Patients with arthralgia who demonstrate subclinical MRI inflammation could have a higher risk of developing PsA. The OMERACT PsA MRI scoring system (PsAMRIS) has been validated in clinical trials to be a sensitive outcome measurement instrument, with good response to change (Table 6.7.2).

MRI in Axial Spondyloarthritis (axSpA)

The most important MRI lesion of active inflammation in the sacroiliac joint (SIJ) includes juxta-articular BME. MRI features of structural damage include peri-articular fat metaplasia, bone erosions, fat metaplasia in an erosion cavity (backfill), bone spurs, ankylosis and sclerosis. The MRI scanning protocols for evaluation of the SIJ along with the latest definitions of inflammatory and structural damage MRI pathologies are highlighted in Table 6.7.3. The volume interpolated breath-hold examination (VIBE) MRI technique is useful in detecting structural changes in the cartilage before they extend into the underlying bone. The same definitions are used for assessing MRI SIJ in patients with PsA.

Table 6.7.3: MRI scanning protocols and definitions of inflammatory and structural lesions in axial spondyloarthritis

MRI scanning protocols for assessment of the sacroiliac joints (SIJ)	
Orientation and sequences • Oblique/semi-coronal (slices parallel to the dorsal surface of S2 vertebra) T1w, T1w gradient echo, STIR, TIRM, T2wFS, T2w Dixon, Proton-density with fat suppression, volume interpolated breath-hold examination (VIBE) 3D turbo gradient echo (slice thickness around 1 mm). • Oblique/semi-axial (slices perpendicular to the dorsal cortex of S2 vertebra) STIR, TIRM, Proton-density with fat suppression. **Slice thickness:** Maximum of 3 mm **Interslice gap:** 0.3 mm	
MRI SIJ inflammation lesion definitions	
Bone marrow edema (Fig. 6.7.5 and 6.7.6)	Hyperintense signal on STIR images and usually hypointense signal on T1 images. Reference for normal signal in the bone marrow is the sacral interforaminal bone marrow signal Inflammation must be clearly present and located in the subchondral bone (typical anatomical area) MRI appearance must be highly suggestive of SpA
Capsulitis	Increased signal on STIR, which is observed at the joint perimeter.
Joint space enhancement	Increased signal in the joint space of the cartilaginous portion of SIJ on contrast-enhanced images (T1FS post-Gd).
Inflammation at erosion site	Increased signal on STIR and/or T1FS post-Gd at the site of erosion.
Enthesitis (Fig. 6.7.5 and 6.7.6)	Increased signal in bone marrow and/or soft tissue at sites of attachment of ligaments and tendons to bone, not including the interosseous ligaments of the SIJ, on STIR and/or T1FS post-Gd.
Joint space fluid	Bright signal on STIR images in the joint space equivalent to the cerebrospinal fluid.
MRI SIJ structural lesion definitions	
Erosion (Fig. 6.7.5 and 6.7.7)	Defect in the subchondral bone associated with full-thickness loss of the dark appearance of subchondral cortex at its expected location, with loss of signal on a T1w non-fat suppressed sequence compared with the normal bright appearance of adjacent bone marrow.
Fat lesion (Fat metaplasia) (Fig 6.7.7)	Homogeneously bright signal, sharply defined along its nonarticular border with normal bone marrow, located in a typical anatomical area (subchondral bone) observed on a T1w non-fat suppressed sequence that is brighter than normal bone marrow.

(Contd.)

Table 6.7.3: MRI scanning protocols and definitions of inflammatory and structural lesions in axial spondyloarthritis (*Contd.*)

Fat metaplasia in an erosion cavity (backfill) (Fig. 6.7.6)	Bright signal on a T1w sequence in a typical location for an erosion or confluent erosions, with signal intensity greater than normal bone marrow, and associated with complete loss of the dark appearance of subchondral cortex at its expected location, clearly demarcated from adjacent bone marrow by an irregular band of dark signal (sclerosis) at the border of the original erosion.
Ankylosis	Abnormal bright signal on a T1w sequence with the same signal intensity as bone marrow, which is in the expected location of the SIJ space and bridges the joint with continuity of bone marrow signal between the ilium and sacrum. Associated with full-thickness loss of the dark appearance of subchondral cortex on both sides of joint.
Bone bud	Abnormal bright signal on T1w sequence with the same signal intensity as bone marrow, which is in the expected location of the SIJ space but does not bridge the joint so that it is continuous with the subchondral bone of either the ilium or the sacrum, but not both.
Sclerosis	Very low signal on all the MRI sequences, located in a typical anatomical area (subchondral bone).
MRI spine inflammation lesions	
Spondylitis (anterior or posterior corner inflammatory lesions) (Fig. 6.7.8)	
Enthesitis (Fig 6.7.6)	
Andersson lesion–aseptic spondylodiscitis (Fig. 6.7.8)	
Facet joint arthritis	
Costovertebral and costotransverse joint arthritis	
Inflammation of pedicles and spinous processes	
Inflammation of spinal ligaments	
MRI spine structural lesions	
Syndesmophytes	
Ankylosis/bone bridging	
Erosions	
Sclerosis	
Ligament calcifications	
Fat metaplasia over vertebral corners	

Adapted from: Sudol-Szopinska I, et al. Semin Musculoskeletal Radiol. 2015;19:396–411; Maksymowych WP, et al. Ann Rheum Dis 2019; 78:1550–8

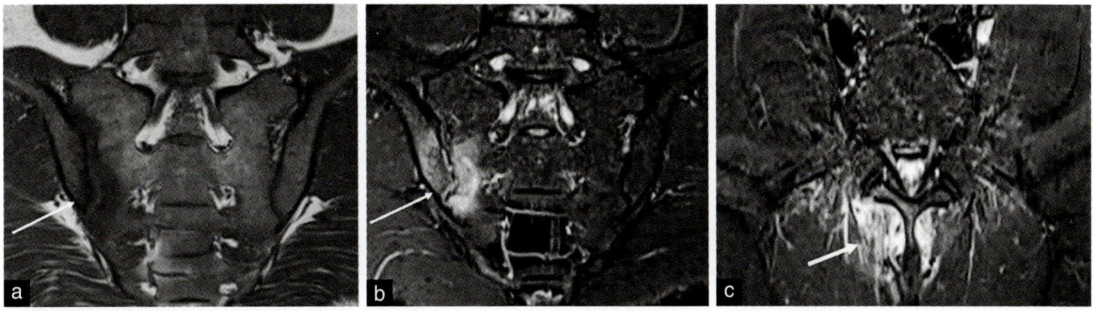

Fig. 6.7.5: Unilateral inflammatory sacroiliitis and active enthesitis: (a) T1W oblique and (b) STIR oblique coronal of the SI joints demonstrating articular surface erosions with bone marrow edema along either side of the right SI joint (thin white arrow). The left SI joint is normal. (c) STIR axial of the lumbar spine demonstrates extensive active enthesitis along the paraspinal muscle (thick white arrow).

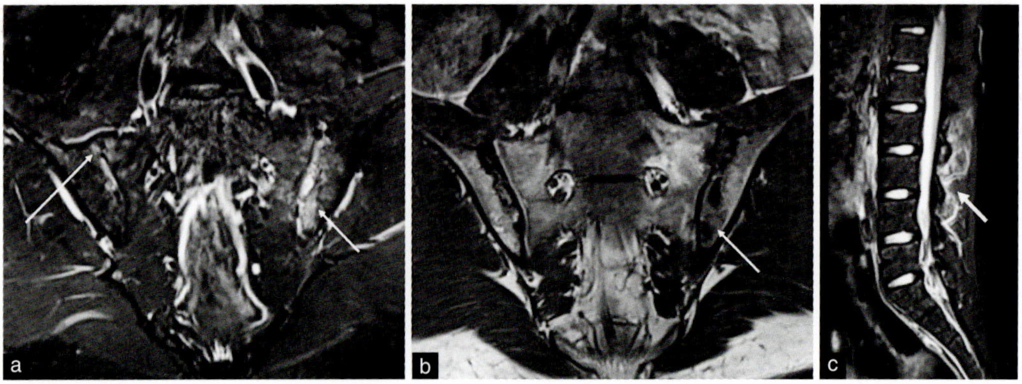

Fig. 6.7.6: Bilateral acute on chronic inflammatory sacroiliitis with active enthesitis: (a) STIR oblique MR image demonstrating BME on the left (thin white arrow) and subtle BME on right side (thin long white arrow). (b) T1W oblique coronal MR image showing articular surface erosions on the left side (thin long white arrow); fat metaplasia in erosion cavity (thin short arrow) and (c) STIR sagittal MR image of the lumbar spine demonstrating extensive active enthesitis along the paraspinal muscle (thick white arrow).

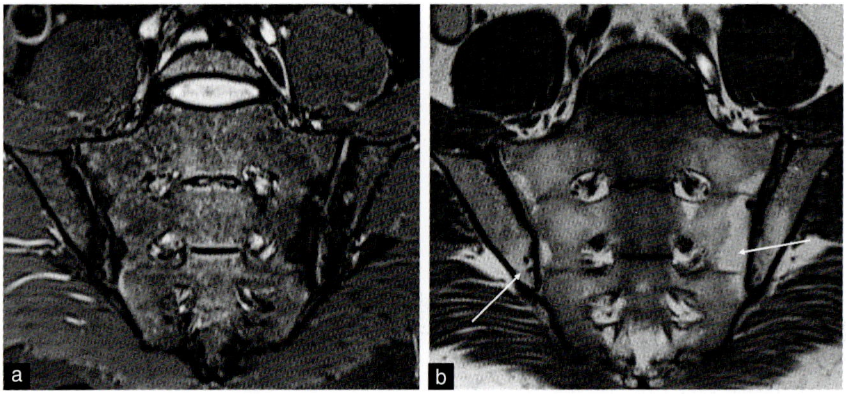

Fig. 6.7.7: Bilateral chronic inflammatory sacroiliitis: (a) STIR oblique and (b) T1W oblique coronal of the SI joints demonstrate bilateral articular surface erosions with juxta-articular fatty marrow replacement (thin white arrows). No bone marrow edema, no synovitis or capsulitis.

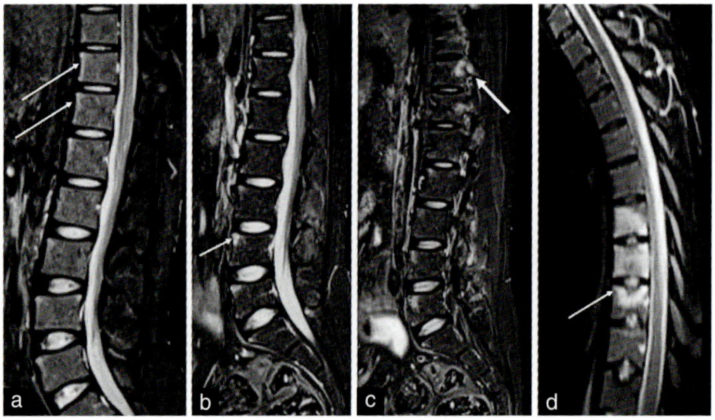

Fig. 6.7.8: Inflammatory lesions in spine: STIR sagittal images of thoracolumbar spine of four different patients—(a) Demonstrates active edema (thin long white arrows) along the anterior vertebral body; (b) Active edema (thin short white arrow) along the anterosuperior corner of the vertebral body; (c) Active edema (thick short white arrow) along the posterosuperior corner of the vertebral body; (d) active edema (yellow arrow) in the intervertebral disc and the vertebral bodies suggesting Andersson lesions

Role of MRI in Diagnosis, Prognostication and Disease Activity Monitoring of axSpA

Inclusion of MRI in the ASAS classification criteria has enhanced its utility in early detection of disease. Including structural MRI lesions, particularly erosions in the criteria along with BME 'highly suggestive of axSpA' improves the diagnostic utility of MRI. BME should never be interpreted in isolation of the clinical context or overinterpreted in the absence of structural changes. SIJ BME has been reported in athletes and postpartum women, more over lower posterior ilium and upper anterior sacrum regions, and should be reported with caution. Fat metaplasia, sclerosis and erosions can be present in normal healthy individuals. Ankylosis, nonetheless, is quite specific for axSpA. It is very important to be cognizant of the differential diagnoses of axSpA while reading an MRI (Table 6.7.4).

Studies on MRI of the spine have demonstrated association of BME at the anterior corners of vertebrae with subsequent development of radiographic syndesmophytes.

The ankylosing spondylitis spine magnetic resonance imaging-activity (ASspiMRI-a), the Berlin modification of the ASspiMRI-a score, the Spondyloarthritis Research Consortium of Canada (SPARCC) and Canada-Denmark (CANDEN) scoring systems have been validated in clinical trials with good responsiveness and reliability.

Table 6.7.4: Differential diagnoses of axSpA in MRI of sacroiliac joint (SIJ) and spine
SIJ
Anatomical variants–accessory SIJs (8–40%), iliosacral complex (ilium opposite posterolateral sacrum, ligamentous portion; mostly in women), bipartite iliac bony plate (mostly in women; posteroinferior segment), transitional vertebrae, hemisacralization, blood vessels (ligamentous portion of SIJ, lower ilium), accessory iliac joints (between iliac and sacral surfaces at posterior joint), isolated ankylosis (mid-third of SIJ)
Other inflammatory sacroiliitis–Behcet's disease, gout, brucellosis, Whipple's disease
Synovitis, acne, pustulosis, hyperostosis, osteitis (SAPHO syndrome), gouty arthritis (Fig. 6.7.9)
Degenerative changes in SIJ, osteoarthritis
Infectious sacroiliitis (Fig. 6.7.10 and 6.7.11)
Osteitis condensans ilii (Fig. 6.7.12)
Diffuse idiopathic skeletal hyperostosis (DISH)
Tumors
Paget's disease
Hyperparathyroidism
Sarcoidosis
Fractures
Chronic recurrent multifocal osteomyelitis (CRMO)
Normal marrow changes (lower iliac bone)
Healthy individuals, sports related (anterior upper sacrum, posterior lower ilium)
Postpartum (structural lesions are rare)
Spine
Schmorl nodes (lower thoracic and upper lumbar vertebrae)
Block vertebrae—congenital (cervical segments), acquired (degenerative disc, advanced axSpA)
Transitional vertebrae
Spina bifida occulta
Intraosseous pneumatocyst (cervical or lumbar spine)

Adapted from: Østergaard M. Curr Opin Rheumatol. 2020;32:357–64; Caetano AP, et al. Front Med (Lausanne) 2021;8:658538

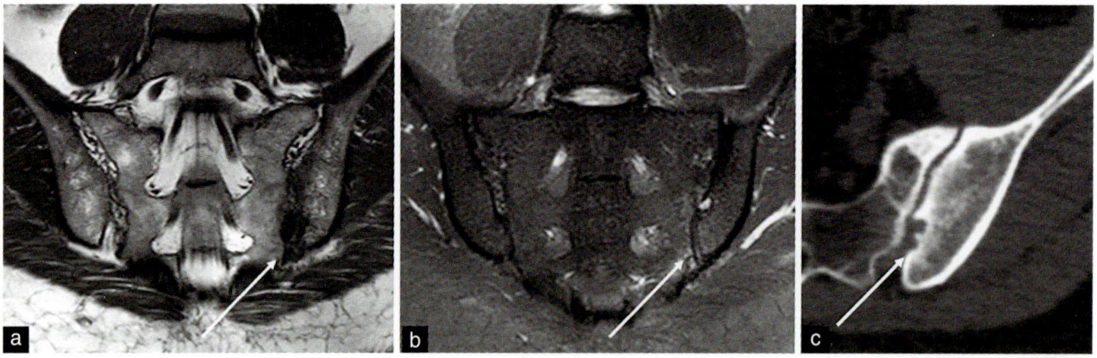

Fig. 6.7.9: Gouty sacroiliitis: (a) T1W, (b) STIR oblique coronal of the SI joints demonstrate articular surface erosions with subtle bone marrow edema and hypointense soft tissue in the left SI joint (long white arrow) and (c) CT axial sections demonstrates high dense soft tissue with deep excavating articular surface erosions with sclerotic margin and overhanging edges along the iliac side of the posterior aspect of the inferior part of the left sacroiliac joint. No joint-space narrowing.

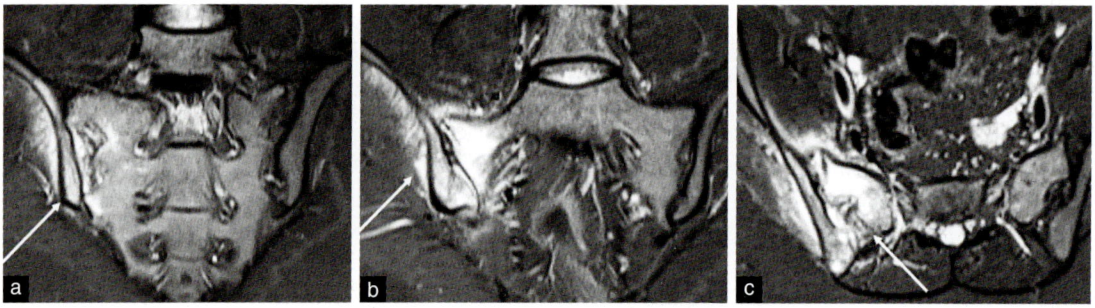

Fig. 6.7.10: Infective sacroilitis: STIR oblique coronal (a and b) and (c) STIR axial of the SI joints demonstrate large articular surface erosions with profound bone marrow edema of the right SI joint (white arrow) with synovitis, capsulitis and edema of the adjacent muscles.

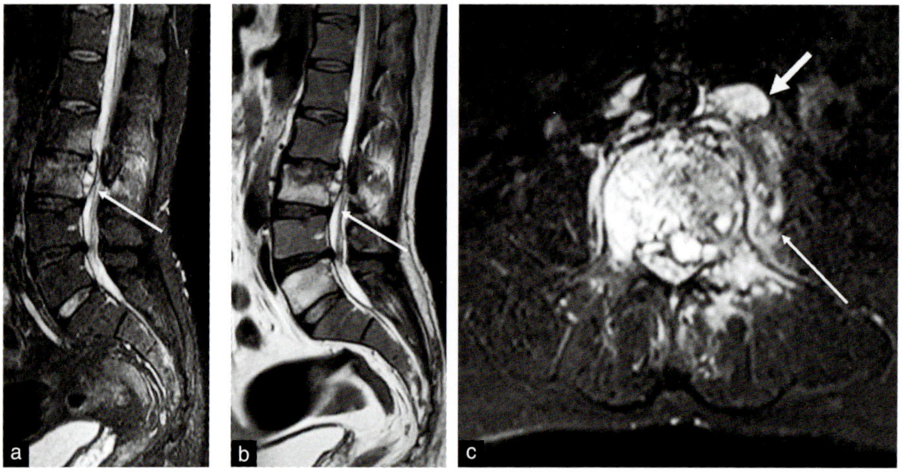

Fig. 6.7.11: Infective spondylodiscitis: (a) STIR, (b) T2W sagittal of the lumbar spine demonstrate fluid signal in the L2–3 intervening disc space with end plate irregularity and destruction and anterior epidural collection (thin white arrow). (c) STIR axial demonstrates pre- and paravertebral edema and inflammatory changes (long white arrow) and para-aortic lymph nodes (short white arrow).

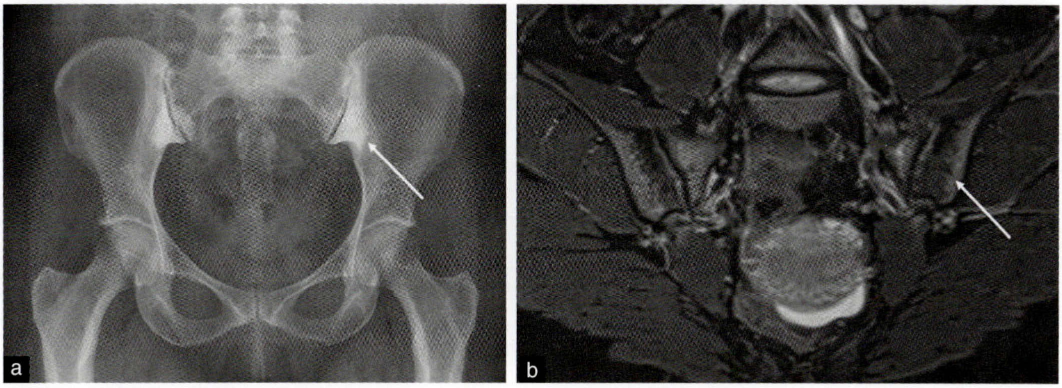

Fig. 6.7.12: Osteitis condensans ilii: pelvic radiograph (a) demonstrate sharply defined and dense sclerosis along the inferior aspect of iliac side of the bilateral SI joint and appears as markedly hypointense on the STIR (b) oblique coronal of the SI joints. Joint space is normal.

Utility of MRI in Gout

Synovitis, BME, tenosynovitis, soft tissue inflammation and bony erosions can be assessed with MRI (Fig. 6.7.9). Tophi in T1w sequences appears as low signal with varying degrees of post-contrast enhancement and as medium to high signal on T2w sequences, and can be measured with high inter-reader reproducibility. The RAMRIS has been applied in cross-sectional studies to monitor disease progression in gout. Cartilage damage in gout can be quantified using the gout MRI cartilage score (GOMRICS).

Utility of MRI in Osteoarthritis (OA)

MRI has been extensively used in assessment of knee, hip and hand OA. Inflammatory and structural changes in joints and compositional changes in the cartilage can be visualized with MRI. Staging and monitoring of OA development can be done with direct assessment of thickness and internal architecture of articular cartilage. MRI bone marrow lesions (areas with inhomogeneous, intermediate-low signal on T1w and high signal on STIR/T2FS) represent trabecular microfracture and bone marrow fibrosis. MRI offers better sensitivity than radiographs by assessment of all the structures involved in OA. Structural abnormalities and their changes can be quantified using computer-aided processing with excellent reproducibility. Newer techniques enable quantification of glycosaminoglycan content in the cartilage. Quantitative cartilage volume change and presence of cartilage defects of BME have demonstrated significant association with subsequent total knee replacement. Increase in BML is closely related to increased pain.

ADVANCEMENTS IN MRI TECHNIQUES AND THEIR UTILITY

Technical advancements with newer sequences and MRI applications have led to better qualitative and quantitative MR imaging along with reduction in scan times. These are highlighted in Table 6.7.5.

Table 6.7.5: Newer MRI techniques

Technique/sequence	*Features*	*Utility/advantages*
Diffusion-weighted imaging (DWI)	Based on tissue signal attenuation as a result of thermal motion of water molecules in the tissue. Diffusion of water is obstructed by cell membrane boundaries. Greater the cellularity, the more restricted will be the diffusion. Inflammatory lesions have an altered ratio of intra- to extracellular water, and thus altered signal.	Apparent diffusion coefficient (ADC) identifies patients with axSpA from lower back pain not due to axSpA at baseline. Maybe useful in detecting early spinal cord damage in patients with RA. No need for contrast medium injection.

(Contd.)

Table 6.7.5: Newer MRI techniques *(Contd.)*

Technique/sequence	*Features*	*Utility/advantages*
Dynamic contrast-enhanced technique (DCE)	Based on T1 relaxation characteristics of Gd agents. Investigates the distribution of Gd in vascular and interstitial space, expressed as changes in signal intensity over the scan time.	Distinguishing synovitis in patients with RA and PsA from healthy controls. Evaluation of synovial activity in early phases of inflammatory arthritis.
Chemical shift encoded MRI (CSE-MRI)	Utilizes small difference between precession frequencies of fat protons and water when exposed to a strong external magnetic field.	Quantitative measurement of BME and fat metaplasia in inflammatory arthritis
Whole-body MRI	Visualization of inflammation and structural damage in a single imaging time frame	Psoriatic arthritis–axial, peripheral joints and enthesitis. Inflammatory myositis SAPHO, CRMO
Delayed gadolinium-enhanced MRI of cartilage (dGEMRIC)	Based on negatively charged Gd-based contrast agent, allowing evaluation of cartilage glycosaminoglycan content.	Assessment of cartilage damage in OA, PsA and RA.
T2 mapping	Based on fast spin echo 3 Tesla MRI unit and advanced knee coil is required By increasing the time-to-echo, T2 mapping can identify areas of early injury in cartilage.	Useful in assessing cartilage damage in OA
3D volume-interpolated breath-hold examination (VIBE)	Gradient echo sequence Higher spatial resolution with lower partial volume effects. Multiplanar reconstruction.	Better visualization of erosions, e.g. SIJ in axSpA (high contrast between joint cavity, cartilage and cortical bone).
MRI based synthetic computed tomography (Bone MRI)	Deep learning-based technology CT-like images from 3D T1w multiple gradient echo sequence (3DT1MGE)	Visualization of osseous morphology Could be useful in SIJ structural lesions

CONCLUSION

MRI plays a pivotal role in early diagnosis and monitoring of disease activity in inflammatory arthritis. Recognizing its advantages and limitations, being aware of the differential diagnoses and interpreting MRI findings within the clinical context are of paramount importance.

LEARNING POINTS

- MRI permits visualization of intra- and peri-osseous pathologies with considerable soft tissue resolution.
- Bone marrow edema is a sensitive biomarker for aggressive erosive disease in rheumatoid arthritis.
- The OMERACT MRI scoring systems define inflammatory and structural damage MRI pathologies observed in various inflammatory arthritis and have been used in clinical trials.
- Periarticular sacroiliac bone marrow edema should always be interpreted in the background of clinical context and presence of structural changes.
- Newer MRI techniques like dGEMRIC and T2 mapping allow better characterisation of cartilage damage in osteoarthritis, and VIBE sequence enables better visualization of erosions in the cartilage in early spondyloarthritis.

FURTHER READING

1. Baraliakos X, Østergaard M, Lambert RGW, et al. MRI lesions of the spine in patients with axial spondyloarthritis: an update of lesion definitions and validation by the ASAS MRI working group. Ann Rheum

Dis. 2022 May 24:annrheumdis-2021-222081. doi: 10.1136/annrheumdis-2021-222081.

2. Diekhoff T, Lambert R, Hermann KG. MRI in axial spondyloarthritis: understanding an 'ASAS-positive MRI' and the ASAS classification criteria. Skeletal Radiol 2022; 51:1721–30.
3. Maksymowych WP, Lambert RGW, Østergaard M, et al. MRI lesions in the sacroiliac joints of patients with spondyloarthritis: an update of definitions and validation by the ASAS MRI working group. Ann Rheum Dis 2019; 78:1550–8.
4. Mathew AJ, Østergaard M. Magnetic resonance imaging of enthesitis in spondyloarthritis, including psoriatic arthritis-status and recent advances. Front Med (Lausanne) 2020;7:296.
5. McQueen F. Bone marrow edema and osteitis in rheumatoid arthritis: the imaging perspective. Arthritis Res Ther 2012;14:224.
6. Østergaard M, Peterfy CG, Bird P, et al. The OMERACT Rheumatoid Arthritis Magnetic Resonance Imaging (MRI) Scoring System: Updated Recommendations by the OMERACT MRI in Arthritis Working Group. J Rheumatol 2017;44:1706–12.
7. Østergaard M, McQueen F, Wiell C, et al. The OMERACT psoriatic arthritis magnetic resonance imaging scoring system (PsAMRIS): definitions of key pathologies, suggested MRI sequences, and preliminary scoring system for PsA hands. J Rheumatol 2009; 36:1816–24.

Chapter 6.8

PET Scan in Rheumatology

Debanjali Sinha, Geetabali Sircar

INTRODUCTION

Positron emission tomography (PET) is a functional imaging technique which is an established tool in oncology and is based on the ability to detect enhanced glucose uptake from high glycolytic activity of inflammatory cells. The role of PET is increasingly being popular in the field of rheumatology over the last few years.

MECHANISM

PET utilizes molecules labeled with isotopes that emit positrons from their nucleus. The most commonly used radiolabeled probe is 2-deoxy-2-(18F) fluoro-d-deoxyglucose (FDG) in which one of the hydrogens has been replaced by 18F radioisotope. 18F-FDG is an analog of glucose and after administration it is taken up by cells according to their level of glucose metabolism. 18F-FDG is transported through the cell membrane via glucose transporters into the cytosol and is phosphorylated by the enzyme hexokinase into 18F-FDG-6-phosphate. In contrast to glucose, 18F-FDG-6-phosphate cannot proceed further in the glycolytic pathway; it is not further dephosphorylated and accumulates in the cell. 18F decays by emitting a positron from its nucleus, which collides with a nearby electron, resulting in an annihilation event where two 511-keV photons in the form of gamma rays are emitted 180° apart. These photons are detected by a ring array of detectors around the patient. Detection of a single annihilation event results in activation of detectors opposing one another, which is recorded as a "coincident event." Mathematical analysis of the coincident events yields the location of cell populations or tissues that have accumulated 18F-FDG.

RHEUMATOLOGICAL INDICATIONS

PET scan can be used in rhematological conditions listed in Table 6.8.1.

Patient Preparation before FDG-PET

A. Patients should fast for at least 6 hours prior to FDG administration and the blood glucose levels should preferably be <126 mg/dL.

B. Strenuous physical activity should be avoided 24 hours prior to PET scan.

C. Images should be acquired at least 60 minutes after FDG administration.

D. Glucocorticoids may reduce vascular wall uptake of FDG, so it is preferred to withdraw or delay therapy until after PET. In case of GCA with temporal artery or ocular involvement, steroids have to be started urgently. In such situations, FDG-PET should be done within 3 days of starting steroids.

Interpretation of PET Report

A. Standardized visual grading system (Fig. 6.8.1):

0 = no uptake (≤ mediastinum);

1 = low-grade uptake (< liver);

2 = intermediate-grade uptake (= liver), possibly positive

3 = high-grade uptake (> liver), positive for active LVV.

Total Vascular score may be calculated in 7 different arterial regions, each graded 0–3 (Range 0–21).

Table 6.8.1: Rheumatological conditions and PET scan patterns

Rheumatological conditions	*Typical PET uptake patterns*
1. Large vessel vasculitis	Uptake in arterial walls. The hybrid PET/CT or PET/MRI can be of particular interest because MRI and CT can give additional information about the changes in the wall structure or luminal blood flow.
2. Polymyalgia rheumatica	Increased metabolic activity of the scapular and pelvic girdles, knee bursae and capsule and cervical and lumbar interspinous bursae.
3. Sarcoidosis	Oligoarticular involvement in medium to large joints (e.g. ankles, knees, and wrists) with typical sarcoidosis findings such as mediastinal and hilar lymphadenopathy and granulomas.
4. Rheumatoid arthritis	Symmetrical intense uptake in multiple (small or large) joints (avoiding DIP joints). 18F-FDG uptake in rheumatoid wrists has been found to correlate with gadolinium uptake evaluated by MRI and with swollen and tender joint counts, ESR, CRP, 28-point disease activity score [DAS28] and simplified disease activity index [SDAI]), and ultrasound parameters like cumulative synovial thickness and number of Doppler-positive joints.
5. Systemic lupus erythematosus	For CNS involvement
6. IgG4 related disease	Multifocal uptake, commonly in salivary glands, pancreas, aorta, retroperitoneum
7. Amyloidosis	Amyloid deposition (typically in shoulders). FDG uptake in large joints (e.g. shoulders, wrists, and hips)
8. Remitting seronegative symmetrical synovitis with pitting edema, RS3PE syndrome	Marked tenosynovitis, depicted as FDG-avid tendons in the hand causing edema
9. Inflammatory myopathy	Mostly to detect underlying neoplasms
10. Adult onset Still's disease	FDG uptake in bone marrow, spleen, and various lymph nodes accompanying polyarthritis
11. Relapsing polychondritis	Symmetrical FDG uptake in two or more cartilages. May involve aortic wall
12. Spondyloarthropathy	Sacroiliitis and enthesitis; FDG predominantly accumulates in the entheses rather than the synovium.
13. SAPHO syndrome (synovitis, acne, pustulosis, hyperostosis and osteitis)	Arthritis in sternoclavicular joints. FDG uptake in sacroiliac joints with sclerosis on iliac side
14. Chronic recurrent multifocal osteomyelitis (CRMO)	Multifocal FDG uptake in bone marrow, predominantly at femur, tibia, fibula, or clavicle
15. Multicentric reticulohistiocytosis	FDG uptake in multiple joints (including DIP joints) and subcutaneous tissue (characteristic papulonodular skin lesions)

B. Semiquantitative analysis (relevant for recurrence or follow-up evaluation):

a. Standardized uptake values (SUV):

$$SUV = \frac{\text{activity concentration in tissue}}{\text{injected activity / body size}}$$

SUVs can be falsely decreased by weight loss, glucose loading, small size of lesion, short uptake time and respiratory motions. These errors can be limited by the use of target-to-background ratios.

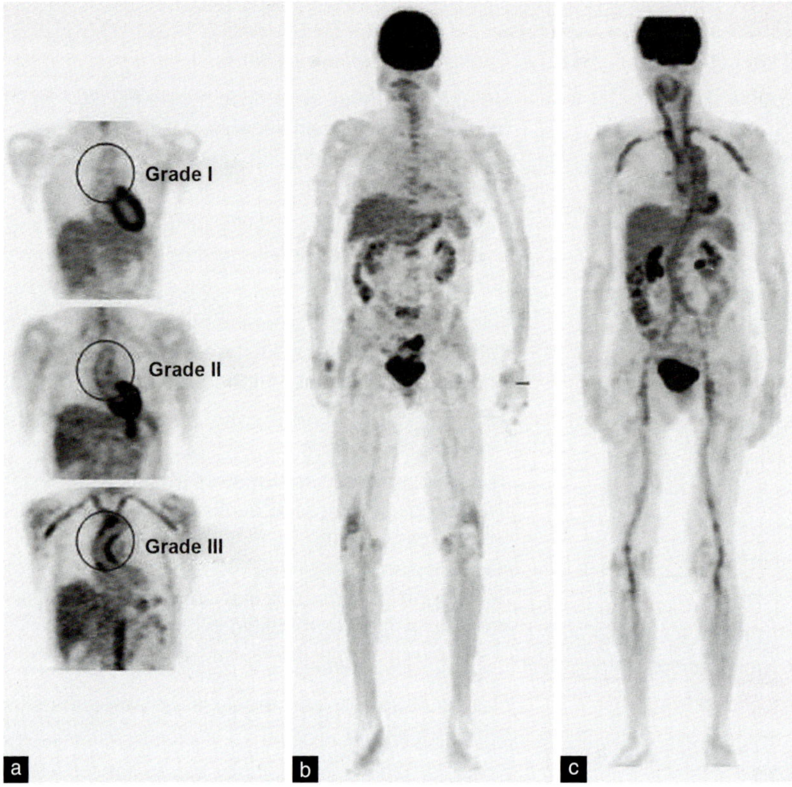

Fig. 6.8.1: Examples of visual grading of [18 F]FDG uptake. Normal whole-body PET scan; Wholebody scan showing extensive large-vessel arteritis (From Malik D et al., Indian J Nucl Med. 2020 Jan-Mar; 35(1):6–12, for non-commercial use)

b. Target-to-background ratios-Target-to-blood pool and Target-to-liver ratios of SUVs.

ADVANTAGES OF FDG-PET SCAN OVER OTHER IMAGING MODALITIES

- It can show inflammation of peri- and extra-articular synovial structures if there is associated polymyalgia rheumatica (PMR), which is present in half of GCA patients. Also, 20% of patients with PMR have GCA.
- It may help in diagnosis of LVV even in the setting of negative temporal artery biopsy, ultrasonography or MRI, when there is a strong clinical suspicion.
- Different large vessels may be involved in a particular patient, e.g. cranial and aortic vessels. FDG-PET by virtue of its whole body scan nature, can detect all such vessels.
- 18F-FDG-PET can quantitatively evaluate the response to treatment
- In patients with fever of unknown origin when systemic LVV is ruled out, FDG-PET helps in identification of other inflammatory or malignant causes.

DISADVANTAGES OF FDG-PET SCAN

1. Difficult to image temporal arteries, due to the high physiological FDG uptake in the brain and limited resolution of the camera.
2. Atherosclerosis may interfere with FDG-PET signal in patients with LVV (Table 6.8.2).
3. Morphological changes in arterial walls found in advanced disease, like aneuryms, stenosis and calcifications cannot be described well by PET.
4. Radiation hazards
5. Expensive.

LEARNING POINTS

- FDG PET/CT can accurately demonstrate whole-body active inflammatory lesions of various

Table 6.8.2: Differentiating factors between large vessel vasculitis and atherosclerosis in PET scan

Large vessel vasculitis	*Atherosclerosis*
More intense inflammation; Grade II or III uptake	Less intense inflammation; Grade I uptake
Linear and continuous uptake pattern; may become patchy in late Takayasu disease.	Patchy uptake pattern
Thoracic vessels are most frequently affected, followed by abdominal vessels. Pulmonary arteries may be affected in Takayasu's arteritis.	Iliofemoral arteries mostly affected
Absence of calcification	Calcification often present

rheumatological diseases, most commonly large vessel vasculitis.

- Not suitable for temporal arteries. Atherosclerosis may hinder interpretation.
- FDG-PET should be done before or within 3 days of starting steroids.
- Addition of CT/MRI to FDG-PET provides high-resolution imaging of vascular morphology.

FURTHER READING

1. Hotta M, Minamimoto R, Kaneko H, Yamashita H. Fluorodeoxyglucose PET/CT of Arthritis in Rheumatic Diseases: A Pictorial Review. Radiographics. 2020; 40:223–40.
2. Slart RHJA; Writing group; Reviewer group; Members of EANM Cardiovascular; Members of EANM Infection and Inflammation; Members of Committees, SNMMI Cardiovascular; Members of Council, PET Interest Group; Members of ASNC; EANM Committee Coordinator. FDG-PET/CT(A) imaging in large vessel vasculitis and polymyalgia rheumatica: joint procedural recommendation of the EANM, SNMMI, and the PET Interest Group (PIG), and endorsed by the ASNC. Eur J Nucl Med Mol Imaging. 2018; 45:1250–69.

Chapter 6.9

Joint Injection Procedures

Rasmi Ranjan Sahoo, BV Harish, Gadde Sudhish, Pradeepta Sekhar Patro

INTRODUCTION

Joint injections are frequently used in the management of various musculoskeletal diseases. Adequate knowledge of the technique is of utmost importance for its appropriate use and in avoiding complications. Intra-articular corticosteroids are effective in controlling disease activity in systemic inflammatory arthritis who have a flare or inadequate response to disease-modifying antirheumatic drugs (DMARDs). Bursitis, tendonitis and enthesitis often respond to local corticosteroid injections rather than oral NSAIDs. Joint injections can be given either conventionally or with ultrasound guidance. In this chapter, we will describe the conventional methods of injection of joints in both upper and lower limbs.

INDICATIONS AND CONTRAINDICATIONS

The indications and contraindications of joint injections are summarized in Table 6.9.1.

Table 6.9.1: Indications and contraindications of joint and soft tissue injections

Indications	*Contraindications*
Inflammatory arthritis Rheumatoid arthritis, spondyloarthritis, juvenile idiopathic arthritis, and gout Osteoarthritis Bursitis Subacromial, olecranon, ischiogluteal, anserine, retrocalcaneal Tendonitis Bicipital deQuervain's tenosynovitis Baker's cyst Plantar fasciitis* Trigger point injections Carpal tunnel syndrome	Cellulitis of the affected limb Psoriasis or eczema at the injection site Septic arthritis Sepsis Fracture Prosthetic joint Anticoagulation therapy Bleeding disorders Known allergy to injection constituents

*Risk of plantar fascia rupture, so best avoided

PREPROCEDURE REQUIREMENTS

Before performing any invasive intervention, the patient must be explained the procedure, its indication and probable complications. Risks and benefits should be adequately explained in the vernacular and patients must be given the choice to decide without any undue pressure. Once a decision is made, it should be documented in written informed consent. Even though intra-articular procedures are safe, one needs to be aware of the certain contraindications as listed in Table 6.9.1.

The patient should be able to maintain the required position for the procedure. Antiseptic solutions (iodine or chlorhexidine-based scrub), alcohol spirit, clean drapes to cover the area, local anesthetic agent, glucocorticoid solution, syringes, and needles should be prepared prior to the procedure. Strict aseptic precautions are mandatory to avoid iatrogenic infections.

CORTICOSTEROID PREPARATIONS

Crystalline corticosteroid preparations are effective in alleviating synovial inflammation and reducing pain. Both methylprednisolone acetate and triamcinolone preparations (acetonide and hexacetonide) are equally effective. Shoulder, hip, and knee joints are injected with 40–80 mg of methylprednisolone acetate or 20–40 mg of triamcinolone acetonide whereas elbow, wrist and ankle joints require 40–60 mg methylprednisolone acetate or 20–30 mg for triamcinolone acetonide. For tendon sheaths, metacarpophalangeal and proximal interphalangeal joints, 10–20 mg of methylprednisolone acetate is often adequate.

TECHNIQUES

Upper Limb Joints

The upper limb joint injection procedures are shown in Figures 6.9.1 to 6.9.12.

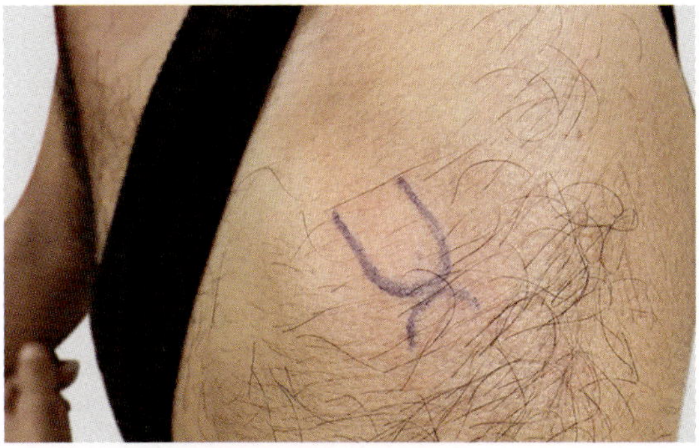

Fig. 6.9.1: Injection of the acromioclavicular joint. The joint is felt as a groove between the lateral end of the clavicle and the tip of the acromion process. A 25-gauge needle is inserted perpendicular to the skin and slightly posteriorly, into the joint space

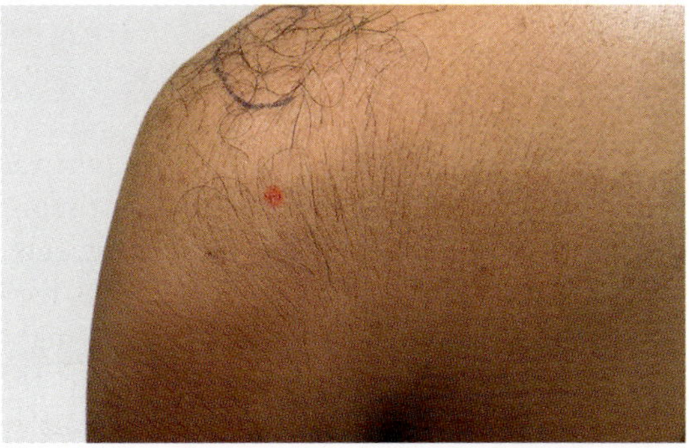

Fig. 6.9.2: Shoulder (glenohumeral) joint injection. The posterior approach is preferred as there are no overlying neurovascular bundles. A mark is made about 2 inches below the acromion process and a 21-gauge needle is directed anteriorly towards the coracoid process, into the joint space

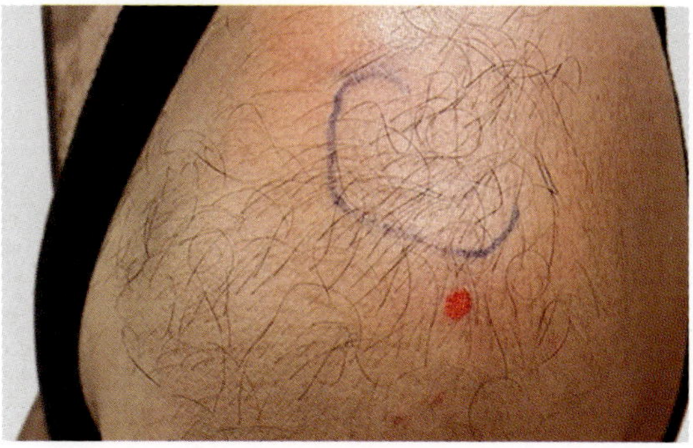

Fig. 6.9.3: Subacromial bursa injection. The bursa is palpated about 1 cm below the acromial process, posteriorly and laterally. A 21-gauge needle is inserted into the bursa, aiming towards the coracoid process

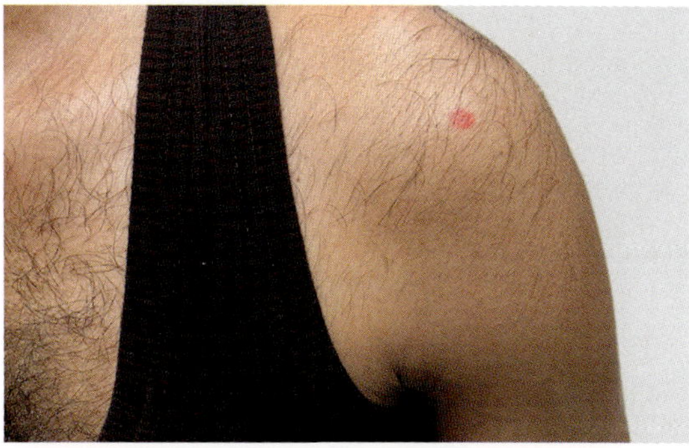

Fig. 6.9.4: Bicipital tendon injection. The tendon is palpated over the anterior shoulder in the bicipital groove with the shoulder externally rotated. A 22-gauge needle is inserted (30–45° angle) into the tendon sheath at the point of maximal tenderness

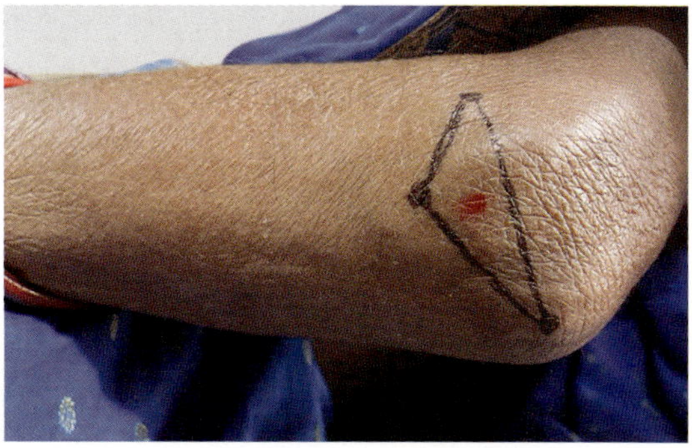

Fig. 6.9.5: Elbow joint injection. Patient lies supine, the elbow is flexed at 45°, the lateral epicondyle, the head of the radius, and the olecranon process tip are marked and connected to form a triangle. A 23-gauge needle is inserted at the center of the triangle, parallel to the imaginary line connecting the medial and lateral epicondyles. The radial approach is preferred as the ulnar nerve is located on the ulnar groove medially

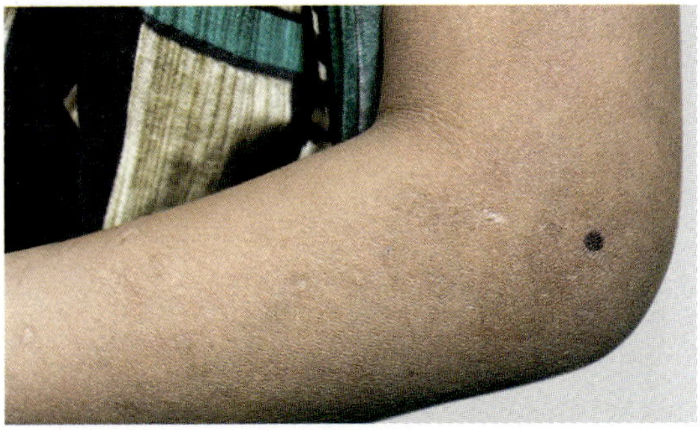

Fig. 6.9.6: Lateral epicondyle injection. The most tender point at the common extensor tendon origin (usually 1 cm distal to the lateral epicondyle) is palpated with the elbow flexed at 90°. A 25-gauge needle is inserted until the needle hits the bony surface, then slightly withdrawn and corticosteroid injection is given

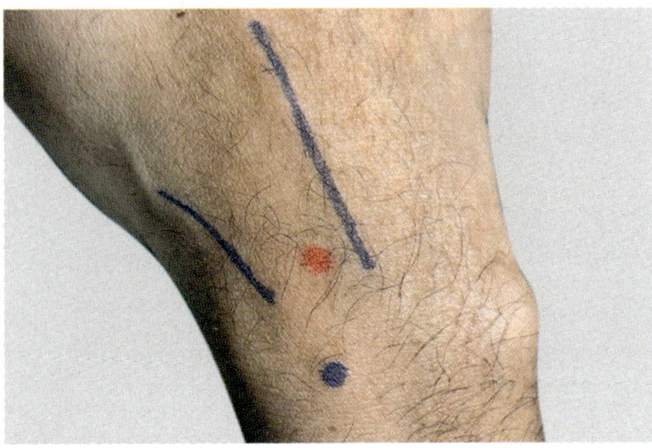

Fig. 6.9.7: Wrist joint injection. The joint space is palpated distal to the Lister's tubercle by flexing and extending the wrist. A 25-gauge needle is inserted perpendicular to the skin into the joint space between the extensor pollicis longus radially and extensor digitorum on the ulnar aspect

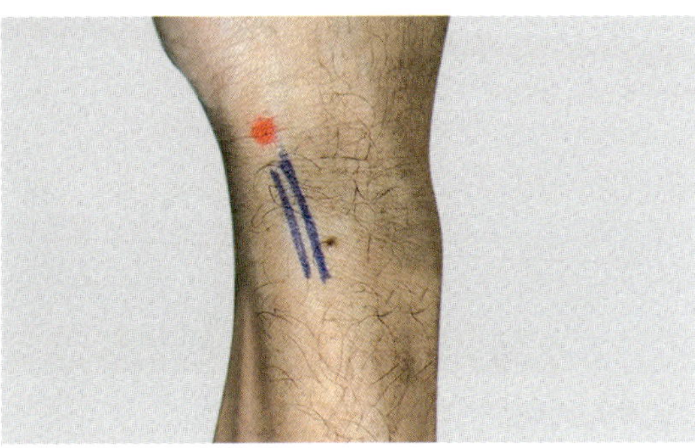

Fig. 6.9.8: deQuervain's tenosynovitis injection. The abductor polices longus and the extensor polices brevis common sheath is palpated with the thumb in abduction and extension. A 25-gauge needle is inserted near the base of the thumb along the tendon sheath towards the radial styloid process

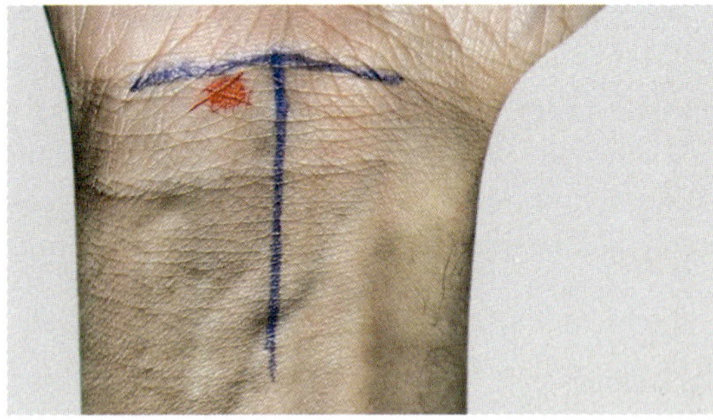

Fig. 6.9.9: Carpal tunnel syndrome injection. A 25-gauge needle is introduced at the distal palmar crease below the palmaris longus tendon towards the index finger. The needle is slightly withdrawn in case the patient complaints of paresthesia

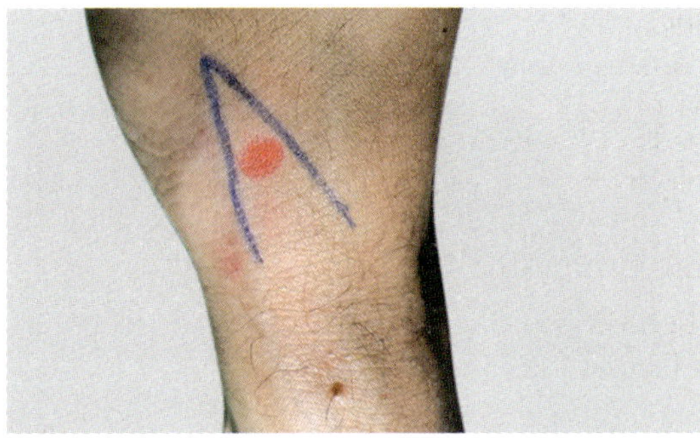

Fig. 6.9.10: Thumb capometacarpal joint injection. The first carpometacarpal joint is palpated at the distal anatomical snuff box with the thumb in flexion and across the palm. A 25-gauge needle is inserted perpendicular to the skin adjacent to the extensor policis brevis tendon with caution for injury to radial artery

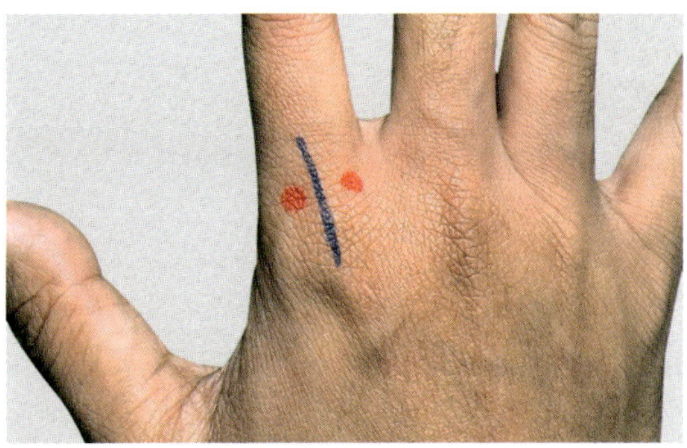

Fig. 6.9.11: Metacarpophalangeal and proximal interphalangeal joints injection. The proximal interphalangeal (PIP) joint is palpated on the dorsal aspect of the finger, either medial or lateral to the extensor tendon. A 25-gauge needle is inserted obliquely to the skin into the joint space below the extensor tendon. The metacarpophalangeal joints are similarly injected below the extensor tendon, either through medial or lateral approach

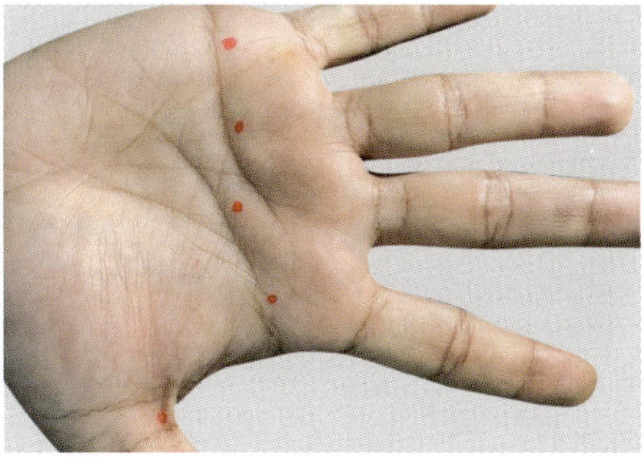

Fig. 6.9.12: Trigger finger injection. A 25-gauge needle introduced at 30° angle, directing the needle distally along the course of the tendon. For the thumb needle is inserted just proximal to the digital crease. For the index finger it is just distal to the proximal palmar crease and just distal to the distal palmar crease for the ring and little fingers. For the middle finger a needle is inserted between the proximal and distal palmar creases

Lower Limb Joints

The lower limb joint injection procedures are shown in Figures 6.9.13 to 6.9.22.

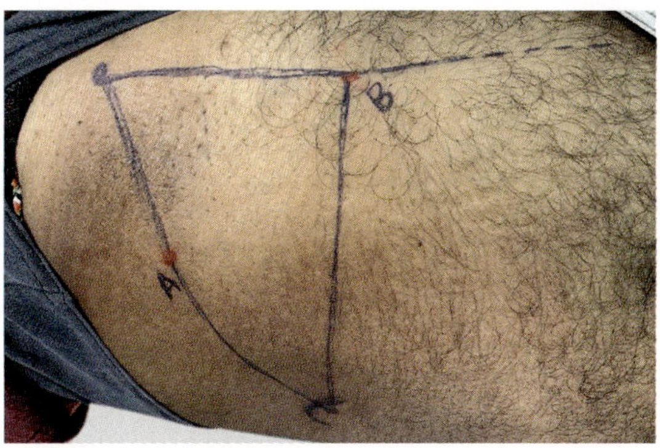

Fig. 6.9.13: Hip joint injection. The lateral approach is preferred because with the anterior approach there is a risk of injury to the femoral neurovascular bundles. The patient lies in supine with the affected limb in neutral rotation. A line is drawn between the anterior superior iliac spine and greater trochanter, and the junction of upper one-third and lower two-thirds is marked (point A, needle entry point). Line 1 connects the anterior superior iliac spine to the upper pole of the patella and line 2 is perpendicular line from the greater trochanter to the line 1. Point B connects line 2 with the line 1. A 18- or 20- gauge spinal needle is inserted at point A towards point B until it hits the bony surface, then slightly withdrawn and corticosteroid is injected.

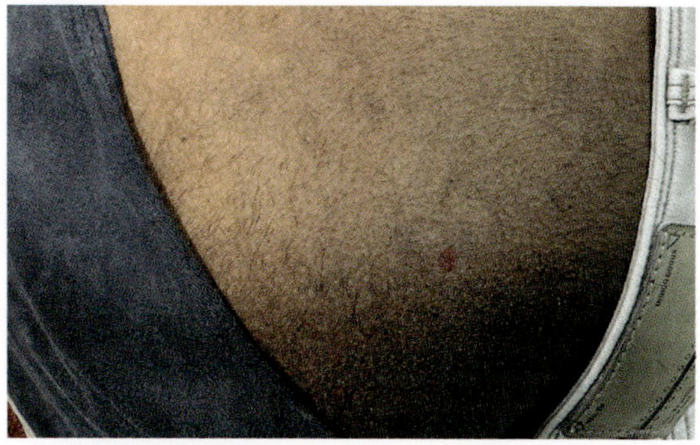

Fig. 6.9.14: Ischiogluteal bursa injection. The bursa is palpated directly over the ischial tuberosity at the buttock region with the patient lying on the unaffected side and knees flexed. A 23-gauge needle is inserted perpendicular to the skin till the bony surface is reached. The needle is slightly withdrawn and the injection is given

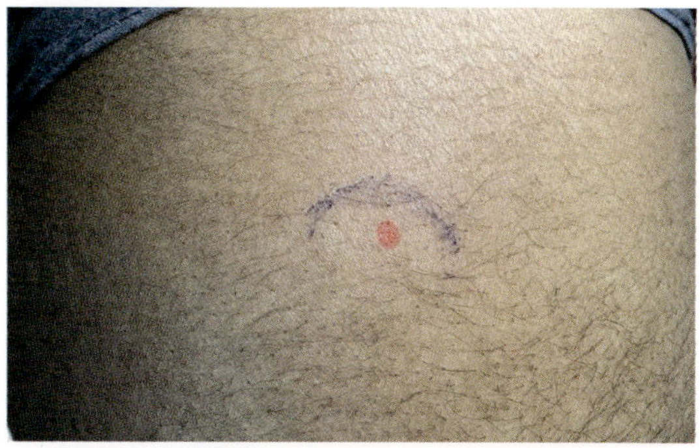

Fig. 6.9.15: Trochanteric syndrome. With the patient affected side facing upwards, the point of maximum tenderness is palpated over the greater trochanter. A 23-gauge needle is then inserted perpendicular to the skin till it reaches the bony surface, slightly withdrawn and the injection is given

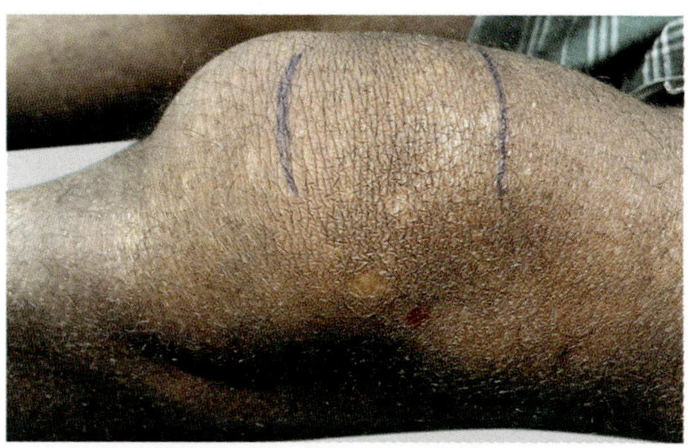

Fig. 6.9.16: Knee joint injection. The patient lies supine and with the knee slightly flexed, a 21-gauge needle is inserted laterally underneath the patella at the junction of proximal one-third and distal two-thirds toward the suprapatellar pouch. A medial approach can be similarly performed

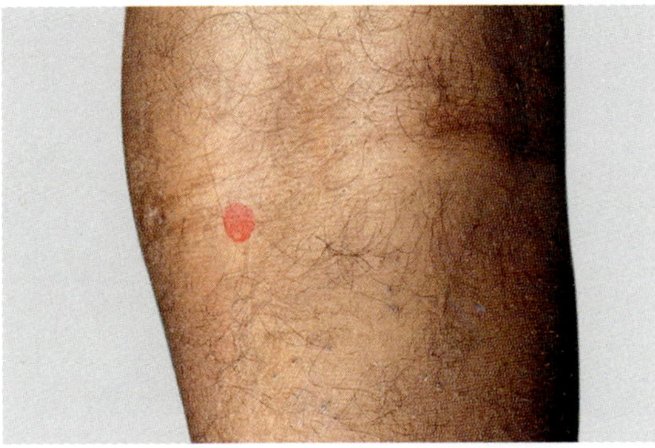

Fig. 6.9.17: Baker's cyst injection. The bursa is palpated on the posteromedial aspect of the knee joint between the medial head of gastrocnemius and semimembranosus tendons. A 21-gauge needle is inserted directly into the bursa and corticosteroid is injected

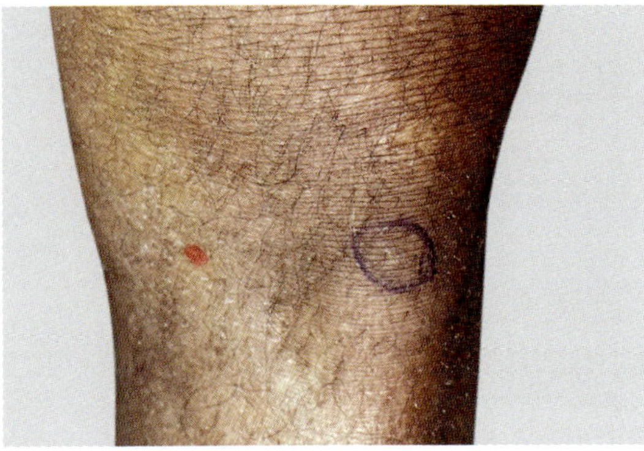

Fig. 6.9.18: Anserine bursa injection. The bursa is located at the level of the tibial tuberosity on the anteromedial aspect of upper tibia. A 23-gauge needle is directed to the point of maximal tenderness close to the bony surface and corticosteroid is injected

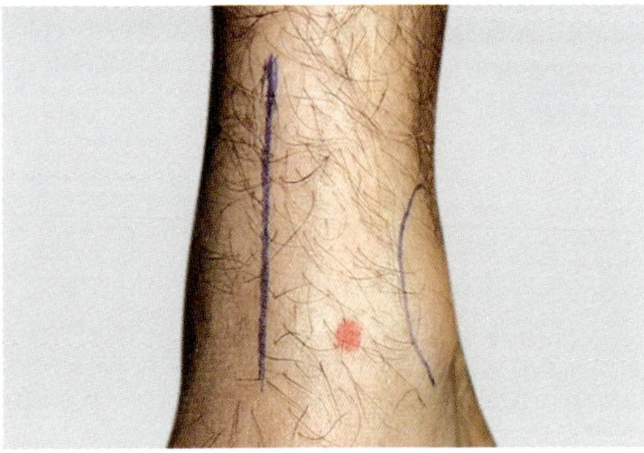

Fig. 6.9.19: Ankle joint injection. The anterior approach is simple and less painful. A 23-gauge needle is inserted between the tibialis anterior and medial malleolus into the joint space, directed posterolaterally

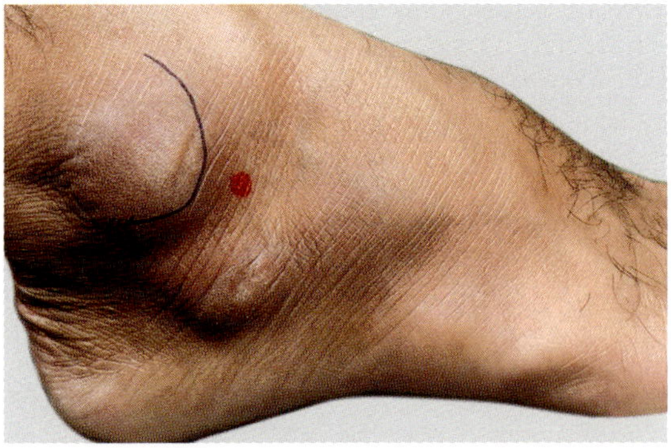

Fig. 6.9.20: Subtalar joint injection. The joint space is palpated anterior and inferior to the lateral malleolus. With the patient lying supine and ankle joint in inversion, a 23-gauge needle is directed perpendicular towards the medial malleolus

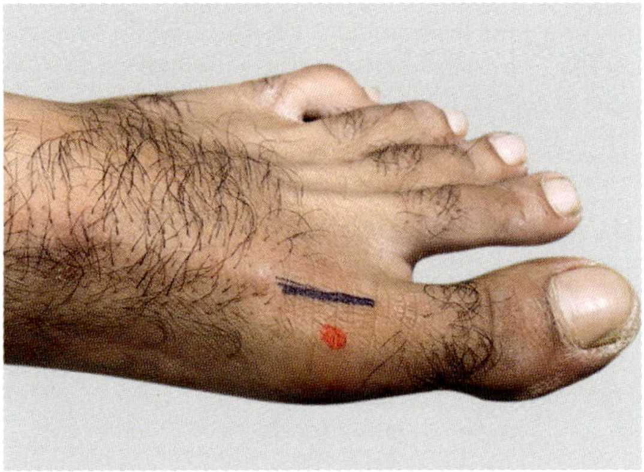

Fig. 6.9.21: Metatarsophalangeal joint injection. A 25-gauge needle is inserted perpendicularly into the joint space, either medial or lateral to the extensor tendon on the dorsal aspect

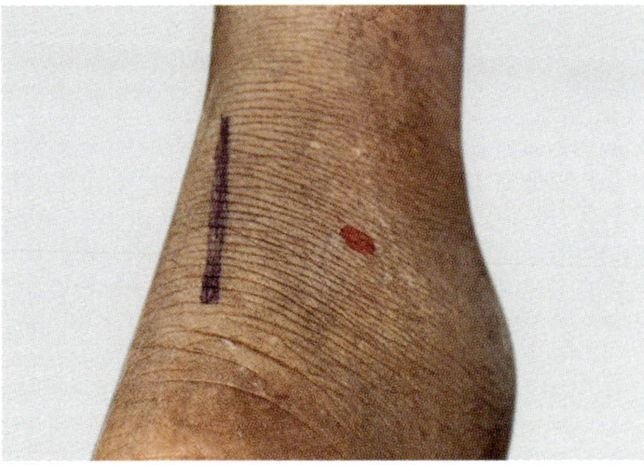

Fig. 6.9.22: Retrocalcaneal bursa injection. Conventional injection of retrocalcaneal bursa is performed when ultrasound is not available. The bursa is injected using a 23-gauge needle inserted perpendicular to the skin anterior to the Achilles tendon

COMPLICATIONS

The complications associated with intra-articular injections are summarized in Table 6.9.2.

Table 6.9.2: Complications associated with intra-articular injections

Iatrogenic infection
Post-injection flare
Tendon rupture
Neurovascular damage
Local skin changes or fat atrophy
Allergy
Transient hyperglycemia
Suppression of hypothalamic-pituitary-adrenal axis
Neuropathic joint (mainly with multiple injections)

LEARNING POINTS

- Appropriate use of joint injection procedures is warranted for improving patient outcomes.
- Intraarticular corticosteroid injections are safe and effective in controlling synovial inflammation.

FURTHER READING

1. Lawry G, Kreder H, Hawker G, Jerome D. Fam's Musculoskeletal Examination and Joint Injection Techniques. 2nd edition. Philadelphia: Mosby; 2010.
2. Wise, CM. Aspiration and injection of joints in soft tissue. In: Firestein GS, Budd RC, Harris ED, McInnes IB, Rudy S, Sergent JS, editors. Kelley's Textbook of Rheumatology. 8th Edition. Philadelphia: WB Saunders; 2009.
3. Zayat AS, Matteo AD, Wakefield RJ. Arthrocentesis and injections of joints and soft tissues. In: Firestein G, Budd RC, Gabriel SE, Koretsky GA, McInnes IB, O'Dell JR, editors. Firestein and Kelley's Textbook of Rheumatology. 11th edition. Philadelphia: Elsevier; 2021. p. 859–74.

Ultrasound-guided Procedures in Rheumatology

Gurjit S Kaeley

INTRODUCTION

Sonography improves the accuracy of accessing target tissues, especially when obtaining fluid for diagnostic purposes is important, and it is also associated with less procedural pain. The following brief section will outline basic principles of interventional sonography, followed by a regional approach to injection guidance.

BASIC PRINCIPLES

A. **Verify diagnosis and injection target:** Even though the indication for local injection may be regional pain, it is essential to clinically correlate sonographic findings to determine the therapeutic injection target. Careful evaluation will also aid in planning the injection route to avoid structures such as blood vessels or nerves. Contraindications to injections include.
   1. Skin damage at the site of injection
   2. Underlying fracture
   3. Prosthetic joint unless coordinating with orthopedics to aspirate joint
   4. Allergy to injectate

B. **Determine the length and size of the needle:** For injections only, smaller bore needles afford less pain than larger bore needles. A summary of needle sizes and typical steroid injection doses by joint size is given in Table 6.10.1.

C. **Injectate for therapeutic injections:** Table 6.10.1 lists common injectates according to joint size. Although it is common practice to mix injectates with local anesthetic agents, one limitation is the

Table 6.10.1: General guidelines for needle size and injectate by size of joint

Joint	*Needle length*	*Needle gauge for injection**	*Typical doses of corticosteroid*	*Typical volume of 1% or 2% lidocaine*
Small e.g. finger joints or tendon sheaths	1–1.5 inches	25–30 G	5–20 mg methylprednisolone**	0.1–0.25 mL
Intermediate e.g. elbow, ankle	1–1.5 inches	22–25 G	10–40 mg methylprednisolone or triamcinolone acetonide	0.5–1 mL
Large e.g. shoulder, knee	1.5–3.5 inches	22–25 G	40 mg methylprednisolone or triamcinolone acetonide	1–2 mL
Very Deep–e.g. Hip	3.5–5 inches	22 G Spinal needle	40 mg methylprednisolone or triamcinolone acetonide	1–2 mL

*For aspiration, 21–22 G needles should be considered. Avoid 18 G needles for routine aspiration due to patient morbidity and pain.

**For tendons and small joints closer to the skin, triamcinolone acetonide/hexacetonide is avoided due to the risk of skin depigmentation and tissue atrophy

flocculation of the mixture, which may block thinner needles. Generally, the author combines lidocaine 2% with Depo-Medrol and prefers to use triamcinolone on its own.

D. **Local anesthesia:** For brief injections utilizing a mixture of lidocaine and Depo-Medrol®, cryoanesthesia is preferred for the skin when available. When the procedure may take time to direct the needle, such as when aspirating, local anesthesia using lidocaine 1–2% without epinephrine is utilized, anesthetizing the skin and the needle track. Of note, some practitioners also mix longer-acting anesthetic agents such as bupivacaine to allow for more prolonged anesthesia. Large volumes of bupivacaine are associated with chondrocyte death and the risk of progression to end-stage osteoarthritis.

E. **Selection of puncture point and preparation of injection site:** Large joints such as the knee and shoulder can be accessed by placing the puncture point well away from the probe. The puncture point is cleaned by using locally available chlorhexidine or iodine as well as isopropyl alcohol. A no-touch technique is utilized to keep the needle sterile. For very deep joints such as the hip, sterile gloves should be utilized to manipulate the spinal needle. Sterile gel or iodine may also be used as a coupling agent to minimize risk of infection. This is especially important for joints or structures where the probe is adjacent to the puncture point. (If iodine is utilized as a coupling agent use of a probe cover will avoid damage to the probe).

F. Determine how to visualize the needle. It is preferable to always visualize the needle during the injection. Figure 6.10.1 demonstrates the difference of in plane and out of plane visualization of the needle. Generally, in plane visualization is preferred and out of plane views can be complimentary to confirm needle position. Best practices for in plane technique include staying perpendicular and parallel to the needle by heel–toing the probe or using beam steering or trapezoid view options if available. The author prefers manipulating the probe to stay parallel and perpendicular to the needle. For out of plane views, it is essential to determine where the needle tip is always. The probe can be moved as the needle is advanced so that the tip is always under the probe (Fig. 6.10.2).

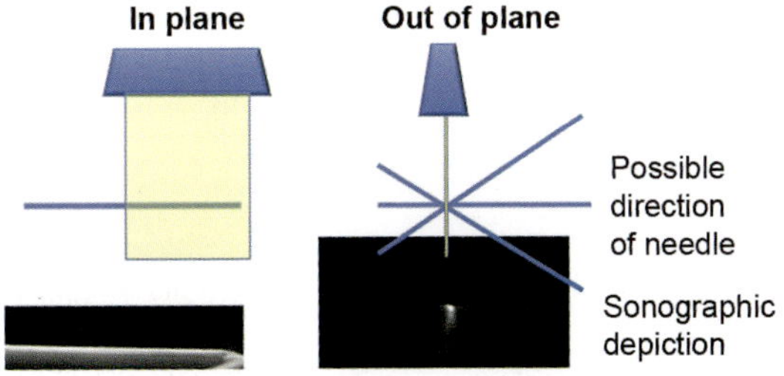

Fig. 6.10.1: Direct needle visualization

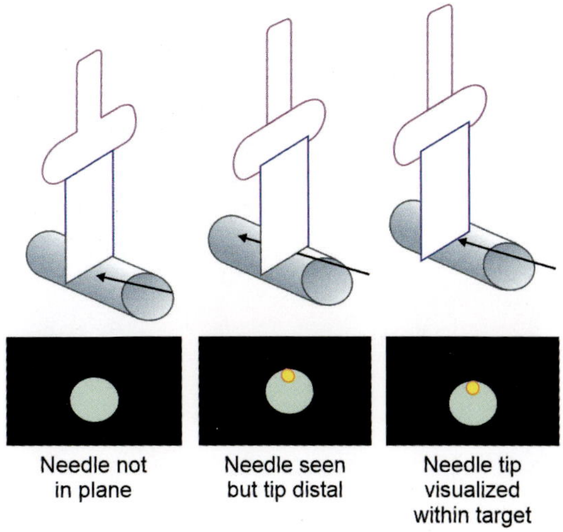

Fig. 6.10.2: Out of plane needle visualization

REGIONAL INJECTION TECHNIQUE

In the following section, a table will summarize the target, patient position as well as needle approach to each anatomic target. Injectate and needle size guidelines are given in Table 6.10.1.

SHOULDER

Subacromial Subdeltoid Bursa

The subacromial subdeltoid bursa is a common target for injection for shoulder pain.

Subacromial Subdeltoid Bursa Injection (Fig. 6.10.3)

Anatomic target	Subacromial subdeltoid bursa under peribursal fat stripe
Patient position	Sitting with arm in neutral position
Approach	In plane, 1. Lateral coronal—inferior to superior. 2. Anterior transverse—lateral to medial.

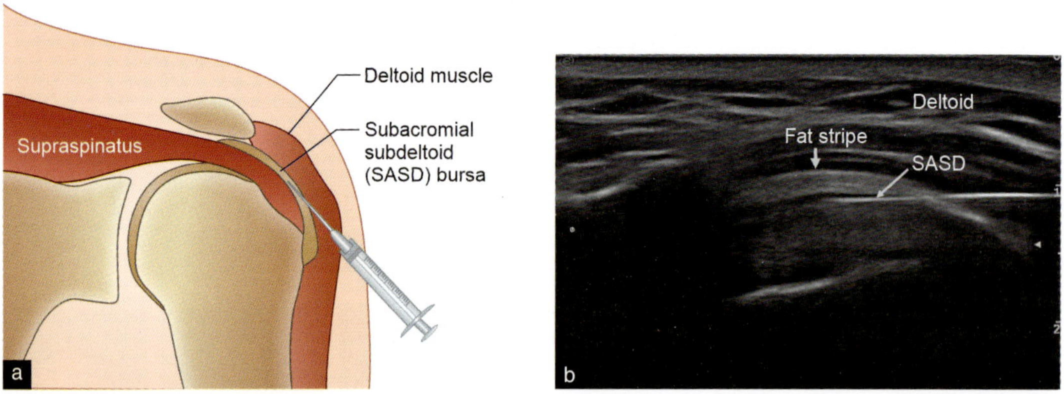

Fig. 6.10.3: Lateral access to subacromial subdeltoid bursa injection. Schematics (a) depicts needle approach, while sonographic image (b) shows in plane visualization of needle in the subacromial subdeltoid (SASD) bursa. Note that the bursa is found under the peribursal fat stripe.

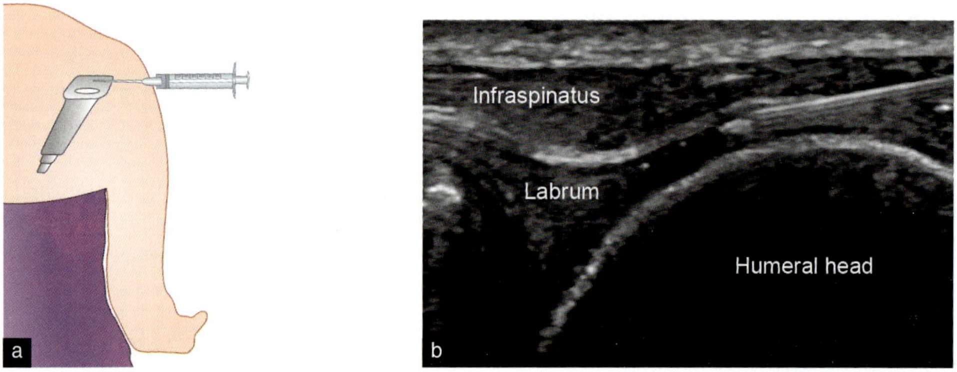

Fig. 6.10.4: Posterior recess injection. Schematic image (a) depicts lateral to medial positioning. Sonographic image (b) shows access to the recess. Due to the deep nature of the joint and angulation in subjects with higher BMI, the needle may need a steeper angle.

Posterior Recess (Fig. 6.10.4)

Anatomic target	Joint recess under infraspinatus Can aim under labrum
Patient position	Sitting with arm in neutral position or prone
Approach	In plane, 1. Lateral to medial transverse. 2. Medial to lateral transverse.
Tips	In large individuals, a spinal needle may be needed to access the recess.

ELBOW

Elbow procedures include elbow joint and bursal injections. The author does not inject the common extensor origin with corticosteroids as recent evidence suggests the injection is not better than conservative care and may worsen pain.

Elbow Posterior Recess Injection

Anatomic target	Olecranon recess
Patient position	Sitting with elbow flexed, rested on pillow
Approach	In plane (Fig. 6.10.5) 1. Short axis lateral to medial oblique. 2. Long axis through triceps tendon.
Tips	Avoid medial posterior approach due to the proximity of the ulnar nerve.

WRIST AND HAND

The wrist and hand injections are a common occurrence in a rheumatology unit to treat flares of inflammatory disease as well as regional pain disorders and nerve entrapments.

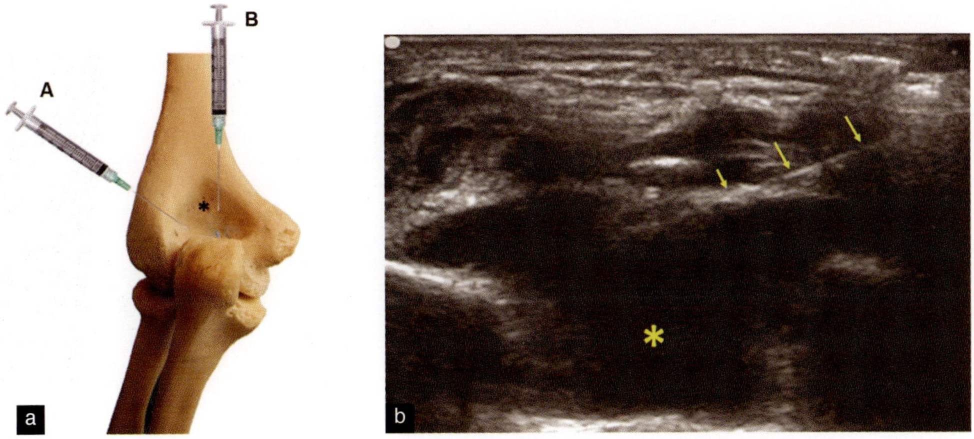

Fig. 6.10.5: Posterior recess injection. Image (a) depicts lateral to medial oblique (A) approach and the midline (B) approach through the distal triceps tendon. Sonographic image (b) depicts the needle (arrows) entering from a lateral oblique approach to access fluid in the olecranon recess (*).

Dorsal Wrist Joints

Anatomic target	Radiocarpal joint, intercarpal joint
Patient position	Sitting with hand on table
Approach	In plane, (Fig. 6.10.6), 1. Transverse in short axis to joint. 2. Midline, long axis to joint.
Tips	If available, **sterile** gel may be used as a standoff to allow needle visualization prior to penetration of skin.

Distal Radioulnar Joint

Anatomic target	Distal radioulnar joint
Patient position	Sitting with hand on table
Approach	In plane, short axis to joint (Fig. 6.10.7).
Tips	If available, **sterile** gel may be used as a standoff to allow needle visualization prior to penetration of skin.

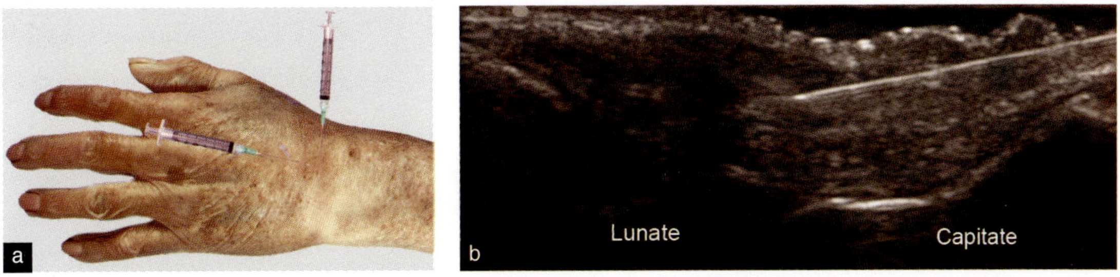

Fig. 6.10.6: Radiocarpal/intercarpal joint injections. Image depicts (a) long and short axis approaches into the wrist joint. Sonographic image (b) depicts targeting of the needle towards the radiocarpal joint.

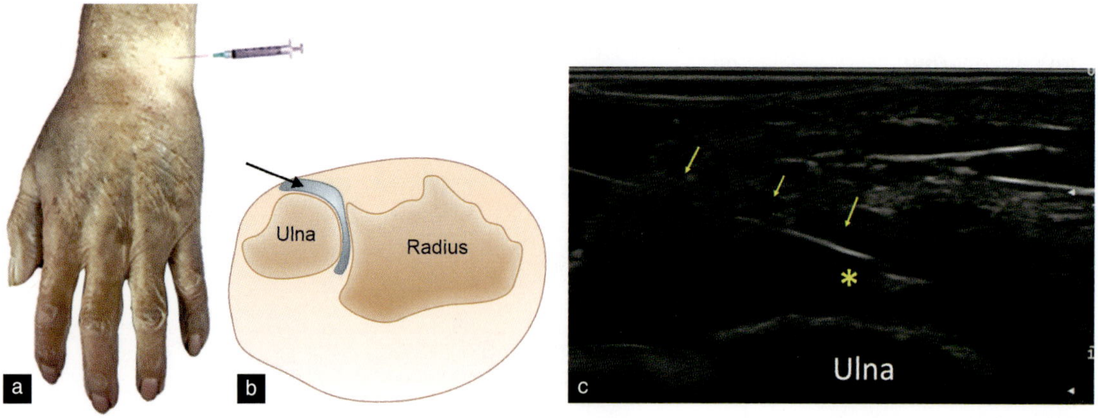

Fig. 6.10.7: Distal radioulnar joint injection. Image (a) indicates clinical landmarks for access into the distal radioulnar joint, which is also shown diagrammatically on the right (b). Sonographic image (c) needle (arrows) accessing the joint recess (*).

Dorsal Wrist Compartment

Anatomic target	Sonographically confirmed compar-tments 1, 2, 3, 4
Patient position	Sitting with hand on table
Approach	In plane, short or long axis to tendon sheath. Identify and avoid radial sensory nerve (Fig. 6.10.8).
Tips	If available, **sterile** gel may be used as a standoff to allow needle visualization prior to penetration of skin.

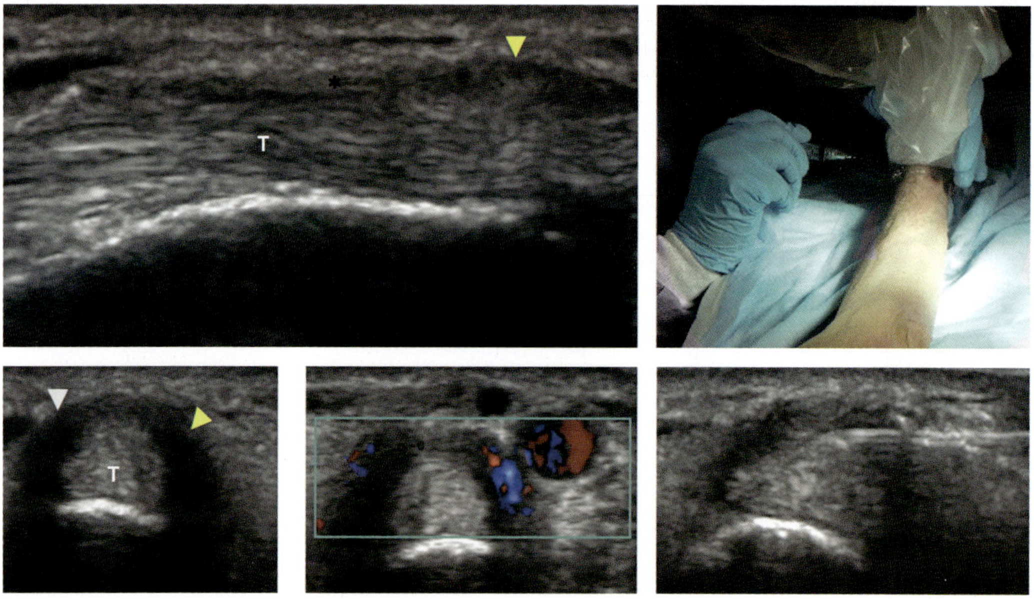

Fig. 6.10.8: Dorsal compartment 1 injection. Composite images depict features of DeQuervain's tendinopathy showing a thickened retinaculum (arrow heads) encasing the extensor pollicis brevis and abductor pollicis longus tendons (T). The local injection can be performed adjacent to the retinaculum or into it as above on the right. Image at the top right in a cadaveric specimen indicates probe placement and needle approach.

Carpal Tunnel Injection

Anatomic target	Carpal Tunnel
Patient position	Sitting with hand on table
Approach	In plane, short axis to carpal tunnel, lateral to medial (Fig. 6.10.9).
Tips	Care needs to be exercised in always visualizing the nerve and being careful not to inject into the nerve. Some practitioners only inject 20 mg Depo-Medrol® without lidocaine into the carpal tunnel to monitor nerve damage.

Metacarpophalangeal Joint Injection

Anatomic target	Proximal recess over the metacarpal neck
Patient position	Sitting with hand on table
Approach	In plane, short axis to metacarpal neck (Fig. 6.10.10).
Tips	If available, sterile gel may help with needle placement.

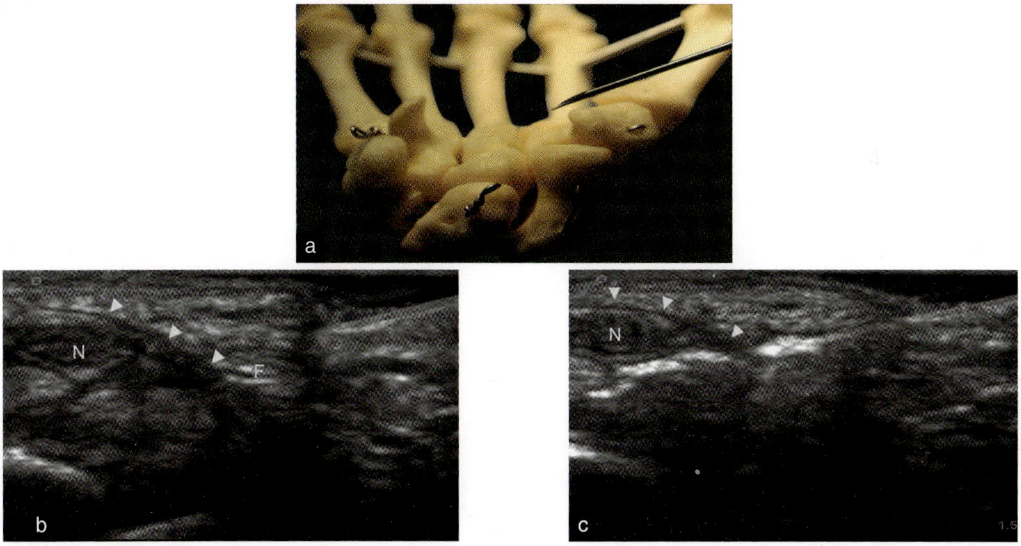

Fig. 6.10.9: Carpal tunnel injection. Carpal tunnel injection from the lateral to medial approach. Image of carpal tunnel and (a) sonographic images (b) and (c) show the access just before the carpal tunnel, targeting the needle above the flexor carpi radialis (F), entering the carpal tunnel lateral to the median nerve (N) and injecting under the retinaculum (arrow heads). In figure (c), the white linear area indicates the injectate which ends under the median nerve.

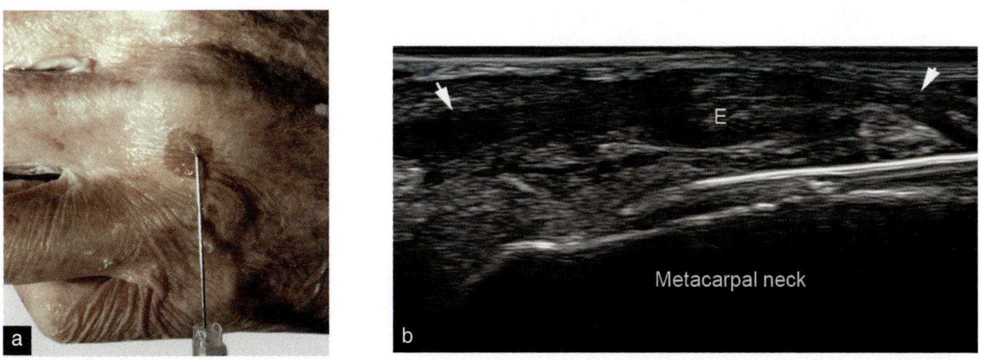

Fig. 6.10.10: Metacarpophalangeal joint injection. Image (a) shows needle placement to access the dorsal recess of the metacarpal phalangeal joint at the level of the metacarpal neck of a cadaveric hand. Ultrasound image (b) shows needle within the recess. The extensor tendon (E) and dorsal hood (arrows) are also visualized at this level.

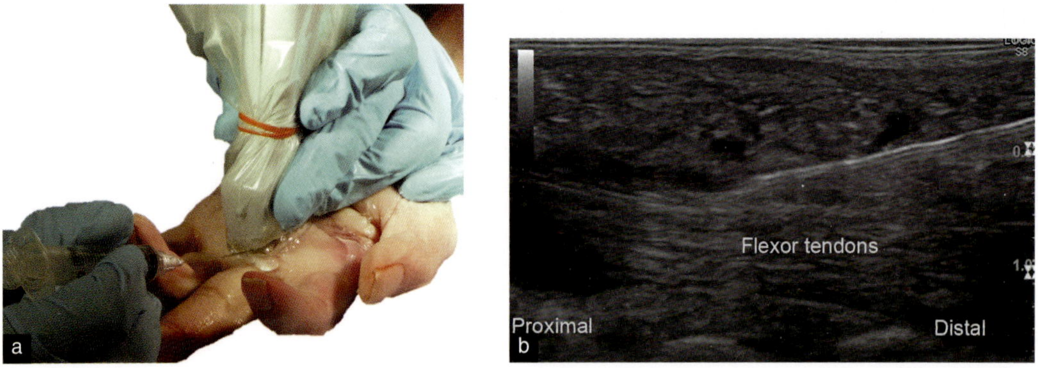

Fig. 6.10.11: Flexor tendon sheath injection. Image (a) depicts use of a sterile probe cover and gel and in plane approach to needle injection of the flexor tendon sheath in a cadaveric specimen. In the sonographic image (b), the needle is seen in the superior tendon sheath.

Flexor Tendon Sheath Injection

Anatomic target	Flexor tendon sheath
Patient position	Sitting with hand on table
Approach	In plane, long axis to the tendon (Fig.6.10.11).
Tips	If available, sterile gel may help with needle placement. Consider confirming needle position in short axis.

HIP JOINT

The hip joint is a deep target and extra-precautions need to be taken so as not to infect the joint.

Anatomic target	Anterior hip joint recess
Patient position	Supine with leg in 15° external rotation.
Approach	In plane, long axis to the joint, distal to proximal (Fig. 6.10.12).
Tips	Recommend using sterile gloves, probe cover and sterile gel since puncture point is close to the probe. Use Doppler to look for the anterior circumflex artery to plan an approach to avoid it. A spinal needle is guided under sonographic visualization into the recess. Aim for the neck of the femur. Doppler may be used to document the injection.

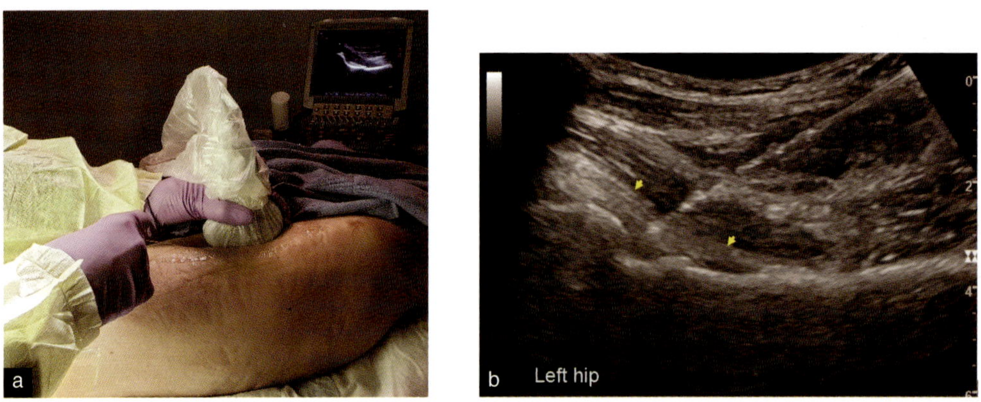

Fig. 6.10.12: Hip joint injection. Cadaveric specimen (a) depicts probe and needle placement to access the hip joint. In the sonographic picture (b), note that the needle is aimed at the femoral neck and that the tip is below the ischiofemoral ligament/capsule (arrows).

KNEE JOINT

Anatomic target	Suprapatellar recess
Patient position	Supine with knee flexed at 30°.
Approach	In plane, short axis to the joint, lateral to medial (Fig. 6.10.13).
Tips	Recommend keeping puncture point below patellar margin to keep needle parallel.

ANKLE JOINT

Anatomic Target	Anterior tibiotalar recess
Patient position	Supine with ankle in a relaxed position.
Approach	In plane, short axis to the joint, either medial or lateral approach under the tendons and neurovascular structures (Fig. 6.10.14).
Tips	Ensure needle track is perpendicular and parallel to the probe.

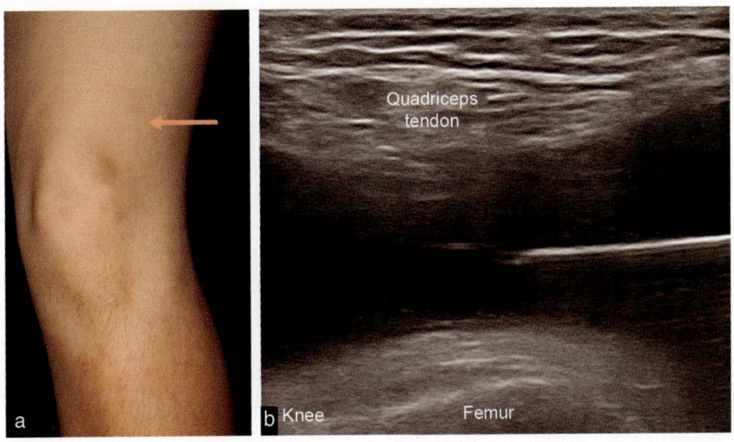

Fig. 6.10.13: Knee joint injection. Image (a) depicts the left knee flexed at 30° and arrow indicating needle approach into the suprapatellar recess. Sonographic image (b) shows needle in suprapatellar recess approaching from the lateral aspect of the knee.

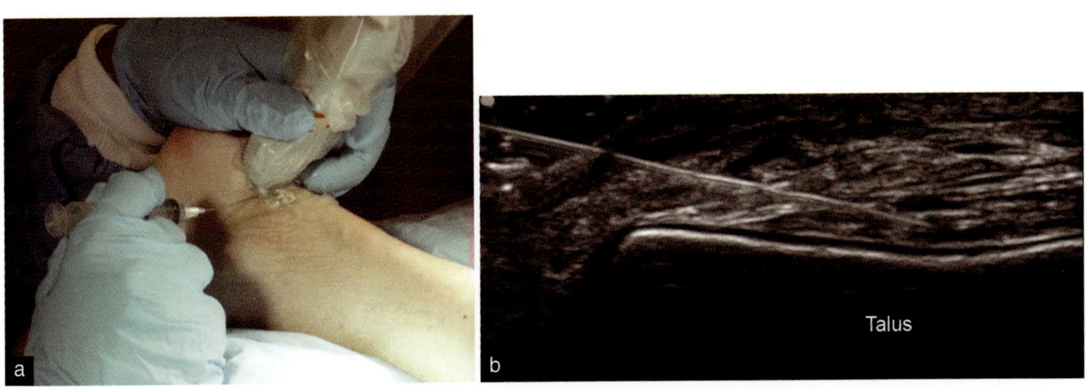

Fig. 6.10.14: Ankle joint injection. Image (a) shows probe placement in a cadaveric specimen for medial to lateral short axis approach to access the tibiotalar joint. Sonographic image (b) shows needle placement underneath the tendons into the recess just superficial to the talar plafond.

Metatarsophalangeal Joint

Anatomic Target	Dorsal Recess
Patient position	Supine or foot placed on bed.
Approach	In plane, dorsal transverse or oblique (Fig. 6.10.15).
Tips	If available, sterile gel may help with needle placement.

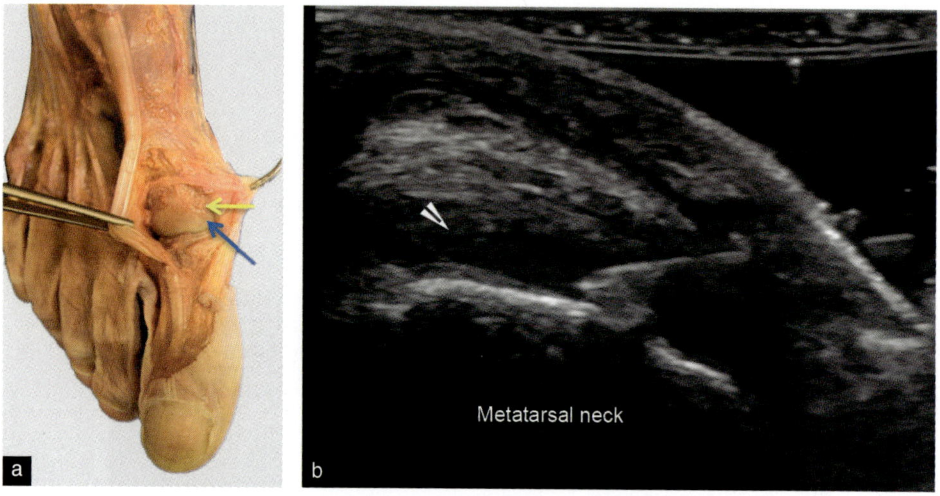

Fig. 6.10.15: Metatarsophalangeal joint injection. Dissection on the image (a) demonstrates the dorsal recess as well as transverse (yellow arrow) and oblique (blue arrow) approaches into the recess. Sonographic image (b) depicts medial to lateral needle access into the recess with hypoechoic injectate (arrow head).

LEARNING POINTS

- First the diagnosis and indications for injection needs to be confirmed.
- Second, the needle size and length should be decided along with the injectate.
- The puncture point should be selected and prepared for sterile injection.
- In plane visualization of needle is preferred. If out of plane, care should be taken to ensure that the tip of the needle is always under the probe.

FURTHER READING

1. Foster ZJ, Voss TT, Hatch J, Frimodig A. Corticosteroid Injections for Common Musculoskeletal Conditions. AFP 2015; 92:694–9.
2. Stephens MB, Beutler AI, O'Connor FG. Musculoskeletal injections: a review of the evidence. Am Fam Physician. 2008; 78:971–6.
3. Tortora S, Messina C, Albano D, et al. Ultrasound-guided musculoskeletal interventional procedures around the elbow, hand and wrist excluding carpal tunnel procedures. J Ultrason 2021; 21:e169–76.
4. Wittich CM, Ficalora RD, Mason TG, Beckman TJ. Musculoskeletal injection. Mayo Clin Proc. 2009;84:831–7.

Section

VII

LABORATORY INVESTIGATIONS

Chapter 7.1

Techniques of Biomarker Detection

Christina Mary Mariaselvam, Vaidehi Chowdhary

INTRODUCTION

A biomarker is a medical indicator that signals a change in physiological state or pharmacologic responses to an intervention. Biomarkers can be nucleic acids, proteins, metabolites, images, clinical and epigenetic features that can be measured consistently and objectively. Biomarkers can be predictive, diagnostic, prognostic, treatment guiding and monitoring tools.

TECHNIQUES FOR BIOMARKER DETECTION

Immune and genetic biomarkers are generally detected in the laboratories using conventional techniques like enzyme-linked immunosorbent assay (ELISA), western blotting, immunofluorescence (IF), flow cytometry and polymerase chain reaction (PCR) etc.

Antigen (Ag) is any substance that can elicit an immune response. **Antibodies (Ab)** or immunoglobulins are glycoproteins produced by activated B cell, in response to an antigen. The interaction between the binding site of Ag (epitope) and binding site of Ab (paratope) is mediated by many non-covalent bonds between them. The Ag-Ab interaction is very specific i.e. an antigen can react only with antibodies produced against the specific antigen or closely related antigens (Fig. 7.1.1).

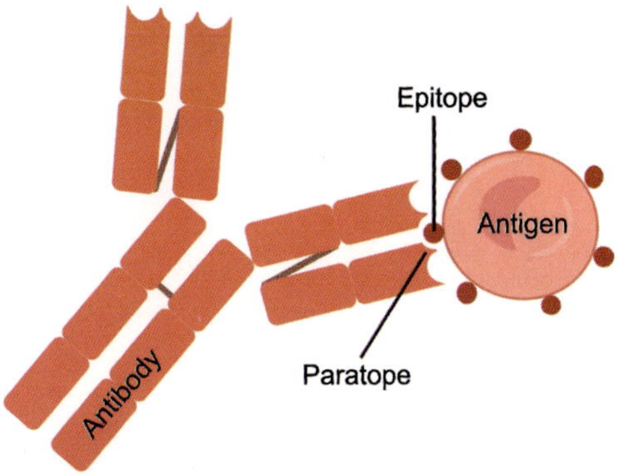

Fig. 7.1.1: Illustration of an epitope and paratope

a. **Affinity and Avidity:** The strength of binding between antigen and antibody is measured by affinity and avidity. Affinity refers to the strength of a single interaction between one epitope on the antigen and one paratope of the antibody while avidity refers to the overall strength of binding between all epitopes and paratopes (Fig 7.1.2).
b. **Specificity and cross reactivity:** Specificity refers to the ability of paratopes to recognize and interact with only a single epitope on the corresponding antigen. When an antibody generated against one specific antigen can bind with another different antigen, cross-reactivity between antigens occurs. Cross-reactivity greatly reduces specificity.

1. **Antigen-antibody reactions:** Ag-Ab interaction is optimal only when both the antigen and antibody are in equal proportions (zone of equivalence). If there is an excess of either the antibody (prozone) or antigen (postzone), precipitation does not occur. The physical form of the antigen influences how the antigen-antibody reactions are detected in vitro. If the antigen is particulate, the antigen and antibody agglutinates but if it is soluble the antigen and antibody precipitates. When the precipitate remains suspended as

floccules, instead of sediment, the reaction is known as flocculation. In general, agglutination is more sensitive than precipitation and is better visualised and interpreted in vitro.

Venereal disease research laboratory (VDRL) test is a slide flocculation test for detection of antibody (reagin) against treponemal infection causing syphilis.

Latex agglutination to detect rheumatoid factor is an example of agglutination. Multiple antibody molecules are coated on latex beads so that there are many sites for antigen binding. In the presence of antigen in a sample, a visible clump is formed as a result of cross linking of antigen and antibody (Fig. 7.1.3). Latex beads can also be coated with antigens for testing the presence of antibodies in a sample.

Coombs' or Direct antiglobulin test is an agglutination test used to check for antibodies that are attached to red blood cells and can destroy them prematurely causing haemolytic anaemia (Fig. 7.1.4) while indirect antiglobulin test looks for antibodies in the serum that can act against certain red blood cells so as to detect Rh incompatibility during blood transfusion for example (Fig. 7.1.5).

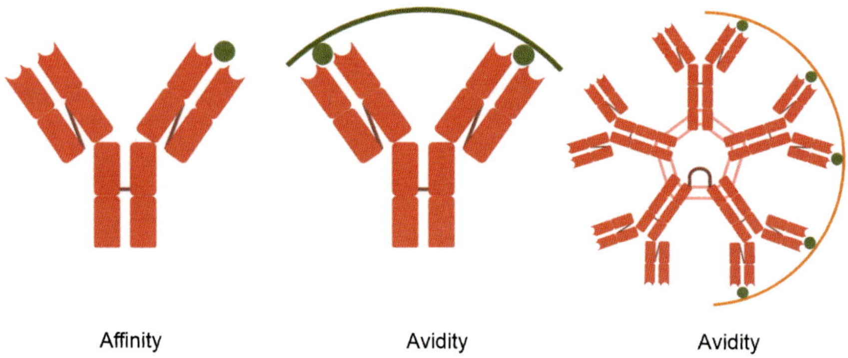

Fig. 7.1.2: Illustration of affinity and avidity

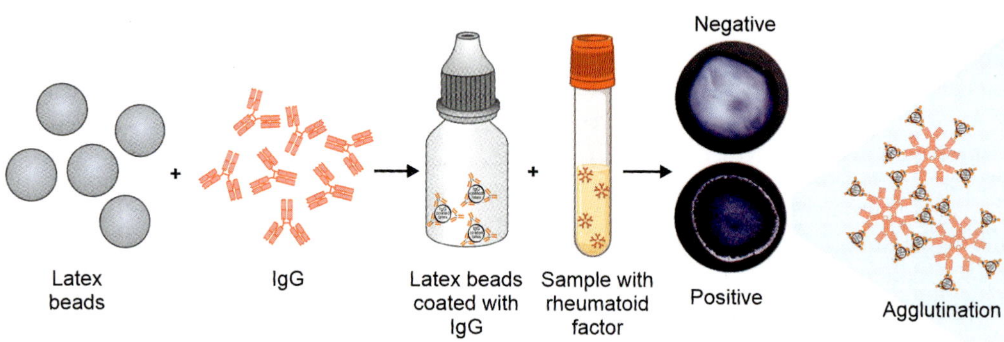

Fig. 7.1.3: Latex agglutination to detect rheumatoid factor

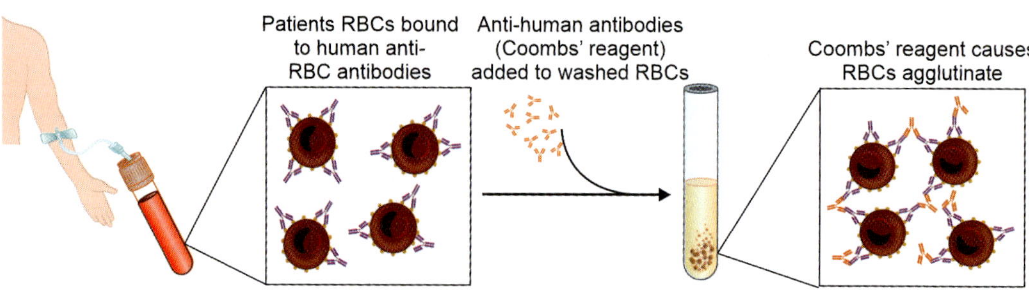

Fig. 7.1.4: Direct Coombs' test

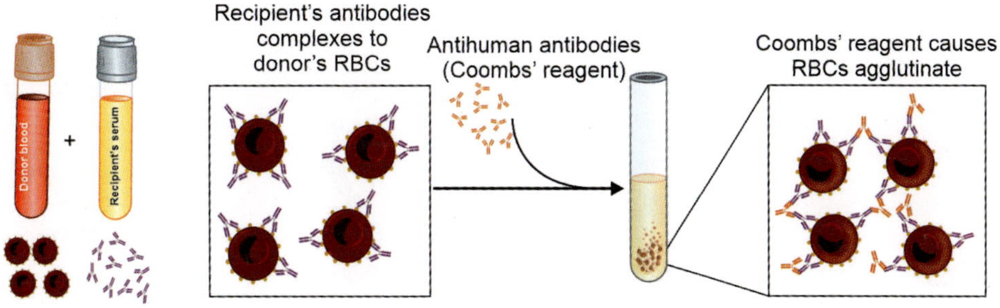

Fig. 7.1.5: Indirect coombs' test

2. **Enzyme-linked immunosorbent assay (ELISA):** ELISA is used to detect and quantify either the antigen or antibody present in biological samples. It relies on analysis of proteins immobilized in microplate wells using specific antibodies. The primary antibody is a specific antibody that only binds to the protein of interest, while a secondary antibody is a second antibody tagged with an enzyme that binds a primary antibody. The Ag-Ab interaction is detected by using a chromogen/substrate system where the enzyme activity produces colour that can be read in a spectrophotometer (Fig. 7.1.6). Depending on the method of antigen capture and/or signal detection, different types of ELISAs exist.

   Direct ELISA: The antigen is attached to a solid support and an antibody that is tagged to an enzyme is added. The Ag-Ab binding is detected by the addition of a chromogen/substrate to produce a color change. The amount of color developed is directly proportional to the amount of antigen (Fig. 7.1.7).

   Indirect ELISA: The antigen is attached to a solid support and antibody specific for the antigen is added. The antibodies that are bound to the antigen are detected by the addition of an enzyme conjugated secondary antibody. Addition of a chromogen/substrate activates the enzyme to produce color that is directly proportional to the amount of antigen (Fig. 7.1.8).

   Sandwich ELISA: Contrary to the above two methods, here the antibody is attached to the solid support and are of two forms. In direct sandwich ELISA, antibody attached to the solid support captures the antigen. The captured antigen is then detected by a second enzyme conjugated antibody specific for the antigen. In indirect sandwich ELISA the captured

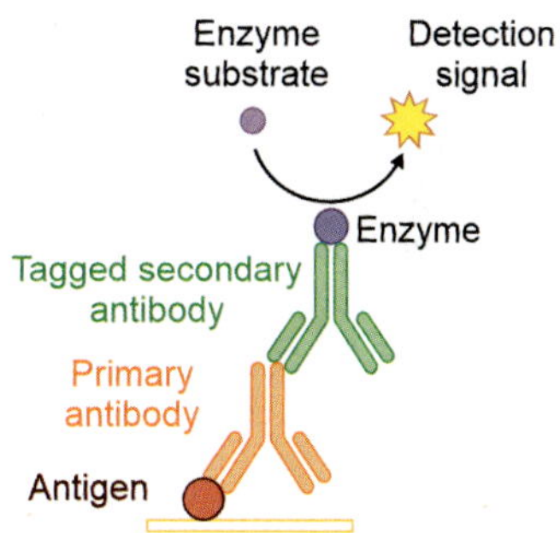

Fig. 7.1.6: Primary and secondary antibody

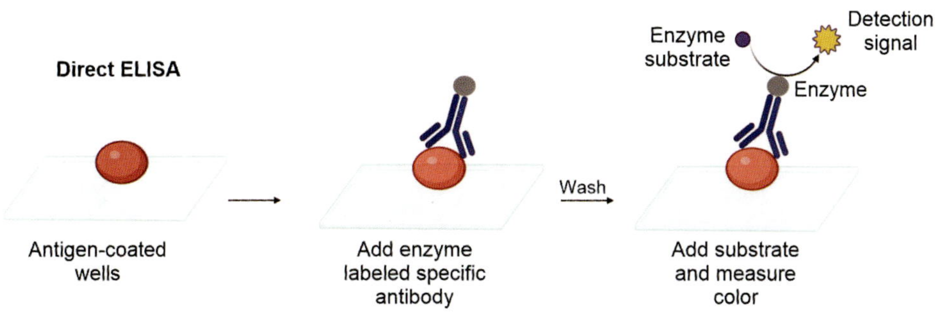

Fig. 7.1.7: Direct ELISA

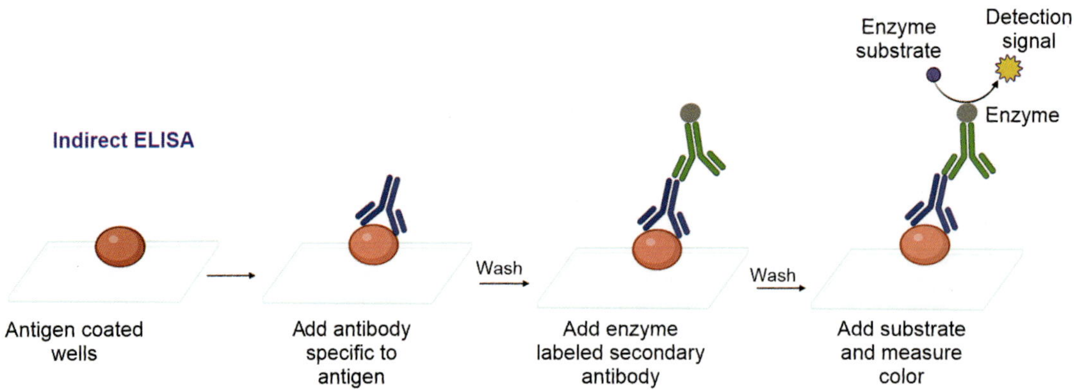

Fig. 7.1.8: Indirect ELISA

antigen is detected with a second antibody (untagged) specific for antigen. This bound second antibody is in turn detected using a third enzyme conjugated antibody. The color thus developed by addition of chromogen/substrate is directly proportional to the amount of antigen (Fig. 7.1.9).

Competitive ELISA: Also known as an inhibition or blocking ELISA, unlabeled primary antibodies are first complexed with antigens in the sample. These are added to wells coated with antigens. After washing, only free, unbound antibodies will bind to antigens coated on the solid support. Then an enzyme conjugated secondary antibody is added. Color developed by addition of chromogen/substrate is inversely proportional to the amount of antigen, i.e. the greater the amount of antigen in the sample, the lesser the signal. A variant of this ELISA uses primary antibodies to coat the solid support. Unlabeled antigen from samples and the labeled purified recombinant antigen is added and they compete with each other for binding to the capture antibody. Chromogen/substrate is added and the resulting color is inversely proportional to the amount of antigen in the sample (Fig. 7.1.10).

3. **Immunofluorescence (IF):** IF detects a wide variety of antigens in different type of tissues or cells. It uses antibodies labeled with fluorescent dyes to visualize molecules under a fluorescent

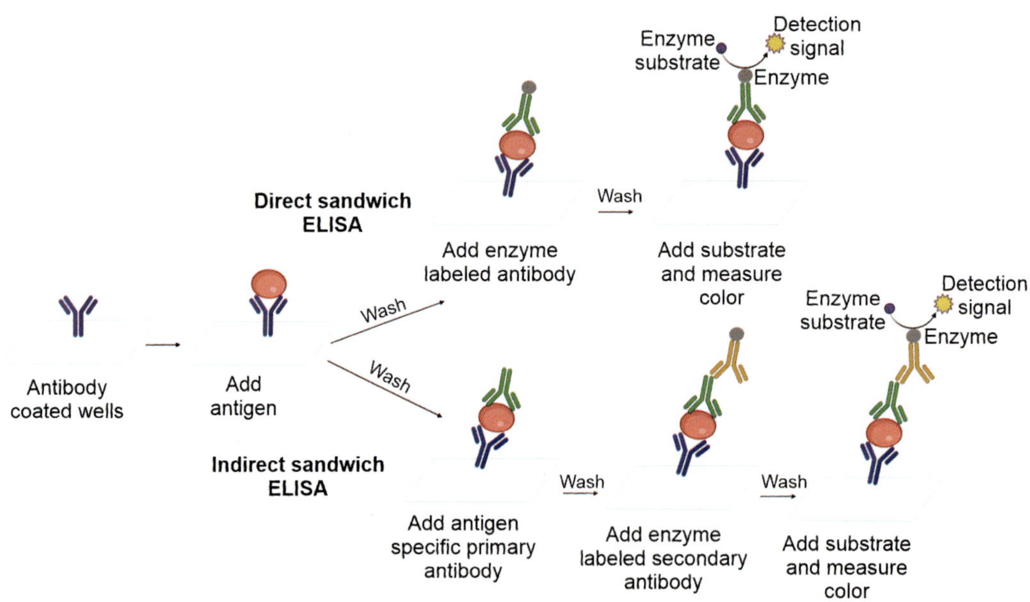

Fig. 7.1.9: Sandwich ELISA

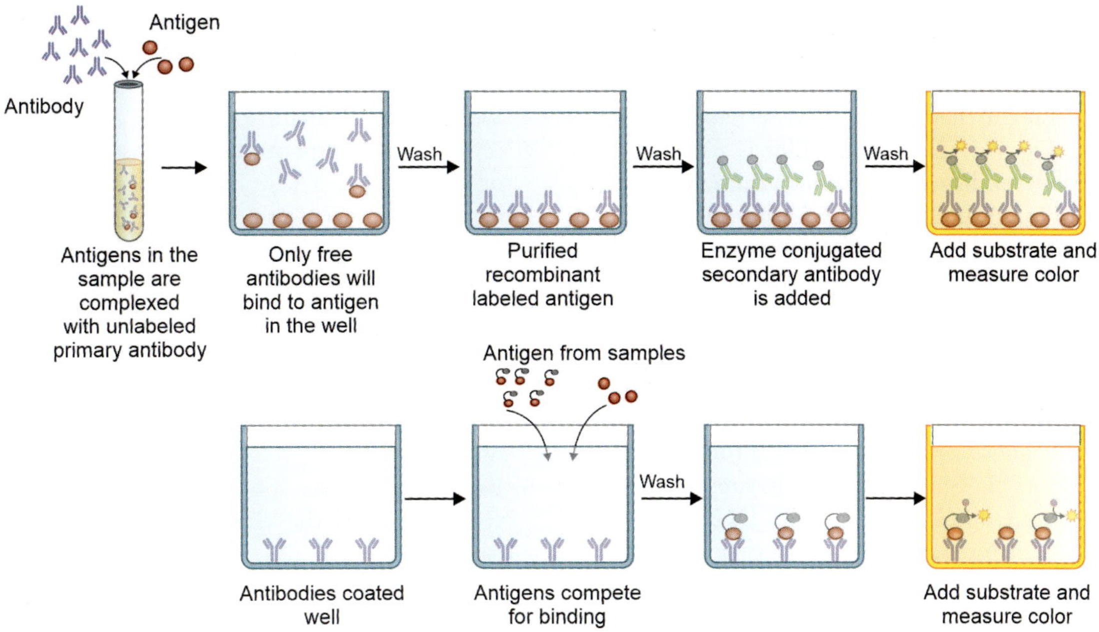

Fig. 7.1.10: Competitive ELISA

microscope. Fluorescent dyes can absorb light of a particular wavelength and emit light of a longer wavelength as it loses energy before fluorescing. In direct IF, fluorescent dye is conjugated to the primary antibody that binds to the target antigen while in indirect IF a primary antibody (untagged) first binds to the target antigen and then a secondary antibody conjugated to fluorescent dye binds to the primary antibody. The fluorescent signal is detected using a fluorescent microscope.

Anti-nuclear antibody assay (ANA) is an indirect IF test to detect nuclear antigens involved in many systemic autoimmune rheumatic diseases. Patient samples are usually incubated on a slide coated with a monolayer of human epithelial type 2 (HEp-2) cells. Antinuclear antibodies if present in patient sample binds to antigens in the HEp-2 cells and this Ag-Ab interaction is detected by fluorescent labelled secondary antibody, which are then visualized using a fluorescent microscope (Fig. 7.1.11).

4. **Western blot:** Western blotting is performed to detect a specific protein from a complex mixture of proteins in a blood or tissue sample. It relies on size separation of proteins by gel electrophoresis. The proteins thus separated is then electrically transferred onto the surface

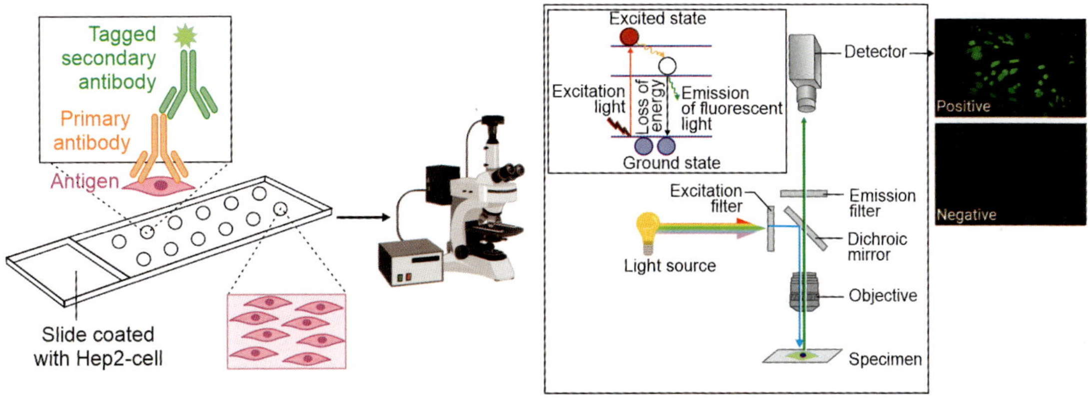

Fig. 7.1.11: Immunofluorescence

of a membrane. An antibody specific to the target protein on the membrane is added. Antigen-antibody interaction is detected using a chemically tagged secondary antibody (Fig. 7.1.12). Western Blot is a confirmatory test for diagnosis of Human Immunodeficiency Virus, Feline Immunodeficiency Virus, Hepatitis B Virus infections and Bovine Spongiform Encephalopathy (mad cow disease) after a positive ELISA test.

5. **Polymerase chain reaction (PCR):** PCR is an in-vitro technique to copy/amplify small segments of DNA/RNA yielding enough material for diagnosis and disease monitoring (viral load) from biological samples. In its simplest form, the DNA sample is mixed with a DNA polymerase, nucleotides, primers and other chemicals to facilitate the copying process using the following three steps: first step called denaturation where sample DNA is heated to >90°C to break them into two separate strands. PCR primers (short pieces of synthetic DNA) marks the starting point for copying the DNA in the second step called annealing at 40–60°C. Two primers-one each for the separated single DNA strands is used. During the third step called extension, the temperature is increased to 72°C and DNA polymerase adds nucleotides in the solution to the annealed primers to create a new strand of DNA that is complementary to the single DNA strands. Thus two identical copies of the original DNA are made and these three steps are repeated several times to exponentially increase the copies of DNA (Fig. 7.1.13). The amplified DNA is visualised by gel electrophoresis at the end of PCR.

   PCR tests are used to diagnose infectious diseases; identify a genetic change that can cause disease [e.g. inflammatory arthritis (Fig 7.1.14)], paternity testing and find small amounts of cancer cells that might be missed in other types of tests, etc.

6. **Real-time PCR:** This technique allows visualisation of the accumulated DNA as it is copied in real time by using fluorescent dyes, whereas conventional PCR requires gel electrophoresis to visualise the product at the end of the process. Total amount of copied DNA is directly proportional to the amount of measured fluorescence. There are two phases of amplification: an exponential phase and a non-exponential phase. In the exponential phase, there is doubling of the PCR product after every cycle. As PCR continues, reagents used for copying are consumed, and become limited. As a result, the reaction slows down to enter a non-

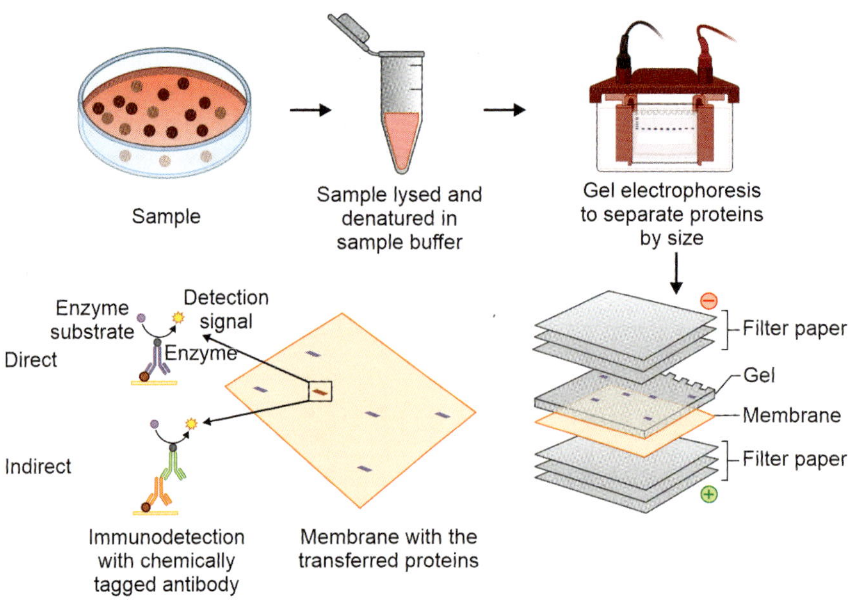

Fig. 7.1.12: Western blotting

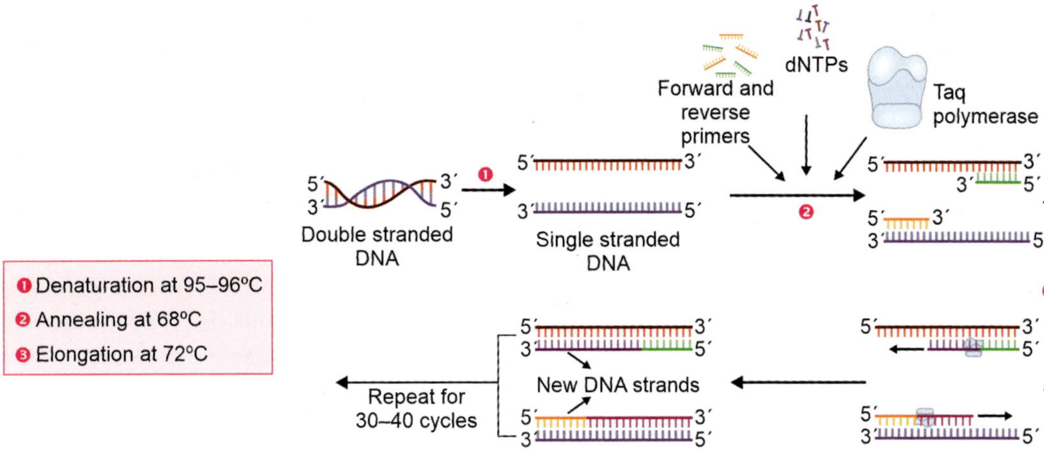

Fig. 7.1.13: Conventional PCR

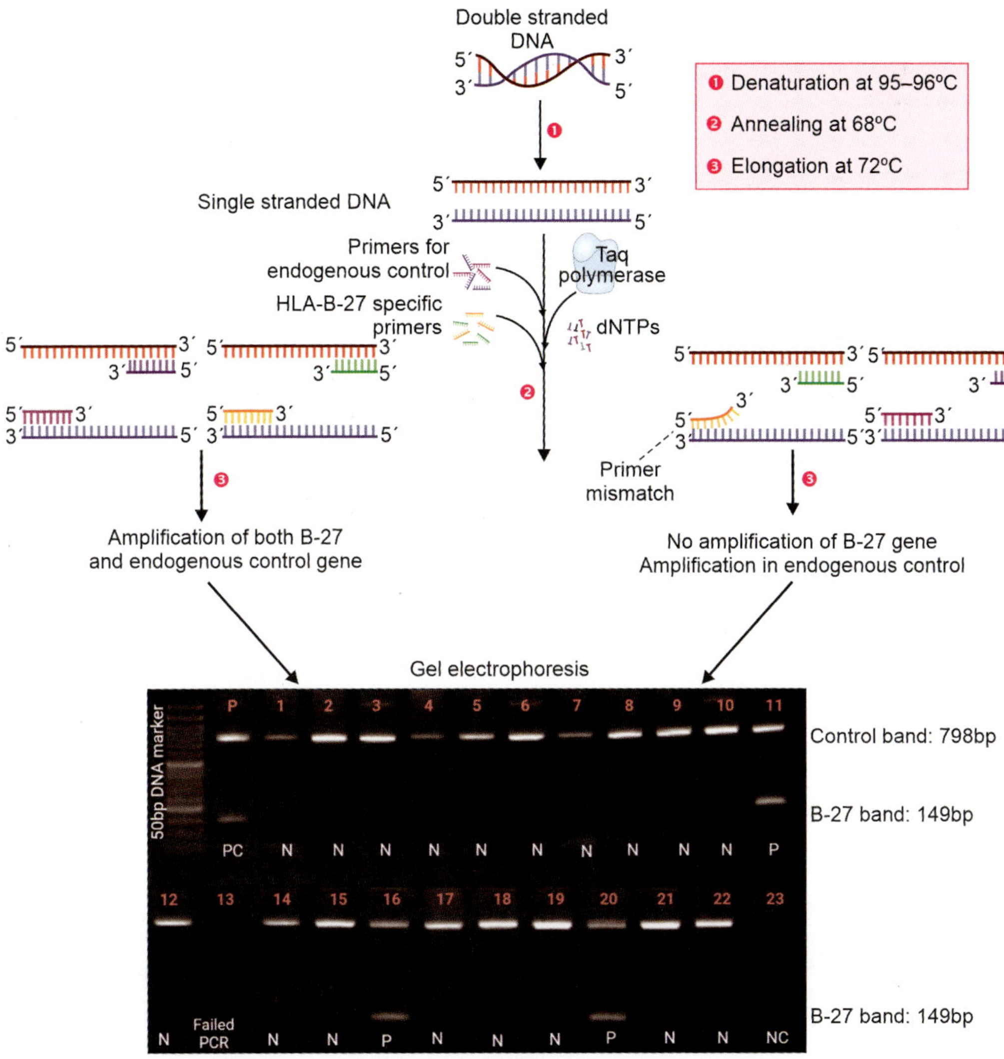

Fig. 7.1.14: HLA-B*27 PCR

exponential/plateau phase. During the initial cycles of amplification, although there is increase in fluorescence and PCR product accumulates exponentially, the signal remains undetectable. A detectable signal is produced after accumulation of sufficient amplified products. The cycle number at which the fluorescence is detected is called cycle threshold (Ct) and is inversely proportional to the quantity of DNA present.

Commonly used fluorescence dyes are SYBR Green I and TaqMan probes. SYBR Green is a fluorescent dye that binds non-specifically to any double stranded DNA. SYBR Green, when free in solution emits low fluorescence but when bound to double stranded DNA can emit many folds greater signal. Annealing and extension steps during PCR generates double stranded DNA with SYBR Green bound to it, causing a net increase in fluorescence for detection (Fig. 7.1.15).

TaqMan probes are designed to bind in between the target DNA marked by primers for amplification. A probe usually has a fluorescent reporter (R) on the 5' end and a quencher (Q) on the 3' end that are in close proximity. When the probe is intact, this proximity reduces the fluorescence emitted by the reporter dye by a mechanism called fluorescence resonance energy transfer (FRET). However, during each annealing and extension cycles of the PCR process, Taq DNA polymerase cleaves the reporter dye of the probe away from the quencher, leading to the emission of fluorescence by the reporter dye (Fig. 7.1.16).

Real-time PCR can be qualitative or quantitative and is used in the diagnosis of cancer, genetic abnormalities, infectious diseases, and emerging diseases like the new strains of flu and coronavirus (Fig. 7.1.17).

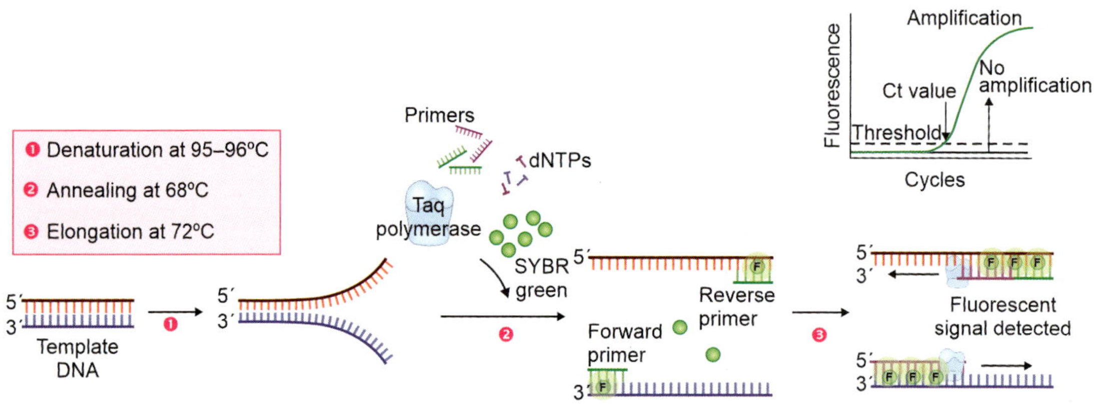

Fig. 7.1.15: Rreal-time PCR: SYBR green

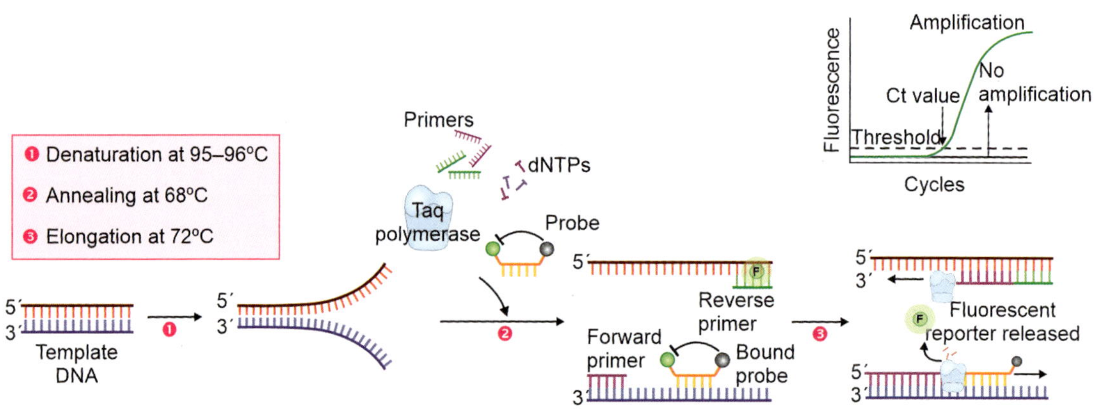

Fig. 7.1.16: Real-time PCR: TaqMan probe

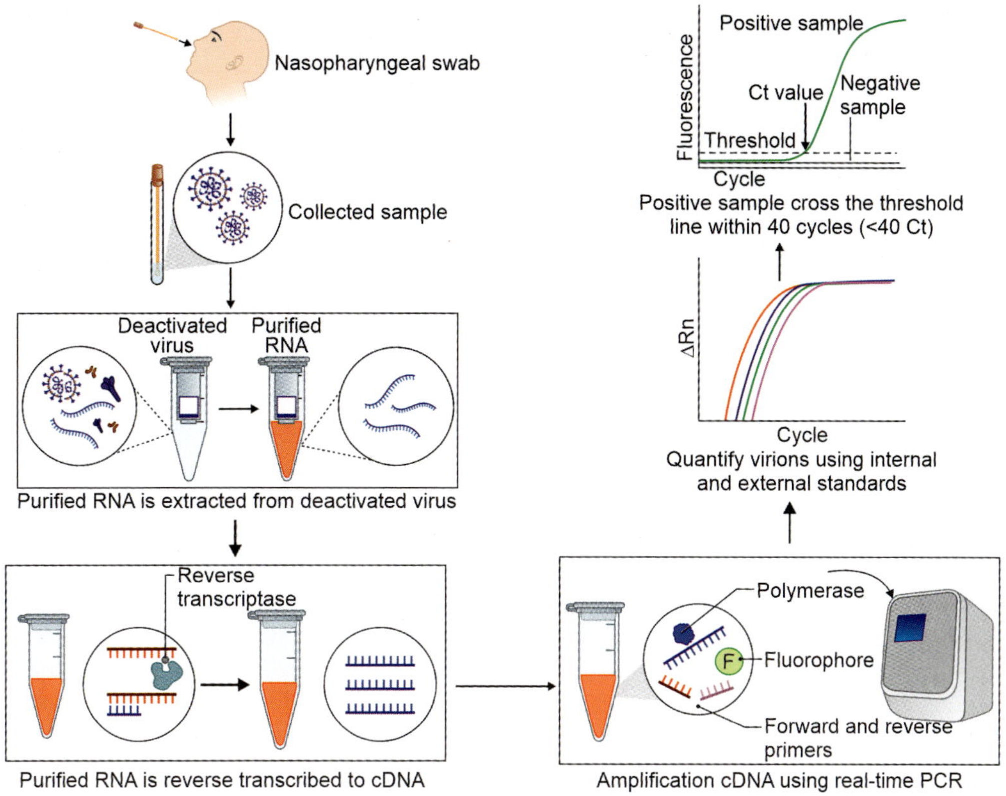

Fig. 7.1.17: Real-time PCR for detection of coronavirus

LEARNING POINTS

- Biomarkers can be anything that can be measured consistently and objectively
- Antigen-antibody reactions, enzyme-linked immunosorbent assay, immunofluorescence, western blotting are serological methods used for detection of immune markers
- Polymerase chain reaction and real-time PCR are molecular techniques used for detection of genetic biomarkers
- Methods used for biomarker detection should be highly specific and reproducible

FURTHER READING

1. Armstrong B. Antigen-antibody reactions. ISBT Science Series 2008; 3 (2): 21–32. https://doi.org/10.1111/j.1751-2824.2008.00185.x
2. Karst SM, Albertsen M, Kirkegaard RH, et al. Molecular Methods. In: van Loosdrecht MCM, Nielsen PH, Lopez-Vazquez CM, Brdjanovic D, editors. Experimental methods in wastewater treatment. ISBN: 9781780404752 (eBook). London UK: IWA Publishing; 2016. pp. 285–317.
3. Fineberg S. Antigen-antibody Reactions: An Overview. Immunochem Immunopathol 2022; 8:133. [cited June 15, 2023]. Available from chrome-extension://efaidnbmnnnibpcajpcglclefindmkaj/https://www.hilarispublisher.com/open-access/antigenantibody-reactions-an-overview.pdf
4. Willis JC, Lord GM. Immune biomarkers: the promises and pitfalls of personalized medicine. Nat Rev Immunol. 2015;15:323–9.

Chapter 7.2

Synovial Fluid Analyses for Crystals

Avinash Jain, Anuj Sharma

INTRODUCTION

Synovial fluid (SF) is an imperfect ultrafiltrate of blood plasma combined with hyaluronic acid produced by the synovial cells. It is imperfect as it allows small ions and molecules (e.g. sodium, potassium, glucose, urea) to readily pass into the joint space; however, large molecules are absent or present in trace amounts. Analysis of synovial fluid, a gold standard, is useful not only for diagnosing a multitude of joint diseases but is valuable for addressing a number of research questions. The focus of the chapter is SF analyses for crystals. Crystals are formed due to a process named supersaturation. In simple words, the synovial fluid contains more dissolved compounds than can ordinarily be accommodated which can lead to crystallization. Synovial fluid findings are inflammatory or non-inflammatory based on the total leukocyte count (Table 7.2.1).

NEED OF SYNOVIAL FLUID ANALYSIS FOR CRYSTALS

Synovial fluid analysis is the gold standard test for the diagnosis of crystals arthritis. The presence of monosodium urate (MSU) crystals is considered a sufficient criterion for diagnosing gout in a patient with at least one episode of arthritis or bursitis. This improves the sensitivity and specificity of classification criteria. The analysis is even more relevant in patients with mono- or oligoarthritis or patients with symmetrical arthritis with negative serology for rheumatoid and often low acute phase reactants.

INDICATIONS

The indications are patients presenting with monoarthritis suggestive of gout classically the metatarsophalangeal joint (MTP), or multiple joint involvements in case of tumor lysis/hematological malignancy, or symmetrical arthritis with waxing

Table 7.2.1: Types of synovial fluid effusion on basis of white blood cell (WBC) counts

Type of effusion	*WBC count*	*Example*
Non-inflammatory	<2000/mm^3	Osteoarthritis
Inflammatory	>2000/mm^3 WBC counts can be >50,000 in crystal arthropathy	Septic arthritis Reactive arthritis Spondyloarthritis Crystal arthropathy
Septic	> 50,000/mm^3	Bacterial
Hemorrhagic	Large number of red blood cells (RBCs)	Bleeding diathesis Trauma Tumor

and waning of articular inflammation independent of other joints and often negative for rheumatoid factor or anticitrullinated peptide antibodies. Other indications are acute exacerbation of knee osteoarthritis to rule out pseudogout. The presence of chondrocalcinosis, well-demarcated erosions with/without overhanging edges are some imaging clues of crystal arthritides. SF analysis aids in confirming gout and calcium pyrophosphate crystal deposition (CPPD) disease, pseudogout when during the evaluation of arthritis there are sonographic findings of chondrocalcinosis, snowstorm appearance, and double contour sign.

TIMING OF SYNOVIAL FLUID ANALYSIS

Ideally aspiration can be done during the flare or acute episode but MSU and calcium pyrophosphate (CPP) crystals can be detected even in asymptomatic individuals, particularly from the joint that was symptomatic previously or from tophi. This allows for diagnosis even in intercritical gout.

JOINT ASPIRATION PROCEDURE AND SAMPLE COLLECTION

Depending on clinical presentation and type of joint to be aspirated, the joint is aspirated either through blind approach or using ultrasound guidance. On the basis of a number of white blood cells, differential counts, gram stain, AFB stain, culture, crystals and cytology, and type of effusion, etiology of arthritis can be ascertained (Fig. 7.2.1).

Aspiration should be done under aseptic conditions using talc-free gloves using blind or ultrasound guidance depending on the joint and transferred to purple-top tube for cell count and a heparin tube for crystals. The gauge of the needle for aspiration depends on joint size, e.g. 21G and 25G needles are appropriate for knee and MTP joints respectively. Analysis of SF should be performed immediately preferably over a centrifuged sample for best results within 6 hours. The examination can be done for up to 24 hours if the fluid is kept at 4°C. This prevents the dissolution of crystals and cells.

EXAMINATION OF SYNOVIAL FLUID

This consists of physical examination, chemical examination, and microscopy examination.

Physical Examination

Parameters assessed include volume, colour, appearance, viscosity, clot and mucin clot test. Cloudy appearance can be an indicator presence of crystals as well as inflammatory infiltrate. The viscosity of the synovial fluid, a non-newtonian fluid, can change in different diseases. To check for viscosity, a string test is performed. Normal synovial fluid will form a "string" approximately 5 cm long before breaking. The presence or absence of a clot can lead to erroneous protein estimation along with cell count. Lastly, the mucin clot test is one of the best indicators of the integrity of the hyaluronate. Crystal arthropathies can result in decreased viscosity and a negative mucin clot test.

Chemical Examination

Synovial fluid protein estimation is generally not recommended as it does not add to the diagnostic value. However, increased synovial fluid protein levels are seen in ankylosing spondylitis, arthritis, and arthropathies that accompany Crohn's disease, gout, psoriasis, reactive arthritis, and ulcerative colitis.

Microscopy

There are various methods available to examine crystals. These include light microscopy, polarized light examination, phase-contrast microscopy, DiffQuik staining and Fourier transform infrared spectroscopy. Commonly light microscopy and polarized light examination are used.

Slide preparation: A very important step here is wet mount preparation. First, the sample should be centrifuged at 1500 G for 10 min. The supernatant should be separated (for a biochemical test) and centrifuged deposits should be taken on a pre-cleaned glass slide and a pre-cleaned cover slip is placed over it. Ensure that there is no air bubble or talc from gloves or dirt . It is essential to examine all areas on the microscope slide, and possibly to prepare a second wet mount to exclude or confirm the diagnosis particularly if CPPD is suspected as load of crystals is low, unlike in gout.

Light Microscopy

It is used to calculate white blood cell (WBC)/total leucocyte count and differential count. Crystal

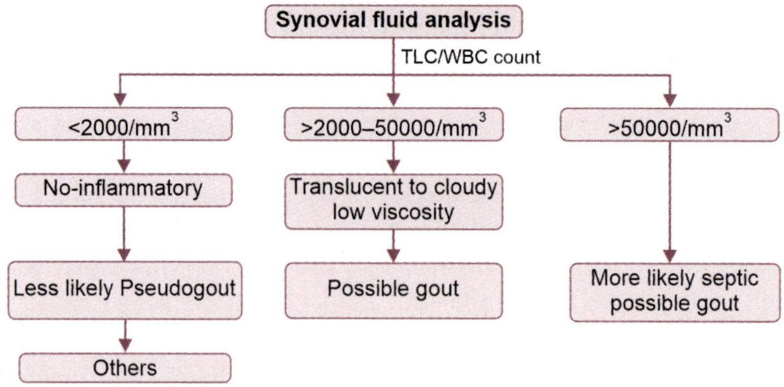

Polarizing microscopy			
Crystals	*Birefringence*	*Shape*	*Disease*
MSU	Strong negative*	Needle (intracellular and extracellular)	Gout
CPP	Weak positive*	Rhomboid (intracellular and extracellular)	CPPD disease Occasionally in OA, Milwaukee
Calcium hydroxyapatite*	Non-birefringent		OA Milwaukee
Calcium oxalate dihydrate	Variable	Bipyramidal octahedral	Chronic kidney disease, dialysis, and primary oxalosis
Cholesterol	Positive and negative	Flat, plate like with notched comers	Not believed to be pathogenic
Lipids	Positive	Maltese	
Corticosteroid	Highly birefringent		Mimic urate or CPPD
Glove crystals	Strongly birefringent	Maltese	
Other crystals	Monoclonal Ig crystals or cryoglobulins, Charcot–Leyden crystals, amyloid fragments, cartilage fragments, collagen fibrils and fibrin strands, hematoidin crystals from prior hemorrhage, crystals from certain anticoagulants, nail polish, prosthetic fragments, and dust particles		

*Compensated polarized microscopy–yellow or blue if long axis is parallel or perpendicular to axis of compensator, respectively

Fig. 7.2.1: Approach to crystal arthritis based on total leukocyte count (TLC)/white blood cell (WBC) count of synovial fluid. Different types of crystals are appreciated under a polarizing microscope

arthropathy can have high WBCs with predominant neutrophils (Table 7.2.1). Though not the standard, light microscopy at 600–1000× magnification can help identify needle-shaped MSU crystals and different shapes of CPP crystals (rhomboid, needle, rod, and parallelepiped).

Polarized Microscopy

Simple and compensated polarised microscopy allows the distinction of crystals by their birefringence. The latter uses a red compensator and is considered the standard for crystal identification. Halogen light is preferred as the source of light. MSU crystals appear yellow when its long axis is parallel to the compensator axis and red when it is perpendicular to the compensator axis (Fig. 7.2.2). CPP crystals show weak birefringence and appear blue when the long axis is parallel. Thus MSU crystals show strong birefringence shining brilliantly against a dark background while CPP crystals are weakly birefringent. MSU and CPP can co-occur but clinical relevance is not clear. It is important to identify intracellular crystals, particularly for MSU and CPP.

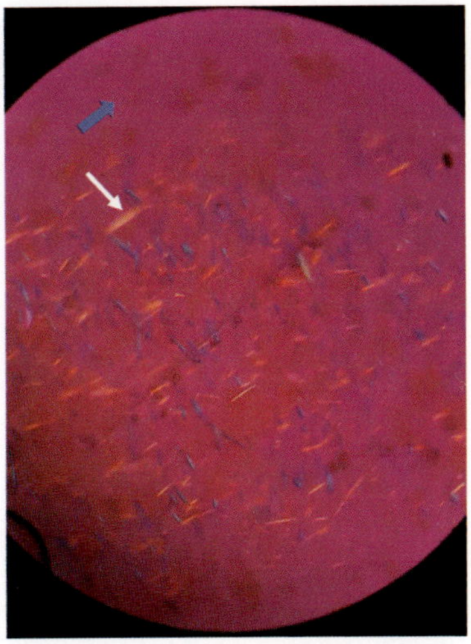

Fig. 7.2.2: Needle-shaped monosodium urate (MSU) crystals visualized under compensated polarized microscopic view. The blue arrow indicates the axis of the compensator. MSU crystals appear yellow is seen as indicated when the long axis is parallel to the compensator axis and blue when perpendicular

TYPES OF CRYSTALS

Figure 7.2.1 lists different types of crystals, shapes, and disease associations. In practice, the most commonly encountered crystals are MSU and CPP crystals. Intracellular MSU and CPP crystals can be present in gout/pseudogout patients during the asymptomatic phase as well. The presence of MSU crystals is considered a sufficient criterion for gout but needs to be done on a fresh sample by a trained observer.

LEARNING POINTS

- Synovial fluid analysis for crystals is the gold standard for the diagnosis of crystal arthritis and helps in confirming the diagnosis particularly in cases where the manifestations are not typical.
- This can even be done bedside for prompt recognition and institution of treatment.
- Compensated polarizing microscope is the standard tool but light microscopy can be useful too.
- MSU crystals show strong birefringence shining brilliantly against a dark background while CPP crystals are weakly birefringent when visualized under polarising microscope.

FURTHER READING

1. Lumbreras B, Pascual E, Frasquet J, et al. Analysis for crystals in synovial fluid: training of the analysts results in high consistency. Ann Rheum Dis. 2005; 64:612–5.
2. Neogi T, Jansen TLTA, Dalbeth N, et al. 2015 Gout classification criteria: an American College of Rheumatology/European League Against Rheumatism collaborative initiative. Ann Rheum Dis. 2015; 74:1789–98.
3. Pascual E, Batlle-Gualda E, Martínez A, et al. Synovial Fluid Analysis for Diagnosis of Intercritical Gout. Ann Intern Med. 1999; 131:756–9.

Interpretation of Antinuclear Antibodies

Dipendra Nath Ghosh, Parasar Ghosh

INTRODUCTION

Antinuclear antibodies (ANA) are a serological hallmark of systemic lupus erythematosus (SLE). They are found also in many other autoimmune rheumatic diseases such as systemic sclerosis (SSc), Sjogren's syndrome, and in non-rheumatic diseases such as type 1 autoimmune hepatitis (AIH).

ANA binds to various components of the nucleus namely DNA, histone, and/or complexes of DNA or RNA with proteins. The gold standard test to detect ANA is indirect immunofluorescence (IIF) assay using human epithelial cell line (HEp2) as a substrate (Fig. 7.3.1). HEp-2 cells grown as a semi-confluent monolayer are the substrate of choice because the cells and nuclei of HEp-2 are larger and easier to read for nuclear patterns compared with other substrates. Thus HEp2 cells have become the standard substrate in almost all commercially available ANA kits since the early 2000s.

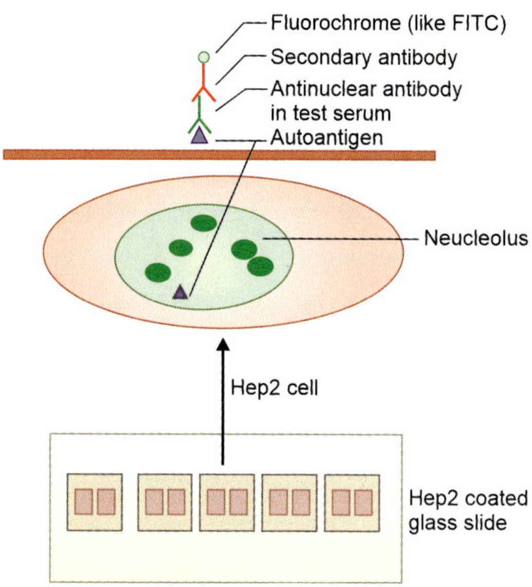

Fig. 7.3.1: ANA detection by indirect immunofluorescence using Hep2 cells as substrate

HEp2 IIF

ANA by HEp2 IIF assay is reported as a titer and pattern. The ACR/EULAR recommends evaluating HEp-2 ANA at a dilution of ≥1:80. A 1:80 titer has high sensitivity (97.8%) to detect SLE, albeit with the specificity of 74.7%.

Patterns on HEp2 IIF

HEp2 IIF assay not only detect antibodies directed to nuclear antigens (ANA) but they also detect antibodies that bind to cytoplasmic antigens and various mitotic structures. So in reality HEp2 IIF assay actually detects 'anti-cell antibodies' and not only antinuclear antibodies. Recently non-nuclear patterns are also considered clinically relevant.

While evaluating ANA by IIF assay various patterns are observed depending on the expression of antigens during specific phases of the cell cycle: interphase, prophase, metaphase, anaphase and telophase cell cycle (Fig. 7.3.2).

There are three major categories of ANA patterns by HEp2 IIF: (1) Nuclear patterns; (2) Cytoplasmic patterns, and (3) Mitotic patterns. However in clinical practice (for example in cases SLE), several autoantibodies may be present in a sample, and the image may appear as a mixed pattern.

The International Consensus on ANA Patterns (ICAP) formed in 2014 established the nomenclature and definitions of HEp-2 IIF assay patterns.

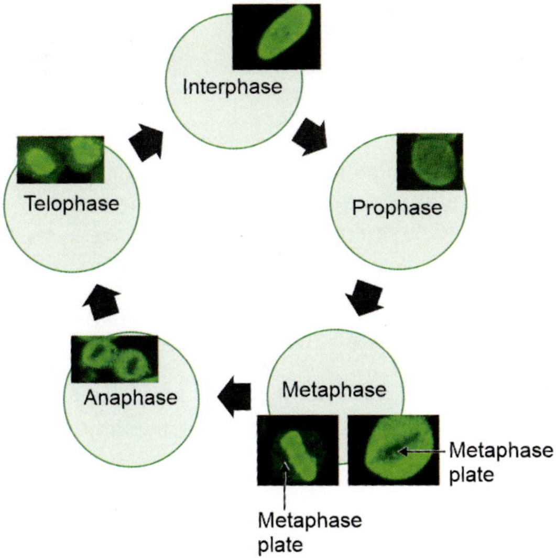

Fig. 7.3.2: Appearances of Hep2 cells in different phases of cell cycle. This helps in differentiation of patterns seen under fluorescent microscope

To date 29 patterns are described that are available on-line at the ICAP website: www.ANApatterns.org. Each HEp-2 IIF pattern is alphanumerically coded from AC-1 to AC-29.

I. Nuclear Pattern

The most commonly observed nuclear patterns are homogeneous, speckled, centromere, nucleolar, and nuclear dots. Table 7.3.1 lists the clinical associations with nuclear patterns. For example, the dense fine speckled pattern (DFS) is negatively associated with autoimmune disease.

a. **Nuclear homogeneous pattern:** This pattern indicates the presence of antibodies to dsDNA or histone. The resting HEp2 cell nucleus (interphase) exhibits a diffuse and homogeneous fluorescent staining, while in the dividing cell (metaphase) the chromatin shows solid homogeneous fluorescence staining (Fig. 7.3.3).

Table 7.3.1: Nuclear patterns by indirect immunofluorescence according to International Consensus on ANA Pattern (ICAP)

Nuclear patterns	*Clinical associations*
Homogeneous pattern *Antigens:* dsDNA, nucleosomes, histones	• SLE, AIH, JIA • Drug-induced lupus
Centromere pattern *Antigen:* CENP-A/B (C)	• Limited cutaneous SSc, also PBC
Fine speckled pattern *Antigen:* SS-A/Ro, SS-B/La, Mi-2, TIF1γ, TIF1β, Ku	• ANA-associated rheumatic diseases, particularly SLE, subacute cutaneous lupus erythematosus, neonatal lupus, congenital heart block, sjogren's syndrome, dermatomyositis and SSc. • Anti-La/SSB are usually found in association with anti-Ro/SSA, and samples with anti-La/SSB without anti-Ro/SSA reactivity are rare. • Anti-SS-A/Ro (Ro60) autoantibodies may be undetected in HEp-2 IIF (HEp-2010 has better sensitivity to detect Anti-SS-A/Ro).
Coarse speckled pattern *Antigen:* hnRNP, U1RNP, Sm, RNA polymerase III	• SLE, SSc, MCTD, UCTD. • Anti-Sm antibodies are predominantly directed against the Sm B/B' and SmD1 proteins. SmD1 is regarded as the most specific ENA in SLE. • If MCTD is suspected, it is recommended to perform a follow-up test for anti-U1RNP antibodies.
Dense fine speckled pattern *Antigen:* DFS70	• Apparently healthy individuals. • Negative association with autoimmune diseases.
Nucleolar homogeneous pattern *Antigens:* PM/Scl-75, PM/Scl-100, Th/To, etc.	• SSc, SSc/Polymyositis overlap syndrome. • Anti-PM/Scl antibodies produce diffuse nuclear fine speckled staining in addition to the nucleolar pattern.

(*Contd.*)

Table 7.3.1: Nuclear patterns by indirect immunofluorescence according to International Consensus on ANA Pattern (ICAP) *(Contd.)*

Nuclear patterns	*Clinical associations*
Nucleolar clumpy pattern *Antigen:* U3-snRNP/fibrillarin	• SSc • Anti-U3RNP/fibrillarin antibodies is associated with diffuse SSc, pulmonary arterial hypertension, skeletal muscle disease, severe cardiac involvement, and gastrointestinal dysmotility.
Nucleolar punctate pattern *Antigen:* RNA polymerase I, hUBF/NOR-90	• SSc, Sjogrens, and Raynaud's phenomenon. • Anti-RNApol I almost always coexist with anti-RNApol III antibodies.
Multiple Nuclear Dots pattern *Antigens:* Sp-100, PML proteins, MJ/NXP-2	• Dermatomyositis • Anti-Sp100 antibodies associate with PBC, particularly when associated with AMA.
Topo I pattern *Antigen:* DNA topoisomerase I	• Highly specific for SSc

b. **Nuclear speckled pattern:** There are two types: fine speckled (Fig. 7.3.4a) and coarse speckled (Fig. 7.3.4b).
   - The fine speckled pattern indicates reactivity with Ro (SSA) and La (SSB) antigens. This pattern on the resting HEp2 cells (interphase) shows a uniform distribution of fine speckles throughout the nuclei.
   - In the coarse speckled pattern resting cells exhibit coarse granular fluorescence throughout the entire nucleus. It occurs

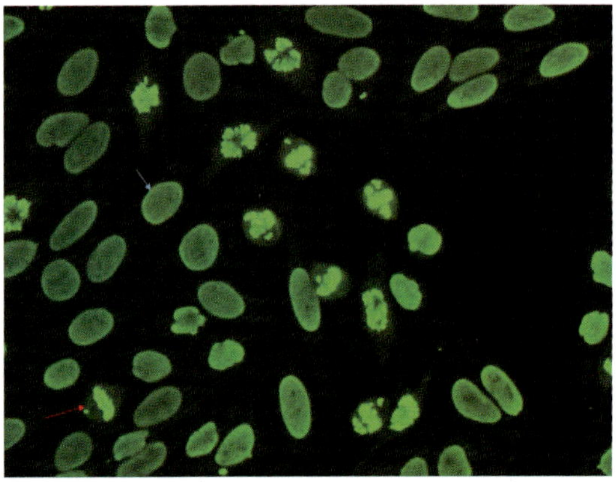

Fig. 7.3.3: Nuclear homogeneous pattern. (AC-1 according to the ICAP nomenclature). Note the diffuse homogeneous fluorescent staining of the nucleus (blue arrow) and the metaphase plate (red arrow).

Source: Chan EK, et al. Report of the First International Consensus on Standardized Nomenclature of Antinuclear Antibody HEp-2 Cell Patterns 2014–2015. Front Immunol 2015;6:412.

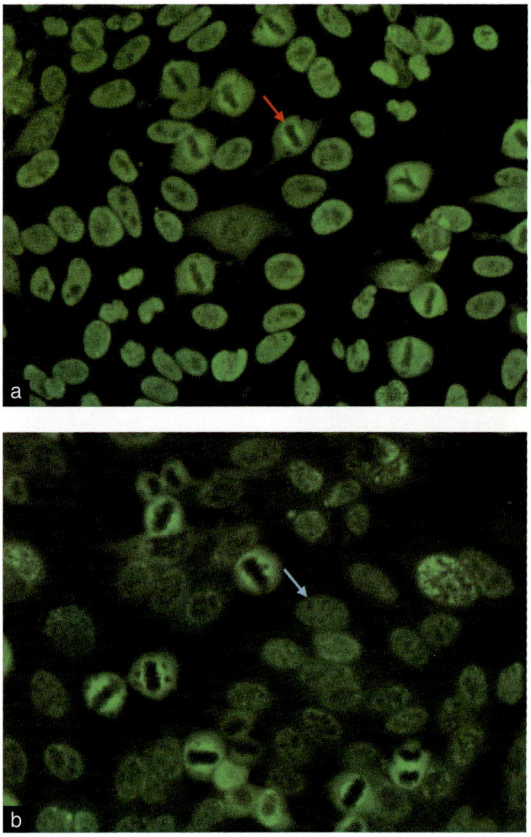

Fig. 7.3.4: Nuclear fine speckled pattern (AC–4) without staining of the metaphase plate red arrow (a); nuclear coarse speckled pattern (AC–5) blue arrow (b).

Source: Chan EK, et al. Report of the First International Consensus on Standardized Nomenclature of Antinuclear Antibody HEp-2 Cell Patterns 2014–2015. Front Immunol 2015;6:412.

when there are antibodies to RNP, Sm antigen, and RNA polymerase III amongst others. In both of the nuclear speckled patterns the condensed chromosomal regions of the mitotic cell are not stained.

- Dense fine speckled (DFS) pattern is increasingly described. There is fine speckling in the nucleus of the resting interphase cell with variable heterogeneity in size, distribution, and intensity of staining. The dividing cells show intense staining of the chromatin (metaphase) plate. DFS is negatively associated with autoimmune diseases.

c. **Centromere pattern:** This is a distinctive pattern due to the reactivity of antibodies to CENP A/B/C and is characteristic of limited cutaneous systemic sclerosis. In this pattern, the nucleus of the resting cell has about 40 to 80 discrete dots (Fig. 7.3.5) that align at the metaphase plate of the mitotic cell.

d. **Nuclear dots pattern:** The HEp2 resting cells show a few discrete (countable) dots in the nucleus of each cell. A few nuclear dots pattern has 1–6 dots/cell in most cells and indicates anti-p80 coilin. Few nuclear dots are also known as Cajal bodies or coiled bodies. Multiple nuclear dots pattern has 6–20 countable dots in each cell of most cells (Fig. 7.3.6). Indicates the presence of anti-SP100. Nuclear dots pattern can also co-exist with cytoplasmic staining (Fig. 7.3.7) and indicates the presence of autoantibodies to mitochondrial antigens.

e. **Nucleolar pattern:** Nucleolar patterns can be homogenous, clumpy, and punctate, identification of which needs a competent (expert) level interpretation (Fig. 7.3.8). The punctate nucleolar pattern was formerly called the nucleolar speckled pattern. In a homogeneous

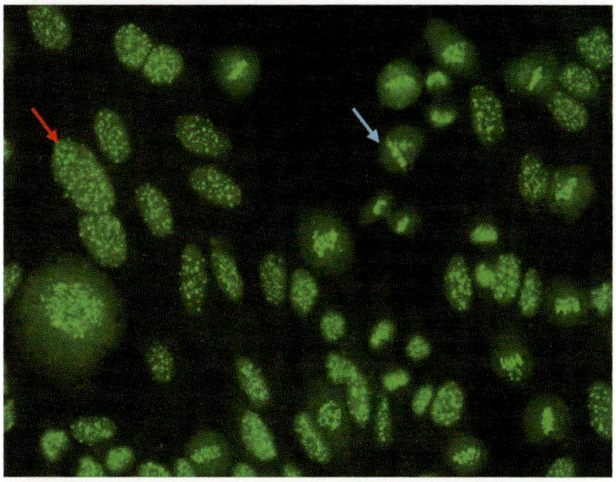

Fig. 7.3.5: Centromere pattern (AC–3). There are discrete dots on the nucleus of the resting cell (red arrow). Note the staining of the metaphase of the dividing cell 'metaphase bar'(blue arrow).

Source: Chan EK, et al. Report of the First International Consensus on Standardized Nomenclature of Antinuclear Antibody HEp-2 Cell Patterns 2014–2015. Front Immunol 2015;6:412.

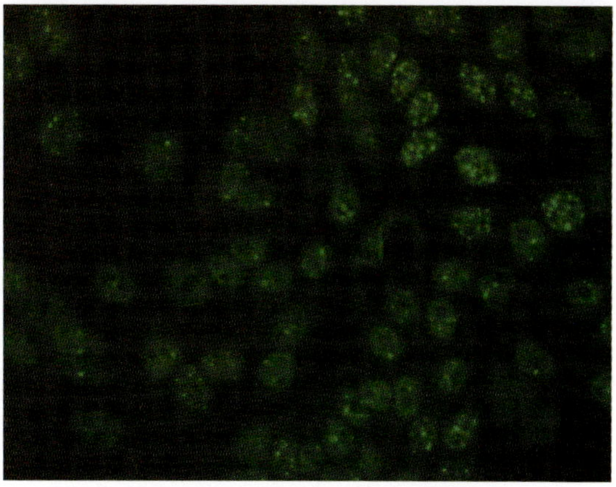

Fig. 7.3.6: Multiple nuclear dots pattern (AC–6)

Source: Chan EK, et al. Report of the First International Consensus on Standardized Nomenclature of Antinuclear Antibody HEp-2 Cell Patterns 2014–2015. Front Immunol 2015;6:412.

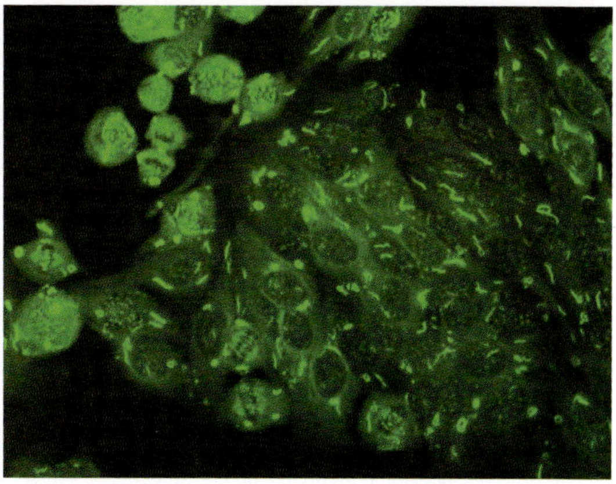

Fig. 7.3.7: Multiple nuclear dots (AC–6) and cytoplasmic rods and rings (AC–23)

Source: Chan EK, et al. Report of the First International Consensus on Standardized Nomenclature of Antinuclear Antibody HEp-2 Cell Patterns 2014–2015. Front Immunol 2015;6:412.

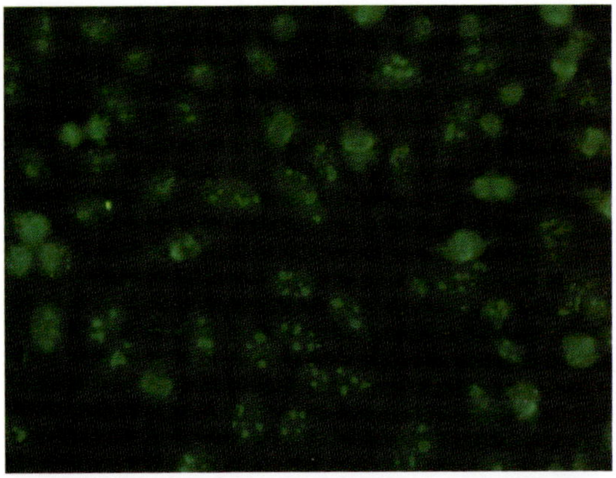

Fig. 7.3.8: Nucleolar pattern: Clumpy nucleolar pattern (AC–10)

Source: Chan EK, et al. Report of the First International Consensus on Standardized Nomenclature of Antinuclear Antibody HEp-2 Cell Patterns 2014–2015. Front Immunol 2015;6:412.

nucleolar pattern, the interphase (resting) cell shows fluorescence staining of the nucleolus. The metaphase plate does not stain. This pattern indicates autoantibodies to PM/Scl-75, PM/Scl-100, Th/To, etc.

There are various other nuclear patterns such as nuclear envelope pattern, PCNA-like, CENP-F like, Topo-1 like that are described in the ICAP website.

II. Cytoplasmic Patterns

There are five major cytoplasmic patterns. These are fibrillar, speckled, AMA, Golgi, and rods and rings.

a. **Cytoplasmic fibrillar patterns** are seen in diseases such as type 1 autoimmune hepatitis, celiac disease, and chronic hepatitis virus C (HCV) infection. They indicate the presence of antibodies to actin and non-muscle myosin. Can be found in MCTD. If the clinical diagnosis is type 1 AIH it is recommended to confirm reactivity with smooth muscle antibodies (ASMA) typically detected by IIF assay on mouse liver, stomach, kidney substrate.
b. **The cytoplasmic speckled pattern** is seen in myositis and antisynthetase syndrome. Anti-PL7, anti-PL-12 and ribosomal P proteins produce a cytoplasmic dense fine speckled pattern (Fig. 7.3.9), while anti-Jo1 produces a cytoplasmic fine speckled pattern.
c. **Cytoplasmic reticular pattern or AMA pattern** due to the presence of anti-mitochondrial antibodies is characterized by coarse filamentous staining throughout the cytoplasm (Fig. 7.3.10). Seen in primary biliary cirrhosis (PBC), systemic sclerosis (SSc), and overlaps of PBC with SSc, PBC with Sjogren's syndrome.
d. **Golgi or polar pattern.** This is a rare pattern indicating presence of antibodies to RNA processing and transport systems such as the Golgi complex. It is visible as a perinuclear ribbon-like staining in the cytoplasm.

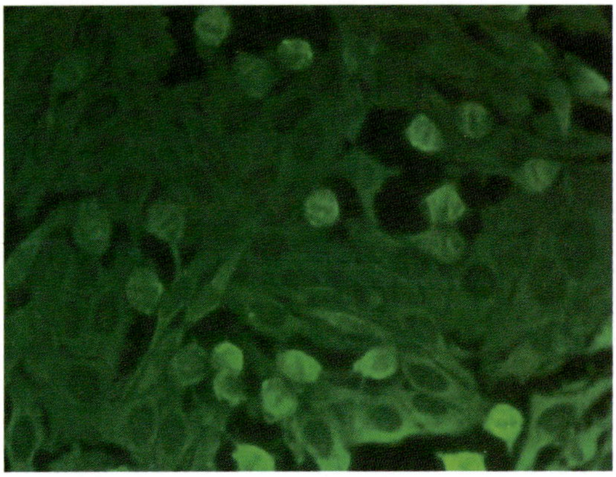

Fig. 7.3.9: Cytoplasmic dense speckled pattern (AC–19)

Source: Chan EK, et al. Report of the First International Consensus on Standardized Nomenclature of Antinuclear Antibody HEp-2 Cell Patterns 2014–2015. Front Immunol 2015;6:412.

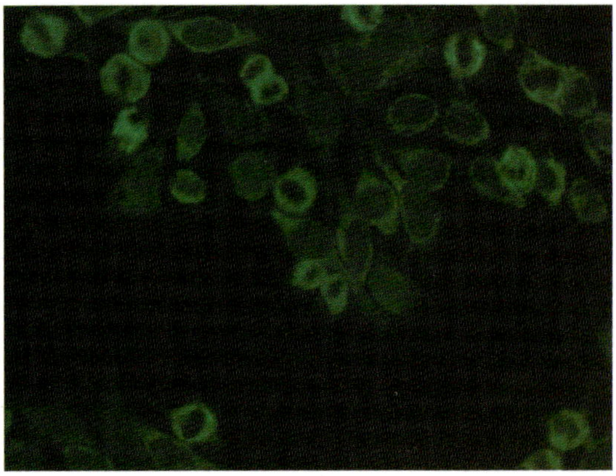

Fig. 7.3.10: Cytoplasmic reticular (AC–21)

Source: Chan EK, et al. Report of the First International Consensus on Standardized Nomenclature of Antinuclear Antibody HEp-2 Cell Patterns 2014–2015. Front Immunol 2015;6:412.

e. **Rods and rings pattern**: This pattern of distinct rods in the cytoplasm (Fig. 7.3.11) is described in patients with chronic HCV infection who have been treated with interferons.

Fig. 7.3.11: Rods and rings (AC–23)

Source: Chan EK, et al. Report of the First International Consensus on Standardized Nomenclature of Antinuclear Antibody HEp-2 Cell Patterns 2014–2015. Front Immunol 2015;6:412.

III. Mitotic Patterns

Antibodies to mitotic spindle apparatus (MSA) are very rare patterns and seen in <0.018% of positive IIF ANA. Their clinical associations are with connective tissue diseases (CTDs), infections, cancer, and PBC. According to the ICAP, there are five mitotic patterns (Table 7.3.2) that are identified at the competent level.

a. **Centrosome pattern:** Mitotic patterns appear as two discrete dots on opposite sides of the metaphase plate of Hep2 cells by IIF assay and they indicate the presence of antibodies to centrosome protein.

b. **Spindle fiber and NuMA pattern:** Another mitotic pattern is the staining of spindle fibers (but not the chromosome plate), due to antibodies to spindle fibers (spindle fiber pattern (Fig. 7.3.12). The NuMA pattern is a sub-pattern of the spindle fibre pattern, which is the staining of the entire Nuclear Mitotic Apparatus (NuMA). In the anaphase and metaphase, there is staining of the spindle poles and proximal part of spindle fibres taking on the shape of a banana.

Both of these are also called MSA2 and MSA1 respectively. Though are found in only 0.3% and 0.4% of positive ANA samples, they are the most frequent mitotic patterns. About 50% of NuMA patterns have clinical associations with CTDs.

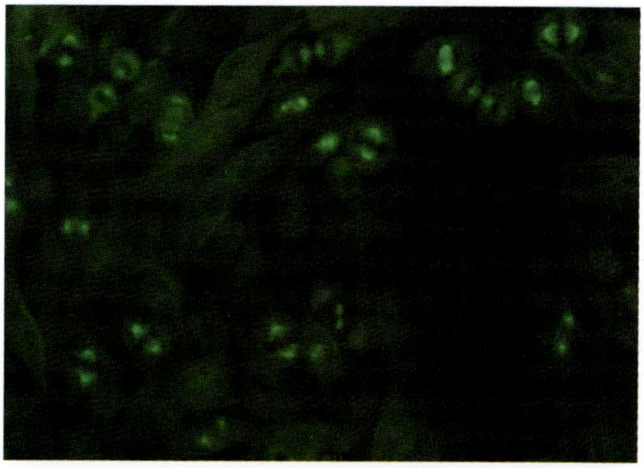

Fig. 7.3.12: Spindle fiber pattern (Non-NuMA) (AC–25)

Source: Chan EK, et al. Report of the First International Consensus on Standardized Nomenclature of Antinuclear Antibody HEp-2 Cell Patterns 2014-2015. Front Immunol 2015;6:412.

Table 7.3.2: Mitotic patterns on HEp2 cells indirect immunofluorescence according to International Consensus on ANA Pattern (ICAP)

Mitotic patterns	*Clinical associations*
Centrosome pattern	Rarely can be seen in UCTD, Raynaud's phenomenon, limited cutaneous SSc, and SLE. Also seen in viral infections
Spindle fibers pattern (MSA1) NuMA pattern (MSA2)	NuMA patterns indicate antibodies to the mitotic spindle apparatus (MSA). They are described in the literature as anti-MSA antibodies. Approximately half patients with MSA patterns have associated autoimmune disease mainly Sjogrens, RA, SLE, UCTD. They can also be found in infections, malignancy and primary biliary cirrhosis.
Intercellular bridge	SSc, Raynaud's, and malignancy
Mitotic chromosomal	Rarely seen in discoid lupus erythematosus, chronic lymphocytic leukaemia, Sjogren's syndrome, and polymyalgia rheumatica.

c. The other mitotic patterns described are intercellular bridge and mitotic chromosome coat.

HEp-2 IIF patterns can predict organ involvement and clinical phenotype in ANA-associated rheumatic diseases.

LEARNING POINTS

- Detection of ANAs by Hep-2 IIF includes endpoint titre and fluorescent patterns.
- ICAP has classified ANA staining patterns into three staining categories: nuclear, cytoplasmic and mitotic patterns. To date, 29 ANA patterns have been identified.
- The nuclear pattern is commonly associated with many systemic autoimmune diseases.
- The cytoplasmic speckled pattern is associated with myositis and antisynthetase syndrome.
- The presence of cytoplasmic pattern on HEp2 IIF assay is also distinctive of organ-specific autoimmune diseases such as type 1 AIH.
- Mitotic patterns are found in <1% of ANA-positive samples. An example of a mitotic pattern is the spindle fibre pattern and NuMA pattern which indicates the presence of antibodies to the mitotic spindle apparatus.

FURTHER READING

1. Andrade LEC, Klotz W, Herold M, et al. International consensus on antinuclear antibody patterns: definition of the AC-29 pattern associated with antibodies to DNA topoisomerase I. Clin Chem Lab Med 2018; 56:1783–1788.
2. Chan EK, Damoiseaux J, Carballo OG, et al. Report of the First International Consensus on Standardized Nomenclature of Antinuclear Antibody HEp-2 Cell Patterns 2014–2015. Front Immunol 2015; 6:412.
3. Chan EK, Damoiseaux J, de Melo Cruvinel W, et al. Report on the second International Consensus on ANA Pattern (ICAP) workshop in Dresden 2015. Lupus 2016; 25:797–804.
4. Ghosh P, Dwivedi S, Naik S, et al. Antinuclear antibodies by indirect immunofluorescence: optimum screening dilution for diagnosis of systemic lupus erythematosus. Indian J Med Res 2007; 126:34–8.

Chapter 7.4

Autoantibodies in Systemic Lupus Erythematosus

Ranjan Gupta

INTRODUCTION

Antinuclear antibodies (ANA) are hallmark serological tests for systemic lupus erythematosus (SLE). SLE is an autoimmune disease with large number of detectable autoantibodies. 2019 European League against Rheumatism (EULAR)/American College of Rheumatology (ACR) classification criteria for systemic lupus erythematosus have made ANA as a mandatory entry criterion for classification of SLE.

ANA TESTS FOR ALL THE POSSIBLE ANTIGENIC SPECIFICITIES IN THE NUCLEUS

ANA are commonly tested by indirect immunofluorescence (IIF) as it has the following advantages over ELISA:

1. Indirect (IIF) has the distinct advantage of testing these antigens in their location within the cell while ELISA tests only some of the antigens on a solid phase assay.
2. IIF assays also provide the information about the probable target antigen(s) and the underlying disease.
3. IIF assays are more sensitive than ELISA and are the test of choice for ANA.
4. With newer technology, IIF can be fully automated to test a particular number of samples.

ANA testing by IIF has been revolutionized after the replacement of the conventional rat liver cells by the human epithelial type-2 (HEp-2) cells as substrate. HEp-2 cells are large cells with its nucleus-occupying almost 80% of the cellular space. Since HEp-2 cells are fixed at various stages of cell cycle, IIF patterns give information not only on nuclear and cytoplasmic antigens within them but also on the mitotic patterns and antigens. A recent modification of HEp-2 cell line with transfected Ro-60 antigen (HEp-2K) expresses Ro much more as compared with the HEp-2 making it more suitable for diagnosis of SLE.

The results with IIF are conventionally reported with 3 parameters: *dilution*, *pattern* and *intensity*, all of which have different relevance. For diagnosing SLE, samples should test positive at a dilution equal/higher to 1:80 (EULAR/ACR 2019 guidelines). Testing at lower dilutions makes it more sensitive but loses specificity traditional testing to endpoint dilutions is not recommended anymore. Pattern of IIF is not specific to any disease but may point to associated antigen, e.g. homogeneous pattern is associated with histones, ds-DNA, nucleosomes and points towards SLE. Intensity informs about the concentration of autoantibodies in the given sample.

Extractable Nuclear Antigen (ENA) Testing

ANA testing do not provide any information about the target antigen that gave the positive result. ENA testing is the next step following ANA to identify which antigens give rise to ANA positivity. ENA testing can either be done by ELISA or by immunoblot assay. Immunoblot assays have the advantage of testing 15–17 antigens in a single assay. Different autoantibodies detected through these assays are of prognostic value as several clinical manifestations have been associated with these autoantibodies (Table 7.4.1).

SLE Specific Autoantibodies

SLE has the highest prevalence of autoantibodies among the rheumatic diseases. However, among the

Table 7.4.1: Prevalence and clinical association of the most common autoantibodies in SLE

S.No.	*Autoantibody*	*Prevalence (%)*	*Clinical association*
1.	Antinuclear antibodies (ANA)	>99	Needed for classifying the patient as SLE; Mandatory entry criteria as per EULAR/ACR 2019 criteria, Must be positive for drug induced lupus.
2.	Antihistone antibodies	70	Diagnostic hallmark of drug-induced lupus.
3.	Anti-ds DNA antibodies	60	95% specific for SLE, Associated with glomerulonephritis, serum levels parallel disease activity of SLE
4.	Anti-Smith antibodies	20–30	99% specific for SLE
5.	Anti-Ro antibodies	30	Associated with cutaneous manifestations like sub-acute cutaneous lupus, photosensitivity in the patient; chances of neonatal lupus and congenital heart block in the fetus.
6.	Anti-La antibodies	20	
7.	Antiphospholipid antibodies	30	Associated with pregnancy morbidity and vascular events and with development of pulmonary artery hypertension.

rheumatic disease. However, among the clinically useful and SLE-specific autoantibodies, anti-ds DNA and anti-Smith (anti-Sm) antibodies are routinely used in clinics. Anti-ds DNA antibodies are commonly measured using ELISA and the levels are considered to be the biomarkers of the clinical disease activity. Anti-Sm antibodies are also highly specific for SLE but unlike anti-ds DNA antibodies, are not recommended for repeated testing to assess disease activity. Both of these antibodies have low sensitivity (60% and 30%, respectively) for diagnosing SLE and therefore, should not be the first antibodies to be tested for this purpose and also, should not be ordered to rule in the diagnosis of SLE if ANA is negative.

Antibodies related to antiphospholipid syndrome (APS), i.e. anticardiolipin antibodies, anti-β2 Gp I antibodies and lupus anticoagulant should be tested in all patients at diagnosis. Testing for them is must in the ones who have history of vascular event (arterial like stroke or venous like deep venous thrombosis) or pregnancy morbidity. Their positivity, only once, is needed to fulfil the immunological criteria of SLE as per the EULAR/ACR 2019 guidelines whereas repeat positivity at a gap of at least 12 weeks is needed to fulfil the classification criteria of APS.

LEARNING POINTS

- The positive predictive value of ANA in the diagnosis of SLE is 20–30% whereas the negative predictive value is almost 100%. Thus a negative ANA test virtually rules out the diagnosis of SLE.
- ANA, once positive by any method, should not be repeated by other methods. Repeated ANA testing should not be used as a biomarker for follow-up of SLE patients.
- In patients with low suspicion of SLE and ANA being negative, specific autoantibody testing for anti-ds DNA and anti-Sm antibodies should not be done.
- It is not recommended to hike up the immunosuppression for high anti-ds DNA levels in an SLE patient who is otherwise in clinical remission. Close observation for the development of clinical flare is suggested in these serologically active clinically quiescent patients.
- All female patients of SLE who test positive for anti-Ro and/or Anti-La antibodies should undergo regular fetal monitoring for heart block during pregnancy.

FURTHER READING

1. Aringer M, Costenbader K, Daikh D, Brinks R, Mosca M, Ramsey-Goldman R, et al. 2019 European League Against Rheumatism/American College of Rheumatology Classification Criteria for Systemic Lupus Erythematosus. Arthritis Rheumatol. 2019; 71:1400–12.
2. Xiao ZX, Miller JS, Zheng SG. An updated advance of autoantibodies in autoimmune diseases. Autoimmun Rev. 2021; 20:102743.

Chapter 7.5

Lupus Anticoagulant: Principles and Interpretation

Prita Pradhan

INTRODUCTION

Lupus anticoagulants (LAC) are essentially anti-phospholipid antibodies (APLA). They are called anticoagulants since they have a prothrombin time prolonging effect *in vitro*. However, they are only prothrombotic *in vivo* and do not cause bleeding. As these were initially detected in patients with systemic lupus erythematosus, hence the name lupus anticoagulant has been used.

These have been detected in various infections ranging from syphilis to COVID-19. These may be IgG or IgM. They may be normally present and prevalence increases with advancing age. LAC detection can be done via tests like kaolin clotting time (KCT), partial thromboplastin time (PTT) or LA sensitive PTT or dilute Russell viper venom test (dRVVT). Of all these, the dRVVT is the most commonly performed. A newer test is the Taipan viper venom test which can be carried out even in the sera of patients on anticoagulation (may cause false-positives in other tests).

dRVVT TESTING

Principle

Dilute Russel viper venom (dRVV) is a direct activator of factor X. So, upon addition of dRVV to normal plasma, there is immediate activation of the common pathway in the presence of phospholipids and calcium. However, when LAC is present in the plasma, they prevent the direct activation of factor X by dRVV due to obscuring of the epitopes of reagent phospholipids by LAC. So the clot formation gets delayed.

Prolongation of dRVVT in a patient's plasma is considered a positive 'screening test'. When the screening test is prolonged, external phospholipids are added to the sera and the test is repeated. On this repeat test, if the dRVVT prolongation is corrected, then it is considered 'confirmatory' evidence of LAC.

Commercial Kits

Commercially available kit has a screen R1 and a confirm R1 reagent which essentially differ only in the concentration of the phospholipids. Confirm R1 contains higher concentrations of phospholipids while both have dRVV. The other reagent needed is calcium chloride to initiate the coagulation cascade. Anticoagulated patient blood is collected in citrated vials and centrifuged to obtain platelet-poor plasma (PPP).

Methods

All reagents are warmed to 37°C. Calcium chloride is first added and then R1 screen is added to the patient's platelet-poor plasma. A stopwatch is used to time till clotting starts. The screen time is generally 24–42s. When screen time is prolonged confirm tests should be done.

The same procedure is repeated with the confirm reagents and the confirm time is noted. The ratio 'R' is calculated by dividing the mean screen time by the mean confirm time. R <1.3 is considered normal while an increase is considered abnormal.

Next control plasma (pooled plasma of healthy people) is added to exclude false positivity due to clotting factor deficiencies.

Interpretation

The screen time is generally 24–42s. When screen time is prolonged confirm tests should be done.

Table 7.5.1: LAC screen test, LAC confirm test and Interpretation

LAC screen test		*LAC confirm test*		*Interpretation*
Patient plasma	*1:1 Mixing with control normal plasma*	*Patient plasma*	*1:1 Mixing with control normal plasma*	
Normal	–	Normal	–	LAC absent
Abnormal	–	Normal	–	LAC present
Abnormal	Normal	Abnormal	Normal	Factor deficiency
Abnormal	Abnormal	Abnormal	Normal	LAC present + Factor deficiency

The ratio 'R' is calculated by dividing the mean screen time by the mean confirm time. R <1.3 is considered as normal while an increase is considered as abnormal. R >1.8 is strongly positive while 1.5 < R <1.8 is moderately positive and 1.3 < R <1.5 is weakly positive or equivocal (Table 7.5.1).

As dRVV is a direct activator of the common pathway the factor deficiencies of the common pathway may also prolong the test. So the mixing studies with normal control plasma will help in resolving the same. Platelets are rich sources of phospholipids, and therefore, platelet-poor plasma preparation should be optimal to avoid errors in interpretation. All tests should be interpreted in appropriate clinical context.

LEARNING POINTS

- 'Lupus anticoagulant' is a misnomer.
- LAC detection is most commonly done with dilute Russel viper venom.
- There are two tests: 'LA screen' and 'LA confirm'.
- If positive, it should be repeated with pooled plasma to exclude clotting factor deficincies.

FURTHER READING

1. Love PE, Santoro SA. Antiphospholipid antibodies: anticardiolipin and the lupus anticoagulant in systemic lupus erythematosus (SLE) and in non-SLE disorders. Prevalence and clinical significance. Ann Intern Med. 1990; 112:682–98.
2. Pengo V, Bison E, Banzato A, Zoppellaro G, Jose SP, Denas G. Lupus Anticoagulant Testing: Diluted Russell Viper Venom Time (dRVVT). Methods Mol Biol Clifton NJ. 2017; 1646:169–76.
3. Simanek R, Panzer S, Lechner K, Pabinger I. Late spontaneous remissions in severe adult autoimmune thrombocytopenia. Ann Hematol. 2007; 86:705–10.

Chapter 7.6

Autoantibodies in Rheumatoid Arthritis

Parshant Aggarwal

INTRODUCTION

Autoantibody testing constitutes an important aspect of clinical evaluation as well as classification process of patients suspected to have rheumatoid arthritis (RA). Demonstration of rheumatoid factor as an autoantibody was the first direct evidence of the autoimmune origins of RA. In addition to being biomarkers for RA, autoantibodies play a role in pathogenesis. The spectrum of autoantibodies in RA is discussed here.

1. **Rheumatoid factor (RF):** The rheumatoid factor is an IgM, IgG, or IgA directed against the Fc component of IgG. It was classically detected by hemagglutination assay using antigens coated on sheep RBC, and subsequently using latex particles. The latex agglutination assay was used widely because of its low cost and ease of performance. It primarily detected IgM-RF and therefore practically RF was taken as the IgM class of RF. The results are expressed as positive or negative. But by dilution of serum, a semiquantitative report can be generated and reported with the positive maximal dilution in which the serum shows agglutination.

   Currently, RF is measured using nephelometry assay and results are quantitatively expressed in IU/mL. Nephelometry can detect low levels of RF, and thus is more sensitive than latex agglutination. Routinely it is the IgM class of RF that is measured.

   RF is not specifically associated with RA but is present in several other autoimmune diseases (Table 7.6.1) including SLE, Sjögren's syndrome, cryoglobulinemia, sarcoidosis, hypothyroidism, and chronic infections thus limiting its diagnostic potential. It can be even found in up to 5% of normal individuals and higher in elderly healthy individuals. At a higher level, the specificity is better for a diagnosis of RA. The sensitivity of RF is in the range of 50–60% but the specificity is only 60%.

2. **Anticitrullinated peptide antibodies (ACPA):** Citrullination is a process of post-translational modification of arginine to citrulline by the enzyme peptidyl arginine deaminase (PAD). Several citrullinated proteins such as citrullinated filaggrin (found in buccal epithelial cells), and citrullinated vimentin (found in esophageal epithelial cells) have been found to be specific targets of autoantibodies in RA. These antibodies were first discovered as antiperinuclear factors and antikeratin antibodies detected by immunofluorescence techniques. Subsequently, synthetic linear citrullinated peptides derived from human filaggrin were developed that could be detected by ELISA. Further, a cyclic citrullinated peptide (CCP) was developed with improved antigen composition and antibody recognition, on the basis of which the first-generation anticyclic citrullinated peptide antibodies (anti-CCP1) were developed.

   Subsequently, more peptides were added and second and third-generation assays were developed called anti-CCP2 and anti-CCP3. Anti-CCP2 has higher sensitivity and better prognostic value in comparison to anti-CCP1. In anti-CCP3 additional citrullinated epitopes are included in the same protein structure but the advantage over anti-CCP2 has not been clearly demonstrated.

Table 7.6.1: Comparison of rheumatoid factor (RF), anticitrullinated peptide antibodies (ACPA) anti-carbamylated P antibodies (anti-CarP Ab)

Properties	*RF*	*ACPA*	*anti-CarP Ab*
Role in the diagnosis of RA	RF is included in 1987 Ameican Rheumatism Association (ARA), and the 2010 EULAR/ACR classification criteria for RA	Included in the 2010 EULAR/ ACR criteria	Not included in any classification criteria for RA. May be helpful in those patients who are RF or ACPA negative
Sensitivity	70–80%	77.5–78.8%	35–46.8%
Specificity	85%	88–97%	93–97%
Other associations	Positive also in autoimmune diseases: Sjogren's syndrome, SLE, sarcoidosis, MCTD, autoimmune hepatitis, etc. Infection such as HCV, TB, etc. and old age	Smoking Mucosal dysbiosis Other inflammatory arthritis, e.g. SLE, Sjogren's syndrome, psoriasis, juvenile idiopathic arthritis Infections: TB, HIV	Autoimmune disease: SLE, Sjogren's, systemic sclerosis, idiopathic inflammatory myositis, autoimmune thyroiditis Renal disease Normal Individuals
Prognosis	High titers associated with severe arthritis, extra-articular manifestations, and cardiovascular morbidity in RA	ACPA is associated with increased risk of progression to RA, severe articular disease, and higher cardiovascular morbidity	Triple positivity may confer higher risk of progression to RA Increased cardiovascular morbidity
Therapeutics	Associated with better response to rituximab, tofacitinib	Associated with better response to abatacept, rituximab, tofacitinib	Associated with better response to abatacept

Anti-MCV is antibodies to mutated citrullinated vimentin. It has been detected in a few anti-CCP2 negative patients and is predictive of poor radiological prognosis, and severe extra-articular manifestations. However, a number of studies have raised issues regarding the diagnostic performance of anti-MCV.

Newer assays detect non-cyclic citrullinated peptides thus anti-CCPs are now named anti-citrullinated peptide antibodies (ACPA). The sensitivity of ACPA is similar to RF while the specificity is >90% (higher than RF).

3. **Anticarbamylated protein antibodies (Anti-CarP Ab):** Proteins resulting from post-translational modifications (PTM) other than citrullination can also trigger autoimmune response. Anti-CarP Ab is the best-studied anti-PTM autoantibody. Anti-CarP Ab can be detected in preclinical RA. In established RA sensitivity is reported to be 27–46% while specificity is more than 90%. The presence of triple positive RF, ACPA, and Anti-CarP Ab in early arthritis patients confers a positive predictive value (PPV) of 96.1% for development of RA. However the role of anti-CarP Ab in routine clinical settings has not been defined.
4. **Other autoantibodies:** Various other autoantibodies have been described in RA which are not in routine clinical use. Some of these are antibodies to anti-p68 (BiP), RA33, Gal 0, alpha-enolase, glucose phosphate isomerase (GPI), ferritin/enzyme peptidyl-arginine deiminase 4 (PADI4).

A summary of RF, ACPA, and anti-Car P antibodies and their utility in clinical practice are given in Table 7.6.1.

ROLE OF RF AND ACPA IN THE DIAGNOSIS OF RA

Autoantibody testing constitutes an important aspect of clinical evaluation as well as the classification of RA for research purposes. RF constituted one of the variables in the 1987 American Rheumatism Association (ARA) classification criteria for RA. The patient could be classified as RA if 4 criteria were fulfilled. Both RF and ACPA are included in the 2010 European League Against Rheumatism (EULAR)/American College of Rheumatology (ACR) classification criteria for RA. In the EULAR/ACR criteria, autoantibodies may contribute up to 50% of the scores needed to classify as definite RA.

Cutoffs are generally described in comparison to healthy controls. For example, the cutoff for RF is generally the level at which 95% of healthy normal controls have negative results. It implies that the proportion of false-positive RF subjects will be much higher than actual RA patients with RF positivity considering that the prevalence of RA in the general population is low. Also, the specificity of the test is likely to be lower in the context of a diseased individual. Similarly, although the specificity of ACPA of about 97% seems very impressive, if the test were to be conducted on randomly selected individuals the proportion of nondiseased false-positives will be much higher than in actual RA patients. It has been found that the probability of RA developing in ACPA-positive individuals is 9% in the general population, 53% if genetic and environmental risk factors were present, 55% in clinically suspect arthralgia subjects, and 80% in undifferentiated arthritis. Hence careful patient selection is of utmost importance before ordering RF or ACPA. RA is a clinical diagnosis. The presence or absence of autoantibodies does not confirm or rule out the diagnosis. Up to 20% of RA patients may remain negative for RF and ACPA throughout the disease course.

The mere presence of RF or ACPA does not make a diagnosis of RA: The following case illustrates this point:

Mr. SK is 65 years old male, a smoker for the past 30 years (pack years 12). He was complaining of low-grade fever, severe fatigue, and arthralgias for 6 months. Acute phase reactants were elevated: Westergren ESR 85 mm in the first hour, CRP 50 mg/L. RF was 280 IU/mL (positive >20 IU/mL), and ACPA was 200 U/mL (positive >15 U/ml). A provisional diagnosis of RA was considered and patient was referred to rheumatology. On evaluation by the rheumatologist, the patient had no objective evidence of synovitis prompting evaluation to rule out other aetiologies. CT chest revealed a lung mass, and a biopsy showed non-small cell lung carcinoma. This case underscores the importance of clinical context in which laboratory tests need to be interpreted and that no test can confirm or rule out the diagnosis of RA.

ROLE IN PREDICTING PROGRESSION TO RA

Cohort studies using biobank samples have demonstrated autoantibodies developing years before the onset of articular symptoms. However, in real-life clinical scenarios testing is performed only in patients experiencing musculoskeletal symptoms. Prospective studies on symptomatic patients evaluating the prognostic value of autoantibodies for the development of RA are few. Some have shown that the presence of autoantibodies confers a higher risk of progression to RA among patients with undifferentiated arthritis, and only 10% of subjects negative for autoantibodies progress to RA within 2 years. ACPA positivity confers a higher risk for RA than RF or anti-CarP Ab positivity. However, it is important to note that 50% of subjects with anti-CCP2 +ve results do not progress to RA. Concurrent ACPA and RF positivity increase the risk. Triple positivity of ACPA, RF, and anti-CarP Ab was found to have significant prognostic value in some studies but few studies did not find any additional advantage of anti-CarP Ab testing.

PROGNOSTIC VALUE

Both RF and ACPA have been demonstrated to be associated with more severe articular disease and higher rates of radiological progression. They have also been associated with a higher incidence of extraarticular manifestations including nodulosis, pleuritis, pericarditis, and vasculitis.

Recent evidence points towards role of autoantibodies in RA cardiovascular comorbidities. RF is associated with increased cardiovascular events, heart failure, and cardiovascular deaths. ACPA is associated with higher incidence of ischemic heart disease, diastolic dysfunction, and valvular disease. Antiphospholipid antibodies are associated with thrombotic events in RA. The presence of anti-CarP Ab, are also associated with higher risk of cardiovascular events in RA.

THERAPEUTIC IMPLICATIONS

RA patients positive for RF and/or ACPA have a more aggressive disease course. Hence it is often necessary to escalate DMARD therapy in seropositive patients. Also there is some evidence for autoantibodies being a biomarker for predicting response to treatment. RF and or ACPA-positive patients are more likely to respond to rituximab as compared to seronegative patients. ACPA and anti-CarP Ab are associated with modestly better response to abatacept. Tofacitinib also works better in seropositive patients.

Serial Measurement of RF and Antibodies is not of Value

While higher autoantibody titers confer better specificity for diagnosis and prognostic value, titre is not a measure of disease activity. Serial monitoring of autoantibody titres is not recommended to measure disease activity or response to treatment.

LEARNING POINTS

- Both RF and ACPA are useful in supporting a diagnosis of RA.
- Both are equally sensitive but the specificity of ACPA is much more than RF.
- Presence of both these autoantibodies predict development of RA in case of undifferentiated arthritis.
- Seropositive for RF and/or ACPA is associated with nodules and extra-articular features and more severe disease.
- Presence of these auta-antibodies favors good response to rituximab.

FURTHER READING

1. Fazeli MS, Khaychuk V, Wittstock K, et al. Cardiovascular Disease in Rheumatoid Arthritis: Risk Factors, Autoantibodies, and the Effect of Antirheumatic Therapies. Clin Med Insights Arthritis Musculoskelet Disord. 2021;14:11795441211028751.
2. Rönnelid J, Turesson C, Kastbom A. Autoantibodies in Rheumatoid Arthritis - Laboratory and Clinical Perspectives. Front Immunol. 2021;12:685312.
3. Sokolova MV, Schett G, Steffen U. Autoantibodies in Rheumatoid Arthritis: Historical Background and Novel Findings. Clin Rev Allergy Immunol. 2022;63:138–51.
4. Wu CY, Yang HY, Luo SF, Lai JH. From Rheumatoid Factor to Anti-Citrullinated Protein Antibodies and Anti-Carbamylated Protein Antibodies for Diagnosis and Prognosis Prediction in Patients with Rheumatoid Arthritis. Int J Mol Sci. 2021;22:686.

Chapter 7.7

Autoantibodies in Inflammatory Myositis

Puja Srivastava

INTRODUCTION

Idiopathic inflammatory myositis (IIM) is classified into four major subgroups: dermatomyositis (DM), anti-synthetase syndrome, immune-mediated necrotizing myopathy (IMNM), and inclusion body myositis (IBM), after which diagnosis of polymyositis becomes a diagnosis of exclusion.

The autoimmune basis of these diseases is reflected by the presence of antinuclear antibodies (ANA) or anti-cytoplasmic antibodies in 70–90% of these patients. Some of these antibodies are termed myositis-specific autoantibodies (MSAs) based on their relatively exclusive expression in patients with IIM, some other autoantibodies also found in patients with other connective tissue diseases are the myositis associated autoantibodies (MAAs). A negative ANA does not rule out the presence of MSAs and MAAs, as the antigenic targets of most of these autoantibodies are cytoplasmic in location, thus producing subtle or absent nuclear immunofluorescence.

Earlier, the detection of MSAs and MAAs was difficult due to the limited availability of the gold standard immunoprecipitation (IP) assay. Recently, techniques such as line immunoassay (LIA) and enzyme-linked immunosorbent assay (ELISA) have been validated as reliable screening tests for MSAs. With the increased availability of commercial LIAs, our knowledge of clinical association of MSA/MAAs among different types of IIM has expanded significantly. The real pathogenic significance of MSAs is still debatable, as to whether they are a by-product of autoimmunity or have a primary pathogenic role. Muscle biopsy still remains crucial for the diagnosis of MSA-negative IIM and IBM sub-groups.

The presence of MSAs supports the diagnosis of IIM in early indeterminate cases and also provides prognostic information regarding the likelihood of future systemic complications and response to therapy. Based on autoantibodies the IIMs can be distinguished from muscular dystrophies, CTD-associated myositis, and cancer-associated myositis.

MYOSITIS SPECIFIC ANTIBODIES

MSA are detected in about 50% of IIM. There are three well-characterised and distinct MSAs:

1. Aminoacyl-tRNA synthetases
2. Anti-Mi-2 antibodies and
3. Anti-signal recognition peptide (SRP) antibodies.

Recently many new antigenic targets are described. Table 7.7.1 shows the list of a few MSA, their antigenic targets, and clinical associations. Certain MSAs are associated with specific clinical manifestations, while others are still under evaluation, and every year newer antibodies are being identified.

Anti-synthetase Antibodies

These antibodies as a group are found in 20–30% of patients, across different subsets of IIM including DM, PM, and juvenile dermatomyositis (JDM). These antibodies are associated with a constellation of symptoms like interstitial lung diseases (ILD), fever, arthritis, mechanic's hands, raynaud's phenomenon, and fever collectively known as

Table 7.7.1: Myositis specific antibodies and their disease associations

Myositis specific antibodies			
Antibody	*Antigen*	*Prevalence (%)*	*Clinical syndrome*
Anti-synthetase Anti-Jo1 Anti-OJ Anti-EJ Anti-PL12 Anti-PL7 Anti-KS Anti-Zo Anti-YRS	**Aminoacyl-t-RNA synthetase** Histidyl-tRNA synthetase Isoleucyl-tRNA synthetase Glycyl-tRNA synthetase Alanyl-tRNA synthetase Threonyl-tRNA synthetase Asparaginyl-tRNA synthetase Phenylalanyl-tRNA synthetase Tyrosyl-tRNA synthetase	15–30 5–15 <5 <5 <5 <5 <5 <1 <1	A clinical syndrome characterised by myositis, arthritis, fever, ILD, raynauds phenomenon and mechanic's hand called the antisynthetase syndrome.
Anti-MDA5 (antiCADM140)	Melanoma Differentiation Antigen 5 (140-kDa protein)	13–35 (DM>PM)	Clinically amyopathic DM (dermato-pulmonary syndrome) ILD associated with MDA-5 antibodies may have a rapidly progressive course
Anti-Mi 2	Nuclear helicase (218/240 kDa)	10–35	DM (adult> children) and classic DM rashes like shawl sign, heliotrope rash, Gottron's papules, etc.
Anti-SRP	Signal recognition particle	4–6	Severe necrotizing myositis
Anti-FHL1	Four and a half LIM domains protein-1	25	Severe muscle weakness and atrophy, dysphagia, without lung or joint involvement, and poor response to treatment.
Anti-TIF1γ	p140/155 kDa protein	14–30	Has strong Association with cancer in patients with IIM
Anti-MJ (Anti-NXP2)	140-kDa protein	<5 (~25 in JDM)	DM associated with cancer and JDM, calcinosis, muscle atrophy, contractures.
Anti-HMGCR	200/100-kd protein	~6	Necrotizing myositis associated or triggered by statins.
Anti-PMS1	DNA repair enzyme	<5	JDM

PM: Polymyositis; *DM:* Dermatomyositis; *JDM:* Juvenile Dermatomyositis; *ADM:* Amyopathic Dermatomyositis; *IBM:* Inclusion body myositis; *OM:* Overlap myositis; Anti-TIF1ϒ: Anti-transcription intermediary factor-1 gamma; *Anti-HMGCR:* Anti-3-hydroxy-3-methylglutaryl-coenzyme A reductase antibodies.

the antisynthetase syndrome. This disease usually follows a relapsing-remitting disease course.

However, most patients have different combinations of the above features. The diagnosis of anti-synthetase syndrome can occur even in absence of myositis which is termed amyopathic dermatomyositis (ADM) or amyopathic antisynthetase syndrome. To date, eight different antisynthetase antibodies have been described (Table 7.7.1). Anti Jo-1 antibody was the first one described and the most prevalent autoantibody in this group. Other antisynthetase antibodies like PL-7, PL-12, EJ, OJ, Zo etc are relatively rare and found in <5% of patients with IIM.

Anti-Mi2 Antibody

This nuclear autoantibody is found in 15–20% of IIM and is almost exclusively associated with adult and juvenile DM phenotypes. Patients positive for this antibody have florid cutaneous rashes classic of DM like heliotrope rash, Gottron's papules, and involvement of both the anterior aspect and posterior surface of the neck and upper back ("V" and "shawl" signs). Further, in contrast to patients with antisynthetase antibodies, patients with anti-Mi-2 antibodies are more likely to develop pharyngeal and respiratory muscle weakness and are very less likely to develop ILD.

Anti-SRP Antibodies

This cytoplasmic antibody is found in 4-6% of patients with IIM, more commonly in PM than in DM. Anti-SRP-associated IIM is characterised by severe and refractory necrotizing myositis with or without cardiac involvement. These patients respond poorly to traditional immunosuppressive agents but often respond well to B cell depletion treatment. Another specific antibody to 3-hydroxy-3-methylglutaryl-coenzyme-A reductase (anti-HMGCoR) is associated with necrotizing myopathy, but patients with anti-SRP and anti-HMGCR antibodies differ in the severity and location of muscle inflammation and atrophy.

Anti-MDA5 Antibodies

They are also known as anti-CADM-140, as they were found to be antibodies directed against a 140-kd polypeptide, in a subgroup of patients suffering from clinically amyopathic dermatomyositis (CADM). Later the antigenic target for this antibody was found to be a distinct RNA-helicase, which is encoded by melanoma differentiation-associated gene 5 (MDA5). The presence of anti-MDA5 is associated with rapidly progressive ILD in patients with amyopathic or hypomyopathic dermatomyositis.

Newer MSAs

Over the last few years, new antigenic targets for MSAs have been described. Autoantibodies directed against the 155/140 kDa doublet or 155-kDa protein are strongly associated with malignancy-associated myositis in adults, and the target antigen of this antibody is 'transcriptional intermediary factor-1 gamma' (TIF1-ϒ). The same p140/155 antibody is also found in 23% of children with JDM and correlates with severe skin disease and cutaneous ulcerations.

Another autoantibody called Anti-NXP2 (also known as anti-MJ) is also directed against 140 kd protein (Nuclear Matrix protein 2) and is associated with aggressive muscle disease, calcinosis, joint contractures and intestinal vasculitis in patients with JDM, and with malignancy in adult DM.

Another antibody known as Anti-FHL1 is directed against four and a half LIM domains protein 1 and has been reported in upto 25% of patients with IIM (PM, DM, IBM, etc.), but not in muscular dystrophies or other autoimmune diseases. These antibodies are again associated with severe myositis with muscle atrophy, pharyngeal muscle weakness, and poor response to treatment.

Figure 7.7.1 illustrates the relationship of various MSAs with muscle, skin, and lung involvement in IIM.

MYOSITIS ASSOCIATED ANTIBODIES

MAAs are found in 20–50% of patients with IIM (Table 7.7.2). These are directed against various nuclear or cytoplamic antigens like Ro-52, PM-Scl, Ku, RNP, and occasionally SS-A (Ro-60) and SS-B (La-48).

Anti-Ro52 is the most commonly detected MAA across all subsets of IIM and seems to be associated with ILD and other antisynthetase syndrome-like clinical features. Further, Ro52 antibodies are frequently found in association with other MSAs, and this association is clearer for anti-Jo-1 antibodies than with other MSAs.

Anti-PM/Scl-75 and Anti-PM/Scl-100 autoantibodies are found in systemic sclerosis and polymyositis overlap. Anti-Ku and anti-snRNP antibodies are found in myositis overlap with other CTDs.

Recently, an antibody called anti-Cytosolic 5'-nucleotidase -1a (CN)-1A has been detected in patients with IBM and other autoimmune disorders such as SLE, Sjogren's etc, hence it has been classified as MAA.

As clinical associations of MSAs have become clearer, several serology-based classification systems have been proposed. In 2018 the EULAR/ACR have incorporated anti-Jo1 antibodies in the classification criteria of IIMs.

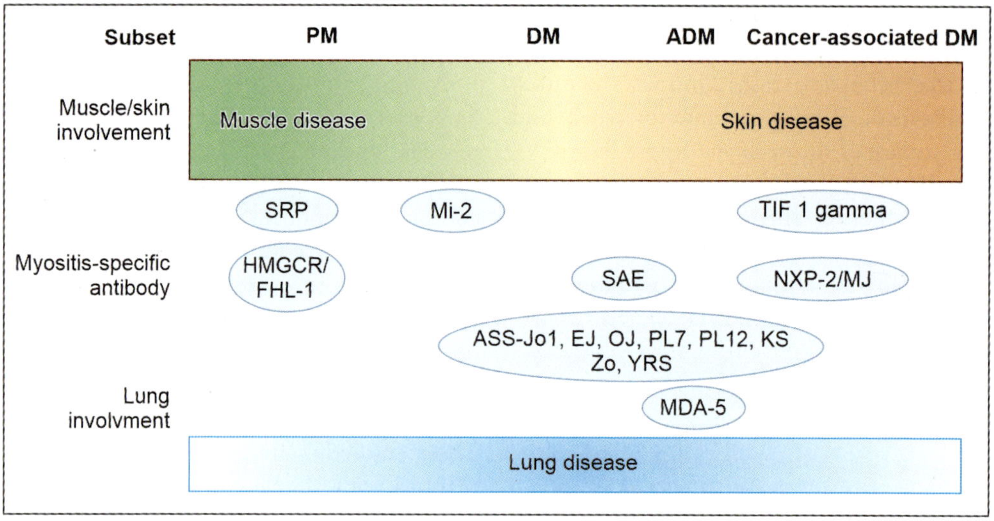

Fig. 7.7.1: An illustration of the association of myositis-specific autoantibodies (MSA) with the spectrum of skin, muscle, and lung involvements in different subsets of idiopathic inflammatory myositis.

PM: Polymyositis; *DM:* Dermatomyositis; *ADM:* Amyopathic dermatomyositis; *ASS:* Anti-synthetase syntdrome

Table 7.7.2: Myositis associated antibodies and their disease associations

Myositis associated antibodies			
Antibody	*Antigen*	*Prevalence (%)*	*Associated clinical syndrome*
Anti-Ro52	TRIM 21	20–35	ILD, Raynauds phenomenon, CTD associated myositis
Anti-Ku	DNA-PK regulatory subunit (70/80 kDa)	8–10	Polymyositis scleroderma overlap, UCTD
Anti-Pm-Scl	11-16 kDa protein nucleolar complex	8–10	Polymyositis scleroderma overlap myositis
Anti-U1RNP	Nuclear U1RNP	10	OM Mixed Connective tissue disease
Anti-SUMO-1	Small ubiquitin-like modifier Enzyme	–	Adult DM, ILD
Anti-cN-1A	Cytosolic 5'-nucleotidase-1A	–	IBM

ILD: Interstitial lung disease; *CTD:* Connective tissue disease; *UCTD:* Undifferentiated connective tissue disease; *OM:* Overlap myositis; *DM:* Dermatomyositis; *IBM:* Inclusion body myositis

LEARNING POINTS

- Autoantibodies help in the early diagnosis, better classification of IIM into homogenous groups, as well as in predicting the outcome
- Presence of TIF1ϒ, NXP2, SAE antibodies and seronegative IMNM phenotype is associated with high risk of malignancy among patients with IIM.
- MDA5 positive DM present as either clinically amyopathic dermatomyositis, cutaneous ulcerations with rapidly progressing ILD or with arthritis
- Anti-synthetase syndrome is a clinical subgroup of IIM with different combinations of arthritis, ILD, mechanic's hand, fever and myositis. Incomplete forms are often present

- The autoantibodies associated with JDM includes TIF1ϒ, NXP2 and MDA 5, and rarely other autoantibodies. TIF1ϒ in JDM is associated with more vasculitic presentations whereas NXP2 is associated with high risk of calcinosis and lipoatrophy

FURTHER READING

1. Cruellas MG, Viana Vdos S, Levy-Neto M, et al. Myositis-specific and myositis-associated autoantibody profiles and their clinical associations in a large series of patients with polymyositis and dermatomyositis. Clinics (Sao Paulo). 2013;68:909–914.
2. Lundberg IE, Miller FW, Tjärnlund A, et al. Diagnosis and classification of Idiopathic Inflammatory Myopathies. J Intern Med. 2016;280:39–51.
3. McHugh NJ, Tansley SL. Autoantibodies in myositis. Nat Rev Rheumatol. 2018;14:290–302.
4. Palterer B, Vitiello G, Carraresi A, et al. Bench to bedside review of myositis autoantibodies. Clin Mol Allergy. 2018;16:5.
5. Srivastava P, Dwivedi S, Misra R. Myositis-specific and myositis-associated autoantibodies in Indian patients with inflammatory myositis. Rheumatol Int. 2016;36:935–943.
6. Tansley SL, Betteridge ZE, McHugh NJ. The diagnostic utility of autoantibodies in adult and juvenile myositis. Curr Opin Rheumatol. 2013;25:772–777.

Chapter 7.8

HLA in Diagnosis and Pharmacogenetics

Christina Mary Mariaselvam, Sonal Mehra

INTRODUCTION

Human Leukocyte Antigens (HLA) are proteins expressed on cell surfaces that are coded by the Major Histocompatibility Complex (MHC) present in chromosome 6. In the human genome they are clustered as MHC-Class I, II and III genes and are highly polymorphic. Majority of these polymorphisms are in the exon 2 and 3 of class I and exon 2 of class II encoding the antigen binding groove. Under normal physiological conditions, HLA molecules are important to initiate and activate the adaptive immune responses towards foreign antigens. Normally, HLA class I processes endogenous antigens and present the antigenic peptides to CD8+ cells while class II processes exogenous antigens to present the peptides to CD4+ cells via the T cell receptors (TCR), thereby generating a T cell repertoire necessary to maintain self-tolerance. Any disturbance in this HLA-peptide-TCR interaction affects the immune homeostasis, leading to disease. Such HLA-associations have been reported in autoimmune diseases, malignancies, infections and organ transplantation etc., although the underlying mechanisms are not clear. Owing to its tendency to be inherited 'en bloc' and extreme polymorphisms that are different among populations, different HLA-disease associations can be observed in different populations for a given disease. HLA-disease associations can have gene dosage effects where the odds ratio is higher if an individual carries two copies of the risk allele compared to one copy of the risk allele. Here we will focus on the role of HLA in conferring risk for certain autoimmune diseases and its diagnostic utility.

ROLE OF HLA IN THE DIAGNOSIS OF AUTOIMMUNE DISEASES

Several population studies and key technological advances had helped to characterize the HLA diversity as well as the HLA-peptide-TCR interactions at greater resolution thus enabling the researchers to get mechanistic insights into its disease associations. Although HLA risk alleles are reported in a variety of autoimmune disorders, a strong association between HLA and autoimmune diseases is well established only in certain autoimmune diseases, thus warranting HLA testing for diagnosis, though not alone.

Ankylosing spondylitis (AS) is an inflammatory arthritis of the spine and large joints that over time can cause fibrosis and ossification of involved sites. Association of HLA-B*27 with AS was first reported in 1973. Being a HLA class I molecule, B*27 presents endogenous peptides to CD8+ T cells. Geographical differences do exist in the prevalence of B*27 and so the risk for AS. Only 4 - 7% of the general population carry the B*27 allele, while over 90% of patients with AS are carriers of B*27, especially Caucasians more than Asians. If a first degree relative of B*27 positive AS patient is also positive for B*27, the odds of them developing AS is higher. But B*27 positivity is not exclusive to AS, as for example, B*27 positivity is 30-80% in reactive arthritis and 30% in psoriatic arthritis. Nevertheless, routine diagnostic work-up of HLA-B*27 for AS is practiced in the clinic.

Beçhet's disease (BD) is characterized by inflammation in the blood vessels affecting the eyes, oral and genital cavities. BD is also called the "silk road disease" because of its marked prevalence in Mediterranean and Asian populations. HLA-B*51 positivity can be observed in around 50–70% of BD patients along this old silk route while its only 10–15% in the other population. HLA-B*51 can activate CD8+ T cells, NK cells and neutrophils. Carriers of B*51 alleles, particularly males, have increased risk of developing genital, oral and skin ulcers. Although HLA-B*51 testing is clinically not recommended, it is performed routinely to aid in the diagnosis of BD. Despite reports of an association between HLA-A*26 positivity and higher risk of iridiocyclitis and retinal chorionitis, testing for A*26 allele is not practiced in clinics.

Celiac disease (CD) is an organ specific disease characterised by damage to the small intestines. It occurs in individuals who have a genetic predisposition. Strong association with HLA-DQ2 and DQ8 heterodimers is reported. HLA-DQ2 is a heterodimer encoded by DQA1*02:01 and DQB1*02:02 (HLA-DQ2.2) or DQA1*05:01 and DQB1*02:01 (DQ2.5) while HLA-DQ8 is a heterodimer encoded by DQA1*03:01 and DQB1*03:02 alleles. DQ8 confers a lower risk to CD compared to DQ2 (DQ2 is present in more than 90% while DQ8 is present only in 5%). First degree relatives of CD patients have a 1 in 10 risk of developing CD. A gene dose effect is reported in CD, where two copies of DQB1*02 (homozygosity) is linked to higher risk and aggressive disease than carrying one copy (heterozygosity). CD diagnosis is primarily based on presence of high amount of auto-antibodies (anti-tissue transglutaminase & anti-endomysium) and findings of small bowel biopsy. Laboratory testing for the presence of these risk alleles merely indicates a risk for CD while its absence excludes CD. In clinical practice, considering the high negative predictive value, typing for HLA should only be used either to clarify uncertain diagnosis or to add strength to diagnosis (e.g. in pediatric patients in the presence of clinical symptoms and autoantibodies where small bowel biopsy may be omitted). In addition HLA typing is warranted in first degree relatives of patients with CD as well as in those with other autoimmune diseases, chromosomal disease, and immunoglobulin deficiency who are likely to develop CD.

Rheumatoid arthritis (RA), is a symmetrical polyarthritis involving multiple joints with other extra articular manifestations. It is characterised by the presence of antibodies to citrullinated proteins and rheumatoid factor even before the onset of symptoms. HLA is the most important genetic risk factor for RA, particularly DRB1 genes encoding the shared epitope (SE). SE is a five amino acid motif in positions 70 to 74 of the DRB1 chain, especially in seropositive RA (Table 7.8.1). HLA alleles with SE associate differently with RA in different populations. For example DRB1*04:01 is associated in Europeans, *04:05 in Eastern Asians while *09:01 a non-SE allele is associated in some populations. Similarly other non-SE alleles such as DRB1*03 (Europeans) and DRB1*14:54

Table 7.8.1: DRB1 shared epitope alleles and RA risk

Allele classification	*AA at position 70–74 of DRB1*	*DRB1 alleles*	*RA Risk*
S1	DERAA	*01:03, *04:02, *11:02, *11:03, *13:01,*13:02, *13:04,*13:36,*13:40	Low
	QARAA	*15:01, *15:02, *15:03	Low
S2	QKRAA	*04:01,*04:09,*04:13,*04:35,04:66	High
	DKRAA	*13:03	High
S3D	DRRAA	*11:01,*11:04,*11:27,*12,*13:05,*13:06, *13:25,*14:22,*16	Low
S3P	QRRAA	*01:01,*01:02,*04:04,*04:05,*04:08,*04:10	Intermediate
	RRRAA	*10:01	Intermediate

Shared Epitope (SE): is a five amino acid sequence motif at positions 70–74 of HLA-DRβ1 chain. *AA:* Amino acid; *RA:* Rheumatoid arthritis

(Asians) are associated with RA patients without antibodies to citrullinated proteins. On the other hand some SE alleles like *13:01 in Europeans and *13:02 in East Asia are protective for RA. Due to the strong association of HLA-DRB1 alleles with positivity to citrullinated protein antibodies in RA, HLA testing is not recommended for RA. Nevertheless HLA testing might guide treatment choice. It has been reported that in the presence of SE alleles, a triple therapy including methotrexate, hydroxychloroquine, and sulfasalazine is more effective than methotrexate monotherapy in RA.

ROLE OF HLA IN PHARMACOGENETICS

Pharmacogenomics is the study of the influence of multiple genetic variations on a person's response to drugs while pharmacogenetics refers to the study of the influence of a single genetic variation on the drug response. These genetic variation(s) among individuals could affect the pharmacokinetics - the way the drug is absorbed, distributed, metabolised and excreted as well as the pharmacodynamics-the way the drug interacts with its target (e.g. via a receptor, ion channel, an enzyme or immune system components).

HLA molecules through their interactions with several drugs can also induce adverse drug reactions i.e. induce hypersensitivity responses through one of the several mechanisms viz. hapten/prohapten (small drug or the toxic metabolites of drugs binds with protein and become immunogenic), pharmacological interaction (p-i) (the drug binds either to peptide binding site of HLA or the CDR3 of the TCR to elicit an immune response), and repertoire alteration (the drug alters the binding chemistry of HLA molecule thereby altering the repertoire of endogenous antigens presented to the TCR). Thus the HLA-drug-TCR interaction activates the cytotoxic T cells and secretion of cytotoxic proteins by immune cells.

Some of the examples of HLA - drug interactions induced adverse events are:

i. Drug reaction (or rash) with eosinophilia and systemic symptoms (DRESS)
ii. Stevens-Johnson syndrome (SJS)
iii. Toxic epidermal necrolysis (TEN)
iv. Drug-induced liver injury (DILI)
v. Maculopapular exanthema (MPE)
vi. Acute generalized exanthematous pustulosis (AGEP)

Today pre-emptive testing of HLA is strongly recommended before prescription of certain drugs (Table 7.8.2) to avoid HLA-drug interaction induced adverse events. In addition caution is warranted before prescribing certain drugs, although the evidence for pre-emptive HLA testing is not strong. For example,

- Lamotrigine can cause SJS, MPE, TEN in those with HLA-A*24:02 allele, prevalent especially in North America
- Flucloxacillin in Caucasians carrying HLA-B *57:01 and Ticlopidine in HLA-A*33:03 carriers of Thai descent can cause DILI.
- Phenobarbital can cause MPE in HLA-A*01:01 carriers (common in Caucasians), DRESS in HLA-B*13:01 positive subjects (common in

Table 7.8.2: Drugs requiring pre-emptive HLA testing

Drug	*Clinical Usage*	*Associated HLA*	*Population*	*ADR*
Abacavir	Anti-viral	B*57:01	South Asians >Europeans	AHS
Carbamazepine	Anti-epileptic	B*15:02	Southeast Asians, Chinese, Taiwanese	SJS & TEN
		A*31:01	European, Japanese, Korean	SJS &TEN
Phenytoin	Anti-epileptic	B*15:02	Thai and Chinese	SJS & TEN
Allopurinol	Hypouricemic agent	B*58:01	widely distributed across all populations	SJS, TEN, DRESS &MPE

ADR: Adverse drug reaction; *AHS:* Abacavir hypersensitivity syndrome; *SJS:* Steven-johnson syndrome; *TEN:* Toxic epidermal necrolysis; *DRESS:* Drug reaction (or rash) with eosinophilia and systemic symptoms; *MPE:* Maculo papular erythema

Thai) and SJS/TEN in carriers of HLA-B*51:01 notably in North Americans.

- Dapsone and salazosulfapyridine can trigger DRESS in individuals of Thai descent carrying HLA-B*13:01.
- Co-trimoxazole causes SJS/TEN in carriers of either of the HLA-B*15:02, B*38:01, B*38:02, C*06:02, C*08:01 alleles.
- Amoxicillin Clavulanate can cause DILI in individuals with HLA-DRB1*15:01 and DQB1* 06:02
- Azathioprine increases the risk of pancreatitis in patients with HLA-DRB1*07:01 and DQA1* 02:01 alleles with inflammatory bowel disease and Crohn's disease.
- More recently, biological (Infliximab and Adalimumab) treatment in Crohn's disease patients carrying HLA-DQA1*05 allele is reported to induce anti-drug antibodies in Europeans leading to treatment failure.

METHODS FOR SCREENING OF RISK HLA ALLELES

PCR based methods utilizing either sequence specific primers (SSP) or sequence specific oligonucleotide probes (SSOP), Real-time PCR (using fluorescent dyes) and sequencing are currently available for screening of HLA risk alleles. The choice of the method is dependent on the volume of samples, the degree of resolution required and the turnaround time.

LEARNING POINTS

- Screening for the presence of HLA-B*27 in spondyloarthritis, HLA-B*51 in Behçet's disease as well as HLA-DQ2/DQ8 in celiac disease has a significant diagnostic utility.
- Screening for HLA-DRB1 shared epitope alleles in RA has no diagnostic utility despite its strong association with seropositive RA.
- Pre-emptive testing of HLA is strongly recommended to avoid the dangerous HLA-drug -TCR interactions. For example Abacavir interacts with HLA-B*57:01; Allopurinol interacts with HLA-B*58:01; Phenytoin interacts HLA-B*15:02; Carbamazepine interacts with HLA-B*15:02 and HLA-A*31:01.
- Association of HLA with autoimmune diseases and HLA-drug-TCR- interactions are different in different populations and necessitates population tailored testing.

FURTHER READING

1. Bodis G, Toth V, Schwarting A. Role of Human Leukocyte Antigens (HLA) in Autoimmune Diseases. Rheumatol Ther. 2018;5:5–20.
2. Kedzierska K, Koutsakos M. The ABC of Major Histocompatibility Complexes and T Cell Receptors in Health and Disease. Viral Immunol. 2020;33:160–178.
3. Kloypan C, Koomdee N, Satapornpong P, et al. A Comprehensive Review of HLA and Severe Cutaneous Adverse Drug Reactions: Implication for Clinical Pharmacogenomics and Precision Medicine. Pharmaceuticals (Basel). 2021;14:1077.
4. Mosaad YM. Clinical Role of Human Leukocyte Antigen in Health and Disease. Scand J Immunol. 2015;82:283–306.

Section

VIII

RHEUMATOID ARTHRITIS, SPONDYLOARTHRITIS, LUPUS, APS, AND SJÖGREN'S SYNDROME

Rheumatoid Arthritis Management

Banwari Sharma

INTRODUCTION

We have witnessed significant improvement in the outcome of rheumatoid arthritis (RA) in the last two decades, which has been made possible by a paradigm shift in the treatment approach.

PRINCIPLES OF MANAGEMENT

Important factors that have contributed to improved outcomes of RA are summarized in Table 8.1.1.

Early Diagnosis and Treatment

Utility of anticitrullinated peptide antibodies (ACPA) and application of the 2010 ACR/EULAR classification criteria for RA made it possible to diagnose these patients early. In early disease, inflammation is at its peak, rate of progression is very high which leads to irreversible damage in the first few years. At this point in time the disease is more responsive to DMARDs which leads to better clinical, functional, and radiological recovery, and reduces long-term mortality. This is called "the window of opportunity period".

Table 8.1.1: General principles of management of RA

1. Early diagnosis
2. Early use of DMARDS
3. Treat to target (T2T) treatment strategy: Remission or low disease activity (LDA)
4. Use of NSAIDs and corticosteroids as adjuncts to DMARD therapy

Optimum Use of Methotrexate (MTX)

MTX is the anchor drug for RA, starting with a 15 mg weekly dose in moderate to severe RA patients, rapidly escalating to 25 mg/week, with use of a subcutaneous route when the dose is above 15 mg/week. This is the first-line standard of care treatment for RA nowadays.

Monitoring Disease Activity

We now have reliable instruments to monitor disease activity such as simplified disease activity index (SDAI), clinical disease activity index (CDAI) or disease activity score 28 joints (DAS 28) (Table 8.1.2). Monitor activity of disease by one of these composite measures at each visit and titrate the dose of medications according to the aim of therapy.

Treat-to-target Approach

The goal of treatment is remission or low disease activity, which is possible by tight control of symptoms and prompt treatment adaptation. Any new treatment (increase in the existing dose or addition of new drug) should show at least a 50% improvement in disease activity within 3 months and the treatment target should be reached within the subsequent 3 months.

Availability of Newer Drugs

Biologics/biosimilars and small molecules: Biologic DMARDs have shown significant efficacy and safety in the last two decades. Cost was the major issue with biologics in our country. With the development of

Table 8.1.2: Measures of disease activity in RA

	Formula	*Remission*	*Low/minimal*	*Moderate*	*High/severe*
CDAI	SJC28 + TJC28 + PGA + EGA	<2.8	2.8–10.0	>10.0–22.0	>22.0
DAS28	Complex formula including the TJC28, SJC28, ESR (or CRP) and GH	<2.6	2.6–<3.2	3.2–5.1	>5.1
SDAI	SJC28 + TJC28 + PGA + EGA + CRP	<3.3	>3.3–11.0	>11.0–26	>26

CDAI: Clinical disease activity index; DAS28: 28-joint disease activity score (with either erythrocyte sedimentation rate or C-reactive protein level); *SDAI:* Simplified disease activity index; *SJC:* Swollen joint count; *TJC:* Tender joint count; *EGA:* Evaluator global assessment (on a 0–10 cm scale); *GH:* Global health (that is, patient global assessment); *PGA:* Patient global assessment (on a 0–10-cm scale)

biosimilars and a nearly similar efficacy and safety profile as compared to original biologics, the cost issue was solved to a great extent. Recent approval of generic small molecules (JAK inhibitors) in India for RA treatment will further improve the outcome of these patients.

Practical and Common Issues of RA Management

At the time of Diagnosis

Before starting DMARDS a baseline workup is required (Table 8.1.3). This would also include vaccination in these patients (Table 8.1.4). Once a patient is diagnosed, patient education about the nature of disease, role of exercise, and physiotherapy is to be given in order to enable the patient's participation in his/her disease management. Encourage the patient to stop smoking. Explain in detail about chronic nature, remission, and relapses, need of frequent monitoring, adverse effects of drugs, and the long-term complications of untreated disease. Importance of physiotherapy and smoking cessation should be explained at baseline and every visit.

Table 8.1.3: Pretreatment evaluations

Routine tests	ESR, CRP, CBC, ALT, serum creatinine, urine complete, X-ray chest PA, X-ray both hands and feet
HCQ: within the first year of treatment	Eye examination: Automated visual field testing and retinal examination
Biologics and JAK inhibitors	Screening for latent TB: Chest X-ray + Mantoux test using 10 tuberculin unit (TU) strength + Interferon-gamma release assays (QuantiFERON®-TB Gold. Hepatitis B screening (HbsAg and HBc antibody) Lipid profile

Table 8.1.4: Pretreatment vaccinations

Vaccine	*Frequency*	*Ideal time*
Pneumococcal vaccination • 13-valent pneumococcal vaccine (PCV13) and the 23-valent polysaccharide vaccine (PPSV23) • They should be given at separate time points to help ensure that protective antibodies to each vaccine develop • When possible, PCV13 should be given before PPSV23	Baseline and PPSV23 every 5 years	Two weeks prior to starting immunosuppressive therapy or when immunosuppression is low
Seasonal influenza vaccination • Quadrivalent influenza vaccine	Annually	Same as above

Selection of DMARD

Selection of DMARDs in RA depends upon many factors (Table 8.1.5). As depicted in Figure 8.1.1, patients with mild disease can be started on monotherapy, however, those with moderate to severe disease based on either DAS28 or CDAI (Table 8.1.2), and those patients with poor prognostic markers (Table 8.1.6) usually require more aggressive therapy from the beginning.

Table 8.1.5: Factors determining the selection of DMARDs

1. Severity of disease (Mild/moderate/severe)
2. Early/advanced/late disease
3. DMARD naïve/inadequately treated/refractory
4. Extra-articular features
5. Comorbidities
6. Cost
7. Patients preferences

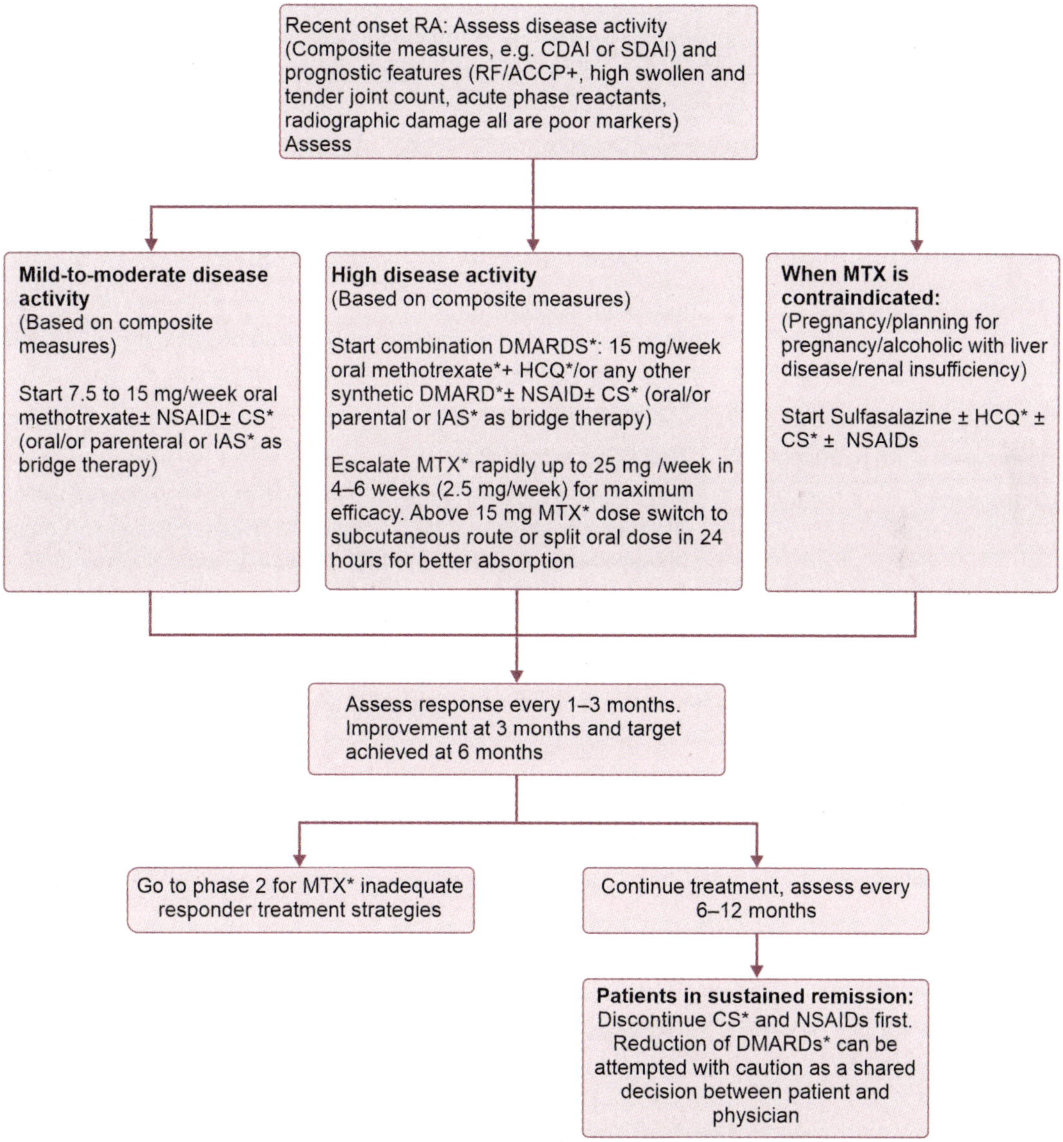

Fig. 8.1.1: Treatment strategies for recent onset RA. *MTX:* Methotrexate; *Lef:* Leflunomide; *HCQ:* Hydroxychloroquine; *CS:* Corticosteroids; *IAS:* Intra-articular steroid; *DMARD:* Disease modifying antirheumatic drug

Table 8.1.6: Poor prognostic features of RA
• Persistently moderate or high disease activity despite conventional synthetic DMARD (csDMARD)
• Failure of two or more csDMARDs
• High acute phase reactant levels
• High swollen joint count
• Presence of RF and/or ACPA, especially at high levels
• Presence of early erosions

It is important to know that the DAS28 score has some limitations. A significant emphasis has been given to tender joint count rather than swollen joint count and acute phase reactant levels in the DAS28. It has been documented in several studies that DAS28 remission may not be associated with true remission; these patients may have active swollen joints when scores show that they are in the remission. Similarly, drugs that reduce acute phase reactants rapidly e.g. IL-6 inhibitors and JAK inhibitors may show an exaggerated remission rate.

MTX is the anchor drug for RA, but when there are contraindications to its use, other conventional synthetic DMARDs (Table 8.1.7) are used. Best efficacy of MTX is achieved when it is used in the full recommended dose of 25 mg/week subcutaneously. MTX inadequate responders (Fig. 8.1.2) usually require the addition of another

Table 8.1.7: Conventional synthetic DMARDs

DMARD	*Dose*	*Remark*
Methotrexate	7.5–25 mg every week	Starting dose in the majority of patients is 7.5–15 mg every week. Escalate rapidly up to 25 mg/week in 4–6 weeks (2.5 mg/week) for maximum efficacy If the dose is >15 mg dose prefer SC route or split dose in 24 hours once weekly dose for better absorption
Hydroxychloroquine	5 mg/kg/day	Maximum 400 mg dose
Leflunomide	20 mg/day	Risk of hepatotoxicity
Sulfasalazine	2–3 g/day	500 mg once daily or 1 g/day in 2 divided doses; increase weekly to maintenance dose: 2 g/day in 2 divided doses; maximum: 3 g/day (if response to 2 g/day is inadequate after 12 weeks of treatment

SC: Subcutaneous

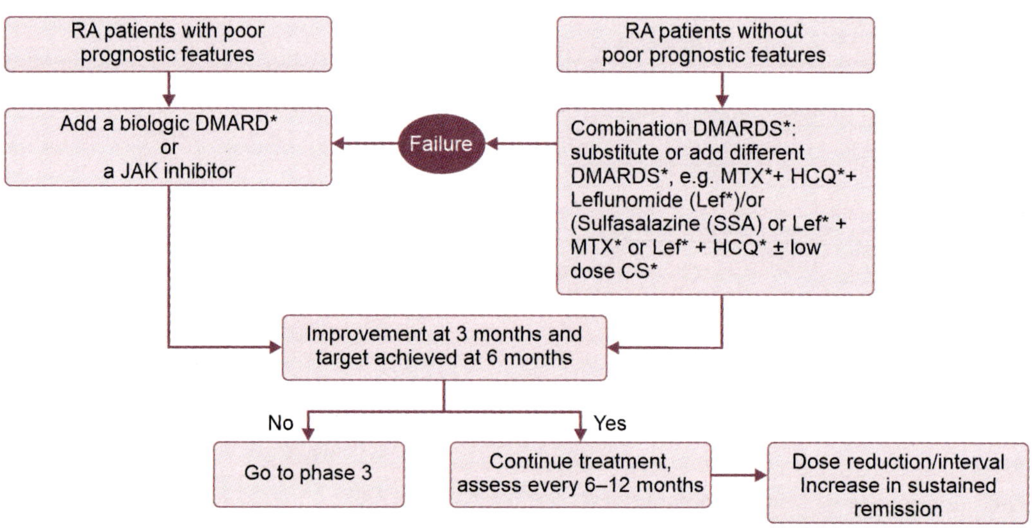

Fig. 8.1.2: Phase 2 treatment strategies for MTX inadequate response in RA

conventional synthetic DMARDs + low dose steroids for short periods or biologic DMARDs (Tables 8.1.8 and 8.1.9) or JAK inhibitors (Table 8.1.10).

If even after adding a biologic DMARD or JAK inhibitor, the target is not achieved then change in biologics from the same or different class or JAK inhibitor is recommended (Fig. 8.1.3). Some RA

Table 8.1.8: Biologic/biosimilar DMARDs: TNF inhibitors

Biologic DMARD	*Dose*	*Remark*
Infliximab	3 mg/kg at 0, 2, and 6 weeks by IV Infusion over at least 2 hours This induction regime is followed by a maintenance regimen of 3 mg/kg every 8 weeks	Temporarily discontinue or decrease infusion rate with infusion-related reactions. Antihistamines (H1-antagonist +/– H2-antagonist), acetaminophen and/ or corticosteroids may be used to manage reactions Always used with MTX
Etanercept	50 mg once a week or 25 mg twice a week, by subcutaneous (SC) injection	Prefilled syringe Can be given as monotherapy
Adalimumab	40 mg SC every 2 weeks	Prefilled syringe
Golimumab	50mg every month SC injection, or 2 mg/kg IV at weeks 0, 4, and then every 8 weeks thereafter	By infusion or SC
Certolizumab pegol	400 mg SC initial dose, repeat dose 2 and 4 weeks after initial dose; Maintenance: 200 mg every other week	Safe throughout pregnancy

Table 8.1.9: Biologic/biosimilar DMARDs other than TNF inhibitors

Biologic DMARD	*Dose*	*Remark*
Abatacept (T-cell costimulation blocker)	500–750 mg (<60 kg: 500 mg, 60–100 kg: 750 mg) IV infusion Repeat IV infusion at 2 weeks and 4 weeks after the initial infusion, and every 4 weeks thereafter	Not available in India
Rituximab (anti-CD20 B-cell depleting monoclonal antibody)	1 g on day 1 and 15, then every 4–6 months (based on clinical evaluation)	Available in India
Tocilizumab (IL-6 receptor antagonist)	4 mg/kg IV infusion over 1 hour once every 4 weeks; may be increased to 8 mg/kg once every 4 weeks based on clinical response (maximum dose: 800 mg)	Available in India
Anakinra (IL-1 receptor antagonist)	100 mg SC daily	Not available in India

Table 8.1.10: Targeted synthetic DMARDs (JAK inhibitors)

JAK inhibitors	*Dose*	*Remark*
Tofacitinib (JAK3 and 1 inhibitor)	5 mg twice a day	JAK inhibitors should not be used in combination with biologic DMARDs or other JAK inhibitors or with strong immunosuppressants such as azathioprine or cyclosporine
Baricitinib (JAK1and JAK2 inhibitor)	2–4 mg once a day (2 mg in the USA)	Available in India
Upadacitinib (JAK 1 inhibitor)	15 mg once a day	Not available in India

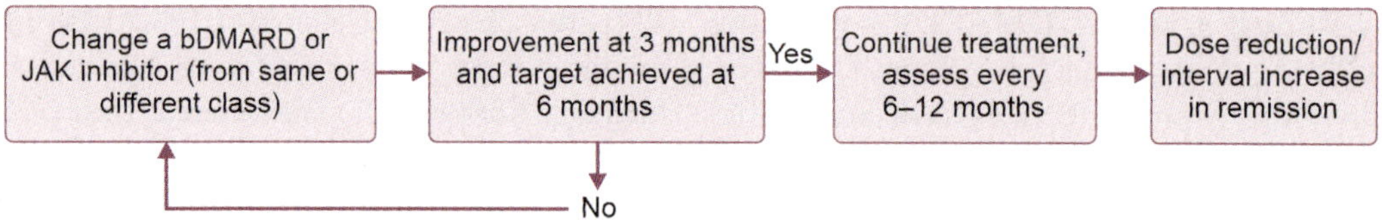

Fig. 8.1.3: Treatment strategies for biologic inadequate response RA

patients have a lot of comorbidities, it is important to assess these comorbid conditions before selecting DMARDs. Monoarticular or oligoarticular flares can be managed by addition of intra-articular corticosteroids after carefully excluding infections.

Once remission is achieved and maintained for 6 months medications may be carefully tapered after discussion with the patient. Most patients require minimum maintenance drugs for a very long period, so it is always better to continue some maintenance drugs even after many years. It has been shown in various reports and in my personal experience that some patients maintain remission even on 5 mg MTX fortnightly. Once a patient discontinues it or stops completely, the majority will relapse.

LEARNING POINTS

- Making a correct diagnosis particularly in early disease is important, after excluding mimickers. In those with palindromic onset disease, presence of other systemic features, or patients with predominant subjective symptoms of arthritis without any objective clinical findings and lab workup it is better to observe rather than labelling the patient as RA.
- Assess the disease activity and damage at baseline and at every visit. Fibromyalgia, depression, secondary pain syndromes, and mechanical pain are quite common in practice. It is important to identify these associated factors and address them accordingly.
- Use of composite measures to assess disease activity and health assessment questionnaires (HAQ) at every visit makes a significant difference in better outcome.
- Assess extra-articular features, prognostic features, comorbidities, financial aspects, and patient preference before starting treatment. Shared decision making in this chronic disease treatment improves compliance and outcome.
- Vaccination is an important advancement for RA patients, and vaccinations are to be given before starting immunosuppressives.
- RA is a heterogeneous disease, every patient is different, and guidelines are made for general understanding. Use your clinical sense and discuss with patients frequently particularly when a patient has very aggressive disease, refractory disease or iatrogenic complications.

FURTHER READING

1. Fraenkel L, Bathon JM, England BR, et al. 2021 American College of Rheumatology Guideline for the Treatment of Rheumatoid Arthritis. Arthritis Care Res (Hoboken). 2021; 73:924–39.
2. Handa R, Rao UR, Lewis JF, et al. Literature review of rheumatoid arthritis in India. Int J Rheum Dis. 2016; 19:440–51.
3. Smolen JS, Landewé RBM, Bijlsma JWJ, et al. EULAR recommendations for the management of rheumatoid arthritis with synthetic and biological disease-modifying antirheumatic drugs: 2019 update. Ann Rheum Dis. 2020; 79:685–99.

Chapter 8.2

Management of Rheumatoid Arthritis with Comorbidities

Chandrashekara S

INTRODUCTION

Comorbidity is the occurrence of multiple chronic disorders other than the index disease. The presence of comorbidities adversely influences the disease outcome, treatment approach, and quality of life of patients with rheumatoid arthritis (RA). Approximately 30–70% of RA depending on the age group will have comorbidity. The persistent inflammation in such cases may lead to the progression of comorbidities, so it is imperative to assess comorbidities, consider drug interactions, and identify a target for treatment (Fig. 8.2.1).

Here we shall discuss the management of a few comorbidities with reference to disease-modifying antirheumatic drugs (DMARDs) prescription in RA. The comorbidities commonly encountered in practice typically are hypothyroidism, hypertension, diabetes, atherosclerotic cardiovascular disease and stroke, heart failure, liver disease including hepatitis B and C, and tuberculosis. Osteoporosis is often a consequence of active disease and inflammation and is discussed in another chapter.

DIABETES, HYPERTENSION, CHRONIC LIVER DISEASE, AND RENAL DISEASE

Prior to treatment with DMARDs assess the status of diabetes and hypertension, enquire about the history of previous cardiovascular diseases, and investigate with a baseline ECG and echocardiography. This baseline evaluation will determine the choice of DMARDs (Table 8.2.1). It is important to monitor patients receiving hydroxychloroquine (HCQ) for hypoglycemia, as it has potential for hypoglycemic effects. Metformin is safe and confers favorable benefits in RA. Pioglitazone is potentially hepatotoxic so when using it with methotrexate (MTX) one should be watchful for liver toxicity. Patients may develop steroid-induced diabetes that is managed in general lines of diabetes.

Most DMARDs are metabolized by the liver hence one should have baseline normal liver function tests before beginning treatment. This is especially applicable to the introduction of MTX and leflunomide (Lef) as both are hepatotoxic. If there is evidence of CLD, the status of liver disease

Comorbidity	• Grade or stage the comorbidity • Assess the impact of the disease on quality of life
Drugs	• Consider the interaction of drugs to be prescribed with DMARDs
Rheumatoid arthritis	• Consider safe target for RA management • Prioritize the therapy and interdisciplinary communications

Fig. 8.2.1: Choice of DMARDs based on baseline evaluation

should be classified using the Child-Pugh-Turcotte system. MTX is contraindicated in patients with all stages of CLD, while Lef is contraindicated in Child C status, while others need dose modification (Table 8.2.1).

Among conventional synthetic DMARDs (csDMARD), MTX are contraindicated in those with significantly poor renal function (Table 8.2.1), while Lef and sulfasalazine (SSZ) can be given with caution in moderately impaired renal function. There is an increased risk for ophthalmic toxicity with hydroxychloroquine (HCQ) in the presence of renal impairment, so HCQ also needs dose adjustment. Biologic DMARDs (etanercept) have been given successfully to patients on hemodialysis but in practice, we tend to avoid prescribing biologic DMARDs (bDMARD) in patients with significantly poor renal function due to fear of infections.

CARDIAC DISEASES

The treatment needs to be customized according to the cardiac comorbidity. HCQ should be introduced with utmost caution in patients with reduced ejection fraction, arrhythmia, and congestive

Table 8.2.1: Management of RA in the presence of diabetes, hypertension, chronic liver disease, or renal disease

Comorbidity	*Caution to be exercised/drugs to avoid*	*Comments*
Hypertension	• Lef, CsA, and Tac are associated with development of hypertension or poor control of hypertension	Replace Lef and Tac, if possible, especially if there is new-onset hypertension
Diabetes	• It is preferable to avoid steroids. However, it can be given for a short term in certain situations for example active RA at diagnosis • MTX, Lef has drug interaction especially with pioglitazone, increasing its serum concentration due to CYP2C8 inhibition • HCQ can induce hypoglycemia	No specific precautions are required for other drugs
Chronic Liver disease (CLD)	• MTX is contraindicated in CLD • Lef, SSZ are contraindicated in Child C status • It is also preferable to avoid Lef in mild and moderate impairment (Child A and B) • Half dose of tofacitinib can be used with caution in Child B status • NSAIDs like diclofenac can precipitate hepatorenal syndrome	• HCQ and steroids are safe • SSZ safe in Child A status • CsA can be given CLD
Renal disease		
eGFR <15	MTX and Tac are contraindicated Lef and SSZ use with caution HCQ 25% of standard dose is allowed	HCQ accumulates in renal failure hence dose adjustment is required Steroids are safe Tofacitinib: According to the manufacturer no dose adjustment for mild impairment. In mild or moderate impairment, reduce the dose by 50% Biologics need no dose modifications, however biologics are avoided in advanced renal failure because of fear of infections. Thus assessment of infection is a priority
eGFR 15–29	MTX contraindicated Lef and SSZ use with caution HCQ 50% of standard dose Tofacitinib dose reduction by 50%	
eGFR 30–60	MTX 50% and HCQ 75% of standard dose allowed Lef and SSZ normal dose	

Lef: leflunomide; *Tac:* Tacrolimus; *MTX:* Methotrexate; *SSZ:* Sulfasalazine; *CsA:* Cyclosporine A; *HCQ:* Hydroxychloroquine; *eGFR:* Estimated glomerular filtration rate in mL/min/m^2

failure (Table 8.2.2). Angina may not be obvious in most cases due to impaired mobility. It is preferable to evaluate when there is a clinical possibility.

TUBERCULOSIS

Screening for latent tuberculosis prior to the use of TNF inhibitors (TNFi) and targeted synthetic-DMARDs (tsDMARDs) is mandatory. In patients with active tuberculosis, the use of MTX and Lef if possible should be deferred (Table 8.2.2). The risk-to-benefit should be carefully weighed prior to the prescription of biologics. There is general agreement that bDMARD can be given after the intensive phase of antitubercular treatment is completed.

CHRONIC VIRAL INFECTIONS

Screening for hepatitis B virus (HBV) infection must include HBsAg, anti-HBc IgM and IgG, anti-HBs, and anti-HCV when biologicals are contemplated. This is necessary because HBV is known to reactivate with immunosuppressive therapy unless appropriately treated with antiviral agents.

The risk of reactivation of HBV in patients taking immunosuppressants differ depending on the DMARDs used and the baseline HBsAg status (Table 8.3.3). Reactivation is defined as transaminitis and increased HBV DNA levels. A study from Thailand on reactivation of HBV among

Table 8.2.2: Management comorbidities in RA: Cardiac disease, cerebrovascular disease, peripheral vascular disease and others

Comorbidity	*Drugs to be avoided*	*Precautionary measures*	*Remarks*
Cardiac disease			
Congestive heart failure	TNFi and HCQ	DMARDs need careful introduction considering the reduction in renal clearance and the drug interaction with amiodarone and other antiarrhythmic drugs	Combination DMARDs need careful adjustment. Non-TNF biologics can be used. Tofacitinib is another alternative
Coronary artery disease	None	Tofacitinib should be carefully introduced since it is associated with excess cardiac events in older people	Other DMARDs like MTX, HCQ and biologics are expected to reduce the incidence. Drug interaction should be considered
Deep vein thrombosis (DVT)			
DVT and thrombophilia	None	Preferable to avoid tofacitinib. Avoid MTX in those with homocysteinemia	Both tofacitinib and MTX can be used, but need to be accompanied with an anticoagulation strategy. Drug interaction should be considered
Other comorbidities			
Erosive gastric ulcers or previous perforation	NSAIDs	Prefer parenteral MTX. SSZ should be carefully introduced	Parenteral biologics are preferred if there are no contraindications
Tuberculosis (TB)	In active TB avoid Lef, bDMARDs, tofacitinib	Introduce MTX after 2–3 months of ATT In LTBI, bDMARDs and tofacitinib can be started after one month of ATT for LTBI	Drug interaction, especially hepatotoxicity

(Contd.)

Table 8.2.2: Management comorbidities in RA: Cardiac disease, cerebrovascular disease, peripheral vascular disease and others (*Contd.*)

Comorbidity	*Drugs to be avoided*	*Precautionary measures*	*Remarks*
Hyperlipidemia	None	Need a careful introduction of tofacitinib The IL-6 blocker tocilizumab causes hyperlipidemia	HCQ and TNFi improve lipid profile Treat hyperlipidemia as per standard recommendations
Fibromyalgia	None	Fibromyalgia interferes with assessment of RA disease activity. Thus escalation of DMARDs should be carefully considered.	None
Depression	None	Check for drug interactions with antidepressants	None

DMARDs: Disease modifying antirheumatic drugs; *TNFi:* Tumor necrosis factor inhibitors; *MTX:* Methotrexate; *LTBI:* Latent tuberculosis infection; *Lef:* Leflunomide; *SSZ:* Sulfasalazine; *HCQ:* Hydroxychloroquine; *ATT:* Antitubercular treatment; *bDMARD:* Biologic DMARD

Table 8.2.3: Risk of HBV reactivation with various DMARDs

Therapy	*HBsAg positive*	*HBsAg negative, anti-HBc positive (occult HBV infection)*
Rituximab	Very high**	Moderate
High dose corticosteroids*	High	Low
Anti-TNF	Moderate	Low
IL-6 inhibitors	Moderate	Low
IL-17 inhibitors	Moderate	Low
Abatacept	Moderate	Low
JAK inhibitors	Moderate	Low
Cyclophosphamide	Moderate	Low
Methotrexate	Low	Low
Sulfasalazine	Low	Low
Leflunomide	Low	Low

*Doses of corticosteroids in excess of 20 mg of prednisone (or equivalent) have been reported to have a high risk of HBV reactivation; **Although reported rates of HBV reactivation vary, rough estimates of very high risk are considered to be >20%, high is 11–20% range, moderate between 1 and 10% and low <1%; Evidence for HBV reactivation with JAK inhibitors is limited. *HBV:* Hepatitis B virus; *TNF:* Tumor necrosis factor

RA who are on MTX, showed that at baseline 95 of 173 (55%) had negative HBV markers; 65 (37%) anti-HBc+ve, 67 (38%) anti-HBs+ve, and one (0.6%) was HBsAg +ve. None of the anti-HBc+ve reactivated after 9 years of MTX therapy. In general reactivation with MTX is rare, but reactivation of HBV is up to 35% when HBsAg is positive and patient receiving TNFi (Table 8.2.3). But when antivirals are given together, reactivation of HBV with the traditional csDMARD and bDMARDs is significantly reduced.

Prophylactic antivirals are recommended when there is occult HBV especially before bDMARD and rituximab and cyclophosphamide (Table 8.2.4).

Table 8.2.4: Managing RA in the presence of HBV, HCV and HIV

HBV status	*Management*	*Remarks*
Hepatitis B Virus (HBV)		
HBsAg+ve	Risk of HBV reactivation with different DMARDs is summarized in Table 8.2.3. Start antivirals (entecavir or tenofovir) at least 2 weeks before or simultaneously at the time of beginning biologic DMARDs Risk of reactivation is low in those who receive traditional csDMARDs. Choice of csDMARDs for RA is based on liver function status (Table 8.2.1)	*ACR guideline:* Low dose steroids, MTX, TNFi, anti-IL-6, and RTX can be given in RA with chronic hepatitis B, with antiviral and regular monitoring
*Occult HBV infection	Cases of occult HBV infection also need antivirals before biologic DMARDs particularly RTX or other immunosuppressive such as cyclophosphamide Monitor with ALT and HBV DNA every 3–6 months	Continue prophylactic antivirals during the entire treatment period, and for at least 12 months after RTX treatment.
Hepatitis C Virus (HCV)		
Anti-HCV+ve	Refer to a hepatologist for management of HCV infection. Available evidence suggests that TNFi therapy of RA in patients with concomitant HCV infection (who are on antivirals) using ETN or IFX with MTX does not lead to rise in viral loads or transaminitis Preliminary data also suggest that tofacitinib can be given along with antiviral treatment Monitor with ALT and HCV RNA	Low to moderate doses of glucocorticoids can be used MTX is safe TNFi is safe in HCV-positive patients, if treatment with antiviral therapy is used Minimize immunosuppression and consider using other DMARDs such as SSZ or HCQ
Human Immunodeficiency Virus (HIV)		
HIV +ve	HIV in RA patient may lead to remission Treatment must be individualized and similar to any RA patient Careful surveillance on drug interactions with ART and adverse effects	Monitor for comorbidities Lacunae for evidence regarding biologic DMARDs

*Occult HBV: HBsAg-ve and antiHBc IgG+ve. If HBV DNAalso +ve it is true occult HBV

DMARDs: Disease modifying antirheumatic drugs; *bDMARD:* Biologic DMARD; *TNFi:* Tumor necrosis factor inhibitors; *ETN:* Etanercept; *IFX:* Infliximab; *MTX:* Methotrexate; *SSZ:* Sulfasalazine; *HCQ:* Hydroxychloroquine; *ART:* Antiretroviral therapy

Reactivation can occur even after 6 months of the last rituximab infusion, hence antiviral prophylaxis in such cases is longer. Treatment of HBV should be in close coordination with a gastroenterologist or infectious disease specialist.

In HCV infection low dose steroids, and MTX are safe. TNFi therapy is also safe provided the patient is on antiviral treatment. But as a principle one should minimize the level of immunosuppression in chronic viral infections.

MALIGNANCY

In a patient with a past history of treated solid organ malignancy, all DMARDs can be used. However, in presence of skin cancers avoid biologics and tofacitinib (Table 8.2.5).

Table 8.2.5: Management of RA with history of malignancy, and previous infections

Malignancy	*Management of RA*
Previously treated or untreated skin cancer (non-melanoma or melanoma)	• Avoid biologics and tofacitinib • Use csDMARDs
Previously treated lymphoproliferative disorder	• Avoid TNFi and tofacitinib • Use rituximab, combination csDMARD or abatacept or tocilizumab
Previously treated solid tumors	• All biologics and csDMARDS drugs can be used
Previous serious infection(s) or tendency for repeated infections	
Previous serious infections and susceptibility to infections	• Use csDMARD over biological and tofacitinib • Use abatacept over TNFi • A careful analysis on infection and disease activity is necessary • Choose the drug with least immunosuppressive property

RA: Rheumatoid arthritis; *DMARDs:* Disease modifying anti-rheumatic drugs; *TNFi:* Tumor necrosis factor inhibitor

LEARNING POINTS

- It is imperative to customize the medications and other supportive therapy based on the comorbidity. DMARDs prescription varies in different scenarios.
- A shared decision-making with patients is key to managing the associated comorbidity.

FURTHER READING

1. Fraenkel L, Bathon JM, England BR, et al. 2021 American College of Rheumatology Guideline for the Treatment of Rheumatoid Arthritis. Arthritis Care Res (Hoboken). 2021; 73:924–39.
2. Padjen I, Crnogaj MR, Anić B. Conventional disease-modifying agents in rheumatoid arthritis—a review of their current use and role in treatment algorithms. Reumatologia. 2020; 58:390–400.
3. Perrillo RP, Gish R, Falck-Ytter YT. American Gastroenterological Association Institute technical review on prevention and treatment of hepatitis B virus reactivation during immunosuppressive drug therapy. Gastroenterology. 2015; 148: 221–44.
4. Smolen JS, Landewé RBM, Bijlsma JWJ, et al. EULAR recommendations for the management of rheumatoid arthritis with synthetic and biological disease-modifying antirheumatic drugs: 2019 update. Ann Rheum Dis 2020; 79:685–699.

Pregnancy and Lactation in Rheumatoid Arthritis

S Rajeswari, Koshy Nithin Thomas

INTRODUCTION

Rheumatoid arthritis (RA) like most autoimmune diseases predominantly affect women. Unlike in SLE pregnancy often has a favorable effect on RA. Nevertheless the physician has a role in ensuring that the patient has a low disease activity preferably remission before planning pregnancy so that the pregnancy outcomes are favorable.

PREGNANCY IN RA

Pregnancy is an example of a natural model for immune tolerance. An initial proinflammatory state is required for implantation, which is followed by an anti-inflammatory state for maintenance of pregnancy, and a return to a pro-inflammatory state during parturition. In RA the postpartum period is characterized by a flare of the disease.

Decreased Fertility in Rheumatoid Arthritis

An increase in 'time to pregnancy' of more than twelve months is considered as subfertility. The prevalence of subfertility in RA is around 25%. Various factors are associated with subfertility in RA, one of which is older age. Women older than 35 years often have subfertility due to low ovarian reserves. Another cause of subfertility in RA is the presence of anovulatory cycles which are mainly associated with drugs used to control disease namely NSAIDs, and corticosteroids. And as expected women with high disease activity (DAS-ESR >5.1) have increased time to pregnancy due to pain, disability, and reduced libido.

Impact of Pregnancy on Rheumatoid Arthritis

Pregnancy has a favorable outcome on RA disease activity. Prospective studies have shown that disease activity significantly improved in the third trimester compared to the first trimester as well as compared to preconception. Similar results were confirmed in a recent systematic review and meta-analysis, which showed an improvement in 60% of pregnancies. In modern times because of good disease control with biologics and nonbiologic DMARDs, increasing proportion of women who enter into pregnancy are in low disease activity state or remission, and significantly more enter into remission during pregnancy.

Pregnancy Outcomes

Pregnant women with RA are at an increased risk for preeclampsia, maternal hypertension, and caesarean section delivery compared to the general population, albeit only marginally. Preterm delivery rates as high as 23% have been reported. Risk factors include high disease activity and corticosteroids. Other reported maternal complications are a higher frequency of infections, premature rupture of membranes, and gestational diabetes.

Fetal Outcomes

The various fetal outcomes of pregnancy in RA include increased odds of intrauterine growth restriction (IUGR) babies, OR=1.93. The frequency of small for gestational age babies varies from 10 to 22%. High disease activity and corticosteroids are risk factors for small gestational-age babies.

Postpartum Period

Upto half of RA patients flare in the postpartum period. The risk is maximum at 12 weeks. Nearly 40% experience a moderate flare by 6 weeks postpartum. Women may also have an increased risk of developing new onset RA after a pregnancy as per retrospective series showing incidence rate ratio of 1.73 (1.1–2.7).

TREATMENT CONSIDERATIONS

During Pregnancy

Teratogenicity remains the primary concern with usage of DMARDs during pregnancy, but an increased time to conception, miscarriages and prematurity have all been variably described with this group of drugs.

NSAIDs: These drugs are associated with delayed time to conception. The association of NSAIDs with abortions is controversial and they are generally considered safe in the first and second trimesters. However, it is advised to discontinue NSAIDs at 32 weeks, to avoid premature closure of the ductus arteriosus. NSAIDs may also impair labor. As data on selective COX inhibitors are lacking, it is generally recommended to use nonselective COX inhibitors during pregnancy.

Glucocorticoids: They can be used for both maternal as well as fetal indications during pregnancy. Non-fluorinated glucocorticoids such as prednisolone are preferred as they are metabolized by the placenta. However, glucocorticoids come at the cost of IUGR, short gestational age, and premature rupture of membranes. Doses greater than 10 mg of prednisolone are associated with increased adverse effects.

Methotrexate: It should be discontinued in all women planning to conceive. The teratogenicity associated with methotrexate is nearly 10% of live births. Methotrexate is also associated with an increased risk of miscarriages (40%).

Sulfasalazine: It crosses the placental barrier but is considered safe during pregnancy. It is important to supplement patients with folic acid in these patients during pregnancy.

Leflunomide: Use after the first trimester, after cholestyramine washout, has not been associated with definite teratogenicity, However, it is still strongly recommended against during pregnancy.

TNF inhibitors (TNFi): They are capable of crossing the placenta by fetal Fc receptor-mediated transport. Transfer increases steadily after 13 weeks. Beyond 30 weeks, cord blood levels are equal to or higher than maternal levels. IgG antibodies have a longer half-life of 48 days in newborns and may persist for up to 6 months of age. Live vaccines in the newborn should be avoided for 6 months if the mother has received biologics after 22 weeks of gestation. The TNFi infliximab, adalimumab, and golimumab can be given up to 20 weeks of pregnancy, while etanercept, a soluble TNFR/Fc fusion protein, is considered safe till 32 weeks. Certolizumab pegol is considered safe throughout pregnancy due to the lack of the Fc portion.

Rituximab: It is an anti-CD20 monoclonal antibody used in refractory RA should be discontinued at least 6 months before conception. However, the recent American College of Rheumatology (ACR) guidelines recommends that rituximab be continued in patients trying to conceive. Rituximab is initiated during pregnancy only in life-endangering situations.

Due to the lack of evidence, the use of abatacept and tocilizumab during pregnancy is not recommended. These drugs can however be continued while trying to conceive.

Evidence is still insufficient for JAK inhibitors. Since these molecules are of low molecular weight, it is expected that these molecules cross the placenta. No formal recommendations have been put forward by the ACR at present. Treatment recommendations for patients planning for pregnancy have been summarised in Tables 8.3.1 and 8.3.2.

During Lactation

Lack of proper counseling during the postpartum period results in a tendency to avoid breastfeeding. Methotrexate and leflunomide are present in breast milk and contraindicated throughout lactation. Sulfasalazine, especially its metabolite, is present in breast milk. Though it is not contraindicated in lactation, it should be avoided in preterm babies and in the setting of neonatal hyperbilirubinemia. Corticosteroids are considered safe during lactation. The only consideration is the dose, there must be a gap of at least 4 hours between the steroid dose and feeding if the dose of prednisolone exceeds 20 mg.

Table 8.3.1: Summary of treatment recommendations in individuals with rheumatoid arthritis (RA) planning for a family

Men	**Strongly recommend continuing** • Hydroxychloroquine (HCQ) • TNF inhibitors (TNFi) **Conditionally recommend continuing** • NSAIDs • Methotrexate (MTX) • Leflunomide • Sulfasalazine: Semen analysis in case of delayed conception **Strongly recommend discontinuation** • Cyclophosphamide: 12 weeks prior to conception
Women	**Discontinue before conception and counsel about the teratogenicity** • MTX • Leflunomide • Cyclophosphamide **Adjustment of DMARDs before conception** • Maximum suppression of disease activity. • Reduce NSAIDS: Stop when conception planned. • To decrease to lowest possible steroid dose (prednisolone <7.5 mg/day) **Unplanned pregnancy while on MTX** • Stop MTX immediately. Give folic acid supplementation **Leflunomide** • Ideally to be avoided in patients of childbearing age • It is to be discontinued at least 2 years before planned conception or eliminate the drug by interrupting its enterohepatic circulation by giving a washout with cholestyramine 8 g TID for 11 days. Serum levels <0.02 mg/L at two weeks apart is safe for pregnancy.

Adopted from: Götestam Skorpen C, et al. Ann Rheum Dis. 2016; 75:795-810; Sammaritano LR, et al. Arthritis Care Res (Hoboken). 2020;72:461–88.

Table 8.3.2: Summary of treatment recommendations during pregnancy

Strongly recommended • **Prednisolone:** Taper to <20 mg/day • **Hydroxychloroquine** • **Sulfasalazine** • **Tacrolimus:** Monitor blood pressure • **Certolizumab:** Can be given throughout pregnancy
Conditionally recommended • **Nonsteroidal anti-inflammatory drugs (NSAIDs):** Contraindicated in 3rd trimester-due to premature closure of foetal ductus arteriosus. Ibuprofen has decreased placental transfer and short t1/2. • **Azathioprine** • **TNF inhibitors:** Preferably to avoid after 20 weeks of pregnancy due to increased fetal absorption. Avoid live vaccines in infants for first 6 months.
Noncompatible with pregnancy • **Methotrexate:** Stop and give folic acid 5 mg/day • **Leflunomide:** Stop and give cholestyramine washout • **Cyclophosphamide:** In case of life or organ threatening disease can be given in 2nd and 3rd trimesters

(Contd.)

Table 8.3.2: Summary of treatment recommendations during pregnancy (*Contd.*)

Insufficient data
- Anakinra
- Abatacept
- **Rituximab:** Can be considered in life-threatening disease
- Tocilizumab
- JAK inhibitor

Adopted from: Götestam Skorpen C, et al. Ann Rheum Dis 2016; 75:795-810; Sammaritano LR, et al. Arthritis Care Res (Hoboken) 2020; 72:461–88.

NSAIDs, hydroxychloroquine, azathioprine, TNF inhibitors, rituximab, abatacept, and tocilizumab are considered safe during lactation (Table 8.3.3).

Table 8.3.3: Summary of treatment recommendations during lactation

Strongly recommended
- Hydroxychloroquine
- Sulfasalazine: Warning for bloody diarrhea in neonate
- All TNFi

Conditionally recommended
- NSAIDs: Ibuprofen preferred
- Prednisolone: After a dose of >20 mg, delay breastfeeding for 4 hours
- Tacrolimus
- Azathioprine

Not compatible with lactation
- Methotrexate
- Leflunomide
- Cyclophosphamide

IS THERE AN IDEAL TIME FOR PLANNING A PREGNANCY IN RHEUMATOID ARTHRITIS?

Prospective studies have shown that the ameliorative effect of pregnancy on RA is seen predominantly in those with low or moderate disease activity and not with high disease activity. Active disease and high doses of corticosteroids during pregnancy are associated with intrauterine growth restriction and preterm delivery.

While a patient has active RA contraceptive advice should be given in consultation with an obstetrician, this is to avoid inadvertent pregnancy while on fetotoxic medicines such as methotrexate. The choice of contraceptives depends on antiphospholipid antibody status (Fig. 8.3.1). With the wide availability of TNF inhibitors and their proven safety in the initial trimester of pregnancy, many patients are achieving good disease control, and those who wish to conceive can do so. However, these drugs continue to be beyond the reach of the majority of patients. Considering these

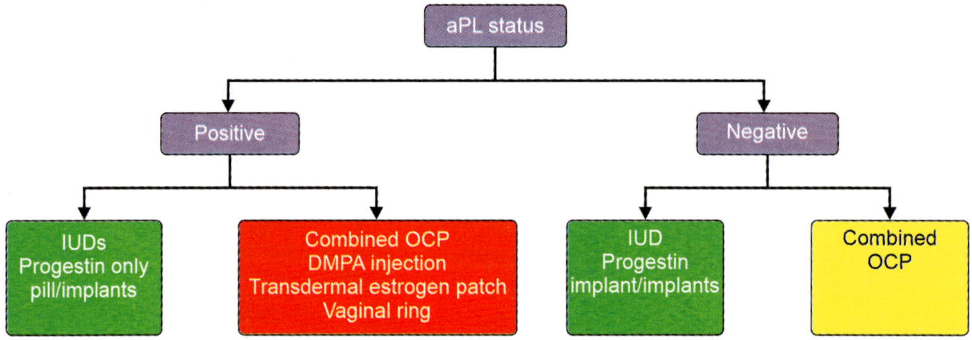

Fig. 8.3.1: Choice of contraceptives in a patient with RA depends on the antiphospholipid antibodies (aPL) status. Green: safe contraceptive choice; Red: Not recommended; Yellow: Is not preferred. *APLA:* Antiphospholipid antibody; *IUD:* Intrauterine device; *OCP:* Oral contraceptive pill; *DMPA:* Depot medroxyprogesterone acetate

points, pregnancy in RA should ideally be deferred till the patient has attained low disease activity.

LEARNING POINTS

- Pregnancy is associated with an improvement in disease activity in rheumatoid arthritis
- A suppressed Th1 state during pregnancy in rheumatoid arthritis rather than a transition to Th2 profile is responsible for the immunotolerant state seen in pregnancy
- The treating physician should enquire about the patient's plans for pregnancy and appraise them of the importance of optimising medications prior to pregnancy to avoid drug related toxicity
- Active disease is a predictor of pregnancy morbidity and thus it would be ideal to time pregnancy at the time of low disease activity
- The physician should allay fears of drug toxicity during breastfeeding when lactation compatible drugs are prescribed
- Postpartum flare of disease is seen in 40% cases

FURTHER READING

1. de Man YA, Dolhain RJ, van de Geijn FE, et al. Disease activity of rheumatoid arthritis during pregnancy: results from a nationwide prospective study. Arthritis Rheum. 2008;59:1241–8.
2. de Jong PH, Dolhain RJ. Fertility, Pregnancy, and Lactation in Rheumatoid Arthritis. Rheum Dis Clin North Am. 2017;43:227–37.
3. Förger F, Villiger PM. Immunological adaptations in pregnancy that modulate rheumatoid arthritis disease activity [published correction appears in Nat Rev Rheumatol. 2020 Mar;16(3):184]. Nat Rev Rheumatol. 2020;16:113–22.
4. Götestam Skorpen C, Hoeltzenbein M, Tincani A, et al. The EULAR points to consider for use of antirheumatic drugs before pregnancy, and during pregnancy and lactation. Ann Rheum Dis. 2016; 75:795–810.
5. Jethwa H, Lam S, Smith C, et al. Does Rheumatoid Arthritis Really Improve During Pregnancy? A Systematic Review and Metaanalysis. J Rheumatol. 2019; 46:245–50.
6. Smeele HTW, Dolhain RJEM. Current perspectives on fertility, pregnancy and childbirth in patients with Rheumatoid Arthritis. Semin Arthritis Rheum. 2019; 49:S32–S35.
7. Sammaritano LR, Bermas BL, Chakravarty EE, et al. 2020 American College of Rheumatology Guideline for the Management of Reproductive Health in Rheumatic and Musculoskeletal Diseases. Arthritis Care Res (Hoboken). 2020; 72:461–88.
8. Zbinden A, van den Brandt S, Østensen M, Villiger PM, Förger F. Risk for adverse pregnancy outcome in axial spondyloarthritis and rheumatoid arthritis: disease activity matters. Rheumatology (Oxford). 2018; 57:1235–42.

Nonradiographic Axial Spondyloarthritis

Himanshu Pathak

INTRODUCTION

Our understanding of axial spondyloarthritis (axSpA) spectrum diseases has improved significantly in the last three decades. The classical term Ankylosing Spondylitis (AS) has been used since the early twentieth century to describe patients with typical clinical and radiographic features of spondyloarthritis (SpA).

Prospective cohort studies in the decades of 1990–2000 using magnetic resonance imaging (MRI) of sacroiliac joints (SIJs) and spine showed subset of patients with typical clinical and laboratory manifestations of SpA without radiographic changes in the SIJs. These patients had describable inflammatory changes on MRI. These studies suggested that reliance only on radiographic SIJs features led to a delayed diagnosis of axSpA. Therefore the concept of *non-radiographic* axial spondyloarthritis (nr-axSpA) was incorporated in the 2009 Assessment of SpondyloArthritis International Society (ASAS) classification criteria for axSpA.

DEFINITION OF NR-AXSPA

By applying the ASAS criteria, in a patient with age less than 45 years and inflammatory back pain for more than three months, axSpA can be classified in two disease subgroups according to radiographic changes at sacroiliac joints, HLA-B27 positivity and characteristic clinical features (Fig. 8.4.1). Patients having *x*-ray changes of sclerosis and erosions at sacroiliac joints (SIJs) are considered having radiographic axial spondyloarthritis (r-axSpA) or AS while the term nr-axSpA is used to describe patient

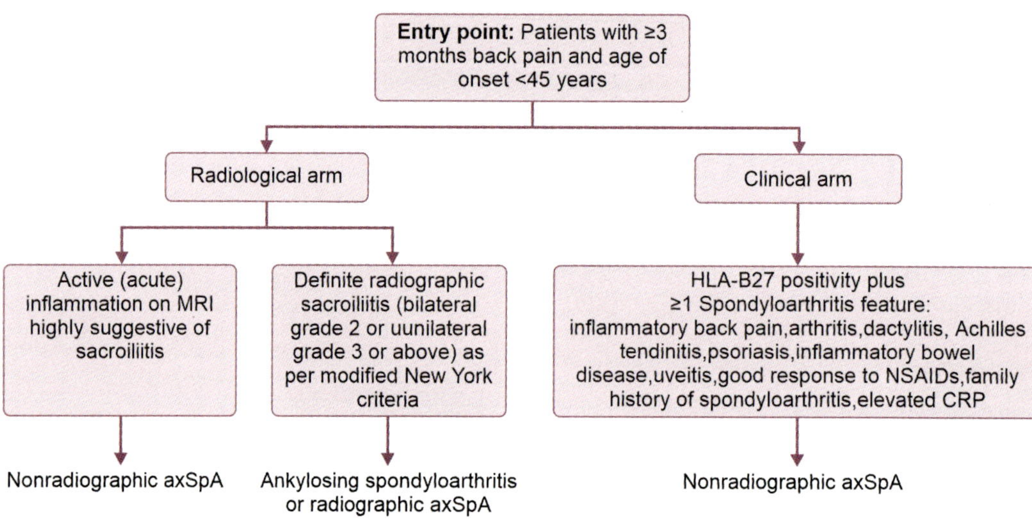

Fig. 8.4.1: ASAS classification criteria for axial spondyloarthritis

subset who has normal SIJs x-ray but has definite features of inflammation on the MRI (imaging arm) OR the patient is HLA B-27 positive with typical clinical features of SpA (clinical arm).

DIAGNOSIS OF NR-AXSPA: CHALLENGES

There remain several challenges in diagnosis of axSpA as there are no biomarkers for diagnosis. The 2009 ASAS criteria were developed to classify patients' groups for clinical research and it is to be understood that diagnosis of axSpA should be clinical, supported by available laboratory and imaging information. Nr-axSpA denotes early disease while AS is a later stage with significant irreversible structural damage. About 10–20% of newly diagnosed nr-axSpA patients will progress to the radiographic stage in the next 2–3 years. Male gender, HLA B-27 positivity, high CRP, and longer disease duration are risk factors of progression to radiographic stage from non-radiographic stage.

AS VS NR-AXSPA: ARE THEY SIMILAR?

Several observational and randomized control studies have shown similar disease burden in patients with radiographic and non-radiographic spondyloarthritis. Nr-axSpA is more common in women while r-axSpA is more prevalent in men. The classical manifestations of axSpA like arthritis, enthesitis and dactylitis occur in comparable frequencies in both r-axSpA and nr-axSpA. The occurrence of extra-articular manifestations like psoriasis, anterior uveitis, inflammatory bowel disease is similar in both disease entities. All available evidence suggests similar patient reported disease activity indices (BASDAI, BASFI) and severity in patients with either radiographic or non-radiographic disease.

MANAGEMENT OF NR-AXSPA

As per 2019 American College of Rheumatology update on management of AS and nr-SpA, treatment principles are similar in both scenarios.

NSAIDs: For initial stages of nr-SpA, nonsteroidal anti-inflammatory drugs (NSAIDs) are strongly recommended, and advice is to continue them during the active phase of disease. No NSAID is preferred over others however, in the author's experience COX-2 inhibitors (etoricoxib and celecoxib) are effective and very well tolerated. Once symptoms are stable, NSAIDs can be taken on demand basis.

Sulfasalazine (**SSZ**) is used for peripheral arthritis. Use of SSZ in axial disease is not well established in clinical studies, however, in resource constraint settings where biologic therapies are not easily available, trials of SSZ along with NSAIDs can be given.

Methotrexate and Leflunomide can be used in peripheral arthritis and have no role in axial symptoms. Patients, who respond partially or minimally to at least two different NSAIDs in maximal doses over one month intake, need escalation to biologic therapies.

Tumor necrosis factor inhibitors (**TNFi**) are drugs of choice in the biologic category because of their established safety and efficacy profile.

Interleukin-17 inhibitors (**Secukinumab and Ixekizumab**) have also been approved for use in nr-axSpA.

JAK inhibitor (**tofacitinib**) has been approved to be used in AS only.

Tapering of biological therapies after patients achieving disease remission is an area of ongoing research. In patients with persistent remission for 6 months 12 months biologic tapering can be considered either by decreasing dose or increasing interval between doses. Patients with baseline high disease activity and radiographic structural damage have more chances of relapse after biologic tapering.

Physical therapy holds a very important place in management of axSpA. Once disease symptoms are reduced, patients are encouraged to participate in physiotherapy. Supervised physiotherapy programs are shown to be more effective than individual efforts. Physical therapy should be customized according to patients occupational and financial needs and importance should be given in making patients self-reliant for their physical and mental wellbeing.

LEARNING POINTS

- Advances in MRI technology have allowed recognition of inflammation in sacroiliac joints and spine in axSpA. In the correct clinical context, active inflammation in sacroiliac joints without any changes on radiographs, is defined as non-radiographic axSpA.

- Non-radiographic and radiographic axSpA are continuum of the same disease process.
- Not all patients with non-radiographic axSpA will progress to radiographic axSpA (AS).
- Disease burden of non-radiographic and radiographic axSpA is the same with identical treatment options.

FURTHER READING

1. Michelena X, López-Medina C, Marzo-Ortega H. Non-radiographic versus radiographic axSpA: what's in a name? Rheumatology (Oxford). 2020; 59(Suppl4):iv18-iv24.
2. van der Heijde D, Ramiro S, Landewé R, et al. 2016 update of the ASAS-EULAR management recommendations for axial spondyloarthritis. Ann Rheum Dis. 2017;76:978–991.
3. Ward MM, Deodhar A, Gensler LS, et al. 2019 Update of the American College of Rheumatology/ Spondylitis Association of America/Spondyloarthritis Research and Treatment Network Recommendations for the Treatment of Ankylosing Spondylitis and Nonradiographic Axial Spondyloarthritis. Arthritis Care Res (Hoboken). 2019;71:1285–1299.

Chapter 8.5

Ankylosing Spondylitis: Clinical Features, Diagnosis, and Management

Sumantro Mondal, Alakendu Ghosh

INTRODUCTION

Ankylosing spondylitis (AS) is a chronic inflammatory arthritis that predominantly affects the axial skeleton, though peripheral arthritis and other extra-articular manifestations may be present. In the advanced stage of the disease, patients may develop spinal ankylosis resulting in gross restriction of movement and limitation of functional capacity.

CLINICAL FEATURES

Back Pain

Back pain and stiffness are the most common presenting features of AS. The back pain of AS is characteristically inflammatory back pain (IBP) (Box 8.5.1). Alternate buttock pain is usually seen in the early phase.

Joint Involvement

Involvement of the hip, shoulder, and other peripheral joints is also seen in AS. Pain in the chest wall, enthesitis, and dactylitis are the other features of AS (Table 8.5.1).

Box 8.5.1: Assessment of SpondyloArthritis International Society criteria for IBP

1. Age of onset <40 years
2. Pain improves with exercise
3. Insidious onset of back pain
4. Pain at night which improves upon getting up.
5. No improvement of pain with rest

Four out of these 5 criteria should be present to make a diagnosis of IBP.

IBP: Inflammatory back pain

Extra-articular Manifestations

Extra-articular manifestations of AS are summarized in Table 8.5.2.

DIAGNOSIS

The 1984 modified New York criteria (Table 8.5.3) was used for the classification/diagnosis of AS. This criteria includes both clinical and radiological features. AS is now called radiographic axial spondyloarthritis (radiographic ax-SpA) a term

Table 8.5.1: Other clinical features of AS

Clinical feature	*Comments*
Arthritis	Hip (in 50%), shoulder joints. Asymmetric oligoarthritis of lower limb
Enthesitis	Tenderness at the insertion of tendon/ligament with the bone. Common site: insertion of tendo-Achilles
Chest wall pain	Due to the involvement of the thoracic spine and enthesitis of costosternal and manubriosternal joints
Dactylitis	Swelling of an entire digit also known as 'Sausage digit'

Table 8.5.2: Extra-articular manifestations of AS

Manifestation	*Prevalence*
Acute anterior uveitis	25–40%
Gut inflammation	**Subclinical:** 50–60% **IBD:** 5–10%
Lung involvement (bilateral upper lobe fibrosis)	**HRCT abnormality:** up to 61% **X-ray abnormality:** 1–2%
Cardiac	**Aortic incompetence:** 10% after 30 years **Conduction abnormality:** 8.5% after 30 years
Neurological (due to vertebral fracture or subluxation)	**Spontaneous anterior atlantoaxial subluxation:** 2%
Renal (IgA nephropathy, rarely amyloidosis)	**Overall:** 10–35%
Osteoporosis	**Overall:** 15%

Table 8.5.3: Modified New York criteria, 1984

Clinical features	*Radiological features*
1. Low back pain and stiffness persisting for >3 months which improves with exercise but not with rest. 2. Limitation of lumbar spinal motion in both the sagittal and frontal planes. 3. Limitation of expansion of chest in respect to normal values corrected for age and sex.	Radiographic sacroiliitis eiher grade 3–4 unilaterally or grade ≥2 bilaterally.

Diagnosis of AS is made in the presence of the radiological feature and at least 1 clinical feature.

defined by the Assessment of SpondyloArthritis International Society (ASAS) group.

MANAGEMENT

Both the pharmacological and non-pharmacological approaches are equally important to achieve the optimal outcome.

Pharmacological Treatment

1. **Non-steroidal anti-inflammatory drugs (NSAIDs):** NSAIDs are the first-line treatment for the active AS. Nearly 70–80% of AS patients report good responses to NSAID treatment. Continuous treatment with NSAID at the highest tolerated dose has been recommended in the recent guidelines. In AS patients with stable disease status, on-demand NSAIDs should be given.
2. **Corticosteroids:** Systemic corticosteroids are not recommended for the management of AS. Intra-articular corticosteroids can be given in sacroiliac or peripheral joints.
3. **Conventional synthetic disease-modifying anti-rheumatic drugs (csDMARDs):** Sulfasalazine or methotrexate can be used in active AS patients, not responding to NSAID adequately, with peripheral joint involvement, or when an anti-TNF agent is not available. It is important to note that, when an anti-TNF agent cannot be used due to the presence of tuberculosis, other chronic infections, or risk of recurrent infections, sulfasalazine is preferred over other biologic-DMARDs.
4. **Biologics DMARDS (bDMARDs):** Currently 2 types of bDMARDs are approved for the management of AS; anti-TNF agents and anti-IL-17 agents.
   i. **Anti-TNF agents:** These drugs improve pain, function, and other symptoms of AS. After 24 weeks of treatment with anti-TNF agents 39–48% of AS patients achieved ASAS 40 response. The ATLAS trial (using adalimumab) showed sustained maintenance (up to 2 years) of various AS disease activity indices and improvement of physical function and mobility. Anti-TNF agents can retard the radiographic progression of AS, however early initiation of treatment, and

a longer duration of follow-up is required. Current guideline recommends using any anti-TNF agents in adult AS patients not responding to NSAID treatment. Screening for active or latent tuberculosis infection is mandatory before the initiation of an anti-TNF agent.

ii. **Anti-IL-17 agents:** Both secukinumab and ixekizumab showed good efficacy in AS in different clinical trials and are approved for the management of AS.

Anti-IL-17 drugs are also quite effective in retarding the radiographic progression of AS with acceptable tolerability and safety profile. *Candida* infection and new-onset or exacerbations of IBD have been reported in a very small proportion of patients receiving anti-IL-17 agents. Importantly, no increased susceptibility to tuberculosis was reported with anti-IL-17 agents. Anti-IL-17 agents can be used for active AS non-responding to NSAIDs, and who have contraindications to TNF-inhibitors. Doses of bDMARDs used in AS are summarized in Table 8.5.4.

Nonpharmacological Treatment

1. **Patient education:** It is an integral part of the management of AS. Upon diagnosis, the patient should be informed about the disease course, lifestyle modification, and medications. Smoking should be strongly discouraged.
2. **Physical therapy:** Spinal extension and rotation-related exercises are advised in AS patients. Breathing exercises are also important to counteract the decreased chest wall movement. Simple exercises such as lying prone is a useful method for the prevention of contractures of the hip joints. This can be done for 15–20 minutes once or twice a day. Patients should use a firm mattress during sleep with a small neck-support pillow.

Surgery

Surgery is reserved for patients with advanced hip arthritis or spinal disease. Total hip replacement is an option for any AS patients with refractory pain in hip joint/s and disability. Spinal corrective osteotomy is an option in patients with advanced spinal deformity and disability

Management of the Extra-articular Manifestations of AS

Acute anterior uveitis: Adalimumab and infliximab are the preferred drugs for the management of recurrent uveitis in AS.

Inflammatory bowel disease (IBD): NSAIDs should be avoided in active IBD. Anti-TNF agents (infliximab, adalimumab) are the preferred treatment options for the coexistent IBD in AS. Etanercept is not effective.

The choice of treatment in AS depends on the manifestation (Table 8.5.5 and Fig. 8.5.1), outcomes are improved with patient counseling and availability of biologic DMARDs.

Table 8.5.4: bDMARDs approved for use in patients with ankylosing spondylitis

	Name of the bDMARD	*Dose and route*
Anti-TNF agents	Infliximab	5 mg/kg at week 0, 2, 6 then every 6 weekly by IV infusion
	Etanercept	25 mg twice weekly or 50 mg once weekly by subcutaneous (SC) injection
	Adalimumab	40 mg every 2 weekly SC
	Certolizumab pegol	400 mg at week 0, 2, 4 This is followed by 200 mg fortnightly or 400 mg every 4 weeks SC
	Golimumab	50 mg every 4 weekly SC
Anti-IL-17 agents	Secukinumab	**With loading dose:** 150 mg at weeks 0, 1, 2, 3, 4 then every 4 weekly SC **Without loading dose:** 150 mg every 4 weekly SC
	Ixekizumab	160 mg at week 0, followed by 80 mg 4 weekly SC

Table 8.5.5: Summary of treatment modalities for different domains of ankylosing spondylitis

Drug	*Axial manifestations*	*Peripheral manifestations*	*Extra-articular*
NSAID	Yes	Yes	No
CsDMARD	±	Yes	Not the 1st line drug
Corticosteroid	No	Yes (Intra-articular)	Can be used
Anti-TNF	Yes	Yes	Yes (Except Etanercept)
Anti-IL-17	Yes	Yes	No
Nonpharmacological measures for all AS patients			
Surgery: THR or spinal osteotomy for refractory and disabling disease			

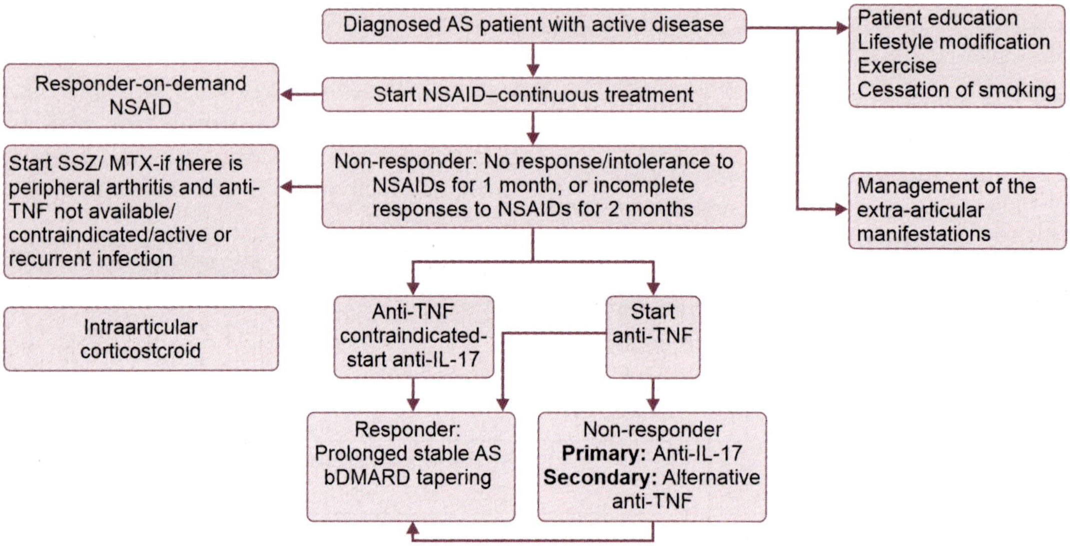

Fig. 8.5.1: Management of ankylosing spondylitis. *AS:* Ankylosing spondylitis; *SSZ:* Sulfasalazine; *MTX:* Methotrexate

LEARNING POINTS

- Back pain and stiffness are the most common presenting features of AS.
- NSAIDs are the first-line treatment for the active AS.
- Anti-TNF agents improve pain, function, and quality of life.
- Sulfasalazine or methotrexate can be used in active AS patients not responding to NSAID adequately with peripheral joint involvement, or when an anti-TNF agent is not available.
- There is no increased risk of tuberculosis with anti-IL-17 agents.

FURTHER READING

1. Maxwell LJ, Zochling J, Boonen A, et al. TNF-alpha inhibitors for ankylosing spondylitis. Cochrane Database Syst Rev. 2015 18;(4):CD005468.
2. Sieper J, Listing J, Poddubnyy D, et al. Effect of continuous versus on-demand treatment of ankylosing spondylitis with diclofenac over 2 years on radiographic progression of the spine: results from a randomised multicentre trial (ENRADAS). Ann Rheum Dis. 2016; 75(8):1438–43.
3. van der Heijde D, Ramiro S, Landewé R, et al. 2016 update of the ASAS-EULAR management recommendations for axial spondyloarthritis. Ann Rheum Dis. 2017; 76(6):978–91.
4. Ward MM, Deodhar A, Gensler LS, et al. 2019 Update of the American College of Rheumatology/ Spondylitis Association of America/Spondyloarthritis Research and Treatment Network Recommendations for the Treatment of Ankylosing Spondylitis and Nonradiographic Axial Spondyloarthritis. Arthritis Care Res (Hoboken). 2019; 71(10):1285–99.
5. Yin Y, Wang M, Liu M, et al. Efficacy and safety of IL-17 inhibitors for the treatment of ankylosing spondylitis: a systematic review and meta-analysis. Arthritis Res Ther. 2020; 22(1):111.

Chapter 8.6

Psoriatic Arthritis

Vinod Chandran

INTRODUCTION

Psoriatic arthritis (PsA) is an inflammatory arthritis, a spondyloarthritis (SpA), associated with cutaneous psoriasis. The prevalence of PsA depends on the prevalence of psoriasis, with about 24% of patients with psoriasis having PsA. The prevalence of psoriasis in adults in India is estimated to be 0.44–2.8%, with only 8.7% of patients with psoriasis having PsA. Nevertheless, patients with PsA have impaired quality of life and function and higher mortality risk, especially from cardiovascular disease.

DIAGNOSIS AND CLASSIFICATION

Most patients with PsA have psoriasis. Psoriasis either precedes or develops simultaneously with PsA in almost 90% of patients. Therefore, the diagnosis of PsA rests on the identification of inflammatory musculoskeletal diseases (peripheral arthritis, enthesitis, dactylitis, inflammatory axial disease) in patients with psoriasis or a family history of psoriasis. Since there are no diagnostic biomarkers and the levels of acute-phase reactants may be normal despite active disease, the diagnosis of PsA is made by careful clinical examination aided by imaging. Most patients with PsA have chronic plaque psoriasis mostly involving extensor surfaces, but flexural psoriasis is also common. Pustular psoriasis is also associated with inflammatory arthritis resembling SpA/PsA and may be a distinct pathophysiologic entity. Psoriatic nail dystrophy is a marker for the presence of current PsA, and a marker for future PsA.

Synovitis of the peripheral joints is the most common manifestation of established PsA. It is often oligoarticular, to begin with and may progress to polyarthritis. The pattern of arthritis is often asymmetric and the joints sustaining significant biomechanical stress such as the joints of the lower extremities, and distal interphalangeal joints are often involved. Enthesitis is a characteristic feature of SpA including PsA and is clinically detected in more than a third of PsA patients. Distinguishing enthesitis from other causes of enthesopathy/entheseal pain such as metabolic syndrome, osteoarthritis and fibromyalgia remains challenging. Imaging with ultrasonography or MRI may provide diagnostic value. Dactylitis, characterized by inflammation of the synovium, enthesis, tendon sheath and soft tissue of the digits is a characteristic feature that has high diagnostic value. Recognition of inflammatory axial arthritis involving any area of the spine or sacroiliac joints also has high diagnostic value, although diagnosing axial disease in patients who are older and have comorbidities such as obesity and metabolic syndrome is challenging. Other features that may be present include tenosynovitis, inflammation of the joints of the chest wall as well as uveitis and inflammatory bowel disease. The most common differential diagnoses include osteoarthritis, gout, and rheumatoid arthritis (Table 8.6.1).

Once the diagnosis is made, patients may be classified as PsA if they satisfy the CASPAR criteria (Table 8.6.2). Given the heterogeneous nature of the disease, it would also be important to determine the degree to which the following

Table 8.6.1: Clinical and imaging features of psoriatic arthritis (PsA) compared to rheumatoid arthritis (RA), osteoarthritis (OA), and gout

Clinical feature	*PsA*	*RA*	*OA*	*Gout*
Joint involved	Classically DIP involvement is present	All joints can be involved, but DIP not involved	PIP, DIP, first CMC	DIP less common
Symmetry	Asymmetrical usually	Symmetrical	Symmetrical	Asymmetrical
Erosion	Marginal and paramarginal erosions	Marginal erosions	Absent	No erosion. Large erosions with overhanging edges in tophaceous gout
Ankylosis	Characteristic	Rare	Rare	Rare
Periostitis	Quite frequent	Uncommon	Uncommon	Rare
Juxta-articular osteopenia	Typically there is lack of periarticular osteoporosis	Common	Rare	Rare
Axial involvement	Common	Axial disease does not occur, except for atlantoaxial involvement in advanced disease	Occurs but it is not inflammatory	Rare
Enthesitis	Common	Uncommon	Enthesopathy	Uncommon
Dactylitis	Frequent	Uncommon	Uncommon	Rare
Skin	Defining feature	Uncommon	Uncommon	Uncommon
Nails	Frequent	Not involved	Not involved	Not involved

DIP: Distal interphalangeal joints; *PIP:* Proximal interphalangeal joints; *CMC:* Carpometacarpal joints

Table 8.6.2: Classification criteria for psoriatic arthritis (CASPAR)

To classify a patient as psoriatic arthritis the patient must have an established arthritis and a minimum of three of the following:

No.	Feature	Score
1	Current psoriasis, or history of psoriasis, or a family history of psoriasis	2
2	Dactylitis	1
3	Periarticular new bone formation	1
4	Rheumatoid Factor is negative	1
5	Nail dystrophy	1

Adapted from: Taylor W, et al. *Arthritis Rheum.* 2006;54:2665–2673. The CASPAR criteria has a sensitivity and specificity of 91.4% and 98.7%, respectively.

domains are affected—peripheral arthritis, axial arthritis, enthesitis, dactylitis, skin, nails, other extra-articular manifestations (e.g. eye, gut) and comorbidities. This helps in treatment planning and disease monitoring.

INVESTIGATIONS

Investigations typically are done to obtain additional evidence on the presence of musculoskeletal inflammation. Acute phase reactants may be normal but if elevated indicate a worse prognosis.

Rheumatoid factor is usually negative and may help differentiate it from rheumatoid arthritis. Plain radiographs of the peripheral and axial joints help identify the erosive disease as well as axial arthritis and helps stratify for more severe disease. Ultrasonography is helpful in identifying synovitis, tenosynovitis, tendonitis and enthesitis. MRI has the most value in evaluating axial arthritis but also synovitis and enthesitis. Other recommended investigations include those to identify comorbidities including diabetes, hyperlipidemia, and fatty liver disease, as well as tests useful to monitor adverse events (liver and renal function test) to therapy.

TREATMENT

Available pharmacotherapeutic agents for the management of PsA include:

1. Non-steroidal anti-inflammatory drugs (NSAIDs): NSAIDs are often used for the management of symptomatic MSK disease including synovitis, enthesitis, dactylitis and axial arthritis.
2. Corticosteroids: Intra-articular, as well as tendon sheath corticosteroid injections, often relieve severe symptoms of PsA and may be the sole treatment for localised disease. Systemic corticosteroids are generally not recommended.
3. Conventional disease-modifying anti-rheumatic drugs (DMARDs) such as methotrexate, leflunomide and sulfasalazine are often used alone or in combination for the management of peripheral synovitis. Methotrexate also improves psoriasis.
4. Targeted biologic DMARDS including anti-TNF agents (infliximab, etanercept, adalimumab, golimumab and certolizumab pegol) are highly effective for the management of all domains of PsA. Biologics targeting IL-17A such as secukinumab and ixekizumab are also highly effective against all domains with efficacy equivalent to anti-TNF agents in the MSK domains and superiority with regard to psoriasis. However, these drugs are avoided if there is significant uveitis and is contraindicated in the presence of inflammatory bowel disease. Biologics targeting IL-23 (guselkumab, risankizumab) are highly efficacious in treating skin domain and has proven efficacy in peripheral PsA. IL23 inhibitors did not improve axial SpA but may have efficacy in axial PsA. This however requires further investigation. Other biologics effective for peripheral PsA include ustekinumab (anti- IL-12/23) and the CTLA-4 immunoglobulin, abatacept.
5. Targeted synthetic DMARDs: Apremilast, a small molecule targeting PDE4 has efficacy against psoriasis, peripheral arthritis, enthesitis and dactylitis but not axial disease. JAK inhibitors tofacitinib (JAK 1, 3 selective) and upadacitinib (JAK 1 selective) are also efficacious in peripheral arthritis, enthesitis, dactylitis, axial arthritis and psoriasis but do not have labels for the treatment of psoriasis alone.

The Group for Research and Assessment of Psoriasis and Psoriatic Arthritis (GRAPPA) have championed the use of a domain-based approach in its treatment recommendations. They recommend that each domain be carefully assessed and treatment decisions are made based on the most active domain while considering other affected domains. GRAPPA also recommends a treat-to-target approach for the management of PsA. The recommended targets include achieving a state of minimal disease activity or a disease activity index for PsA (DAPSA) remission.

LEARNING POINTS

- Psoriatic arthritis is a spondyloarthritis affecting patients with a personal or family history of psoriasis.
- There are no diagnostic biomarkers and hence the diagnosis depends on careful clinical examination to identify inflammatory musculoskeletal disease (synovitis, enthesitis, dactylitis, axial arthritis) and ruling out other inflammatory diseases.
- Assessing the domains affected including peripheral arthritis, axial arthritis, enthesitis, dactylitis, skin and nail disease, other extra-musculoskeletal disease and comorbidities helps in disease assessment and management planning.
- Many DMARDs are now available with varying efficacy in different domains. Each domain should be careful assessed and treatment decisions made based on the most active domain while considering other affected domains.

- A treat-to-target approach leads to better short and long-term outcomes, and the target for treatment could be either MDA or DAPSA remission.

FURTHER READING

1. Alinaghi F, Calov M, Kristensen LE, et al. Prevalence of psoriatic arthritis in patients with psoriasis: A systematic review and meta-analysis of observational and clinical studies. J Am Acad Dermatol. 2019;80:251–65.
2. Coates LC, Kavanaugh A, Mease PJ, et al. Group for Research and Assessment of Psoriasis and Psoriatic Arthritis 2015 Treatment Recommendations for Psoriatic Arthritis. Arthritis Rheumatol. 2016; 68:1060–71.
3. Dogra S, Mahajan R. Psoriasis: Epidemiology, clinical features, comorbidities, and clinical scoring. Indian Dermatol Online J. 2016; 7:471–80.
4. Kumar R, Sharma A, Dogra S. Prevalence and clinical patterns of psoriatic arthritis in Indian patients with psoriasis. Indian J Dermatol Venereol Leprol. 2014; 80:15–23.

Enteropathic Arthritis

Shounak Ghosh, Rajiva Gupta

INTRODUCTION

Enteropathic arthritis is inflammatory arthritis occurring in concert with inflammatory bowel diseases (IBD) namely Crohn's disease (CD) and ulcerative colitis (UC). The most common extraintestinal manifestations (EIM) of both CD and UC are musculoskeletal (axial and peripheral arthritis). Other reported musculoskeletal EIMs are fibromyalgia, osteoporosis and myositis.

Enteropathic diseases like Whipple's and coeliac disease also have arthritis as a manifestation, and therefore have been mentioned in this chapter.

GUT JOINT AXIS

The relation of gut inflammation and spondyloarthritis is like a two-way street. Up to 60% patients with ankylosing spondylitis (AS) or axial spondyloarthritis (ax-SpA) have subclinical intestinal inflammation. And on the other hand, arthritis is a manifestation of IBD. According to a systematic review the pooled prevalence of arthritis in IBD is 13% peripheral arthritis, 10% radiographic sacroiliitis, and 3% AS (1984 modified New York Criteria).

Further altered gut microbes in the form of increased Prevotellaceae and *Ruminococcus* sp. have shown a correlation with SpA disease activity.

In IBD there is damage to the intestinal mucous layer and intestinal epithelial cells which secrete interleukins (IL) IL-1 and IL-6. Gut barrier damage leads to increased intestinal permeability and systemic circulation of microbial antigens, leading to secretion of IL-23 and activation of Th17 pathway, systemic overproduction of IL-22 and IL-17, which in turn helps Th17 T-lymphocytes to migrate to the synovium and other sites, causing enthesitis, synovitis and osteoproliferation.

CLINICAL FEATURES OF IBD-RELATED ARTHRITIS

Arthritis in IBD occurs simultaneously with or after gut inflammation. Both axial and peripheral arthropathy may occur, with substantial amount of overlap between the two.

Peripheral Arthritis

Peripheral arthritis is more common than axial disease in IBD and in CD>UC. Up to 20% of patients with IBD present with peripheral arthritis. Peripheral arthritis has two patterns pauciarticular (type I) and polyarticular (type II) (Orchard et al.) discussed in Table 8.7.1. The recent classification system using the ASAS (Assessment of SpondyloArthritis International Society) criteria does not use the distinction into type I or type II arthritis anymore but this distinction remains of clinical interest. Both patterns are usually nonerosive and more common in female patients.

Axial Involvement

Recent studies (IBSEN cohort) have revealed the presence of IBP, radiographic sacroiliitis, and AS in 11.5%, 14.7% and 4.5% respectively in a cohort of 470 patients. Asymptomatic sacroiliitis on imaging is seen in 5–24% of IBD patients, and these patients are usually HLA-B27 negative and often do not progress to AS.

Table 8.7.1: Features of IBD-associated Arthritis

Feature	*Axial spondyloarthritis*	*Type I peripheral arthritis*	*Type II peripheral arthritis*
Pattern	Axial joints	Pauciarticular (<5 joints)	Polyarticular (>5 joints)
Joints involved	Spine, Sacroiliac joints	Mainly lower limb, asymmetrical, large joints (e.g. knee)	Symmetrical small joints mainly
Symptom duration	Chronic, >3 months	Acute, <6 weeks	Persistent, chronic
Prevalence in IBD	5–22% in CD; 2–6% in UC	6% CD, 3.5% UC	4% CD, 2.5% UC
Correlation with IBD activity	Independent	Parallels activity, especially in UC	Independent
Extra-intestinal manifestations	Variable association	Strong association	Only associated with uveitis
HLA association	HLA B27 in 50–70%	HLA B27, B35 and DRB1*0103	HLA B44
Timing of arthritis	Frequently precede bowel disease	May occur before IBD, but coincide with IBD flares	Usually after IBD onset
Effect of treating IBD	No response	Usually responds	Responds but less than type I

The clinical features are the same as in axial SpA patients. HLA-B27 is present in 50–60% of IBD-related axialSpA, while in idiopathic AS >90% are HLA-B27 positive. The course and severity of IBD and axial disease are usually independent of one another. IBD-related AS has an equal distribution between males and females.

Enthesitis has been reported in 7–50% in IBD-SpA, and these individuals have a higher prevalence of HLA-B27 positivity. Dactylitis is reported in 4–15%.

DIAGNOSIS

The diagnosis of enteropathic arthritis is clinical and supported by imaging. Radiographic evidence of sacroiliitis on plain radiograph of the pelvis, or detection of early disease using magnetic resonance imaging (MRI) are useful to help decide management. The presence of erosions in peripheral joints should raise a red flag for the possibility of a disease other than enteropathic arthritis. Assessment of disease activity using the Bath indices is routinely done for axial disease. Inflammatory markers may be elevated and used as supportive clues for disease activity. HLA-B27 testing is not routinely recommended for diagnosis, as IBD patients have lower prevalence of positivity. Positive HLA-B27 in IBD with axial disease only warrants close follow up, as they may progress to AS over time.

MANAGEMENT OF IBD-RELATED ARTHRITIS/SPA

Because pauciarticular arthritis occurs in parallel to IBD activity, therefore its management rests on control of underlying IBD. However axial disease and polyarthritis occurs independently, so in the management the first step is to assess IBD disease activity (Fig. 8.7.1).

If the bowel is inactive, a short course of NSAIDs forms the first line of management for axial and peripheral arthritis. Most patients with mild IBD-SpA respond well to NSAIDs. NSAID enteropathy develops in 50–83% individuals after 2 weeks of oral daily NSAID but usually these changes resolve on discontinuing therapy. COX-2 selective inhibitors have lesser gut damage in short courses.

Sulfasalazine (SSZ) is used for IBD-related peripheral arthritis. 5-Aminosalicylic acid (5-ASA) the active moiety in SSZ and mesalamine induces and maintains remission in UC, while its role in CD is not as robust.

Local steroid injections or short-term oral steroids are recommended for the management of

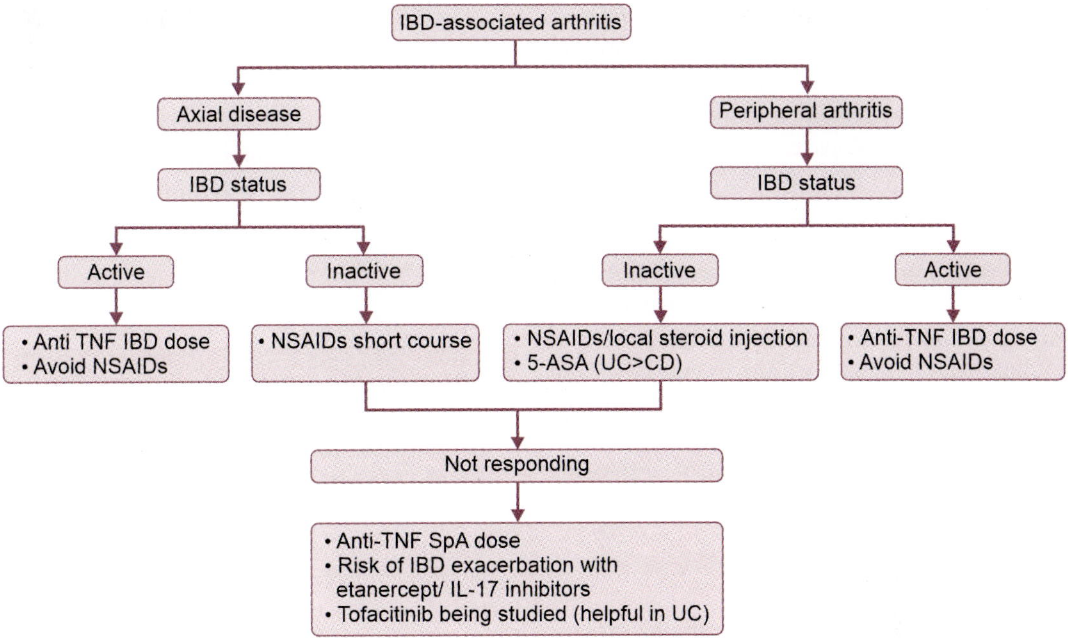

Fig. 8.7.1: Algorithm for treatment of IBD-associated arthritis

arthritis or enthesitis, but oral long-term oral steroid use is not advised in SpA.

DMARDs for Inducing and Maintain Remission of IBD

Corticosteroids are useful for controlling active IBD. Methotrexate in injectable form induces remission in CD, and helps in steroid withdrawal, however not effective for maintenance of remission. Azathioprine (AZA) and 6-mercaptopurine (6-MP) are effective in both inducing and maintaining remission in IBD, but have not shown efficacy for arthritis in SpA.

TNF-α Inhibitors (TNFi)

Infliximab, Adalimumab, Certolizumab pegol, and Golimumab are all effective for inducing and maintaining remission in IBD (including fistulizing CD), and aid to taper steroids. This benefit extends to arthritis and sacroiliitis as well. The dose of TNFi for active IBD is higher (up to 10 mg/kg infliximab per dose or 40 mg adalimumab weekly dosing) than that needed to control arthritis in SpA. Etanercept is not effective in IBD, and some studies have reported flares of IBD after its use. Newer biologics are indicated in CD and UC who have primary or secondary failure to TNFi.

IL-17A/IL-23 Inhibitors

- **Ustekinumab** a human Mab against p40 subunit of Il-12/23 is effective in refractory IBD but ineffective in axial-SpA.
- **Secukinumab and ixekizumab** are not recommended for IBD related SpA, as they exacerbate IBD. Both these agents however are effective and safe in axial-SpA.

Anti-integrin Therapies

Natalizumab and Vedolizumab have definite roles in inducing remission in IBD, but similar outcomes have not been obtained in managing arthritis.

OTHER CAUSES OF ENTEROPATHIC ARTHRITIS

Whipple's Disease

Whipple's disease is caused by *Tropheryma whipplei* and spreads by oral–fecal route. The clinical manifestations are diarrhea, weight loss, fever, arthritis, and abdominal pain. Other manifestations are neurologic, culture-negative endocarditis, lymphadenopathy, or uveitis. Joint symptoms seen in up to 90% cases, are usually migratory large joint non-erosive arthralgias or arthritis. Sacroiliitis has been reported. The diagnosis is by tissue sampling of the intestine or synovium to check for PAS staining, foamy macrophages or PCR identification of the organism. Treatment is IV cephalosporins followed by maintenance with oral cotrimoxazole. Doxycycline and hydroxychloroquine are tried in refractory non-neurologic cases.

Celiac Disease

This gluten-sensitive autoimmune enteropathic disease with a strong association with HLADQ2 or DQ8, is an important cause of malabsorption leading to anemia, hypocalcemia, osteopenia and neuropathy. Inflammatory arthritis may be seen in up to 41%, usually non-erosive and non-deforming. Diagnosis requires intestinal biopsy findings or supportive evidence in the form of anti-tissue transglutaminase antibodies.

Bowel-associated Dermatosis–Arthritis Syndrome (BADAS)

BADAS was identified in the 1970s among patients who underwent jejunoileal bypass procedures; it is identified in patients with IBD as well. A flu-like prodrome precedes the development of arthralgias and skin lesions. The basic pathology is neutrophilic dermatosis, due to circulating immune complexes and complement deposits in skin and joints. Arthropathy may occur in 25–52% patients after intestinal bypass surgeries, characterised by episodic, large joint predominant, nonerosive arthropathy. The condition is usually self-resolving within a week or so, and may be reversed by reversal of the bypass.

MISCELLANEOUS

Microscopic colitis which encompasses both lymphocytic colitis and collagenous colitis, have been noted in several autoimmune diseases.

LEARNING POINTS

- Arthritis in IBD may be axial or peripheral
- Axial disease and polyarthritis are independent of IBD status, while pauciarticular arthritis may parallel IBD activity.
- NSAIDs are to be used with caution in active IBD, while sulfasalazine may be used for both gut and joint complaints.
- TNFi are first line biologics in IBD related SpA, but etanercept is not effective.
- Secukinumab and ixekizumab are also not effective.
- Ustekinumab (IL-12/23 inhibitor) is effective in IBD.

FURTHER READING

1. Colìa R, Corrado A, Cantatore FP. Rheumatologic and extraintestinal manifestations of inflammatory bowel diseases. Ann Med. 2016;48:577–85.
2. Karreman MC, Luime JJ, Hazes JM, et al. The prevalence and incidence of axial and peripheral spondyloarthritis in inflammatory bowel disease: a systematic review and meta-analysis. J Crohn's Colitis. 2017; 11:631–42.
3. Löfberg R, Louis EV, Reinisch W, et al. Adalimumab produces clinical remission and reduces extraintestinal manifestations in Crohn's disease: results from CARE. Inflammatory bowel diseases. 2012 Jan 1;18(1):1–9.
4. Lubrano E, Ciacci C, Ames PR, Mazzacca G, Ordente P, Scarpa R. The arthritis of coeliac disease: prevalence and pattern in 200 adult patients. Rheumatology. 1996; 35:1314–8.
5. Orchard TR, Wordsworth BP, Jewell DP. Peripheral arthropathies in inflammatory bowel disease: their articular distribution and natural history. Gut. 1998; 42:387–91.
6. Ossum AM, Palm Ø, Lunder AK, et al. Ankylosing spondylitis and axial spondyloarthritis in patients with long-term inflammatory bowel disease: results from 20 years of follow-up in the IBSEN study. J Crohn's Colitis. 2018; 12:96–104.
7. Queiro R, Maiz O, Intxausti J, et al. Subclinical sacroiliitis in inflammatory bowel disease: a clinical and follow-up study. Clin Rheumatol 2000; 19:445–9.
8. Sandborn WJ, Hanauer SB, Katz S, et al. Etanercept for active Crohn's disease: a randomized, double-blind, placebo-controlled trial. Gastroenterology 2001; 121:1088–94.

Reactive Arthritis

Sakir Ahmed

INTRODUCTION

Reactive arthritis (ReA) is a spondyloarthritis (SpA) that follows a gastrointestinal or urogenital infection by a minimum of 3 days and a maximum of 6 weeks (Table 8.8.1). ReA is diagnosed only when the infections are caused by specifically recognized organisms (Table 8.8.2). Any eponyms used with this condition are discouraged as such individuals have been convicted of war crimes.

Table 8.8.1: Braun criteria for reactive arthritis

Major criteria	1. Arthritis with at least 2 out of: • Asymmetric • Mono- or oligoarthritis • Lower limb involvement
	2. Known symptomatic infection with either: • Gastroenteritis (defined as diarrhea for at least 1 day, and 3 days to 6 weeks before the onset of arthritis) • Urethritis (dysuria or discharge for at least 1 day, 3 days to 6 weeks before the onset of arthritis)
Minor criteria At least one of	1. Evidence of triggering infection: • Positive urine ligase reaction or urethral/cervical swab for *Chlamydia trachomatis* • Positive stool culture for *enteric pathogens associated* with reactive arthritis
	2. Evidence of persistent synovial infection (positive immunohistology or PCR for Chlamydia)

Table 8.8.2: Organisms recognized to cause ReA

Commonly implicated	*Less frequent agents*
Gastrointestinal tract: *Yersinia* *Salmonella* *Shigella* *Campylobacter jejuni*	*Clostridium difficile* *Campylobacter lari* *Chlamydia psittaci* *Chlamydia pneumoniae*
Urogenital tract: *Chlamydia trachomatis* *Neisseria gonorrhoea* *Mycoplasma genitalium* *Ureaplasma urealyticum*	

CHARACTERISTICS

1. Occurring after an episode of diarrhea/dysentery or genitourinary tract infection.
2. **Genetic predisposition:** Around 60–90% of ReA are associated with the presence of the HLA class I gene B27.
3. **Predominantly affects large joints of the lower limbs:** usually hyperacute or overnight onset.
4. Inflammatory low backache (Table 8.8.3).
5. **Enthesitis:** An enthesis is the site of attachment of a ligament or a tendon on the bone. Entheseal inflammation is a defining feature of SpA. Table 8.8.4 mentions the most common sites.
6. **Dactylitis:** Diffuse painful swelling of digits (toes or fingers) is called dactylitis or 'sausage digits'.
7. **Keratoderma blennorrhagicum:** Skin rash often starts in the soles. The name suggests keratinized skin with mucositis and discharge. If widespread can be difficult to distinguish from psoriasis rash (histopathologically there is no difference from psoriasis).
8. **Circinate balanitis:** It is the formation of serpiginous superficial ulcers in a circle around the glans penis.

Table 8.8.3: Defining Inflammatory Back pain (IBP)
Age at onset <40 years
Associated night pain
Worse when at waking up in the morning
Associated early morning stiffness (at least 30 minutes: the longer, the more severe)
Improves with activity
Worsens with rest
Good response to NSAIDs (Non-steroidal anti-inflammatory drugs)

Table 8.8.4: Common entheseal sites involved in ReA

Achilles tendon	Iliac crest
Plantar fascia	Anterior-superior iliac spine
Costochondral junctions: 4th and 6th most common	Greater trochanter of femur
Tip of spinous process of vertebra: most common lumbar vertebra	Upper and lower poles of patella

9. **Uveitis:** The uveitis in ReA is recurrent, acute anterior uveitis. Sequalae of previous attacks like anterior synechiae, complicated cataract, glaucoma might be seen.

PEARLS

A. Certain cases of acute onset or recurrent peripheral SpA may not have known preceding infection. Technically they do not meet the definition of ReA. The author refers to these as "Undifferentiated peripheral SpA". However, the management and outcomes are not different from classical ReA.

B. Terms that may be confused with ReA are:
   1. Post-streptococcal reactive arthritis: though called "reactive arthritis", these are usually milder, and shorter-lasting than classical ReA. Unlike required in the definition for ReA, these usually occur after a sore throat. Also, streptococcus is not a recognised aetiology of classical ReA.
   2. An entity called "Post COVID-19 reactive arthritis" has been recognized recently. However, it does not meet the definition of classical ReA.

DIAGNOSIS

The diagnosis is purely clinical based on different combinations of presenting features (Fig. 8.8.1). Laboratory tests reveal increased acute phase reactants, with/out the presence of HLA-B27.

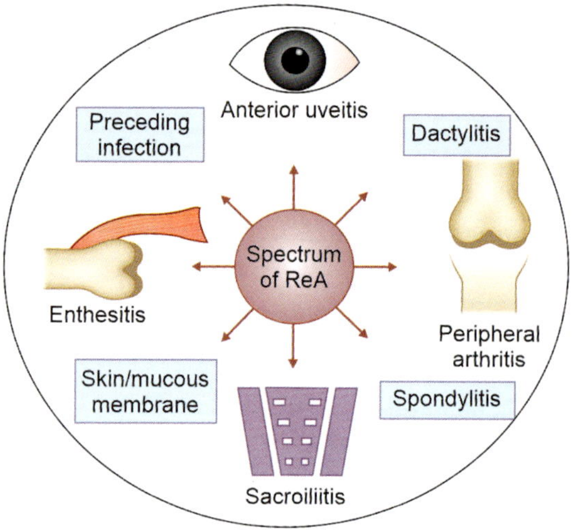

Fig. 8.8.1: Spectrum of reactive arthritis (ReA)

Ultrasound can be used for confirmation of enthesitis while MRI can pick up sacroiliitis or spondylitis in doubtful cases with backache.

OUTCOMES

Two-thirds of ReA is expected to resolve within 3–6 months. This may recur especially with similar precipitating cause (UTI or diarrhea). One-third becomes chronic and 2–10% of these may evolve into ankylosing spondylitis or chronic psoriatic arthritis.

MANAGEMENT

In the lack of clinical trials, management is mostly based on principles carried over from other SpA (Fig. 8.8.2). Meta-analyses have shown that antibiotics have no role in the management of ReA.

LEARNING POINTS

- Post-infectious spondyloarthritis precipitated by symptomatic UTI/diarrhea by specific organisms.
- Spectrum of arthritis, spondylitis including sacroiliitis, acute anterior uveitis, enthesitis, dactylitis and skin/mucous membrane manifestations.
- First line of therapy is NSAIDs and intra-articular (and peri-entheseal) steroid instillation. TNF inhibitors can be used if refractory to first line. Alternatives are methotrexate and sulfasalazine.

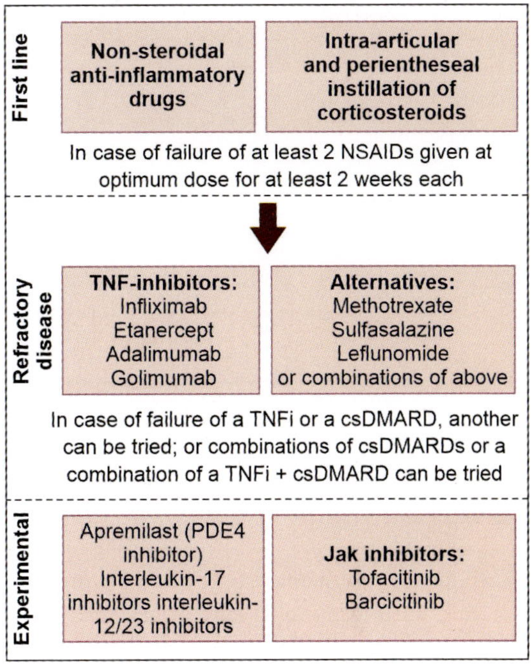

Fig. 8.8.2: Management of ReA

FURTHER READING

1. Ahmed S, Zimba O, Gasparyan AY. COVID-19 and the clinical course of rheumatic manifestations. Clin Rheumatol. 2021;40:2611–9.
2. Selmi C, Gershwin ME. Diagnosis and classification of reactive arthritis. Autoimmun Rev. 2014;13:546–9.
3. Sieper J, Braun J. Reactive arthritis. Curr Opin Rheumatol. 1999;11:238–43.

Systemic Lupus Erythematosus

Vineeta Shobha, Anu Desai

INTRODUCTION

Systemic lupus erythematosus (SLE) is a prototypic systemic autoimmune disease characterized by heterogeneous, multisystem involvement and production of a vast array of autoantibodies. Clinical features in individual patients can be quite variable, ranging from mild joint and skin involvement to severe, life-threatening internal organ disease. Lupus typically affects women (F:M 9:1) in the reproductive age group, the mean age being 35 years. The diagnosis rests on the judgment of an astute clinician based on a constellation of characteristic symptoms, signs, and laboratory findings after excluding all other reasonable diagnoses.

CLINICAL MANIFESTATIONS

Clinical manifestations can vary depending on ethnicity and age of presentation. At onset, patients may have one or several organ involvement and symptoms may accumulate over time resulting in multisystem presentation. Some of the symptoms such as fatigue or myalgia or fever are common though nonspecific.

Constitutional Manifestations

Constitutional symptoms including fever (70–80%), fatigue (67–90%), weight loss, anorexia can be seen in more than three-fourth of the patient and can be presenting manifestation. Fever is more commonly low grade but can go beyond 100°F. Proportion of patients presenting with fever is more common in the Indian setting as compared to western population. Some of the patients may also have generalized lymphadenopathy with hepatosplenomegaly which is the result of activation of the reticuloendothelial system.

Musculoskeletal Manifestations

Arthralgia to arthritis have been described in 76–95% of patients and is usually non-erosive, polyarticular (>5 joints) and symmetrical. They may develop deformity but are usually correctible (Jaccoud's arthropathy). Myalgia is much more common than frank myositis characterized by proximal muscle weakness with creatine phosphokinase often less than 1000 IU/mL.

Mucocutaneous Manifestations

One of the important manifestations are involvement of skin and oral mucosa (Fig. 8.9.1) seen in 90% patients. The most common and classical is butterfly rash which is facial erythema, flat or raised, over malar prominence that tends to spare nasolabial fold and worsens on exposure to sun. The butterfly rash is classified as an acute cutaneous lupus erythematosus (ACLE) rash. There are many other lupus specific and non-lupus specific rashes described. Lupus specific cutaneous lesions includes annular or papulosquamous (psoriasiform) cutaneous eruption, usually photosensitive known as subacute cutaneous lupus erythematosus (SCLE) rash, and discoid lupus rash which manifest as erythematous raised patches with adherent keratotic scaling and follicular plugging. Nonspecific lupus rash included livedo, raynaud, digital gangrene/infarct, chilblain seen in up to half of the patients.

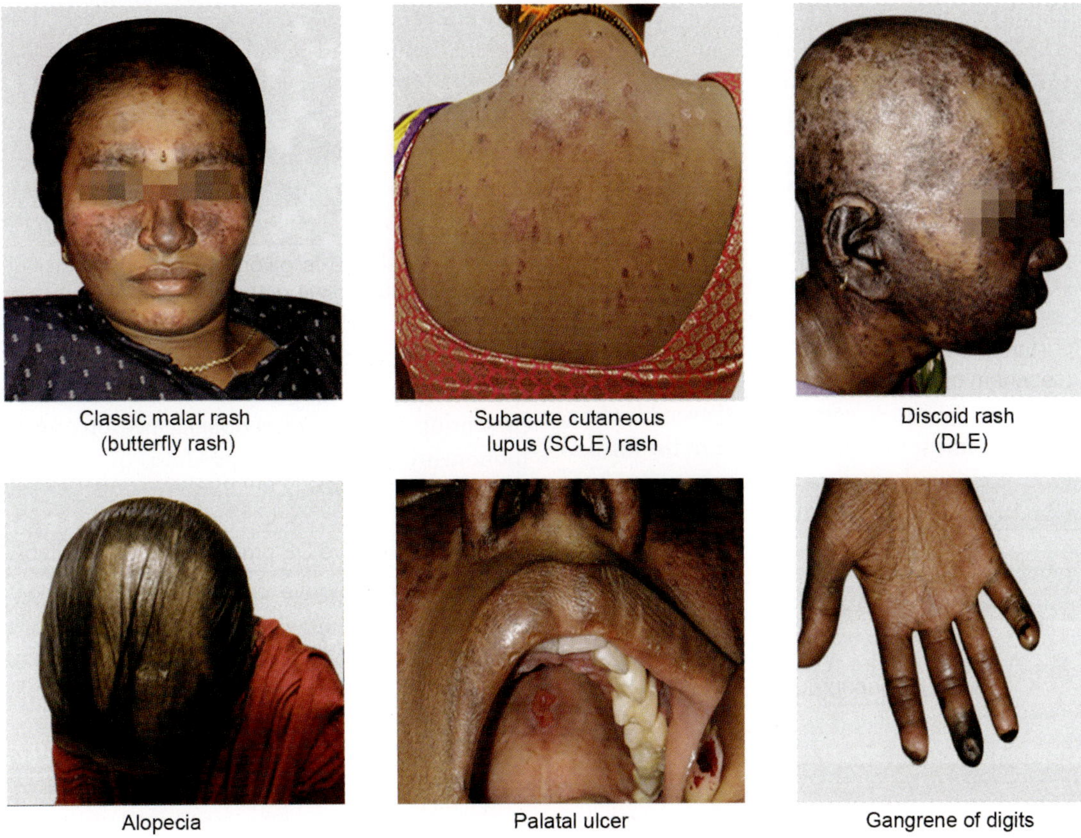

Fig. 8.9.1: Mucocutaneous manifestations

Many patients develop painless oral ulcers (45–50%) and nonscarring alopecia (37–45%). Classical location for oral ulcers is over the palate. Scarring alopecia can develop with DLE rash but is less common.

Renal Manifestations

Patients may have no symptoms or may have hypertension, pedal edema, decreased urine output in varying proportion. Presence of more than 5 RBCs or WBCs or cellular cast and/or more than 0.5 g/24 hours is considered significant and is an indication of renal biopsy and escalation of therapy. For more details, refer to chapter on lupus nephritis.

Cardiopulmonary Manifestations

Patient may develop asymptomatic fluid collection (35–50%) in pericardial or pleural cavity (commonly bilateral) picked up on imaging or can have chest pain, typically pleuritic in nature with pleuritis or substernal chest pain that gets relieved on leaning forward in pericarditis. Patients may develop myocarditis presenting with tachycardia, raised cardiac enzymes with/without heart failure with preserved or reduced ejection fraction. Libman–Sacks endocarditis, seen less commonly now, has been described in up to 10% with involvement of mitral or aortic valve commonly. Lupus patients are at increased risk of cardiovascular events like myocardial infarction due to accelerated atherosclerosis (risk 2–3 times). Other uncommon manifestations include interstitial lung disease (<5%), shrinking lung syndrome, lupus pneumonitis (9%), diffuse alveolar hemorrhage (<25) or pulmonary hypertension (0.5–43%).

Neuropsychiatric Manifestations

There are a wide range of manifestations involving the central nervous system (CNS) more commonly than peripheral nervous system (PNS) (15–85%). American College of Rheumatology has defined 12 and seven manifestations under CNS and

PNS domains including psychosis, cognitive decline, mood disorder, seizure, confusional state, demyelinating disease, mononeuropathy multiplex, plexopathy, polyneuropathy, etc.

Other Manifestations

Gastrointestinal involvement can be associated with high mortality often because of delay in diagnosis and more common mimics including drugs. Pancreatitis, lupoid/autoimmune hepatitis, ascites/peritonitis, mesenteric ischemia, lupus enteris have been reported and can present as abdominal pain, distension, diarrhoea, vomiting and even bleeding. Eye involvement in lupus can occur in the form of uveitis, retinopathy (Cotton-wool spot, correlated with avascular zones on fluorescein angiography) rarely.

INVESTIGATION AND MANAGEMENT

Laboratory tests: The tests listed in Table 8.9.1 are typical of SLE and form part of the ACR and EULAR classification criteria for SLE. Apart from the antibodies listed in Table 8.9.1 there are a host of other antibodies of various significance in SLE.

When to Suspect SLE

It is easy to diagnose SLE in a young patient who presents with fever, malar rash, oral ulcers, arthralgias, pleuritic chest pain, and has low leukocyte count, low platelet count, and urinary abnormalities on routine investigations. A few patients can present as isolated nephrotic syndrome or rapidly progressive renal failure. Other rare presenting features are peripheral neuropathy, or mononeuritis multiplex or psychosis or transverse myelitis or mesenteric vaculitis. In such patients who do not have typical mucocutaneous and musculoskeletal manifestations, subtle laboratory abnormalities such as cytopenias or urinary sediment can often point to the diagnosis.

Past history is equally important such as thrombocytopenia, difficulty to crossmatch

Table 8.9.1: Laboratory investigations in SLE

Coombs + hemolytic anemia	A Coombs positive hemolytic anemia is seen in up to 27% patients. Hemolysis: reticulocytosis, low haptoglobin, elevated indirect bilirubin or elevated LDH and a positive Coombs' direct antiglobulin test (DAT). Sometimes patients only have DAT positive without hemolytic anemia
Leukopenia	Leucopenia is seen in 40–60%, defined as total leukocyte count <4000/mm^3
Thrombocytopenia	Seen in about 50%, thrombocytopenia is defined as platelet <100,000/mm^3
Urinary sediment	Significant proteinuria is >0.5 g/24 hours by 24 hours urine or equivalent spot urine protein-to-creatinine ratio. Other urinary findings are microscopic hematuria, sterile pyuria, cellular casts
ANA	ANA titer of ≥1:80 on HEp-2 cells or equivalent positive test Titer of ≥ 1:160 is generally considered significant
Anti-dsDNA	Anti-dsDNA are present in 30–70% patients. Highly specific, especially associated with renal lupus, higher disease activity
Anti-Sm	Anti-Sm is present in up to 40% patients. They are specific for SLE, Vasculitis, CNS lupus. Higher prevalence in Afro-American patients.
Anti-phospholipid antibodies	The prevalence of aPLs in SLE is 30–40%. Anticardiolipin antibodies (IgA, IgG, or IgM) at medium/ high titer (>40 APL, GPL, or MPL) or positive anti-β2-glycoprotein I antibodies (IgA, IgG, or IgM) or positive lupus anticoagulant.
Serum C3 or C4	Hypocomplementemia occurs in 40–65% due to consumption of complements in the pathogenic process

APLA: Antiphospholipid antibody; *ANCA:* Antineutrophil cytoplasmic antibody; *ANA:* Antinuclear antibody; *APS:* Antiphospholipid antibody syndrome; *LDH:* Lactate dehydrogenase; *APL:* Immunoglobulin (A) phospholipid unit; *MPL:* Immunoglobulin (M) phospholipid unit; *GPL:* Immunoglobulin (G) phospholipid unit

blood transfusion, chronic arthralgia or arthritis, hypertension, unacceptable photosensitivity and such. It is also not unusual to have patients manifesting for the first time with hemolytic manifestations namely autoimmune hemolytic anemia or immune thrombocytopenia.

The classification criteria for SLE are primarily meant to be applied when selecting patients for research. In clinical practice to diagnose SLE, patients need not fulfill the ACR/EULAR classification criteria. We diagnose SLE based on a combination of typical clinical features, routine lab features, ANA positivity by IIF, low complements, positive anti-dsDNA, and renal histological features.

Principle of Management

The goals of therapy for SLE patients are to ensure long-term survival, achieve the lowest possible disease activity, prevent organ damage, minimize drug toxicity, improve quality of life, and educate patients about their role in disease management. Nonpharmacologic therapies include advice regarding photoprotection, diet, exercise, sleep, smoking cessation, de-stressing and prevention of osteoporosis and infections and regular surveillance to take care of long-standing complications and damage.

Treatment is based on the disease activity, the extent and severity of organs involved, any pre-existing chronic damage, comorbidities and adverse events of prior medications (Fig. 8.9.2).

Glucocorticoids: They are the mainstay of treatment both for induction and maintenance. The intensity of glucocorticoids and the choice of *steroid-sparing agents* are titrated as per the lupus disease activity status and organ involvement. Over the past decade, the target has been to decrease steroids burden but at the same time treat to target approach has been emphasised.

Hydroxychloroquine: It reduces overall mortality, risk of flare and disease activity in SLE; it should be given in all SLE patients long-term unless contraindicated. For outcome measures and disease activity assessment, refer to the chapter on outcome measure.

Biologic Agents in SLE

Rituximab is a chimeric monoclonal antibody (mAb) that targets CD20, a transmembrane protein present on all B-lineage cells except the pro-B cells and plasma cells. Experts use rituximab in refractory lupus based on data derived from observational studies. Belimumab is a fully humanised IgG1γ mAb directed against soluble B lymphocyte stimulator (BLyS) also known as BAFF (B cell activation factor). It was approved as add-on therapy in 2011 for moderate to severe non-renal lupus, and for lupus nephritis in the year 2020.

Anifrolumab binds to type 1 interferon receptor and blocks activity of IFN alpha and IFN beta. It received approval in July 2021 for treatment of moderate to severe non-renal lupus. Co-stimulation blockers like abatacept had mixed results in lupus management. Tumor necrosis factor inhibitors are associated with drug induced lupus, and are not recommended.

Other Prophylactic Measures

Assessment of bone strength and risk of fracture especially those on prolonged high dose glucocorticoid therapy should be part of management. Preventive strategies for glucocorticoid-induced osteoporosis include supplementation with vitamin D, calcium and antiresorptive therapies when indicated. Simple exercises such as walking, dancing and low-impact aerobics are useful to maintain bone strength.

Routine immunizations are safe, but their potency may be impaired. Live vaccines should be given with caution in those who are receiving immunosuppressive drugs. COVID-19 vaccination can be safely administered in all SLE patients, however the potency may be lower in those on current treatment with cyclophosphamide or rituximab.

PROGNOSIS

The presence of renal disease, severe lupus disease activity, infection, and cardiovascular disease are the most important contributors to death. However, improved ability to diagnose and treat SLE has contributed to longer survival for patients, currently placed at 5-year survival rates of 95%. This places emphasis on prevention of complications of the disease and its treatments, especially infections.

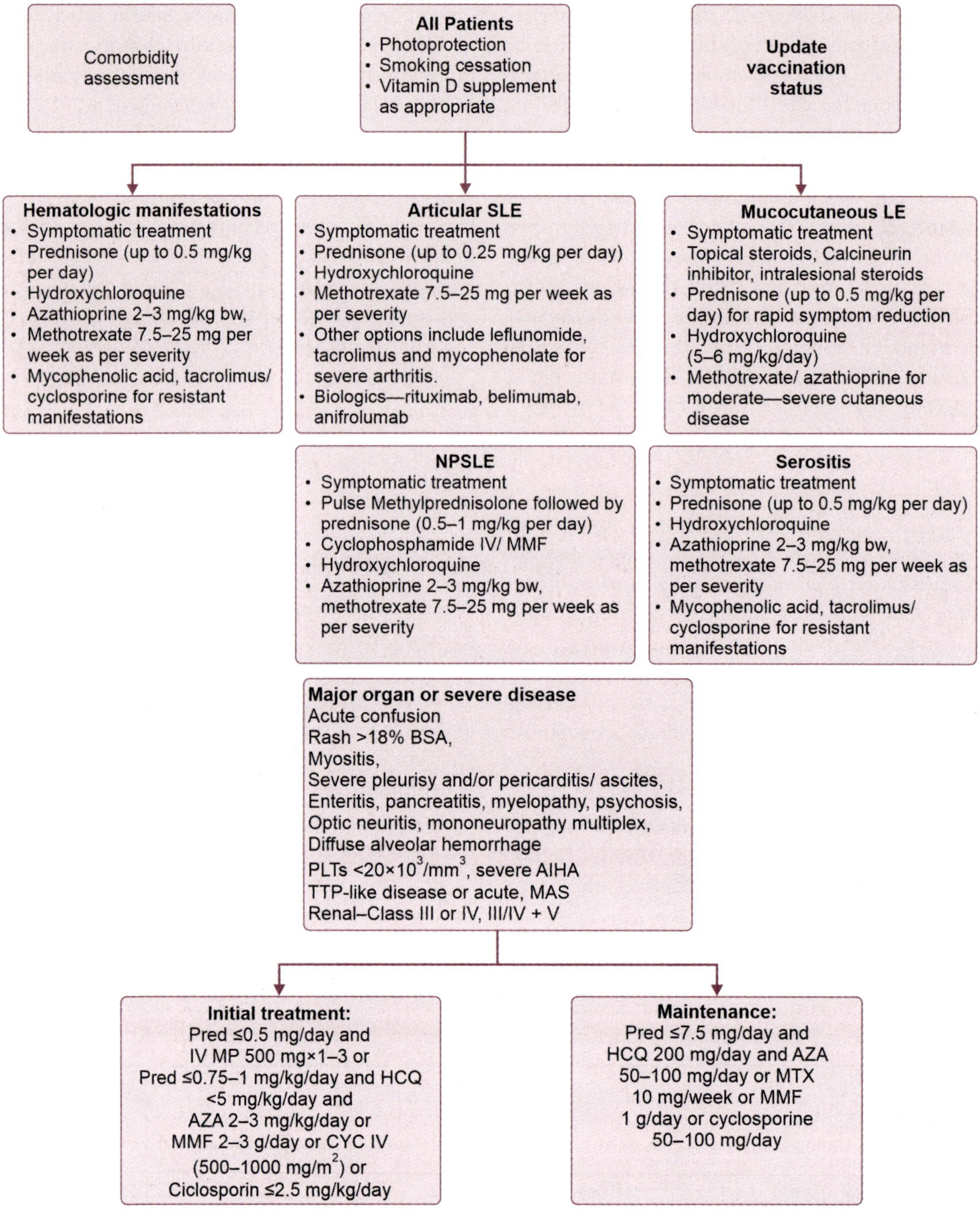

Fig. 8.9.2: Overview of SLE treatment as per organ manifestations

AIHA: autoimmune hemolytic anemia; *AZA:* Azathioprine; *BSA:* Body surface area; *bw:* body weight; *HCQ:* hydroxychloroquine; *IV:* Intravenous; *MAS:* Macrophage activation syndrome; *MMF:* Mycophenolate mofetil; *MP:* Methylprednisolone; *MTX:* Methotrexate; *PLTs:* Platelet; *Pred:* Prednisolone; *TTP:* Thrombotic thrombocytopenia purpura

LEARNING POINTS

- SLE is one of the most clinically and serologically diverse autoimmune disease. It can affect almost any organ/organ system and display a variable spectrum and severity of organ manifestations.
- A high index of suspicion and early referral to a rheumatologist is recommended.

- Remissions and exacerbations are an important feature of SLE, thereby demanding lifelong support and care which includes both non-pharmacologic as well pharmacologic interventions such as photoprotection, glucocorticoids and immunosuppressants.
- Survival and good outcome depend on optimum and continued use of preventive and supportive therapies in addition to immune modulation.

FURTHER READING

1. Doria A, Gatto M, Iaccarino L, Punzi L. Value and goals of treat-to-target in systemic lupus erythematosus: knowledge and foresight. Lupus. 2015;24(4-5):507–15.
2. Fanouriakis A, Kostopoulou M, Alunno A, et al. 2019 update of the EULAR recommendations for the management of systemic lupus erythematosus. Ann Rheum Dis. 2019;78:736–45.
3. Gordon C, Amissah-Arthur MB, Gayed M, et al. The British Society for Rheumatology guideline for the management of systemic lupus erythematosus in adults. Rheumatology (Oxford). 2018;57:e1-e45.
4. Klein RS, Morganroth PA, Werth VP. Cutaneous lupus and the Cutaneous Lupus Erythematosus Disease Area and Severity Index instrument. Rheum Dis Clin North Am. 2010;36:33-vii.
5. Lahita RG. The clinical presentation of systemic lupus erythematosus. In: Lahita RG, editor. Systemic lupus erythematosus. London: Academic press; 2011. pp 525–39.
6. Ruiz-Irastorza G, Ramos-Casals M, Brito-Zeron P, Khamashta MA. Clinical efficacy and side effects of antimalarials in systemic lupus erythematosus: a systematic review. Ann Rheum Dis. 2010;69(1):20–8.
7. Shaban A, Leira EC. Neurological Complications in Patients with Systemic Lupus Erythematosus. Curr Neurol Neurosci Rep. 2019;19:97.
8. Santhosh P, Ajithkumar K. Anti-nuclear antibodies: A practical approach to testing and interpretation. J Skin Sex Transm Dis 2021;3:175–9.
9. Wise LM, Stohl W. Belimumab and Rituximab in Systemic Lupus Erythematosus: A Tale of Two B Cell-Targeting Agents. Front Med (Lausanne). 2020;7:303.

Lupus Nephritis

Amita Aggarwal

INTRODUCTION

Renal involvement in SLE is seen in about 60–65% of patients and has a significant impact on patient outcome. It can be seen at the onset of disease or may develop over time. Renal disease can affect any part of the kidney, i.e. glomerulus, tubules, interstitium or the blood vessels. However, glomerulonephritis is the most common among these.

CLINICAL PRESENTATION

The presentation of renal disease in SLE can vary from asymptomatic urinary abnormalities to rapidly progressive renal failure. The other manifestations include hypertension, pedal edema, nephrotic syndrome and rarely features of azotemia. Every patient with SLE should have regular blood pressure measurement along with review of above symptoms. A simple urine examination can reveal proteinuria, microscopic hematuria, leukocyturia and casts (RBC, hyaline). Urinary protein quantification can be done using 24-hour urine collection or by measuring spot urine protein by creatinine ratio (UPCR). UPCR has the advantage of ease as well as the result can be obtained early. Proteinuria more than 500 mg/day or UPCR> 0.5 suggests significant proteinuria.

Serum complement levels as well as antibodies to dsDNA have a modest correlation with activity of renal disease. The gold standard for diagnosis is renal biopsy. It has been shown that delay in biopsy is associated with a poor prognosis, thus it should be done in all patients with proteinuria >0.5 g with or without active sediment, unexplained rise in serum creatinine unless there is a contraindication. Renal tissue should be sent for histopathology, immunofluorescence and electron microscopy studies.

CLASSIFICATION

Lupus nephritis is classified based on histological findings as Class I–VI; in 2019, the initial ISN/RPS classification has been modified to define the histological features more clearly and further NIH activity and chronicity index was proposed to describe class III and IV disease instead of a or c (Tables 8.10.1 and 8.10.2). A detailed histology helps us in planning therapy as well as predicting the prognosis (Fig. 8.10.1).

Table 8.10.1: ISN/RPS classification

Class	*Characteristic features*
Class I: Minimal mesangial lupus nephritis	Normal glomeruli by light microscopy, but mesangial immune deposits by immunofluorescence.
Class II: Mesangial proliferative lupus nephritis	Presence of any degree of pure mesangial hypercellularity or expansion by light microscopy. On immunofluorescence mesangial depositis are present. Subepithelial or subendothelial deposits are isolated and few.

(*Contd.*)

Table 8.10.1: ISN/RPS classification *(Contd.)*

Class	*Characteristic features*
Class III: Focal proliferative lupus nephritis	Active or inactive focal, segmental or global endo- or extracapillary glomerulonephritis involving ≤50% of all glomeruli, typically with focal subendothelial immune deposits, with or without mesangial alterations.
Class IV: Diffuse proliferative lupus nephritis	Active or inactive diffuse, segmental or global endo- or extracapillary glomerulonephritis involving ≥50% of all glomeruli, typically with diffuse subendothelial immune deposits, with or without mesangial alterations.
Class V: Membranous lupus nephritis	Global or segmental subepithelial immune deposits or their morphologic sequelae by light microscopy and by immunofluorescence or electron microscopy, with or without mesangial alterations.
Class VI: Advanced sclerotic lupus nephritis	≥90% of glomeruli globally sclerosed without residual activity.

Modifications in 2019 classification (Bajema IM, et al. Kidney Int. 2018;93:789–96)

Mesangial hypercellularity has been clearly defined as 4 or more nuclei surrounded by matrix in the mesangial region excluding the hilar region. Endocapillary proliferation has been replaced by the term endocapillary hypercellularity. Crescents have been defined and classified as celluar, fibrocellular and fibrous. Definitions for adhesions and fibrinoid necrosis have been included. Interstitial inflammation, fibrosis and vascular thrombosis to be reported separately.

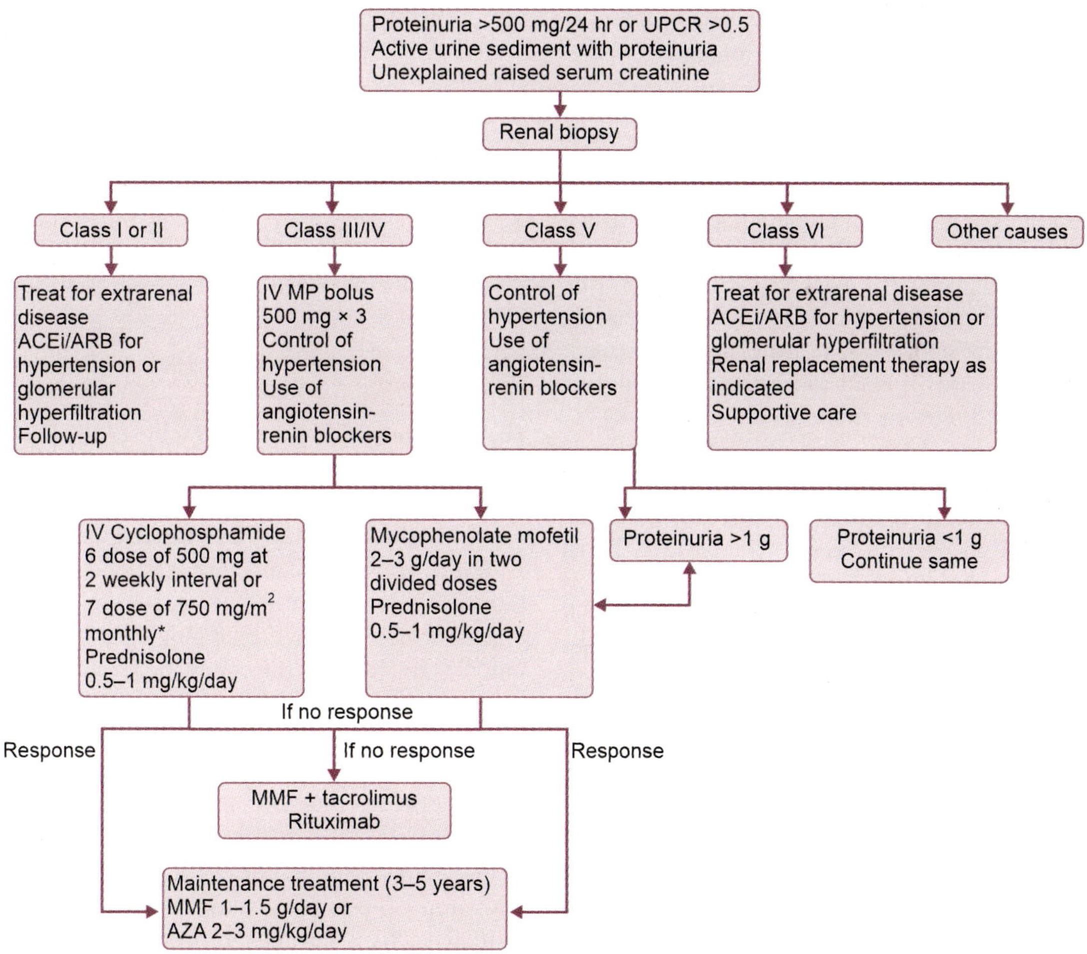

*High risk patients (low GFR, presence of crescents)

Fig. 8.10.1: Approach to management of lupus nephritis

Table 8.10.2: NIH activity and chronicity index

Activity index		*Chronicity index*	
Endocapillary hypercellularity	0–3	Glomerulosclerosis	0–3
Neutrophils/karyorrhexis	0–3	Fibrous crescents	0–3
Fibrinoid necrosis*	0–3	Tubular atrophy	0–3
Hyaline deposits	0–3	Interstitial fibrosis	0–3
Cellular/fibrocellular crescents*	0–3		
Interstitial Inflammation	0–3		
TOTAL (*are scored double)	0–24		0–12

*0–3 is based on % involvement

MANAGEMENT

The aim of treatment is control of symptoms and hypertension, have remission and preserve renal function. The treatment includes general measures like control of blood pressure, use of diuretics and salt restriction to reduce edema and use of angiotensin blockers to reduce proteinuria.

Class I and II LN does not require addition immunosuppressive (IS) drugs and treatment depends on extra-renal disease. Classes III and IV are treated with high dose corticosteroids (CS) with IS agents. There are multiple guidelines available from international societies, a suggested plan is given in Figure 8.10.2. For Class V disease, initially angiotensin blockade should be tried; if proteinuria still remains above 1 g, IS drugs should be used. Class VI patients need to be treated with renal replacement therapy and supportive care.

In patients who do not respond to initial therapy, switching from MMF to cyclophosphamide or *vice versa* is done. In some centers tacrolimus is added to MMF in refractory cases. Rituximab, a B cell depletion therapy not found useful in randomized controlled trials, has been shown to be beneficial in 2/3rd of patients in registry data. The other therapies that can be used are leflunomide, bortezomib (proteasome inhibitor), and low dose IL-2 therapy.

Patients with LN should be initially followed up monthly and then every 3 months. At every visit blood pressure, serum creatinine, UPCR/urine routine as well as screening for drug toxicity needs to be done. Though 3 monthly C3, C4 and anti-dsDNA antibodies are recommended it can be done sparingly in resource constrained situations like at the time of flare, before reducing/stopping IS therapy.

Complete response with resolution of proteinuria, active sediment may take up to 6–8 months. A complete response (proteinuria <500 mg, absence of active sediment and no rise in creatinine) at 6 months is a good prognostic factor for long-term renal outcome.

All patients should receive hydroxychloroquine unless contraindicated. Once induction therapy has been completed maintenance therapy with either azathioprine (AZA) 2–3 mg/kg/day or mycophenolate 1–1.5 g/day should be used for 3–5 years. Monitor patients for disease flare as well as drug toxicity. In addition comorbidities like diabetes, hyperlipidemia, etc. should also be treated adequately.

PROGNOSIS

The outcome of LN has improved over the last 5 decades with use of IS agents. In recent studies from developed countries about 10–15% develop end stage renal disease at the end of 10 years and about 5–7% die. However, results are not as good in India with data from our centre showing 10-year survival with normal renal function of only 69% in adults and 79% in children. Infections and uncontrolled disease activity are the major cause of mortality. The overall results of renal transplant in SLE are almost as good as transplantation for any other cause. The recurrence of LN is rare in the transplanted kidney.

Besides LN, lupus patients can also have renal involvement due to associated anti-phospholipid syndrome, lupus podocytopathy, interstitial nephritis, drug induced injury. Thrombotic thrombocytopenic purpura, real vein thrombosis and rarely amyloidosis.

LEARNING POINTS

- All patient with SLE at diagnosis should have a urine routine examination as well as serum creatinine estimation to look for asymptomatic renal involvement.
- Renal biopsy should be done in all patients with proteinuria more than 500 mg/dL with or without sediment abnormalities or raised creatine unless contraindicated.
- Treat class III and Class IV disease aggressively for early control of disease.
- Keep blood pressure under control and use ARBs to reduce proteinuria.
- Assess response every 1–3 months and titrate therapy accordingly.
- Use hydroxychloroquine and maintenance therapy with AZA or MMF for 3–5 years.

FURTHER READING

1. Bajema IM, Wilhelmus S, Alpers CE, et al. Revision of the International Society of Nephrology/Renal Pathology Society classification for lupus nephritis: clarification of definitions, and modified National Institutes of Health activity and chronicity indices. Kidney Int. 2018; 93:789–96.
2. Dhir V, Aggarwal A, Lawrence A, et al. Long-term outcome of lupus nephritis in Asian Indians. Arthritis Care Res (Hoboken). 2012;64:713–20.
3. Fanouriakis A, Kostopoulou M, Cheema K, et al. 2019 Update of the Joint European League Against Rheumatism and European Renal Association-European Dialysis and Transplant Association (EULAR/ERA-EDTA) recommendations for the management of lupus nephritis. Ann Rheum Dis. 2020; 79:713–23.
4. Gasparotto M, Gatto M, Binda V, et al. Lupus nephritis: clinical presentations and outcomes in the 21st century. Rheumatology (Oxford). 2020; 59:v39-v51.

Chapter 8.11

Pregnancy in Lupus

Shefali K Sharma, Debashish Mishra

Introduction

Systemic lupus erythematosus (SLE), an autoimmune multisystem disease, predominantly affects females in the reproductive age group. With the advances in treatment, survival has improved, and a significant proportion of patients attain remission on treatment.

LUPUS AND PREGNANCY

Multiple hormonal, physiological and immunological changes occur during pregnancy which can have direct or indirect effect on SLE, one of which is shift in lymphocyte predominance from Th1 to Th2 phenotype. Because SLE is Th2 driven, this shift from Th1 to Th2 can result in a flare during pregnancy. However, clinical studies have observed that the majority of flares occur in the postpartum period rather than during pregnancy.

Generally, SLE flare is defined as a measurable increase in disease activity in one or more organ systems involving new or worse clinical signs and symptoms and/or laboratory measurements. It must be considered clinically significant by the assessor and usually, there would be at least consideration of a change or an increase in treatment'.

Prepregnancy Assessment

Since the majority of patients with SLE are women, counselling for pregnancy-related issues should be part of the treatment, to avoid inadvertent pregnancy while on fetotoxic immunosuppressants and while the disease is active. SLE patients who are in remission for the last 6–12 months can plan pregnancy under high-risk obstetric care. But certain contraindications to pregnancy exist (Table 8.11.1). Baseline assessment of SLE patients contemplating pregnancy must include the following:

- Assess disease activity, ensure patient is remission before conceiving.
- Screen for antiphospholipid antibodies (aPLs) and lupus anticoagulant.
- Anti Ro/La.
- Fetotoxic medications that are contraindicated in pregnancy are methotrexate, leflunomide, mycophenolate, and cyclophosphamide should be discontinued at least 3 months earlier.

Table 8.11.1: Contraindications for pregnancy in patients with SLE

Absolute contraindications
1. Moderate-to-severe lupus flare (including renal) in past 6 months
2. History of stroke in past 6 months
3. Pulmonary hypertension (estimated systolic pulmonary artery pressure >50 mm Hg or symptomatic)
4. Left ventricular ejection fraction <40%
5. Severe restrictive lung disease (forced vital capacity <50% predicted or <1L)
6. Chronic kidney disease stage 4–5
Relative contraindications
1. Presence of antiphospholipid syndrome
2. Thrombocytopenia
3. Hypertension
4. Serum creatinine >2.8 mg/dL
5. Increased lupus activity at conception/first trimester
6. Prior pregnancy losses
7. Anti Ro/ La antibodies

- Patients can be switched to safer alternatives like azathioprine, cyclosporine or tacrolimus.
- Low dose steroid and hydroxychloroquine (HCQ) are safe through pregnancy.
- Low dose aspirin (75 mg/day) is started at the beginning of pregnancy to prevent preeclampsia.

ASSESSMENT OF SLE DISEASE ACTIVITY AND FLARES DURING PREGNANCY

The systemic lupus erythematosus pregnancy disease activity index (SLEPDAI) shown in Table 8.11.2, lupus activity index in pregnancy (LAI-P Table 8.11.3), and the modified systemic lupus activity measure (MSLAM) are available for the clinician to assess disease activity in a pregnant lupus patient.

Flares during Pregnancy

The risk of a flare increases in patients with an active disease 6–12 months prior to conception, lupus nephritis (ever), not on hydroxychloroquine therapy, and primigravida. There are challenges to

Table 8.11.2: Systemic lupus erythematosus pregnancy disease activity index (SLEPDAI)

Score	*Descriptor*	*Modified for pregnancy*	*Considerations*
8	Seizure	Yes	Rule out eclampsia
8	Psychosis	No	
8	Organic brain syndrome	No	
8	Visual disturbance	No	Hypertension is already considered an exclusion in SELENA-SLEDAI and SLEDAI
8	Cranial nerve disorder	Yes	Rule out Bell's palsy
8	Lupus headache	Yes	Rule out Bell's palsy
8	Cerebrovascular accidents	Yes	Rule out eclampsia
8	Vasculitis	Yes	Consider palmar erythema
4	Arthritis	Yes	Consider bland knee effusion
4	Myositis	No	
4	Urinary casts	No	
4	Hematuria	Yes	R/o cystitis and vaginal RBC reflective of placental problems
4	Proteinuria	Yes	Rule out eclampsia
4	Pyuria	Yes	Rule out infection
2	Rash	Yes	Consider chloasma
2	Alopecia	Yes	Consider normal postpartum alopecia
2	Mucosal ulcers	No	
2	Pleurisy	Yes	Hyperventilation may be secondary to progesterone, dyspnea secondary to enlarging uterus
2	Pericarditis	No	
2	Low complements	Yes	Complements normally rise during pregnancy
2	Increased DNA binding	No	
1	Thrombocytopenia	Yes	R/o preeclampsia, HELLP syndrome, incidental thrombocytopenia of pregnancy
1	Leucopenia	Yes	Consider normal rise of leucocyte counts during pregnancy
1	Fever	No	

recognize flares because pregnancy in itself leads to a physiological increase in erythrocyte sedimentation rate (ESR), hemodilution-induced anemia, increase in C3, C4 levels (due to increased synthesis in the liver), and an increase in leucocyte count. Certain features help to distinguish between the two (Table 8.11.4).

Table 8.11.3: Lupus activity index in pregnancy (LAI-P)

Group	*Parameter*	*Point values*				*Values to calculate LAI-P*
1	Fever	0	1			(a) Mean
	Rash	0		2		
	Arthritis	0		2	3	
	Serositis	0	1	2	3	
2	Neurologic	0			3	(b) Maximum
	Renal	0		2	3	
	Lung	0			3	
	Hematologic	0	1	2	3	
	Vasculitis	0			3	
	Myositis	0			3	
3	Prednisone, NSAID, HCQ	0	1	2	3	(c) Mean
	Immunosuppressor	0			3	
4	Proteinuria	0	1	2	3	(d) Mean
	Anti DNA	0	1	2		
	C3, C4	0	1	2		

Point value of LAI-P = (a + b + c + d)/4

HCQ: Hydroxychloroquine; *NSAID:* Non-steroidal anti-inflammatory drugs

Table 8.11.4: Features to differentiate physiological alterations in pregnancy from a SLE flare

Feature	*Lupus flare*	*Normal physiological alterations that can mimic a flare*
Clinical	Active rash of lupus Inflammatory arthritis Lymphadenopathy Fever >38°C (not related to infection or drug) Pleuritis Pericarditis	Fatigue Arthralgia Bland effusion of knees Myalgias Malar and palmar erythema Postpartum hair loss Carpal tunnel syndrome Edema of hands, legs and face Mild resting dyspnea
ESR	Increased	18–46 mm/hr <20 weeks gestation 30–70 mm/hr ≥20 weeks gestation
Anemia	Hemoglobin <10.5 g/dL	Hemoglobin >11g/dL first 20 weeks gestation Hemoglobin >10.5 g/dL after 20 weeks of gestation

(Contd.)

Table 8.11.4: Features to differentiate physiological alterations in pregnancy from a SLE flare *(Contd.)*

Feature	*Lupus flare*	*Normal physiological alterations that can mimic a flare*
Thrombocytopenia	Platelet count <95,000 /µL	Mild in approximately 8%
Urine analysis	Hematuria or cellular casts	Rare hematuria from vaginal contamination
Proteinuria	≥300 mg/day	<300 mg/day
dsDNA antibodies	Rising titers	Negative or stable titers
Complements	≥25% drop	Usually increased

Adapted from: Stojan G, Baer AN. Flares of systemic lupus erythematosus during pregnancy and the puerperium: prevention, diagnosis and management. Exp Rev Clin Immun 2012;8(5):439–53.

Effect of SLE on Pregnancy Outcomes

If planned properly, most of the pregnancies are uneventful. But still, adverse outcomes of pregnancy are more prevalent in lupus pregnancy compared to the general population, particularly if the disease is active at the time of conception. The adverse outcomes are as follows:

- **Fetal related:** Intrauterine growth restriction, preterm birth.
- **Fetal wastage:** Spontaneous abortions, fetal death occur more in lupus pregnancies
- **Maternal:** Premature rupture of membrane, pre-eclampsia, eclampsia and abruptio placenta are also increased in SLE patients. A common clinical dilemma is differentiating pre-eclampsia and eclampsia from lupus flare (Table 8.11.5).

Neonatal Lupus

Anti Ro antibodies can cross the placenta between 16–30 weeks of gestation and cause permanent damage to the fetal cardiac conduction system. Neonatal lupus manifests in the first 2 weeks of life as transient erythematous rash resembling subacute lupus rash or complete heart block (CHB). Neonatal lupus occurs in only ~2% of babies born to anti-Ro positive mothers. The risk of CHB is 1–2% in a first pregnancy, which rises to 17–18% in subsequent pregnancies if the firstborn had CHB. In such cases, screening with fetal echo is recommended from 18 weeks onwards. hCG is the only proven therapy that prevents development of cardiac complications. Role of IVIg, plasma exchange, prophylactic steroids or immunosuppressants is refuted.

MANAGEMENT DURING PREGNANCY

Aspirin: Low-dose aspirin should be initiated at <16 weeks of gestation and continued throughout pregnancy.

Presence of aPLs

- If aPLs are positive in moderate titers and there is no prior thrombosis or obstetric morbidity only aspirin would suffice.

Table 8.11.5: Differentiating features between lupus flare and preeclampsia

Features suggestive of preeclampsia	*Features suggestive of lupus flare*	*Features common to both*
Severe headache Visual symptoms (including flashing lights) Epigastric or right upper quadrant tenderness Clonus (>2 beats) Deranged liver function tests Raised uric acid Signs of hemolysis Falling levels of vascular endothelial growth factor and placental growth factor	Onset <20 weeks gestation Active urinary sediment/cellular casts Hematuria Low/falling complement levels High/increasing anti-dsDNA antibodies Evidence of flare in other organs	Hypertension Worsening proteinuria Edema Renal impairment Thrombocytopenia

Adapted from: Knight CL, Nelson-Piercy C. Management of systemic lupus erythematosus during pregnancy: challenges and solutions. Open Access Rheumatol. 2017;9:37–53.

- If aPLs are positive with pregnancy loss (no thrombosis) then prophylactic low molecular weight heparin (LMWH) throughout pregnancy till delivery.
- If antiphospholipid syndrome (aPLs + pregnancy loss + thrombosis) is present then therapeutic LMWH and aspirin throughout pregnancy till 6 weeks postpartum.

Follow-up

Regular follow-up with complete blood count, liver and renal function tests, urine analysis, complement and anti-dsDNA titers to monitor for early evidence of impending flare.

Immunosuppressive Treatment

As in nonpregnant patients, organ involvement guides therapy in pregnant SLE patients. Risk of active SLE to mother is weighed against deleterious effects of medications to the fetus. For a minor flare the dose of oral steroids can be increased while for a major flare intravenous pulses of steroids can be given. IVIG, plasma exchange can be tried in desperate situations. No life/organ salvaging treatment is denied due to pregnancy.

Medications that are avoided during pregnancy and lactation are methotrexate, mycophenolate, leflunomide, cyclophosphamide, and tyrosine kinase inhibitors. Among biologics Rituximab should be discontinued at least 6 months before planning pregnancy but in desperate situations (for example myelitis) it can be given.

Contraception

In the postpartum period, couples must be adequately and enthusiastically counseled regarding contraception. Barrier contraceptives, progesterone only methods and intrauterine devices are safe for these patients. Estrogen-containing pills are contraindicated in SLE due to increased risk of thrombotic events.

CONCLUSION

SLE patients with active disease, lupus nephritis, anti-phospholipid antibodies have an increased risk of pregnancy morbidities. To have safe and successful confinement, achieving and maintaining remission is of utmost importance.

LEARNING POINTS

- Proper prepregnancy counseling, risk assessment and evaluation is the foundation to a successful pregnancy in lupus patients.
- Achieving and maintaining remission for at least 6 months prior and throughout pregnancy, with compatible medications, is most important.
- To differentiate SLE flare from pregnancy related changes or complications is difficult at times.
- No treatment which is organ or lifesaving is denied due to pregnancy.

FURTHER READING

1. Adamichou C, Bertsias G. Flares in systemic lupus erythematosus: diagnosis, risk factors and preventive strategies. Mediterr J Rheumatol. 2017;28(1):4–12.
2. Dalal DS, Patel KA, Patel MA. Systemic lupus erythematosus and pregnancy : A brief review. J Obstet Gynaecol India 2019;69(2):104–9.
3. Knight CL, Nelson-Piercy C. Management of systemic lupus erythematosus during pregnancy : challenges and solutions. Open Access Rheumatol. 2017;9:37–53.
4. Lateef A, Petri M. Management of pregnancy in systemic lupus erythematosus. Nat Rev Rheumatol 2012;8:710–18.
5. Lateef A, Petri M. Managing lupus patients during pregnancy. Best Pract Res Clin Rheumatol. 2013;27(3): 10.1016/j.berh.2013.07.005.
6. Ruiz-Irastorza G, Khamashta MA. Evaluation of systemic lupus erythematosus activity during pregnancy. Lupus 2004;13(9):679–82.
7. Stojan G, Baer AN. Flares of systemic lupus erythematosus during pregnancy and the puerperium: prevention, diagnosis and management. Exp Rev Clin Immun 2012; 8(5):439–53.

Chapter 8.12

Antiphospholipid Syndrome

Amita Aggarwal, Claire Reynolds, Pravin Hissaria

INTRODUCTION

Antiphospholipid syndrome (APS) is a disease characterized by arterial or venous thrombosis, recurrent pregnancy morbidity in association with the presence of antiphospholipid antibodies. APS predominantly affects females in the reproductive age group however no age is bar. APS can also occur in association with other connective tissue diseases like SLE, systemic sclerosis, Sjogren syndrome, etc. when it is called secondary APS.

SPECTRUM OF ANTIPHOSPHOLIPID ANTIBODIES

Antiphospholipid antibodies (aPL) are autoantibodies directed against various phospholipids located on the cell membrane or proteins in circulation. The various targets include phosphatidylserine, phosphatidylethanolamine, annexin V, protein C, protein S, prothrombin, etc. In clinical practice it refers to antibodies to cardiolipin, beta 2 GP1 and lupus anticoagulant (LA). The former two are measured by ELISA and the latter is a functional assay to measure the prolongation of prothrombin dependent coagulation pathways. In the lab we use cardiolipin and beta 2 GP1 as antigens for measuring aPL.

SPECTRUM OF CLINICAL MANIFESTATIONS IN APS

Spectrum of clinical manifestations in APS is very diverse. The two major features are vascular thrombosis and pregnancy morbidity. In a series of 1000 cases, 37.1% had only venous thrombosis, 27% had only arterial thrombosis, 12.1% had both venous and arterial thrombosis and 12.1% had only foetal morbidity and a small proportion, i.e. 8.6% had microcirculatory thrombosis (Table 8.12.1).

Table 8.12.1: Classification criteria for APS

Criteria	*Characteristic features*
Clinical criteria	Venous thrombosis (e.g. deep vein thrombosis, pulmonary embolism, unusual site venous thromboembolism)
	Arterial thrombosis (e.g. coronary artery disease, transient cerebral ischemia or stroke, peripheral artery disease)
	Obstetric complications: Three or more unexplained consecutive spontaneous abortions <10 weeks of gestation. One or more unexplained deaths of a morphologically normal fetus ≥10 weeks of gestation One or more premature births of a morphologically normal neonate <34 weeks of gestation due to eclampsia, severe preeclampsia, or placental insufficiency.

(Contd.)

Table 8.12.1: Classification criteria for APS (*Contd.*)

Criteria	*Characteristic features*
Laboratory criteria*	Lupus anticoagulant, detected according to international guidelines
	Anticardiolipin antibodies, IgG, or IgM isotype, at high titre (>99th percentile of normal controls)
	Anti-β2 glycoprotein-I antibodies, IgG, or IgM isotype, at high titre (>99th percentile of normal controls)

*These tests should be repeated after 12 weeks to see for persistence
A patient can be classified as APS can be made if you have minimum of one criterion from clinical and lab criteria

Table 8.12.2: Noncriteria features of APS

Nervous system	*Skin*	*Heart*	*Blood*	*Kidney*
Multiple sclerosis–like illness	Livedo reticularis	Valve thickening (Libman–Sacks endocarditis)	Thrombocytopenia	Microangiopathy
Seizures	Livedoid vasculopathy	Diastolic dysfunction	Hemolytic anemia	Chronic vaso-occlusive lesions (atherosclerosis, glomerular ischemia, interstitial fibrosis, arterial fibrous intimal hyperplasia)
Dementia				
Chorea				
Myelitis				

Besides this, patients can have neurological, hematological, cardiac and renal manifestations (Table 8.12.2).

LABORATORY TESTS TO DIAGNOSE APS

Prolonged activated partial thromboplastin time (APTT) or mild thrombocytopenia may be observed in routine tests. Antibodies to cardiolipin of both IgG and IgM isotype are measured by ELISA and expressed as IgG phospholipid units (GPL) or IgM phospholipid units (MPL). The test result is reported as mild (20–40), moderate (40–80) and marked (>80) elevation. In addition, total or IgG antibodies to β2 glycoprotein 1 (β2GPI) are also measured by ELISA and value above 99th centile of the general population is taken as significant.

Lupus anticoagulant (LA) is a functional assay, which is done in 3 steps:

1. Demonstration of prolonged coagulation using either dilute RVVT or APTT assay.
2. Failure of correction of the abnormal test by addition of pooled normal plasma.
3. Correction of the abnormal test by addition of excess phospholipids.

The plasma sample should be centrifuged twice to have platelet-poor plasma for the assay otherwise it can be falsely-negative.

In addition, patients should have a thorough evaluation to exclude other associated autoimmune diseases, especially SLE (complete blood count, renal function, urine examination, ANA, anti-dsDNA antibodies). Further co-morbid conditions that increase the risk of thrombosis like hyperlipidemia also need to be evaluated.

The laboratory criteria to diagnose APS is the positivity of any of the aPL antibodies on at least 2 occasions, at least 12 weeks apart. Of note, aCL and β2GPI positivity may be IgG or IgM.

Note: aCL and β2GPI IgG levels have higher clinical correlation than IgM.

IgA levels do not correlate clinically, and should not be used in diagnosis of APS.

Presence of aPLs is not specific for APS. They can occur transiently in healthy individuals and in acute infection. Inter-assay and intra-assay variability is quite significant and can even result in false-negative results in symptomatic patients. When in doubt, repeat the test.

RISK ASSESSMENT BASED ON LABORATORY RESULTS

Highest risk:	Triple positive tests
High risk:	Positive LA; aCL and/or β2GPI positive
Moderate risk:	LA negative; moderate to high titre of either aCL or β2GPI
Low risk:	Negative LA; low titre aCL or β2GPI

CATASTROPHIC APS

Catastrophic APS (CAPS) is a medical emergency characterized by multi-organ small vessel thrombosis. Infections are the major trigger for CAPS. Kidney, heart, lung, brain are the major organs involved. In addition, skin can have skin infarcts, livedo reticularis, digital gangrene, etc. Most patients have either Lupus anticoagulant, IgG anticardiolipin and IgG anti-β2-glycoprotein antibodies, however rarely they may be absent during the event due to consumption of autoantibodies. If not treated it has a high mortality varying from 30–40%. In SLE-related CAPS mortality may reach 50%.

The treatment of choice is anticoagulation, immunosuppressive therapy (Corticosteroids as methylprednisolone IV bolus and IV cyclophosphamide) and plasmapheresis + intravenous immunoglobulin along with treatment of triggering factor. The key for improving outcomes is rapid recognition and prompt therapy.

TREATMENT

Anti-phospholipid antibodies are seen in a proportion of healthy subjects thus mere presence of antibodies does not need any treatment except a detailed history and examination. In patients with low to moderate levels of antibodies or the presence of LA in the setting of SLE, low-dose aspirin is used to prevent preeclampsia though the evidence for this is limited. Global antiphospholipid score (GAPPS) includes hypertension, and hyperlipidemia along with aPLs and assesses the risk of thrombosis. This can be used to tailor therapy.

Venous Thrombosis

Anticoagulation with a vitamin K antagonist aiming for INR of 2–3, indefinitely. High-intensity anticoagulation with INR between 3 and 3.5 may be needed if there is recurrent thrombosis at INR between 2 and 3. Anticoagulation may cease at 3 or 6 months in those with low-risk profiles and clear triggering events for thrombosis.

Direct oral anticoagulants (DOAC) may have a role in patients with absolute contraindications to vitamin K antagonists, or in those unable to achieve adequate INR levels. Bleeding risk is similar with both anticoagulants.

Arterial Thrombosis

Anticoagulation with a vitamin K antagonist aiming for INR of 3–4 indefinitely OR aim for INR 2–3 with aspirin therapy indefinitely. Use of DOAC in arterial thrombosis is associated with an increase in recurrent thrombosis.

In patients with only obstetric APS, low-molecular weight heparin (LMWH) in prophylactic dose is needed throughout pregnancy and 6 weeks postpartum. A simple plan on how to manage patients is given in Figure 8.12.1.

In addition, severe thrombocytopenia, and autoimmune haemolytic anaemia needs treatment with corticosteroids. Rarely IVIG in emergency situations and Rituximab in refractory cases can be used.

LONG-TERM OUTCOME

In a 10-year follow-up study, nearly 15% had recurrent thrombosis in the first and another 15% in the second 5-year period. 73% of pregnancies resulted in a live birth. Mortality was 9.3% with thrombosis and infection contributing to nearly 1/3rd of deaths. Catastrophic APS was seen in about 1% of patients.

LEARNING POINTS

- The key features of APS are recurrent vascular thrombosis and pregnancy loss.
- Anticardiolipin antibodies and lupus anticoagulant are the most often used lab tests.
- Oral anticoagulation using warfarin is the mainstay of therapy.
- In pregnancy LMWH should be given throughout pregnancy as well as 6 weeks postpartum.

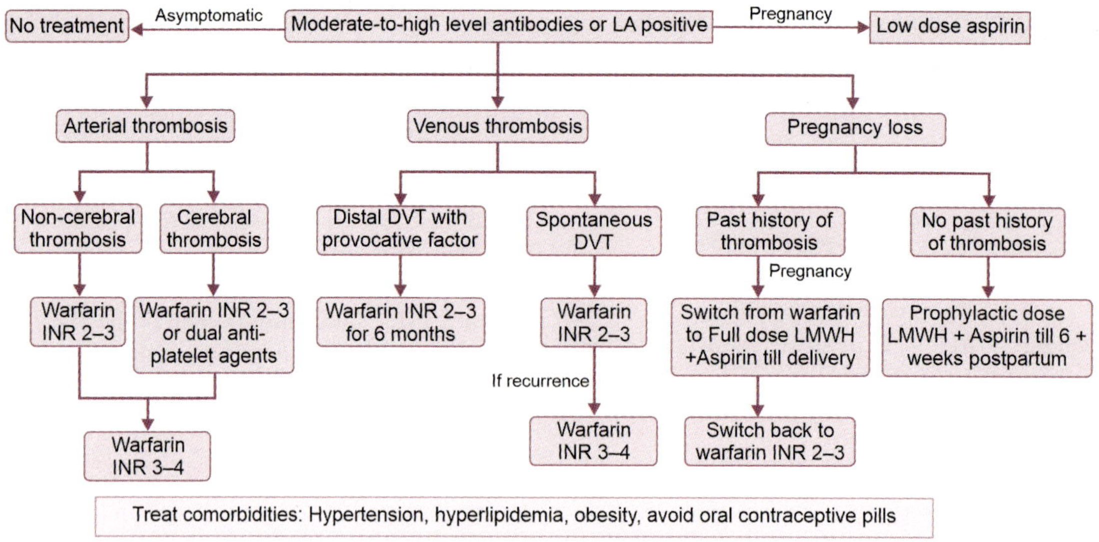

Fig. 8.12.1: Management of APS

- Low-dose aspirin is useful in decreasing risk of preeclampsia.
- Multi-organ dysfunction developing over a week may be due to CAPS.

FURTHER READING

1. Alijotas-Reig J, Esteve-Valverde E, Ferrer-Oliveras R, et al. for EUROAPS Study Group. The European Registry on Obstetric Antiphospholipid Syndrome (EUROAPS): A survey of 1000 consecutive cases. Autoimmun Rev. 2019;18:406–14.
2. Cervera R, Serrano R, Pons-Estel GJ, et al. for Euro-Phospholipid Project Group (European Forum on Antiphospholipid Antibodies). Morbidity and mortality in the antiphospholipid syndrome during a 10-year period: a multicentre prospective study of 1000 patients. Ann Rheum Dis. 2015;74:1011–8.
3. Cervera R, Bucciarelli S, Plasín MA, et al. Catastrophic Antiphospholipid Syndrome (CAPS) Registry Project Group (European Forum On Antiphospholipid Antibodies). Catastrophic antiphospholipid syndrome (CAPS): descriptive analysis of a series of 280 patients from the "CAPS Registry". J Autoimmun. 2009;32: 240–5.
4. Miyakis S, Lockshin MD, Atsumi T, et al. International consensus statement on an update of the classification criteria for definite antiphospholipid syndrome (APS). J Thromb Haemost. 2006;4:295–306.

Chapter 8.13

Sjögren's Syndrome

Pulukool Sandhya

INTRODUCTION

Sjögren's syndrome (SS) is a common but underdiagnosed systemic autoimmune disease. Autoimmune epithelioid and lymphocytic infiltration is the hallmark histopathological feature. Exocrine glands are typically involved resulting in exocrine dysfunction and mucosal dryness. The disease is however not limited to sicca symptoms. Extraglandular features are observed in two-thirds of patients and may vary from mild features like fatigue and polyarthralgia to serious complications like vasculitis, severe renal and neurological involvement, and lymphoma (Table 8.13.1). The disease predominantly affects women. As compared to the Caucasian population where the disease is seen in the peri- and postmenopausal age group, onset at a younger age is seen in India, especially in those presenting with extra glandular features.

Table 8.13.1: Extraglandular features in Sjögren's syndrome

Constitutional
Fever and night sweats
Weight loss
General symptoms
Fatigue*
Musculoskeletal
Arthralgia
Non-erosive arthritis
Myalgia/chronic pain*
Myositis
Reticuloendothelial
Benign lymphadenopathy
Splenomegaly
Lymphoma
Cutaneous
Dry skin*
Annular erythema
Cutaneous vasculitis
Pulmonary
Chronic dry cough
Interstitial lung disease
Cystic lung disease*
Small airway disease*
Bronchiectasis*
Pleuritis*
Renal and urological
Tubulointerstitial nephritis
Renal tubular acidosis
Glomerulonephritis
Interstitial cystitis*
Peripheral nervous system
Axonal sensory/sensorimotor polyneuropathy
Inflammatory demyelinating polyneuropathy
Autonomic neuropathy*
Cranial neuropathies (V, VII and VIII)
Vasculitis-associated neuropathy (mononeuritis multiplex)
Small fiber sensory neuropathy
Ganglionopathy
Central nervous system
Cranial neuropathies of central origin
Cognitive dysfunction
Cerebral vasculitis with cerebrovascular accident
Seizures
Transverse myelitis
Lymphocytic meningitis
Optic neuritis or multiple sclerosis-like syndrome

(Contd.)

Table 8.13.1: Extraglandular features in Sjögren's syndrome (*Contd.*)

Hematological
Anemia
Leukopenia (lymphopenia and/or neutropenia)
Thrombocytopenia
Biological
Hyper- or hypogammaglobulinemia
Hypocomplementemia
Cryoglobulinemia
Cardiovascular*
Raynaud's phenomenon
Pulmonary hypertension
Pericarditis
Gastrointestinal*
GERD
Autoimmune hepatitis/biliary cirrhosis
Pancreatitis
Gynecological/obstetric*
Dyspareunia
Bad obstetric outcome—Fetal heart block

*Not included in ESSDAI (EULAR SS disease activity index)

In many instances, extraglandular features could precede the onset of sicca symptoms and could be the dominant clinical feature as depicted in Figure 8.13.1.

This has been especially seen in patients with neurological and renal manifestations. Such patients with serious systemic and "non-rheumatological" features are more likely to consult specialities other than rheumatology. Different extra glandular features and sicca could be widely disseminated in time and hence the connection may not be apparent either to the patient or the doctor(s). Understandably, in the face of serious systemic features, patients may not be forthcoming about sicca symptoms. Poor awareness about the disease may additionally limit the elicitation of features and/or evaluation of the disease. This can be detrimental as those with serious systemic features are most likely to benefit from immunosuppression if treated early. Therefore, timely diagnosis of SS requires close collaboration with other specialities.

When to Suspect?

As in other rheumatological diseases, suspicion should be based on pattern recognition and not merely based on antibody positivity or sicca symptoms. Sicca symptoms have been hailed as the most common presenting feature of the disease. However, in India, most patients with SS seek medical attention for their extra glandular features and generally do not volunteer sicca symptoms. In these patients, salivary gland enlargement, dental caries, lack of salivary pooling, lobulated tongue with loss of filiform papillae, and erythematous candidiasis are clues for exocrine dysfunction and must be looked for.

Active screening for SS in patients with glandular and characteristic extraglandular features for instance long-standing arthralgia or non-erosive arthritis, renal tubular acidosis with or without hypokalemic paralysis, ganglionopathy, cryoglobulinemic vasculitis, hyperglobulinemic purpura, etc. can be quite rewarding. Lab abnormalities like cytopenia, hyperglobulinemia, hypokalemia, elevated urine pH in metabolic acidosis, and mild proteinuria are important clues.

DIFFERENTIAL DIAGNOSIS

Most patients with sicca symptoms do not have SS. More common causes such as medication-related and diabetes mellitus should be considered in those who present with just sicca features.

Anti-Ro positivity can be seen in other rheumatic diseases like lupus, rheumatoid arthritis, myositis, and scleroderma, and hence these diseases must be included in the differential diagnosis. As a corollary, ANA and RF positivity can be seen in SS, and the mere presence of these antibodies should not lead to the diagnosis of lupus and rheumatoid arthritis, respectively.

In patients with glandular enlargement, sarcoidosis, human immunodeficiency virus (HIV) infection, IgG4-related disease (IgG4-RD) and lymphoma are differentials.

Chronic hepatitis C virus (HCV) infection can have clinical and immunologic abnormalities similar to SS, and it is mandatory to exclude HIV and HCV before diagnosing SS.

DIAGNOSIS

There is no single lab test for diagnosis. Anti-Ro positivity is seen in 60–80% of SS. A broad approach to diagnosis is outlined in Figure 8.13.2. Diagnosis

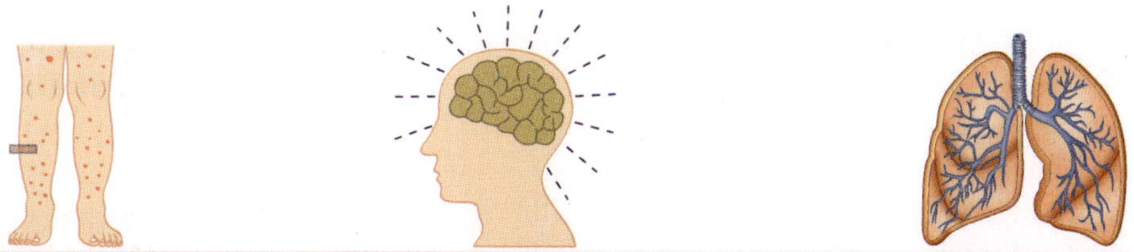

2010	Asymptomatic	2016	Asymptomatic	2020
Purpura Hyperglobulinemia ANA+ ?SLE Short course Steroids		Meningoencephalitis CSF-lymphocytic ?TB meningitis ATT+steroids		ILD Sicca since 2008 Using tear drops Schirmer's+ Anti-Ro+

a

Sjogren's syndrome

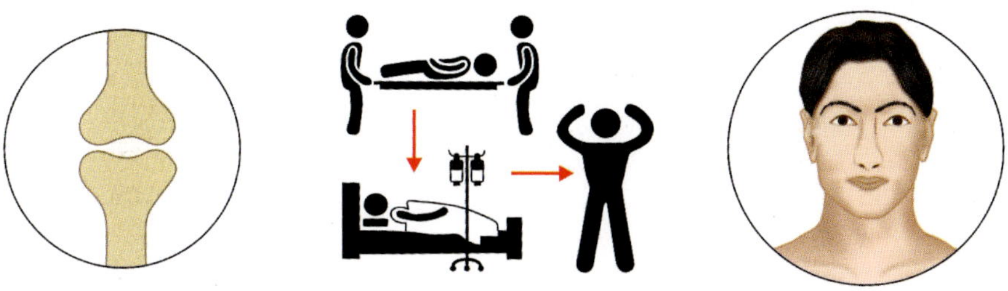

2010–2011	2011–2016	2018	
Mild arthritis-RF+ RA Low WBC count—No MTX intermittent HCQ, NSAIDs "Cured completely"	5 episodes-A/C onset paralysis improved with potassium Hyperchloremic non-anion gap metanolic acidosis	Parotitis carious teeth No sicca	Schirmer's- Anti-Ro+ MSGBx+

b

Sjögren's syndrome

Fig. 8.13.1: Extraglandular manifestations could precede the onset of sicca symptoms and be the dominant clinical feature

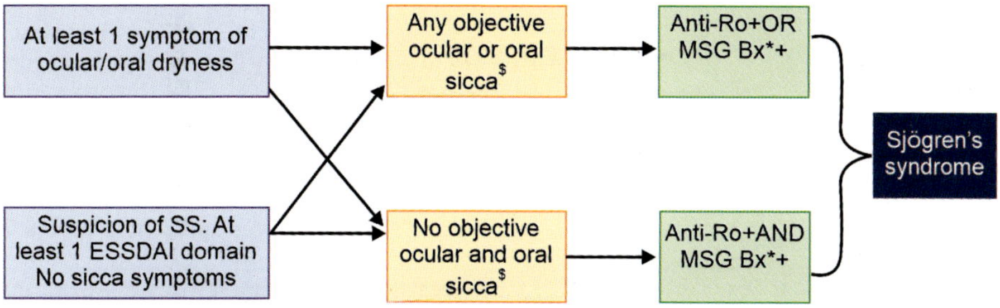

Fig. 8.13.2: Diagnosis of Sjögren's syndrome

$ Unstimulated Salivary Flow rate ≤0.1 mL/min
Schirmer's test ≤5 mm/5 min in any eye
Ocular Staining Score ≥5 or van Bijsterveld score ≥4 in any eye

*MSG Bx(minor salivary gland biopsy)+: Focal lymphocytic sialadenitis with FS≥1 is supportive of a diagnosis of SS

should be based on a constellation of clinical features, one of the oral/ocular signs (Fig. 8.13.3a to 8.13.3c), and the presence of focal lymphocytic infiltration on salivary gland biopsy (Fig. 8.13.3d) and/or anti-Ro positivity. Though not included in any classification criteria so far, salivary gland imaging could have an ancillary role. The presence of hypoechoic areas and hyperechoic bands on ultrasonography could be suggestive of SS in the appropriate clinical setting.

How to Assess Disease Activity?

Sicca, pain and fatigue are assessed by ESSPRI (EULAR SS Patient Reported Index) score. Disease activity is assessed by ESSDAI (EULAR SS disease activity index) score. Sicca symptoms do not correlate with disease severity. Adverse prognostic factors for lymphoma are indicated in Table 8.13.2.

Management

Sicca complex: Management of the sicca complex requires a multidisciplinary approach along with a dentist and ophthalmologist (Fig. 8.13.4 and 8.13.5). The primary goal is to alleviate the symptoms of dryness and prevent complications of dryness. Ensure that sicca-causing drugs are substituted wherever possible. Immunomodulators, systemic steroids, and other immunosuppressants are not indicated. Emphasis should be placed on patient self-care, and general measures such as humidification of the environment and avoiding tobacco.

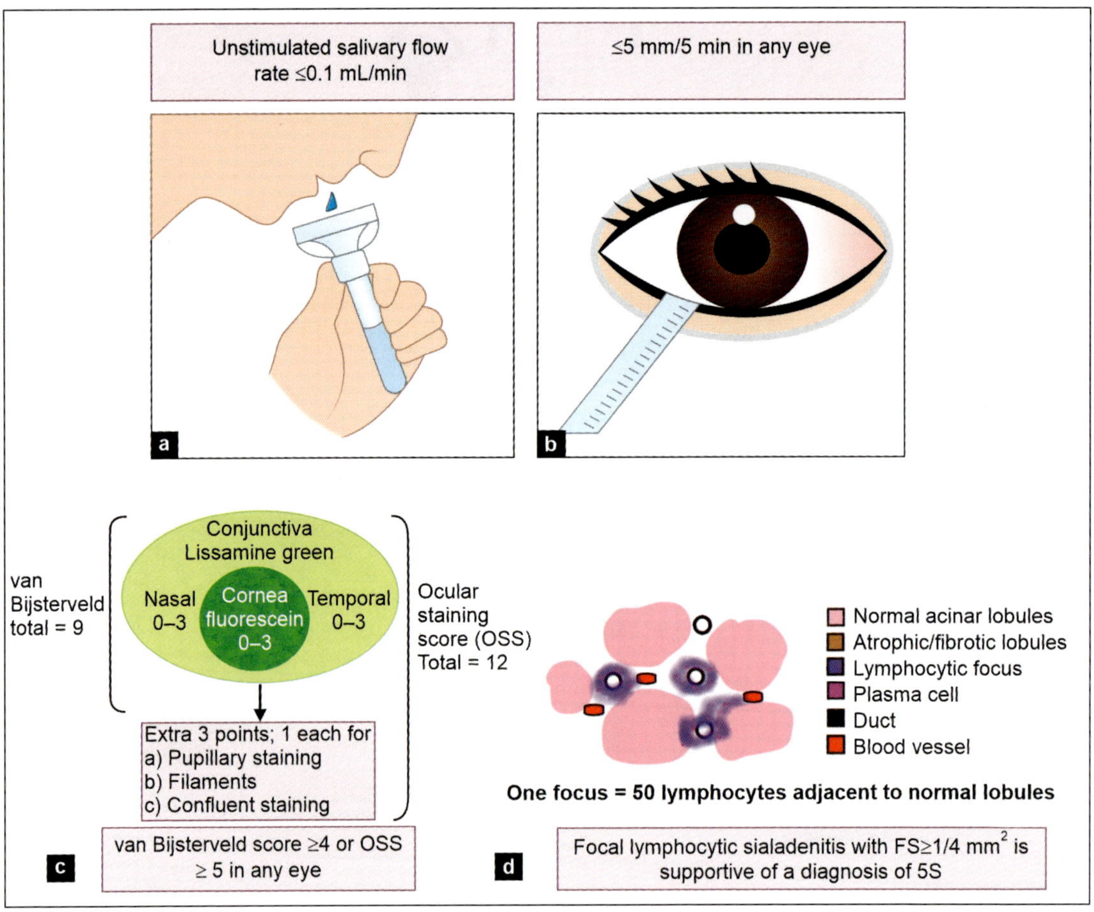

Fig. 8.13.3: Objective tests for Sjögren's syndrome: (a) Salivary flow, (b) Schirmer's test, (c) Ocular staining, *Lissamine green or Rose bengal in van Bijsterveld score; (d) *FS:* Focus score, Reused with permission *from* Chandra Krishnan, MD, Dell Children's Medical Center

Table 8.13.2: Adverse prognostic factors	
Clinical	*Lab*
Parotidomegaly	CD4+Lymphopenia
Lymphadenopathy	Hyperglobulinemia
Splenomegaly	MGUS
Vasculitis	Mixed cryoglobulinemia
High ESSDAI	Low complements
	RF positive
	Anti-Ro positive
	Focus score >3

Non-inflammatory pain and or fatigue- Osteomalacia, small fiber neuropathy, or rarely lymphoma could present with widespread pain and fatigue. However, more common causes like vitamin deficiency, hypothyroidism, degenerative joint disease, depression, or fibromyalgia should not be overlooked. Treatment should be based on underlying etiology. HCQ may have a role in some cases. Aerobic exercise has been shown to improve fatigue in trials.

Systemic disease: Treatment of systemic disease must be guided by the severity of domain involvement as

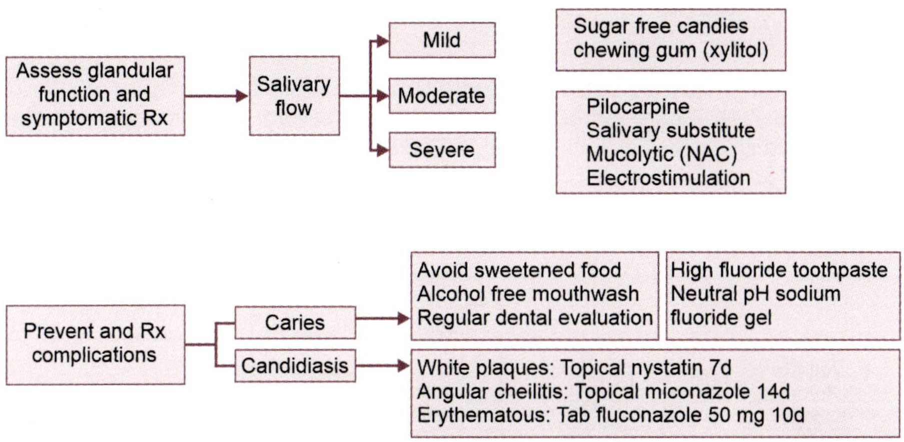

Fig. 8.13.4: Management of oral sicca; Tab Pilocarpine: starting dose of 2.5 mg od and titrate to maximum 5 mg 4 times daily. In case tab pilocarpine is not available, add equivalent dose of Pilocarpine 4% in 100 ml water (3 drops = 5 mg). N acetyl cysteine NAC- 600 mg orally twice daily

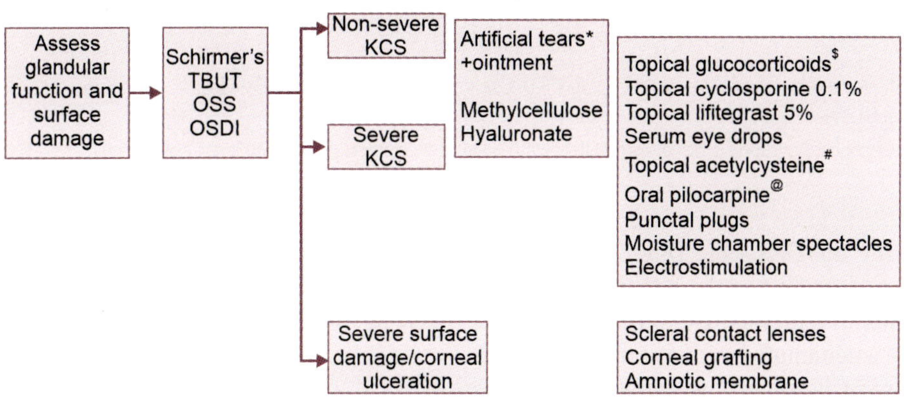

Fig. 8.13.5: Management of ocular sicca; TBUT: Tear break-up time; OSS: Ocular staining score; OSDI: Ocular surface disease index; KCS: Keratoconjunctivitis sicca *Preservative free artificial tears

$Prednisolone 0.5% in moderate, dexamethasone 0.1% in severe cases for short-term (2–4 weeks) only

#Acetylcysteine 5–10% in mucous threads or ocular surface filaments

@Tab pilocarpine: starting dose of 2.5 mg od and titrate to maximum 5 mg 4 times daily

In case tab pilocarpine is not available, add equivalent dose of Pilocarpine 4% in 100 mL water (3 drops = 5 mg)

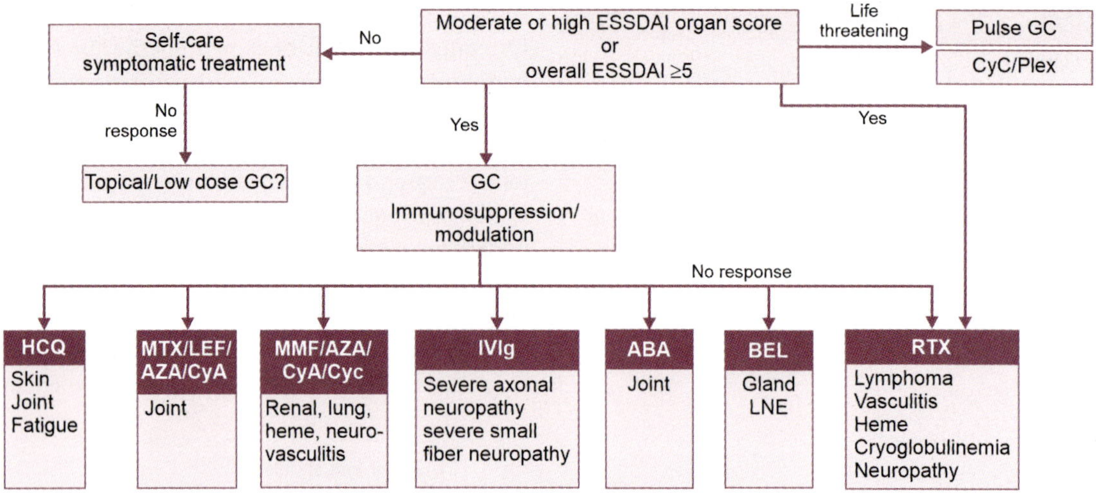

Fig. 8.13.6: Management of systemic disease; *ESSDAI:* (EULAR SS disease activity index); *GC:* Glucocorticoids; *Cyc:* Cyclophosphamide; *Plex:* Plasma exchange; *RTX:* Rituximab; *HCQ:* Hydroxychloroquine; *MTX:* Methotrexate; *Lef:* Leflunomide; *Aza:* Azathioprine; *CyA:* Cyclosporine A; *IVIg:* IV Immunoglobulin; *ABA:* Abatacept; *BEL:* Belimumab; *LNE:* Lymph node enlargement

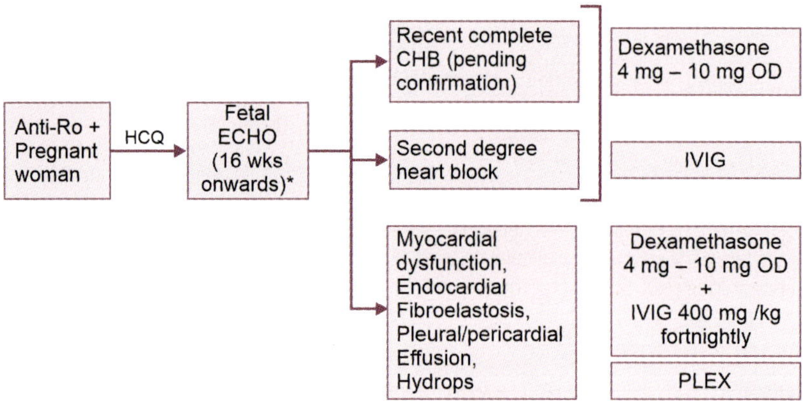

Fig. 8.13.7: Management of fetal heart block; *CHB:* Congenital heart block; *PLEX:* Plasma exchange; *IVIG:* Intravenous immunogloubulins

*Weekly fetal echocardiography is done from 16th to 24th week at most centers and then less frequently till term

given by the ESSDAI score (Fig 8.13.6). In the absence of controlled trials, broad principles of using immunosuppression are to be followed. Use steroids for a minimum duration at the least possible dose to control disease activity. Immunosuppressive agents are to be used as steroid-sparing agents whenever long-term steroid use is indicated. Lymphoma is to be treated as per haematology guidelines. Management of fetal heart block is depicted in Fig. 8.13.7. HCQ has a definite role in the prevention of fetal heart block and fluorinated steroids are (as they cross the placenta) used for treatment. IVIg and plasma exchange could have a role in select scenarios.

LEARNING POINTS

- Sicca symptoms ≠ SS. The absence of sicca symptoms does not rule out primary Sjogren's syndrome nor does the presence of sicca rule in SS.
- Anti-Ro positivity ≠SS. Remember anti-Ro positivity can be seen in other rheumatic diseases

or may be incidental. Anti-Ro can be negative in 20–40% of SS.

- Screen for pSS in patients with characteristic extraglandular features such as renal tubular acidosis, sensory neuronopathy, or cryoglobulinemic vasculitis.
- Ocular/oral signs of dryness, anti-Ro positivity and focal lymphocytic sialadenitis on minor salivary gland biopsy are key to establishing the diagnosis.
- Look for ESSDAI domains in all patients with SS
- Immunosuppression should be tailored to the severity of systemic diseases and is not indicated for the treatment of sicca complex alone.
- Treatment of sicca complex is based on a multidisciplinary approach with a dentist and ophthalmologist and emphasis on patient self-care.

FURTHER READING

1. Mariette X, Criswell LA. Primary Sjögren's Syndrome. N Engl J Med. 2018 8;378:931–9.
2. Price EJ, Rauz S, Tappuni AR, et al.; British Society for Rheumatology Standards, Guideline and Audit Working Group. The British Society for Rheumatology guideline for the management of adults with primary Sjögren's Syndrome. Rheumatology (Oxford). 2017; 56:e24-e48.
3. Ramos-Casals M, Brito-Zerón P, Bombardieri S, et al.; EULAR-Sjögren Syndrome Task Force Group.EULAR recommendations for the management of Sjögren's syndrome with topical and systemic therapies. Ann Rheum Dis. 2020;79:3–18.
4. Shiboski CH, Shiboski SC, Seror R, et al. 2016 American College of Rheumatology/European League Against Rheumatism classification criteria for primary Sjögren's syndrome: A consensus and data-driven methodology involving three international patient cohorts. Ann Rheum Dis 2017;76:9–16.

Section

IX

SYSTEMIC SCLEROSIS, MYOSITIS, MCTD, AND VASCULITIS

Chapter 9.1

Systemic Sclerosis

Vikas Agarwal

INTRODUCTION

The basic pathological signature of systemic sclerosis (SSc) includes endothelial dysfunction and fibrosis in various connective tissues and in organs such as lungs, intestine, and the myocardium. This uncommon disease often has a bad prognosis, with standardized mortality ratio (SMR) of 1.5–7.2 across different cohorts. The mortality occur due to cardiac, respiratory or kidney failure.

PATHOLOGY AND PATHOGENESIS

There is excessive collagen deposition as evident from biopsies from skin or other tissue. There is also a "bland" vasculopathy leading to intimal proliferation of dermal capillaries leading to luminal compromise and finally obliteration.

Characteristics of a lung biopsy is infiltration of macrophages, lymphocytes and mast cells with thickening of the alveolar septa.

Siblings, parents and children of patients have a 13–19 fold higher risk of developing SSc, implicating a strong genetic predisposition (Table 9.1.1). However, concordance is much lower in monozygotic twins. Thus, it is not entirely genetic and environment has a major part to play.

Classification criteria: Various classification criteria have evolved since 1980 onwards and are summarized in Table 9.1.2.

Autoantibodies: SSc is characterized by presence of multiple autoantibodies and different antibodies have different clinical associations (Table 9.1.3)

CLINICAL FEATURES

Beyond skin thickening, tethering and pigmentary changes, patients often present with manifestations of severe Raynaud such as pain and digital ulcers. Another leading presentation is progressive dyspnea on exertion due to lung fibrosis or pulmonary vascular involvement. Most patients have dysphagia with heartburn and altered bowel habits due to gut involvement. Clinical features of SSc are summarized in Table 9.1.4.

Table 9.1.1: Factors important in SSc susceptibility and pathogenesis

Genetic susceptibility	*Epigenetic factors*	*Environmental factors*
Candidate genes: Polymorphisms of STAT4, TNFSF4, TBX21, NLRP1 (T cell signaling) FAM167A-BLK, BANK, IRAK1 (B cell signaling) **GWAS:** HLA DPB1, DPB2, IRF5 and STAT4, CD247, PRORS1C1, RhoB **Immunochip studies:** DNASE1L3, TREX-DDX6, ATG5	DNA hypomethylation (T lymphocytes, fibroblasts) Increased FOXP3 methylation Increased miRNA 21 Decreased miR29a and let7a	Organic solvents, silica, rapeseed oil L-tryptophan Bleomycin Pentazocine Gadolinium

Table 9.1.2: Classification criteria for systemic sclerosis

1980 ACR criteria for classification of SSc		
Major criteria	**Minor criteria**	
Scleroderma-like skin change proximal to MCP or MTP joints.	1. Sclerodactyly 2. Digital pitting scars of fingertips or loss of distal finger pad 3. Bibasilar pulmonary fibrosis	
Either 1 major or 2 or more of the minor criteria had to be fulfilled for a patient to be classified as systemic sclerosis.		
2013 ACR/EULAR criteria for classification of SSc		
Item	**Sub-item(s)**	**Weight/ score**
Skin thickening of the fingers of both hands extending proximal to the metacarpophalangeal joints (*sufficient criterion*)	–	9
Skin thickening of the fingers (*only count the higher score*)	Puffy Fingers	2
	Sclerodactyly of the fingers (distal to the 4 metacarpophalangeal joints but proximal to the proximal interphalangeal joints)	4
Fingertip lesions (*only count the higher score*)	Digital tip ulcers	2
	Fingertip pitting scars	3
Telangiectasia		2
Abnormal nailfold capillaries		2
Pulmonary arterial hypertension and/ or interstitial lung disease (*maximum score is 2*)	Pulmonary arterial hypertension	2
	Interstitial lung disease	
Raynaud's phenomenon		3
SSc-related autoantibodies (*maximum score is 3*)	Anticentromere Anti–topoisomerase I Anti–RNA polymerase III	3

The criterion was tested in a validation cohort and sensitivity and specificity was 0.91 and 0.92, respectively.

Table 9.1.3: Antibodies in SSc and their clinical associations

Antibody	*Prevalence*	*Clinical associations*
Anti-Topoisomerase 1 or Scl-70 antibody (ATA)	Common in diffuse SSc	Increased risk of interstitial lung disease and mortality
Anti-centromere antibody (ACA)	Common in limited SSc	Esophageal dysmotility, calcinosis, pulmonary hypertension
anti-RNA polymerase III (anti-RNAP III)	Common in diffuse SSc	Rapidly progressive, higher risk of scleroderma renal crisis, but lesser risk of interstitial lung disease
Anti- Th/To antibodies	Uncommon	Limited skin involvement with severe interstitial lung disease, scleroderma renal crisis and poorer survival
anti-fibrillarin antibodies	Uncommon	Severe Raynaud and pulmonary hypertension
and anti-U11/U12 RNP antibodies	Uncommon	Severe interstitial lung disease

Patients with early, diffuse disease, tendon crepitations, RNA polymerase III antibodies or rapidly progressive disease are more likely to develop scleroderma renal crisis (SRC). Use of higher doses of steroids may precipitate SRC.

Eighty % of patients with SRC have a classical rise of blood pressure of more than 20% from baseline. The peripheral blood smear shows schistocytes while urine may have bland proteinuria or casts with microscopic proteinuria. Prompt initiation of angiotensin-converting enzyme (ACE) inhibitors have revolutionized the treatment of SRC bringing down mortality from above 80% to below 10%.

Systemic sclerosis sine scleroderma: Less than 2% of patients with SSc may lack skin tightening. They are more likely to be male and have lesser vasculopathy like limited Raynaud and absence of telangiectasias. However, they may have higher prevalence of GERD symptoms and ILD.

Table 9.1.4: Clinical features in systemic sclerosis

Clinical feature and frequency	*Symptoms*
Raynaud's phenomenon, 95% Digital ulcers (Fig. 9.1.1), 50–70% Gangrene, 10–20%	Triphasic color change on exposure to cold
Skin tightening, >90% Depigmentation of skin, 20–25%	**Diffuse SSc:** Proximal to elbow/knee **Limited SSc:** Distal to elbow/knee Salt and pepper appearance (Fig. 9.1.2)
Lung involvement, 80% ILD, 50–55% PAH, 10–17%	 Dry cough, DOE, fatigue DOE, Syncope, loss of weight
Cardiac involvement, 15–25% Arrhythmias, 20–46% Conduction defects, 11% Pericarditis, 5–16% Pericardial effusion, 41% LV systolic dysfunction, 2% LV diastolic dysfunction, 33–72%	 Asymptomatic, palpitations, tachy/bradycardia, Chest pain, ECG changes Asymptomatic, low BP, fatigue DOE, orthopnea, PND, pedal edema Asymptomatic
Gastrointestinal tract involvement, 90% Esophageal, 4–5% Gastroesophageal reflux disease, 70% Gastroparesis, 50% GAVE, 22–24% Bacterial overgrowth syndrome, 43–60% Chronic intestinal pseudo-obstruction, 5–6%	 Dysphagia Retrosternal/epigastric burning Early satiety Asymptomatic, anemia Abdominal pain, diarrhea, malabsorption Constipation, abdominal distension
Arthritis, 15%	Polyarthritis, small and large joints
Renal involvement, 50% Glomerulonephritis, 5% SRC, 5–15% Renal failure, 2–7%	 Proteinuria, periorbital edema Hypertension, MAHA, rise in serum creatinine Azotemic symptoms, oliguria
Tendon friction rubs, 35–40%	Tendon clicks
Myositis, 10–15%	Proximal muscle weakness
Nail fold capillaries alterations, 80–95%	Abnormal capillary patterns

SRC: Scleroderma renal crisis; *ILD:* Interstitial lung disease; *PAH:* Pulmonary arterial hypertension; *DOE:* Dyspnea on exertion; *PND:* Paroxysmal nocturnal dyspnea; *GAVE:* Gastric antral vascular ectasia; *MAHA:* Microangiopathic hemolytic anemia

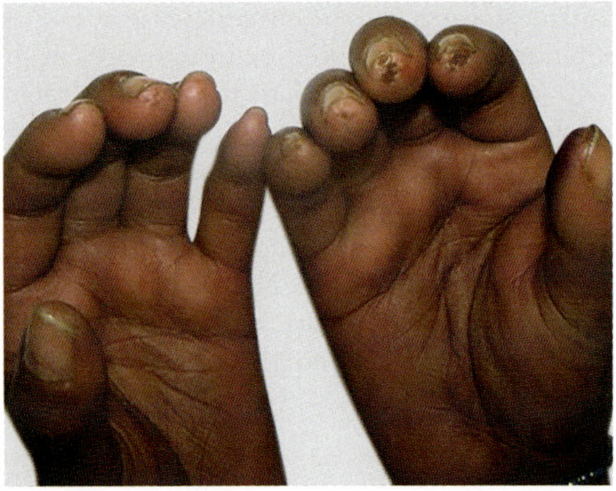

Fig. 9.1.1: Digital ulcer involving right index and middle fingers with digital pits on other fingers and left middle finger

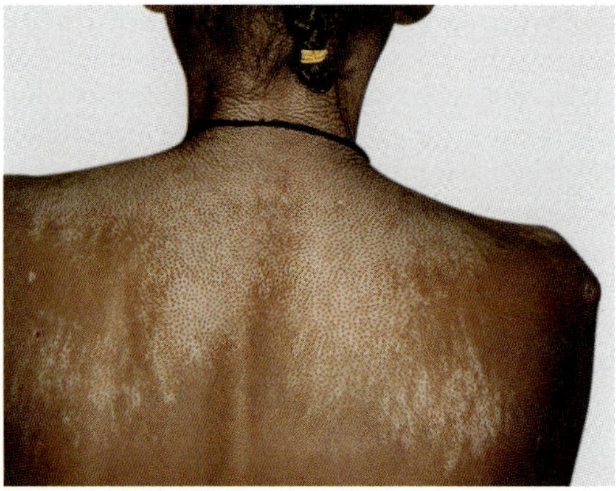

Fig. 9.1.2: Salt and pepper skin appearance over upper back in a patient with diffuse SSc

MANAGEMENT

The management of SSc depends on clinical manifestations (Table 9.1.5). It needs to be individualized for skin involvement, Raynaud phenomenon, lung fibrosis, pulmonary hypertension, or gut symptoms.

Autologous hematopoietic stem cell transplant (HSCT) has a role in selected cases of severe SSc within the first few years of onset. This has been shown in at least three randomized trials. However, the criteria for patient selection for HSCT needs to be strict.

Despite the advances in rheumatology and immunology overall, the SMR in SSc has remained the last in last few decades at 3.5. The leading causes of mortality is lung, heart and kidney involvement.

Table 9.1.5: Management of various manifestations in SSc

Manifestation	*Management*	*Dose*
Raynaud's phenomenon (RP) with/ without DU	Nifedipine Tadalafil (refractory RP or RP with DU as first-line therapy) Losartan Intravenous iloprost (RP/DU non-responsive to oral agents)	10–20 mg three times a day 20 mg alternate day 50 mg/day 0.5–3 ng/kg/min continuous infusion for 3–5 days, repeated at intervals of 6-8 weeks
ILD	Cyclophosphamide Mycophenolate mofetil Rituximab Nintedanib	2 mg/Kg/day oral 2–3 g/day in two divided doses 500 mg weekly ×4 followed by maintenance every 6 months 150 mg twice a day
PAH	Bosentan Ambrisentan Tadalafil Epoprostenol	125–250 mg/day 5 mg/day 20–40 mg/day 2 ng/kg/min over 24–48 hours increased in increments of 2 ng/kg/min every 15 minutes or longer until dose limiting pharmacologic effects are elicited or until a tolerance limit to the drug is established

(Contd.)

Table 9.1.5: Management of various manifestations in SSc (*Contd.*)

Manifestation	*Management*	*Dose*
GERD	Pantoprazole Rabeprazole Domperidone Itopride Metoclopramide	40–80 mg/day 20–40 mg/day 10–30 mg/day 50–150 mg/day 20–60 mg/day
SRC	ACE inhibitors Ramipril Captopril	 5–20 mg/day 25–75 mg/day

DU: Digital ulcerations; *ILD:* Interstitial lung disease; *PAH:* Pulmonary arterial hypertension; *GERD:* Gastroesophageal reflux disease; *SRC:* Scleroderma renal crisis

LEARNING POINTS

- Diagnosis of SSc is clinical and the disease is categorized into 2 subsets, limited cutaneous and diffuse cutaneous with distinctive autoantibodies profile.
- Digital gangrene, GERD , ILD and pulmonary arterial hypertension are major concerns n limited cutaneous disease.
- Besides the above cardiac and scleroderma renal crisis are responsible for poor clinical outcome
- Treatment is largely symptomatic and angiotensin converting enzymes have improved the outcomes of scleroderma renal crisis.
- Autologous hematopoietic stem cell transplantations remains to be explored more to find its utility.

FURTHER READING

1. Elhai M, Meune C, Avouac J, et al. Trends in mortality in patients with systemic sclerosis over 40 years: a systematic review and meta-analysis of cohort studies. Rheumatology (Oxford). 2012;51:1017–26.
2. Galie N, Brundage BH, Ghofrani HA, et al. Tadalafil therapy for pulmonary arterial hypertension. Circulation. 2009;119:2894–903.
3. LeRoy EC, Black C, Fleischmajer R et al. Scleroderma (systemic sclerosis): classification, subsets and pathogenesis. J Rheumatol 1988;15(2):202–5.
4. Preliminary criteria for the classification of systemic sclerosis (scleroderma). Subcommittee for scleroderma criteria of the American Rheumatism Association Diagnostic and Therapeutic Criteria Committee. Arthritis Rheum 1980;23:581–90.
5. Roustit M, Blaise S, Allanore Y, et al. Phosphodiesterase-5 inhibitors for the treatment of secondary Raynaud's phenomenon: systematic review and meta-analysis of randomised trials. Ann Rheum Dis. 2013;72: 1696–9.
6. Tashkin DP, Elashoff R, Clements PJ, et al. Cyclophosphamide versus placebo in scleroderma lung disease. N Engl J Med. 2006;354:2655–66.
7. van den Hoogen F, Khanna D, Fransen J et al. 2013 classification criteria for systemic sclerosis: an American College of Rheumatology/European League against Rheumatism collaborative initiative. Arthritis Rheum. 2013;65:2737–47.

Idiopathic Inflammatory Myositis

Debashis Maikap, Liza Rajasekhar, Ramnath Misra

INTRODUCTION

Idiopathic inflammatory myositis (IIM), are a rare category of acquired autoimmune heterogeneous muscle disorders characterized by muscle inflammation with associated extra-muscular involvement (cutaneous, pulmonary, joints, cardiac and digestive tract) with variable clinical features, therapeutic responses, and prognoses. Currently IIM can be classified into 5 subgroups—dermatomyositis (DM), polymyositis (PM), overlap myositis (OM) (including antisynthetase syndrome), sporadic inclusion body myositis (IBM), and immune mediated necrotizing myositis (IMNM). Excluding IBM, these muscle diseases exhibit progressive muscle weakness as a clinical phenomenon, and muscle tissue has inflammatory infiltrates seen in histopathological examination. This chapter will focus on the different types of myopathies, their clinical profile, the autoantibodies associated and their treatment with long-term prognosis.

EPIDEMIOLOGY

Inflammatory myopathies affect 9–14 cases out of every 100,000 people. The prevalence of overlap myositis (OM) is highest, up to 50% of cases, followed by 33% of cases in dermatomyositis (DM). IMNM is thought to be the third most common group. OM, IMNM, and DM are thought to account for 90% of myositis cases in total. Myositis generally affects women more frequently and juvenile DM (JDM) is seen in both children and adolescents.

ADULT DERMATOMYOSITIS

The pathognomonic cutaneous manifestation of dermatomyositis (DM) is heliotrope rash and Gottron's papules. Photosensitivity, poikiloderma, typical erythematosus rash over neck (V sign), pathognomonic erythematous plaques over knuckles (Fig. 9.2.1) and extensor aspect of the

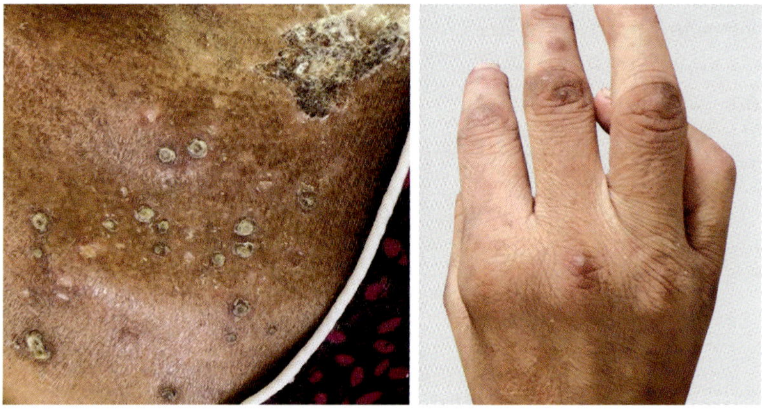

Fig. 9.2.1: Typical skin rash of Dermatomyositis associated with antibodies to Mi-2, papulo squamous crusted lesions over neck (V Sign) and elevated erythematosus lesions over knuckles (Gottron's rash)

elbow (Gottrn's rash) diffuse erythema, palmar papules, and diffuse hair loss are among the other cutaneous abnormalities, as are nail changes such as ragged cuticles and periungual erythema (Fig. 9.2.1). Cutaneous manifestations of DM often precede myopathy by 6 months. Amyopathic DM is a rare type of DM (20%) with typical skin findings without clinically appreciable muscle weakness. Clinically, patients with hypomyopathic dermatomyositis do not have muscle weakness. However, laboratory tests, electromyography, or muscle biopsy show evidence of myositis. According to a prevalence survey, around 70% of dermatomyositis patients have myositis -specific autoantibody, which is associated with a distinct clinical phenotype (Table 9.2.1).

Table 9.2.1: Overview of auto-antibodies and their associated clinical features

Myositis type	*Auto-antibody*	*Frequency (%)*	*Clinical feature*
Antisynthase syndrome	Anti-Jo-1 (histidyl-tRNA synthetase)	15–20	May be clinically amyopathic Associated with fever, constitutional symptoms, ILD, mechanic hand Raynaud's Earlier and more severe ILD with higher rate of mortality seen in non-Jo-1 antibodies (particularly, PL-7 and PL-12)
	Anti-PL-7 (threonyl-)	5–10	
	Anti-PL-12 (alanyl-)	< 5	
	Anti-EJ (glycyl-)	5–10	
	Anti-OJ (isoleucyl-)	< 5	
	Anti-KS (asparaginyl-)	<5	
	Anti-Zo (phenylalanyl-)	<1	
	Anti-Ha-YRS (tyrosyl-)	<1	
CTD myositis	Anti-Ro	19–25	Associated with SLE, Sjogren's syndrome systemic sclerosis if associated with Jo 1 antibody then associated with poor prognosis including malignancy.
	Anti-La	7–12	
	Anti-Pm/Scl	8–10	Associated with systemic sclerosis, severe disease course, poor response.
	Anti-U1-RNP	10	Good prognosis
	Anti-Ku	20–30	Higher rate of ILD, steroid refractory
IMNM	Anti SRP	5–10	Muscle atrophy, 20% develop ILD, dysphagia, severe cardiac involvement, refractory to treatment.
	Anti-HMGCR	20	Higher risk of malignancy, statin naïve patient -resistant to treatment.
DM	Anti-Mi2	5–30	Classical DM, steroid responsive
	Anti SAE	5–10	Often amyopathic, dysphagia and with mild ILD, increased risk of malignancy
	Anti-NXP2	11–24	Malignancy in adult (37.5%), dysphagia, vasculitic skin rash, ulcer, nodule, gi vasculitis distal extensor weakness and oedema Associated with JDM without malignancy and calcinosis
	Anti-TIF1	10–15	Malignancy 75% in adult Most common antibody in JDM without risk of malignancy
	Anti-MDA5/CADM140	15–20	Often amyopathic DM with rapidly progressive ILD, skin/tongue ulceration, palmar papules, alopecia, arthritis poor response, higher mortality.

IMNM: Immune mediated necrotizing myositis; *DM:* Dermatomyositis

ADULT POLYMYOSITIS (PM)

Patients presenting with weakness and high muscle enzymes in the absence of typical cutaneous features of DM offer a more tough diagnostic challenge because of the absence of typical cutaneous findings with no diagnostic serologic test. Most notably, these patients must be recognised from other causes of myopathy that do not have a rash, such as hypothyroid myopathy, muscular dystrophy, and metabolic myopathies. As a result, PM is uncommon, especially "pure PM," and may include IIM mimics, antisynthetase syndrome, OM, or immune mediated necrotizing myositis. As true PM is still a diagnosis of exclusion, patients with PM should undergo regular monitoring for the appearance of new clinical features that may point to other forms of IIM.

CONNECTIVE TISSUE DISEASE-ASSOCIATED MYOSITIS

Myositis that is accompanied by an underlying connective tissue disease (CTD) such as lupus, inflammatory arthritis, scleroderma, or MCTD is referred to as overlap myositis. The clinical presentation is one of an autoimmune CTD despite the possibility that the muscle biopsy may show signs of necrotising myositis, dermatomyositis, or non-specific myositis.

IMMUNE-MEDIATED NECROTIZING MYOSITIS (IMNM)

Patients with necrotising autoimmune myositis are a diverse group who frequently exhibit atrophy in the affected muscles, weight loss, and necrosis on biopsy. Based on serology and clinical picture IMNM are of two types: Statin-associated or statin-naive HMGCR (3-hydroxy-3-methylglutaryl-CoA reductase) antibody and signal recognition particle (SRP) antibody necrotizing myositis. IMNM has also been documented in cases of malignancy, autoimmune diseases, and viral infections like hepatitis C and the human immunodeficiency virus.

ANTISYNTHASE SYNDROME (ASS)

Anti-synthetase syndrome (ASS) is now considered an overlap myositis characterized by antibodies directed against an aminoacycl transfer RNA synthetase (ARS) (most prevalent is Jo1) along with clinical features that can include interstitial lung disease, myositis, mechanic's hands (hyperkeratosis and fissuring of the palmar skin), Raynaud's phenomenon, and arthritis. Antisynthase antibodies can be found in 30–40% of inflammatory myositis patients and 7–10% of idiopathic interstitial pneumonia patients (Fig. 9.2.2). It should be noted that not all patients with antisynthetase syndrome experience muscle weakness. It is important to note that muscle weakness does not occur in all patients with antisynthetase syndrome. Furthermore, while 90% of individuals with anti-Jo1 autoantibodies have ASS, up to 50% of individuals with anti-PL12 autoantibodies have ILD without muscle disease.

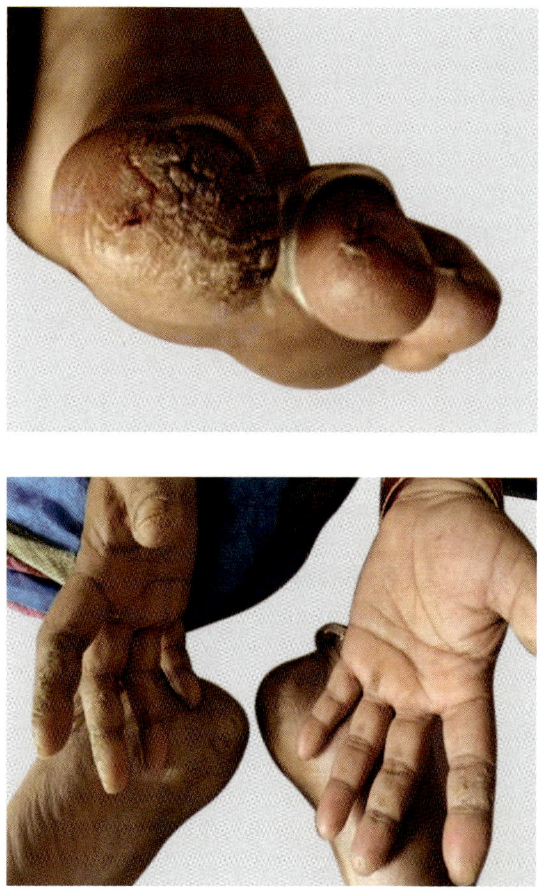

Fig. 9.2.2: Fissuring and Hyperkeratosis of the toes and the radial aspect of the fingers in a patient with anti-Jo-1 positive inflammatory myositis. The patient also has non-specific interstitial pneumonia on high-resolution computed tomography of the chest

CANCER-ASSOCIATED MYOSITIS

The defining features of cancer-associated myositis (CAM) are:

1. Cancer incidence is highest at the time of first presentation and for the initial three years of myositis.
2. Myositis is resistant to standard treatment, but it usually improves when the malignancy is treated.
3. Cancer relapse results in relapse or development of myositis.

Risk factors for cancer include elderly, male gender, pharyngeal muscle involvement, and cutaneous manifestations (such as skin necrosis, vasculitis, periungual erythema, and the shawl sign), resistant disease, low serum complement (C4) levels, presence of the anti-NXP2 or (TIF)-1gamma, muscle biopsy showing capillary damage and absence of other myositis autoantibodies. Concomitant ILD, antisynthetase antibodies, and low lymphocyte counts have seemed to be protective factors. Adenocarcinomas of the breast, lung, ovaries cervix, pancreas, bladder, colorectal and stomach account for approximately 70% of the CAM.

Although there is no universal agreement on the investigation of underlying malignancy, clinicians should be familiar with age and sex pertinent cancer screening tests such as Pap smear, mammogram or ultrasound breast, prostate specific antigen, CA-125, and fecal occult blood screening. In adult IIM subtypes with an increase incidence of malignancy, such as TIF-1 and NXP-2 antibody-association and myositis autoantibody negative necrotising myositis patients within 3 years of diagnosis, more advanced screening methods, such as PET-CT (positron emission tomography–computed tomography) of whole body should be considered.

DIAGNOSIS

Diagnosis should be done in a stepwise manner to exclude mimics as well as to categorize the type of myositis (Fig. 9.2.3).

TREATMENT

Immunosuppressive therapy generally works for polymyositis, dermatomyositis, and the majority of necrotizing myositis, and overlap myositis patients. Muscle strengthening is provided through physical rehabilitation in the form of physiotherapy, occupational therapy, and speech therapy. Adequate dietary guidance is also necessary to achieve favourable outcome.

For the most IIM patients, glucocorticoids remain the cornerstone therapy. Prednisolone dosage is started at one mg per kg and continued

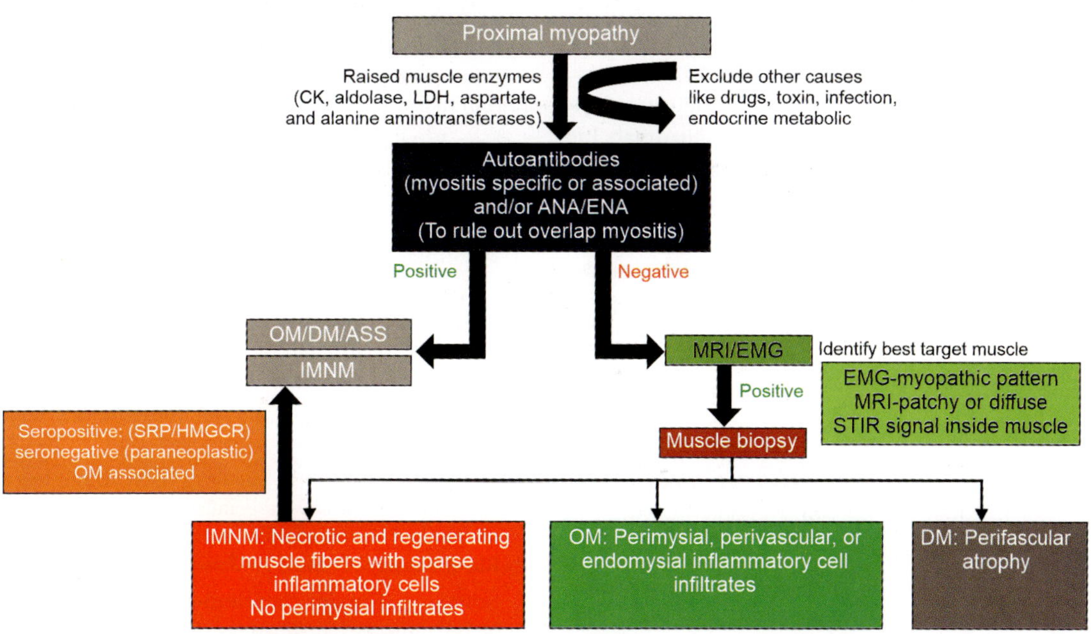

Fig. 9.2.3: Diagnostic algorithm for proximal muscle weakness

for 4–6 weeks before being gradually tapered off, based on the response and recovery of patient and adverse outcomes. There are no established guidelines, but in our practice, this typically takes over 9–12 months.

Intravenous methylprednisolone pulse therapy may be necessary in patients with rapidly progressive severe muscle weakness or muscle involving diaphragm or other respiratory muscles. It is typically given at doses of 0.5–1 g daily for 3–5 days. Immunomodulators such as azathioprine, mycophenolate, or methotrexate are very useful in controlling mild to moderate case of myositis which helpful in tapering corticosteroid. A high dose IVIG treatment may be necessary in patients with severe active myositis (usually 2 g/kg). In diabetes mellitus patients with HMGCR-positive necrotising myositis, IVIG alone has been shown to be effective in preventing glucocorticoid-induced hyperglycaemia and useful in patients with uncontrolled diabetes mellitus. As an alternative, rituximab (one gram given two times, 2 weeks apart) may be taken into consideration for induction therapy. As there is variable response to immunosuppression in different subtypes of IIM, treatment may be individualized for each patient.

RECENT ADVANCES

Abatacept a T-cell modulator, and Lenabasum a cannabinoid receptor type 2 agonist, are both undergoing phase 3 trials for dermatomyositis. According to some case studies, tocilizumab (an interleukin 6 receptor antagonist), anakinra (anti-interleukin 1), and alemtuzumab (anti-CD52) are effective treatments for idiopathic inflammatory myopathies. Additionally, Janus kinase inhibitors have encouraging results in treating severe DM conditions like MDA5 myositis and severe refractory calcinosis.

LEARNING POINTS

- The adult idiopathic inflammatory myositis is a diverse group of disorders that affect muscle and involve extramuscular organs, resulting in significant disability.
- Since each clinical phenotype has a different prognosis and necessitates a different therapeutic strategy, it is important to distinguish between those that have cutaneous and muscular affection as well as those that do not.
- Anti-HMGCR and anti-SRP myositis-specific autoantibodies are hallmark of immune-mediated necrotizing myopathy (IMNM) when muscle biopsy cannot be done.
- We can now diagnose IIM without performing invasive tests like muscle biopsies thanks to the development of newer myositis-specific autoantibodies and exciting advancements in imaging techniques, particularly bedside muscle ultrasound and MRI.
- Treatment guidelines propose a combination of corticosteroids with steroid sparing agents. However, in IMNM with anti-HMGCR antibodies IVIG is preferred while for anti SRP antibodies associated with IMNM Rituximab is preferred.

FURTHER READING

1. Ashton C, Paramalingam S, Stevenson B, et al. Idiopathic inflammatory myopathies: a review. Intern Med J. 2021; 51:845–52.
2. Betteridge Z, McHugh N. Myositis-specific autoantibodies: an important tool to support diagnosis of myositis. J Intern Med 2016;280:8–23.
3. Hsu JL, Liao MF, Chu CC, et al. Reappraisal of the incidence, various types and risk factors of malignancies in patients with dermatomyositis and polymyositis in Taiwan. Sci Rep 2021;11:4545.
4. Khadilkar SV, Dhamne MC. What is new in Idiopathic Inflammatory Myopathies: Mechanisms and Therapies. Ann Indian Acad Neurol. 2020; 23:458–67.
5. Lega JC, Fabien N, Reynaud Q, et al. The clinical phenotype associated with myositis-specific and associated autoantibodies: A meta-analysis revisiting the so-called antisynthetase syndrome. Autoimmun Rev 2014;13:883–91.
6. Lazarou IN, Guerne PA. Classification, diagnosis, and management of idiopathic inflammatory myopathies. J Rheumatol. 2013; 40:550–64.
7. Selva-O'Callaghan A, Pinal-Fernandez I, Trallero-Araguás E, et al. Classification and management of adult inflammatory myopathies. Lancet Neurol. 2018;17:816–28.
8. Svensson J, Arkema EV, Lundberg IE, et al. Incidence and prevalence of idiopathic inflammatory myopathies in Sweden: A nationwide population-based study. Rheumatology (Oxford) 2017;56:802–10.
9. Schmidt J. Current classification and management of inflammatory myopathies. J Neuromuscul Dis. 2018;5:109–29.

Chapter 9.3

Mixed Connective Tissue Disease and Overlap Connective Tissue Disease

Avinash Jain, Arun Hegde, Vaidehi Chowdhary

INTRODUCTION

Mixed connective tissue disease (MCTD) is a rare, systemic autoimmune disease, characterized by overlapping features of SLE, polymyositis, and systemic sclerosis (SSc). The presence of high titer anti-U1RNP antibodies is the sine qua non feature of this disease. It was originally described in 1972 by Sharp et al. as a mild disease, with a low likelihood of renal and nervous system disease, good response to steroids and a favorable prognosis. Published series in the last four decades challenge this concept with significant morbidity and mortality described in many from serious manifestations like pulmonary hypertension and interstitial lung disease.

Debate exists if MCTD represents a distinct disease entity or the intermediate stage of an evolving disease. The argument against MCTD being an independent disease is that over time additional clinical features accrue and 6–12% of patients evolve into another autoimmune rheumatic disease such as SSc more frequently. Moreover presence of antibodies to U1RNP is not unique to MCTD as these autoantibodies are seen in other autoimmune rheumatic diseases as well. Proponents of MCTD being a unique entity cite the genetic association with HLA-DR4 or DR2 (along with the low frequency of DR5 and DR3, HLA genotypes that are associated with SSc and SLE respectively) and a core group of symptoms, namely, "puffy hands", Raynaud phenomenon (RP), esophagal hypomotility, myositis, telangiectasia and sclerodactyly that cluster with anti-U1 70 kD antibodies.

Regardless of the controversies in nomenclature, MCTD identifies a group of patients in whom active surveillance for manifestations or conversion to other autoimmune rheumatic diseases is needed.

Overlap connective tissue diseases or overlap syndromes (OS) on the other hand fulfill the classification criteria of two unique connective tissue diseases (CTDs). They have clinical and serological features consistent with two well-defined CTDs with dominant features of one of the CTDs. MCTD can be considered as one type of overlap CTD with a unique serological profile.

EPIDEMIOLOGY, CLINICAL FEATURES AND DIAGNOSIS OF MCTD

The incidence of MCTD is 0.2–2 per 100,000 population with a lack of large ethnicity-based data with a female: male ratio of 5–10:1. Exact prevalence of overlap syndrome is not known.

CLINICAL MANIFESTATIONS OF MCTD

Clinical presentation may be nonspecific with constitutional symptoms, fatigue and weight loss or involve multiple organs (Fig. 9.3.1). Myositis, pulmonary arterial hypertension (PAH) and interstitial lung disease (ILD) constitute serious manifestations of MCTD and contribute significantly to mortality and morbidity. ILD in MCTD is seen in 50–80% of high-resolution CT scans (HRCT) but many patients are asymptomatic. ILD often clusters with Raynaud's phenomenon, dysphagia, esophagal dysmotility and myositis. Anti-Sm and anti-Ro52 antibodies are common in MCTD-ILD, whereas the presence of arthritis and rheumatoid factor are protective. Radiologic features

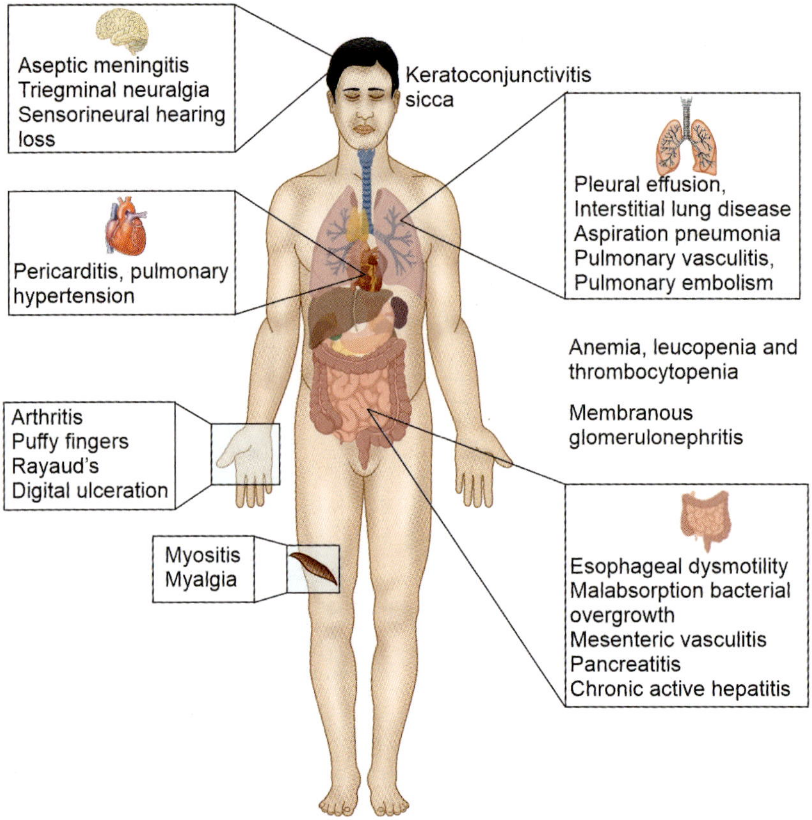

Fig. 9.3.1: Various manifestations are seen in patients with MCTD

include consolidation, ground glass opacities, traction bronchiectasis and honeycombing. Histologically common phenotypes are fibrosing NSIP (especially for myositis overlap) or unclassifiable fibrosis in systemic sclerosis overlap phenotype (Fig. 9.3.2).

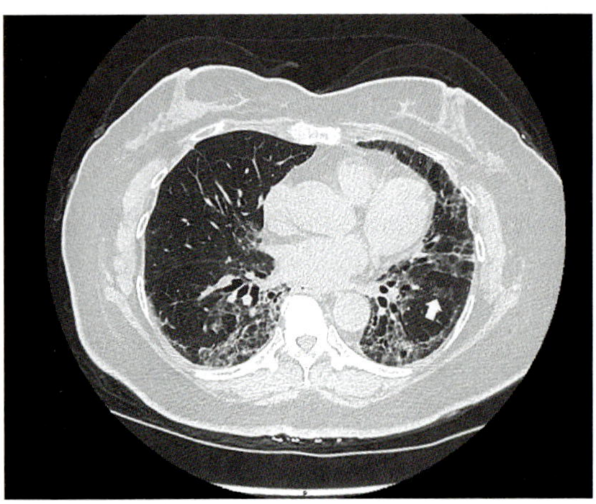

Fig. 9.3.2: Fibrotic interstitial lung disease with an NSIP pattern in MCTD. Ground-glass opacities are noted in the right lower lobes (arrow)

Precapillary pulmonary hypertension (PH, defined as mean pulmonary arterial pressure of ≥20 mm Hg, pulmonary arterial wedge pressure ≤15 mm Hg and pulmonary vascular resistance ≥3 wood units, by right heart catheterisation) is common in MCTD. Frequency is estimated to be from 3–24% over the disease course and most patients have either isolated pulmonary arterial hypertension (PAH, WHO Group 1.4.1) or PH-associated with ILD (WHO Group 3.2). Symptoms include dyspnoea, fatigue, exertional chest pain, syncope and a physical examination demonstrating signs of right heart failure in advanced disease. Because the mortality is high the early detection of PH is important. Annual pulmonary function tests (PFT), diffusion capacity of the lungs for carbon monoxide (DLCO), transthoracic echocardiogram (TTE) and serum N-terminal pro-B-type natriuretic peptide (NT-Pro-BNP) level are recommended for screening.

The presence of additional autoantibodies besides U1RNP may influence disease phenotype.

Anti-endothelial and anticardiolipin antibodies are associated with PAH, Raynaud's phenomenon, and thrombotic events. Erosive arthritis is often seen with anti-CCP positivity. A small subset of patients may develop deforming arthritis called arthritis mutilans.

Clinical Manifestations in Overlap Syndrome

It depends on the dominant CTDs and present with different organ system involvement. Patients with SSc have typical features like Raynaud (Fig. 9.3.3), digital pits (Fig. 9.3.4), skin tightening, visceral fibrosis with features of another autoimmune disease like myositis. Similarly, lupus overlap syndrome may have classical features like malar rash, palatal ulcer, glomerulonephritis, and antibodies to dsDNA and Sm with/without low complements.

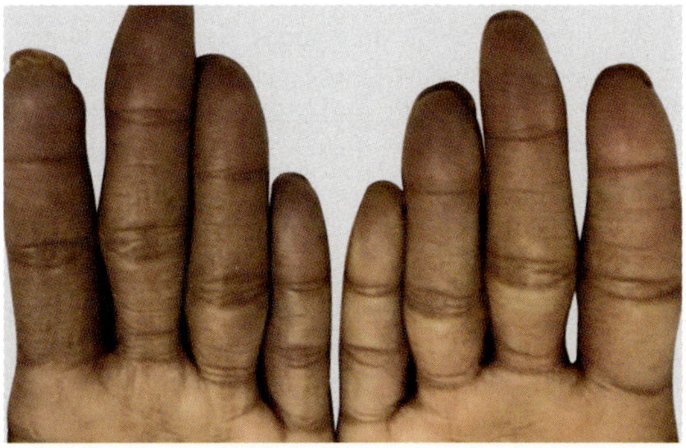

Fig. 9.3.3: Raynaud's phenomenon. Note bluish discoloration of fingers (*Source:* IRA image bank—Chotalia et al.)

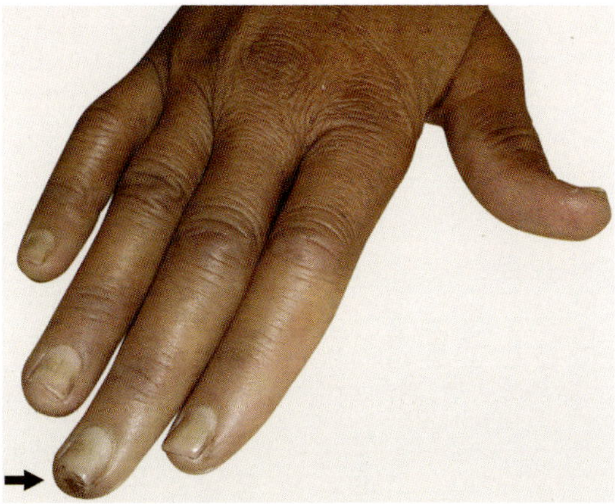

Fig. 9.3.4: Digital ulcer (black arrow) (*Source:* IRA image bank—Nagaprabhu et al.)

DIAGNOSIS OF MCTD

Diagnosis of MCTD is suggested by typical clinical manifestations and supported by serology. Investigations for diagnosis of individual manifestations are summarized in Table 9.3.1. Several criteria are available for the classification of MCTD (Table 9.3.2). The newest set of criteria (2019) are from the Japan committee which states that in presence of CTD-specific antibodies like anti dsDNA, anti-Smith, anti-Scl-70, anti-RNA-polymerase III, and anti-synthetase antibodies, diagnosis of MCTD should be carefully made. This criterion has a sensitivity of 90.6% and a specificity of 98.4% (Table 9.3.3)

Depending on clinical phenotype, OS will have antibodies that are specific to a CTD or antibodies that are classically associated with overlap features like antibodies to PM/Scl seen with an overlap of myositis and scleroderma.

MANAGEMENT

There are no separate guidelines for the management of MCTD and OS. The treatment is governed by the type and severity of organ involvement. Table 9.3.1 highlights the management depending on disease manifestations. The difference lies in the management of PH in a setting of MCTD where the use of immunosuppressive agents has been found to be beneficial in improving outcomes. In the case of OS, depending on underlying pathogenesis–vasculopathy vs vasculitis, management of PH varies. If the class of dyspnea is WHO II or more, use of immunosuppressive agents is recommended in patients with MCTD or overlap with SLE or myositis or multiple autoantibodies other than autoantibodies associated with SSc. Initial therapy is with a phosphodiesterase 5 inhibitor vasodilator agent with the addition of a second vasodilatory agent if there is no improvement or if the patient has dyspnoea WHO Class III or more.

Corticosteroids form the mainstay of MCTD-related ILD. Azathioprine, mycophenolate mofetil, rituximab and cyclophosphamide provide stabilisation of disease and steroid-sparing effect. Antifibrotic agents like nintedanib slow the progression of fibrotic ILD and pirfenidone added to the existing treatment regimen might attenuate disease progression. However, they are not used

Table 9.3.1: Management of MCTD and overlap syndrome

Manifestations	*Diagnosis*	*First line management*	*Second and third line management*	*Monitoring*
Arthritis	Clinical Diagnosis X-rays to look at erosions	NSAIDs HCQ (5 mg/kg) LD	MTX (15–25 mg/week) LEF (10–20 mg/d) bDMARDs tsDMARDs	Periodic CBC and LFT to look for drug toxicity of NSAIDs, DMARDs
ILD	Dry cough, dyspnea, fatigue, velcro crackles PFT with DLCO annually if no e/o ILD on imaging If symptomatic or drop in FVC by 10% or DLCO by 15% in three months, an HRCT chest is indicated	CS (0.5–1 mg/kg) MMF (up to 2 g/d) AZA (2–2.5 mg/kg)	CYC (600 mg/m^2 every 4w for six doses) RTX (750 mg/m^2 * 2 doses) Nintedanib 150 mg twice daily Pirfenidone (titrated to 801 mg three time daily)	6MWT PFT with DLCO 3–6 monthly Quantification by HRCT (lower-lobes % ILD-HRCT score) Repeat imaging every 1–2 year or early if worsening
PH (Elaborate)	Dry cough, dyspnea, fatigue, loud P2 DLCO out of proportionally low when compared to FVC (FVC/DLCO >1.6) ECHO	Vasodilators (VDs)–group 1 PH WHO Class II–single VD WHO Class III-IV–two or more VDs IS agents in MCTD and depending on dominant CTD in overlap		6 MWT Echo PFT with DLCO
Myositis	Clinical CPK, LDH, SGOT, SGPT EMG MRI	CS (1 mg/kg) MTX (15–25 mg/week)/AZA (2–2.5 mg/kg)/tacrolimus (0.075–0.1mg/kg/d)	MMF RTX	Clinical Muscle enzymes–SGOT SGPT CPK LDH Damage vs activity–MRI
Skin involvement**	Clinical	Topical CS LD HCQ	MTX* AZA MMF Dapsone	Clinical
Raynaud Without digital ulcer(s) (DUs)	Clinical NFC	CCBs	PDE5i	Clinical
Raynaud with DUs	Clinical NFC	CCBs, PDE5i	ETA Prostacyclin Others like ARBs, fluoxetine	

(Contd.)

Table 9.3.1: Management of MCTD and overlap syndrome (*Contd.*)

Manifestations	*Diagnosis*	*First line management*	*Second and third line management*	*Monitoring*
Nephritis	Hypertension Edema Lipid profile Urine showing active sediments and proteinuria	Depending on histopathological examination will need CS with CS sparing agents like AZA, MMF, CYC, TAC, RTX		Monitor for proteinuria, urine routine examination for active sediments
GERD	Clinical May need UGIE	PPIs Antiemetics like domperidone Prokinetics like metoclopramide, mosapride		Clinical
Serositis	Clinical Imaging like chest x-ray, ECHO, ultrasound abdomen	NSAIDs	LD	Clinical and imaging
Headache	Clinical Rule out sinister causes if not responding and associated with vomiting, visual disturbances, seizure, or FND using brain imaging	NSAIDs LD		Clinical
Trigeminal neuralgia	Clinical	CBZ 100–200 mg twice per day	Gabapentin Lamotrigine	Clinical

*VDs include PDE5i like Tadalafil (maximum 40 mg/d), ET antagonists (ETA) like ambrisentan (maximum 10 mg/d), macitentan (maximum 10 mg/d), cGMP agonist riociguat and prostacyclin analogs; **for cutaneous vasculitis, upfront higher dose CS with second line therapy. *ARBs:* Angiotensin receptor blocker; *AZA:* Azathioprine; *bDMARDs:* biological DMARDs; *CBZ:* Carbamazepine; *CS:* Corticosteroids; *CYC:* Cyclophosphamide; *FND:* Focal neurological deficit; *HCQ:* Hydroxychloroquine; *LD:* Low-dose steroids (prednisolone equivalent <= 7.5mg/d); *LEF:* Leflunomide; *MTX:* Methotrexate; *NFC:* Nail fold capillaroscopy; *RTX:* Rituximab; *TAC:* Tacrolimus; *tsDMARDs:* targeted synthetic DMARDs

Table 9.3.2: Existing classification criteria for MCTD

Components of the criteria	*Alarcon-Segovia*	*Kahn*	*Kasukawa et al.*	*Sharp*
Serology	Anti RNP titer ≥1:1600	Anti-RNP with speckled ANA ≥ 1:1200	Anti-snRNP antibody positive	U1RNP positive, negative anti-Sm
Clinical criteria				
Clinical	Anti-U1RNP is must and 2 of the following:	Raynaud with 2 out 3	At least 1 common symptom plus snRNP plus >1 symptoms in at least 2 out 3 disease categories from mixed symptoms	At least 4 major with U1-RNP titer ≥1:4000 or ≥2 major from 1, 2 and 3 plus 2 minor with U1-RNP of atleast 1:1000; Exclusion–positive anti-Sm
Swollen hands	Yes	Yes	Common symptoms 1. RP 2. Swollen fingers or hands	Major criteria 1. Severe myositis 2. Pulmonary involvement (a) Dico <70% (b) PH (c) Proliferative vascular lesions on lung biopsy 3. RP or esophageal dysmotility 4. Swollen hands or sclerodactyly 5. ENA ≥1:10,000 and U1RNP positive and negative anti-Sm
Myositis	Yes	Yes	Mixed symptoms 1. SLE like findings (a) Polyarthritis (b) Lymphadenopathy (c) Facial erythema (d) Pericarditis or pleuritis (e) Leuko- or thrombocytopenia 2. SSc-like findings (a) Sclerodactyly (b) Pulmonary fibrosis,restrictive changes of lung, or reduced diffusion capacity (c) Hypomotility or dilatation of esophagus 3. PM like findings (a) Muscle weakness (b) Elevated Muscle enzymes (c) Myopathic patter on EMG	Minor criteria 1. Alopecia 2. Leukopenia 3. Anemia 4. Pleuritis 5. Pericarditis 6. Arthritis 7. Trigeminal neuropathy 8. Malar rash 9. Thrombocytopenia 10. Mild myositis 11. History of swollen hand
Sclerodactyly/ Acrosclerosis	Yes	No		
Raynaud	Yes	Must be present		
Arthritis	Yes	No		

EMG: Electromyography; *RNP:* Ribonuclear protein; *RP:* Raynaud's phenomenon; *Sm:* Smith; *snRNP:* small nuclear RNP; *SSc:* Systemic sclerosis

Table 9.3.3: Diagnostic criteria for mixed connective tissue disease 2019, from the Japan research committee of the ministry of health, labor, and welfare for systemic autoimmune diseases

I. Common manifestations 1. Raynaud's phenomenon 2. Puffy fingers and/or swomen hands
II. Immunological manifestation • Positivity for anti-U1 ribonucleoprotein antibody
III. Characteristic organ involvement 1. Pulmonary arterial hypertension 2. Aseptic meningitis 3. Trigeminal neuropathy
IV. Overlapping manifestations
A. Systemic lupus erythematosus-like manifestations 1. Polyarthritis 2. Lymphadenopathy 3. Malar rash 4. Pericarditis or pleuritis 5. Leukopenia (4,000/μL or less) or thrombocytopenia (100,000/μL or less)
B. Systemic sclerosis-like manifestations 1. Sclerodactyly 2. Interstitial lung disease 3. Esophageal dysmotility or dilatation
C. Polymyositis/dermatomyositis-like manifestations 1. Muscle weakness 2. Elevated levels of myogenic enzymes 3. Myogenic abnormalities on electromyogram

Mixed connective tissue disease is diagnosed when a patient meets all the following: at least one common manifestation, immunological manifestation, and at least one characteristic organ involvement; or when a patient meets all the following: at least one common manifestation, immunological manifestation, and at least one feature each in 2 or more from items A, B, and C in overlapping manifestations (from children, one feature from at least one item A, B or C)

as first-line agents. Gastrointestinal side effects of diarrhea, weight loss, nausea, vomiting and anorexia are common and can be dose-limiting. Liver enzyme monitoring is required during therapy.

NATURAL COURSE AND PROGNOSIS

Evolution of MCTD is infrequent (6.3–12% over 10 years) and the disease phenotype remains relatively stable with mortality similar to the general population highlighting the benign nature of the disease. A most common reason for reduced life expectancy is PH.

ILD in the setting of MCTD, is usually mild and has a more benign course than IPF or scleroderma ILD. Severe disease is seen in 19% and the mortality is 6–8%. Patients at risk of disease progression are males, having anti-Ro52, or high tire U1RNP antibodies , extensive fibrosis on chest CT, and poor lung function. Presence of these features warrants need for close monitoring.

LEARNING POINTS

- MCTD is U1RNP mediated autoimmune diseases with features common to Rheumatoid arthritis (erosive arthritis), lupus (rash, oral ulcer), myositis and systemic sclerosis (raynaud, digital ulcers, sclerodactyly, and ILD) and with few characteristic features like trigeminal neuralgia.
- Overlap syndrome is a constellation of clinical symptoms and serology which cannot be explained by one CTD and meets the classification criteria for two or more CTDs.
- Management is guided by the type and severity of organ involvement.
- Prognosis of MCTD and overlap syndrome is better than well-defined CTDs except in the case of severe PH and ILD.

FURTHER READING

1. Alarcón-Segovia D, Cardiel MH. Comparison between 3 diagnostic criteria for mixed connective tissue disease. Study of 593 patients. J Rheumatol. 1989;16:328–34.
2. Chaigne B, Scirè CA, Talarico R, et al. Mixed connective tissue disease: state of the art on clinical practice guidelines. RMD Open. 2018;4 (Suppl 1):e000783. doi:10.1136/rmdopen-2018–000783.
3. Sharp GC, Anderson PC. Current concepts in the classification of connective tissue diseases. Overlap syndromes and mixed connective tissue disease (MCTD). J Am Acad Dermatol. 1980;2:269–79.
4. Tanaka Y, Kuwana M, Fujii T, et al. 2019 Diagnostic criteria for mixed connective tissue disease (MCTD): From the Japan research committee of the ministry of health, labor, and welfare for systemic autoimmune diseases. Mod Rheumatol. 2021;31:29–33.
5. Tani C, Carli L, Vagnani S, et al. The diagnosis and classification of mixed connective tissue disease. J Autoimmun. 2014;48–49:46–9.

Chapter 9.4

Takayasu Arteritis

Debashish Danda

INTRODUCTION

Takayasu arteritis (TAK) is a chronic, granulomatous, large-vessel panarteritis, characterized by stenosis, occlusion, and sometimes aneurysm of the aorta and its main branches and pulmonary arteries.

CLINICAL FEATURES

TAK predominantly affects young females with insidious onset and is detected in some asymptomatic individuals because of absent pulses during medical check-up. The clinical manifestations (Table 9.4.1) vary based on the arteries involved and the severity of inflammation. Males have more abdominal aorta involvement and complications than females. Both IL-6 driven systemic inflammation and Th1 cell-mediated vascular granuloma formation have been proposed (Fig. 9.4.1) as possible pathogenesis of TAK.

TAK is classified angiographically (Numano classification) into six types based on involvement of arch of aorta and its branches, ascending aorta, thoracic aorta, abdominal aorta, and renal arteries with type 5 being more common in India (Fig. 9.4.2).

Table 9.4.1: Clinical presentations of Takayasu arteritis

System involved	*Symptoms/signs*
1. Constitutional	Fever, weight loss, loss of appetite, fatigue, headache
2. Musculoskeletal	Arthralgia, Arthritis, myalgia
3. Cutaneous	Pyoderma gangrenosum, erythema nodosum
4. Vascular	Diminished or absent pulses, bruit
Aorta	Aortic root dilatation leading to aortic regurgitation, Aneurysm
Carotid arteries	Syncope, TIA/stroke, visual loss, seizures, carotidynia
Vertebral arteries	Vertigo
Subclavian arteries	Most common artery involved: Claudication of upper limbs, ischemia or gangrene, asymmetric blood pressure between two arms
Pulmonary arteries	Dyspnoea, chest pain, pulmonary hypertension and hemoptysis
Mesenteric arteries	Abdominal pain, anorexia, diarrhea, gastrointestinal hemorrhage
Renal arteries	Hypertension
Iliac arteries	Claudication in lower limbs
Coronary arteries	Angina, heart failure

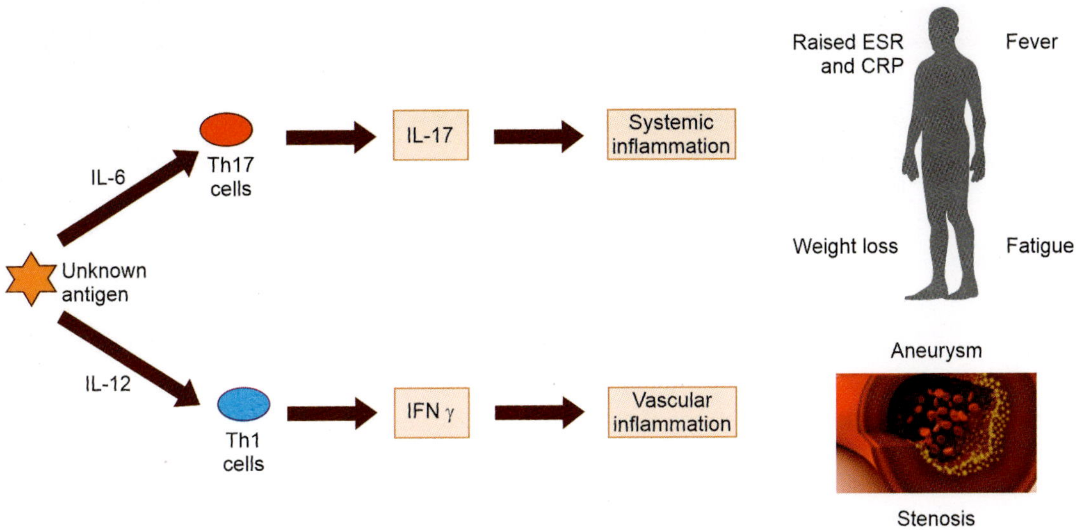

Fig. 9.4.1: Schematic representation of proposed pathogenesis in Takayasu arteritis. Unknown antigen triggers the activation of antigen presenting cells (not shown in figure) which produces cytokines that direct differentiation of T helper cells in to two different pathways. IL-6 causes stimulation of Th 17 cells which produces IL-17 which resulted in systemic inflammatory response. IL-12 stimulates Th1 cells to produce IFN γ which resulted in granular in vessel wall leading to vascular inflammation

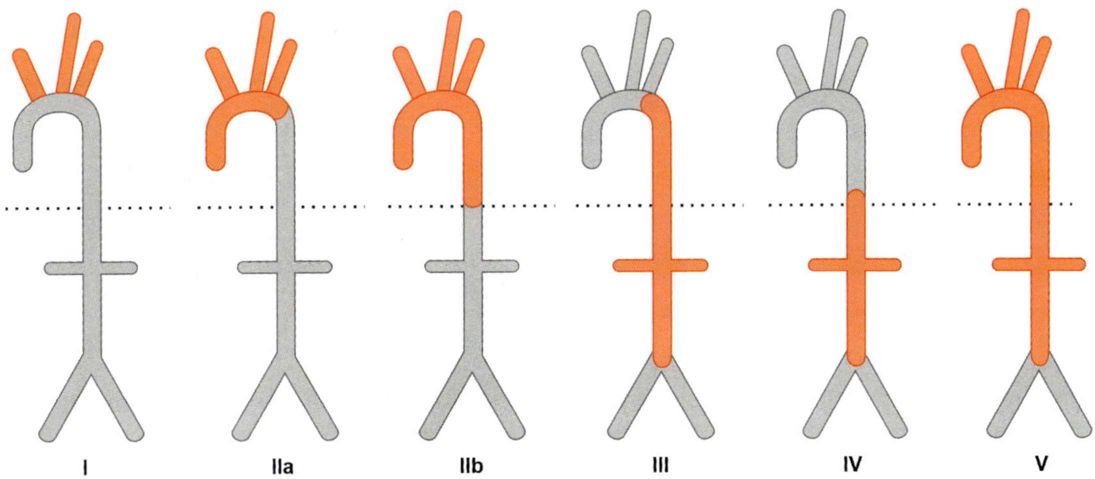

Fig. 9.4.2: Numano classification of Takayasu arteritis based on sites of involvement of aorta and its primary branches. The involvement of pulmonary or coronary arteries are designated as P^+ or C^+, respectively

DIAGNOSIS

The diagnosis of TAK is challenging as there are no gold-standard imaging or laboratory tests with adequate sensitivity or specificity. The American College of Rheumatology (ACR) classification criterion (1990) is being followed till now but with certain nuances (Table 9.4.2).

Ishikawa proposed a diagnostic criterion with age <40 years as obligatory criteria and clinical, laboratory, and angiographic parameters that rely mainly on aortic arch involvement for diagnosis. Sharma's modification of Ishikawa criteria increased the sensitivity from 60 to 92.5% preserving the specificity. In children less than 18 years EULAR/PRES/PRINTO developed a classification criterion with a sensitivity of 100% and specificity of 99.9%.

Table 9.4.2: The 1990 American College of Rheumatology (ACR) classification for Takayasu arteritis (TAK)

Item	*Definition*
Age	Symptoms or findings related to TAK at age <40 years
Claudication	Fatigue and discomfort in muscles of one or more extremity while in use, especially upper limbs
Brachial artery pulse	Decreased pulsation of one or more of brachial arteries
Bruit	On auscultation bruit over abdominal aorta or one/both subclavian arteries
Blood pressure	Blood pressure (systolic) difference of >10 mm Hg between arms
Arteriogram abnormality	Occlusion or narrowing of the entire aorta, its branches, or large arteries in the proximal upper or lower extremities. The narrowing must not due to arteriosclerosis, or similar causes. The vascular changes are usually focal or segmental

A patient is classified as TAK, in the presence of at least 3 of these 6 criteria. Sensitivity 90.5% and specificity 97.8%

ASSESSMENT OF DISEASE ACTIVITY

Markers such as ESR and CRP cannot be used accurately to assess disease activity in TAK. The Kerr criteria or NIH criteria are simple and widely used to detect active TAK. The currently established criteria for measuring disease activity are the NIH criteria, ITAS-2010 (Table 9.4.3). Recently 18-FDG PET CT has been used to assess disease activity. A PET vascular activity score (PETVAS) >20 indicates active disease (Fig. 9.4.3).

Table 9.4.3: Disease activity measures in Takayasu arteritis (TAK)

Criteria	*Essential features*	*Advantages*	*Disadvantages*
NIH criteria	Based on clinical features, angiographic abnormalities and ESR	Simple four category system Inclusion of angiography findings	New onset abnormalities on clinical examination or angiogram alone can suggest active disease irrespective of the value of ESR
ITAS 2010	There are 44 items in six categories. Measures symptoms that occurred or worsened over last 3 months. Cardiovascular involvement have increased weightage. ITAS-A includes ESR/CRP.	Good interrater agreement and better than PGA Validated in adult TAK Numerical score, so comparison easy	CRP and ESR had weak correlations with ITAS2010 Angiography not included Abnormal physical findings had poor sensitivity (14–50%) 30% of arteriographic lesions missed when ITAS2010 was used alone
PETVAS	PET-based parameter created by integrating the visual 0–3 scores (relative to liver FDG uptake) of nine main susceptible arteries, which can quantitatively reflect the global inflammatory burden Total score >20 suggest active disease	Suitable for precise monitoring of TAK even when ESR and CRP are normal Strong correlation of PETVAS and ITAS-2010 scores Combination of PET/CT with PTX-3 added value in assessing activity	PET/CT is more expensive Involves radiation exposure Not validated

NIH: National institutes of health; *ITAS2010:* Indian T'akayasu's clinical activity score 2010; *PET:* Positron emission tomography; *PETVAS:* PET vascular activity score; *PTX-3:* Pentraxin 3

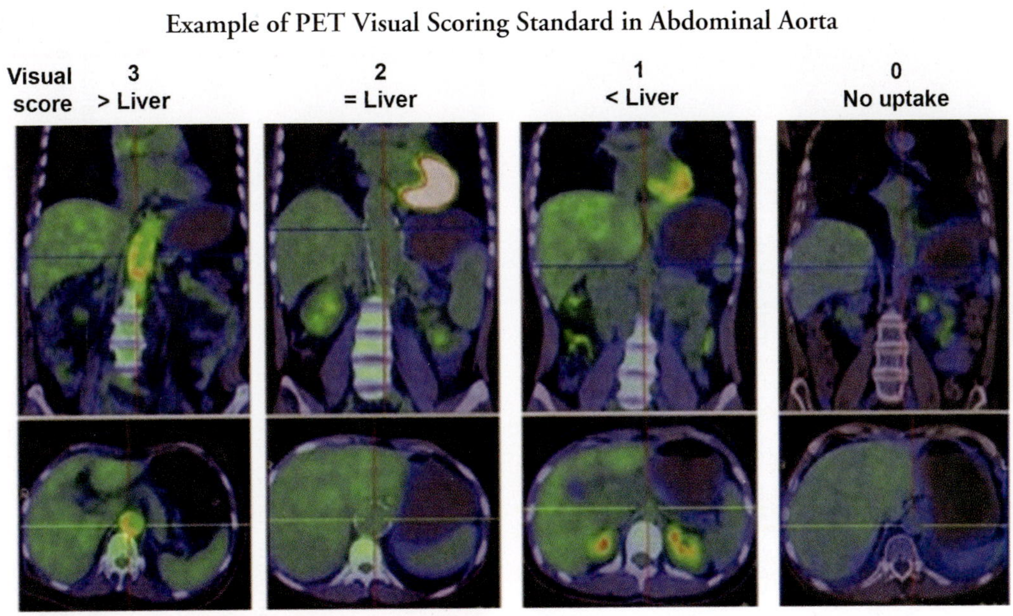

Arterial territory	Qualitative score
Ascending aorta	0, 1, 2, 3
Aortic arch	0, 1, 2, 3
Descending thoracic aorta	0, 1, 2, 3
Abdominal aorta	0, 1, 2, 3
Right carotid artery	0, 1, 2, 3
Left carotid artery	0, 1, 2, 3
Right subclavian artery	0, 1, 2, 3
Left subclavian artery	0, 1, 2, 3

Note:

1. To calculate PETVAS: Add the qualitative scores from each of the above specified 9 arterial territories. PETVAS range = 0–27.
2. Qualitative visual assessment of FDG uptake is performed in each arterial territory relative of FDG uptake in the liver; 0 l= no FDG uptake; 1 = less than liver;p 2 = equal to liver; 3 = greater than liver.
3. FDG uptake is not scored within areas of stent or graft placement but can be scored an arterial territory containing a stent or graft if portions of the native artery can be visualized within the territory.

Fig. 9.4.3: PETVAS: Assessing disease activity using PET/CT with the use of visual score from 0 to 3.

LABORATORY INVESTIGATIONS

A complete blood count reveals normocytic normochromic anaemia, with leukocytosis and thrombocytosis. ESR and CRP are currently recommended to be used to assess disease activity Several other biomarkers like Pentaxin 3, IL-6, IL-18, MMP (matrix metalloproteinase)-2, MMP3, MMP-9, SAA, BAFF APRIL, sHLA-E are currently under investigation (Table 9.4.4). The problem of course is inaccessible vessels to document inflammation.

IMAGING

Conventional angiography is considered the gold standard for the diagnosis of TAK. There is no single imaging modality that can provide all the information required and each method has distinct benefits and complementary roles (Table 9.4.5). The most commonly used imaging modality for diagnosis of TAK is CT angiography, and MR angiography for follow-up. There is no consensus on when to do follow-up imaging in TAK as the course is variable from one patient to the other but is recommended if relapse is suspected as per 2018 EULAR guideline.

MANAGEMENT

The management of TAK includes control of disease activity with immunosuppressive agents and revascularization procedures for specific circumstances (Table 9.4.6).

Table 9.4.4: Biomarkers in assessing disease activity in Takayasu arteritis

Biomarker	*Utility*	*Advantages*	*Disadvantages*
ESR	Reveal systemic inflammation	ESR higher than CRP in TAK patients with vascular inflammation in the absence of anti-cytokine therapies	Not correlated with vascular inflammation
CRP	Reflects the burden of systemic inflammation	Cheap, easily available test	Not correlated with vascular inflammation
Upcoming and investigational biomarkers			
PTX3	PTX3 are influenced by arterial inflammation and progression. Most reliable of the new markers available for disease activity.	PTX3 reflects TAK activity better than CRP or ESR Not affected by prednisolone dose	Not specific for TAK as the plasma levels are higher in many autoimmune diseases
IL-18	Higher in active TAK assessed by ITAS2010	Useful for monitoring	Only cytokine correlated with CRP
IL-6	A good biomarker associated with active disease	Useful for monitoring Best	
MMP-2	Helpful in diagnosing TAK	Higher levels in TAK patients when compared to controls	No correlation between MMP-2 level and disease activity
MMP-3	Could be used as a marker for TAK activity	Positive correlation between MMP-3 and disease activity	Affected by prednisolone dose
MMP-9	Could be a sensitive marker for TAK activity	Not affected by prednisolone Suggest prior existence of TAK	Different studies show conflicting results
SAA	A promising biomarker of disease activity	SAA decreased during follow-up in treatment responders	SAA not decreased in non-responders
BAFF and APRIL	APRIL–levels elevated in active TAK		BAFF–not raised in TAK patients Neither BAFF nor APRIL correlate with disease activity or damage
sHLA-E	Useful as a biomarker of disease activity in TAK	sHLA-E levels higher in active disease, and increased in those with persistently active or relapsing more than in those with stable course.	Polymorphism of HLA-E was not associated with susceptibility to TA and did not affect sHLA-E levels

PTX3: Pentraxin-3; *MMP-2:* Matrix metalloproteinase 2; *MMP-3:* Matrix metalloproteinase-3; *MMP-9:* Matrix metalloproteinase-9; *SAA:* Serum amyloid A; *BAFF:* B cell activating factor; *APRIL:* A proliferating inducing ligand; *sHLA-E:* Soluble human leukocyte antigen-E.

Table 9.4.5: Imaging modalities in Takayasu arteritis

Modality and findings	*Sensitivity and specificity*	*Role in disease activity*	*Advantages*	*Disadvantages*
CT angiography: Stenosis Aneurysm Circumferential wall thickening Contrast enhancement	95% and 100%	± Double ring pattern on delayed phase imaging has been described in active disease in small studies	1. Wide vascular assessment 2. Minimally invasive 3. Ability to evaluate stenotic and aneurysmal lesion 4. Detect complications	1. Exposure to radiation 2. Contraindicated in case of allergy to contrast agents and impaired renal function 3. Limited resolution for small vessels
MRI angiography: Can assess patency of artery lumen Circumferential wall thickening Wall edema (with no contrast) Contrast enhancement	100% and 100%	± Vessel wall edema poorly correlated with disease activity	1. No radiation 2. Vessel wall evaluation (thickening, edema and degeneration)	1. Expensive 2. Contrast studies with gadolinium cannot be given if renal functions are impaired 3. Long acquisition time needed 4. Overestimate degree of stenosis 5. Limited resolution for medium/small vessels
PET/PET-CT: Increased FDG uptake in areas of inflammation	70–87% and 73–87%	± Possible PETVAS–good correlation with other disease activity measures	1. Wide vascular evaluation 2. Minimally invasive 3. Almost whole-body assessment 4. Localizes active vessel wall inflammation 5. Documents the intensity of inflammation	1. Radiation exposure 2. Expensive 3. Not widely available 4. Cannot assess lumen 5. Poor resolution for medium/small vessels
CDUS: Lumen patency assessment Hypoechoic wall thickening (Macaroni sign)	77% and 96%	± Macaroni sign	1. Ability to evaluate localised areas of stenosis or aneurysm 2. Vessel wall evaluation 3. Inexpensive, no radiation, or contrast exposure 4. Good resolution for small arteries	1. Unable to provide a road-map of vascular lesions. 2. Interobserver variation 3. Not suitable for structures below air or bone
Conventional angiography: Lumen patency assessment Central aortic pressure measurement possible	100% and 100%	Considered gold standard modality for diagnosis of Takayasu arteritis	1. Severity of stenotic arterial lesions are evaluated precisely 2. Measurement of central aortic pressures possible 3. Therapeutic intervention 4. High resolution for medium vessels	1. Radiation exposure 2. No information about vessel wall status 3. Invasive 4. Contraindicated if allergy to iodine and poor kidney functions

(Contd.)

Table 9.4.5: Imaging modalities in Takayasu arteritis *(Contd.)*

Modality and findings	*Sensitivity and specificity*	*Role in disease activity*	*Advantages*	*Disadvantages*
Echocardiography: Transoesophageal and/or transthoracic to assess aortic root and cardiac involvement	NA	NA	1. Noninvasive 2. Can be useful to demonstrate circumferential aortic mural wall thickening 3. Good modality for surveillance of ascending aorta dilatation or aneurysm 4. Pulmonary hypertension	1. Roadmap of arterial lesions not possible 2. Operator dependant

CDUS: Color-duplex ultrasonography; *CTA:* Computed tomography angiography; *PETVAS:* PET vascular activity score

Table 9.4.6: Treatment options in Takayasu arteritis

General measures	*Medical*	*Surgical*
• Hypertension • Adequate exercise • Low salt diet • Aspirin (75 mg/day) • Statins	I. Glucocorticoids: Starting dose 40–60 mg/day II. Glucocorticoid sparing agents (a) Immunosuppressive agents 1. Mycophenolate mofetil (2–3 g/day) 2. Methotrexate (15–25 mg/week) 3. Azathioprine (2 mg/kg/day) 4. Leflunomide (10–20 mg/day) 5. Cyclophosphamide (iv or oral) 6. Cyclosporine or tacrolimus (b) Biological DMARDs/targeted synthetic DMARDs 1. Tocilizumab (8 mg/kg iv monthly or 162 mg s/c weekly 2. Tumor necrosis factor inhibitors 3. Rituximab 4. Janus kinase inhibitors	1.Endovascular interventions 2. Open repair

Glucocorticoids (GC) are the mainstay for induction of remission in TAK. Traditionally, a dose of 1 mg/kg prednisolone daily (or equivalent) had been used for the initial 3–6 months with tapering once the inflammation has been controlled. Tapering of GC to a dose of 15–20 mg/day within 2–3 months and to <10 mg/day within 1 year is recommended. GC monotherapy resulted in failure in >70% of TAK patients. Therefore, early initiation of GC-sparing therapy is recommended (Fig. 9.4.4).

Conventional Immunosuppressives

- Methotrexate was the first disease-modifying antirheumatic drug (DMARD) that was used as a GC-sparing agent owing to its safety profile. There is evidence that remission occurred in about 80% of patients, which was sustained in half of the patients after 18 months.
- Mycophenolate mofetil is also useful as a steroid-sparing maintenance agent with a good safety profile.
- Azathioprine in a few uncontrolled studies had uniform effectiveness in ameliorating symptoms and is the agent of choice in pregnant TAK patients.
- Cyclophosphamide was mostly studied in refractory or life-threatening or organ-threatening TAK patients and showed good response but with increased incidence of side effects especially infections.
- Recent studies with leflunomide in refractory TAK led to a quick induction and sustained remission, especially in cyclophosphamide refractory cases with lower reproductive toxicity.
- Cyclosporine had a good response in TAK patients complicated with pyoderma gangrenosum. The Turkish study group issued a definition of refractory TAK as shown in Table 9.4.7.

Biological Agents

TNF inhibitors (TNFi) represent a promising agent in the treatment of refractory cases. Most of the observational studies with TNFi showed at least partial remission in >80–90%. Over 40% patients were able to fully discontinue prednisolone.

Tocilizumab, an anti-IL-6 agent was studied in the TAKT study, the first and only double-blind RCT in 36 refractory TAK patients. The primary endpoint of time to relapse was not met, but the open-label extension found that almost half of

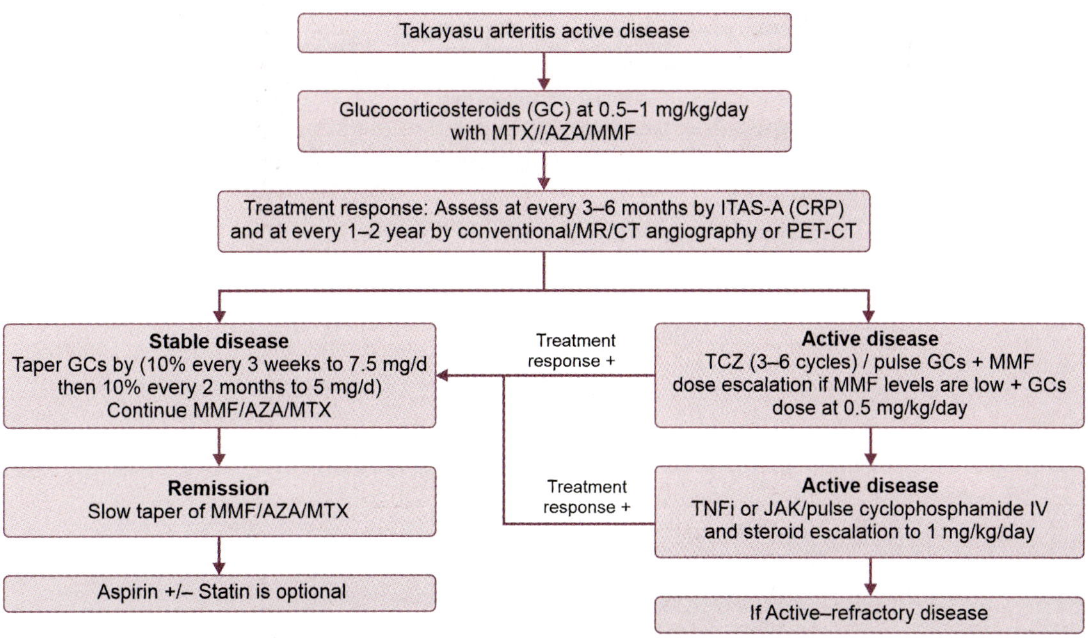

Fig. 9.4.4: PETVAS: Assessing disease activity using PET/CT with the use of visual score from 0 to 3.

MMF: Mycophenolate mofetil; *AZA:* Azathioprine; *MTX:* Methotrexate; *LEF:* Leflunomide; *TNFi:* Tummour necrosis factor inhibitor; *Jaki:* Janus kinase inhibitor; *ISA:* Immunosuppressant agent; *ITAS:* Indian takayasu activity score

Table 9.4.7: Refractory Takayasu arteritis: Turkish Takayasu arteritis study group's definition

Angiographic or clinical progression despite treatment *Or* *Presence of any of the following characteristics*
1. Prednisolone >7.5 mg/day even beyond 6 months of treatment, despite steroid sparing agents (conventional immunosuppressives)
2. Requirement of new surgery due to persistent disease activity
3. More than 3 attacks per year
4. Death due to disease activity

the patients achieved a GC dose <0.1 mg/kg/day by 96 weeks with a good safety profile. Pooled data from all observational studies showed at least partial clinical response in 87% of patients and normalization of inflammatory markers in nearly all patients, but relapse is seen in almost one-quarter of patients after stopping tocilizumab.

Studies on **rituximab** in refractory TAK had conflicting results. Initial case series on subcutaneous Ustekinumab in TAK patients reported good clinical response and safety, which when continued for 3 years had marginal effects in reducing steroid dosage and inflammatory markers. An RCT with Abatacept did not provide a longer duration of relapse-free survival when compared to steroids alone.

JAK inhibitors in TAK refractory to DMARDs as well as biological agents had shown possible efficacy in clinical studies with at least 80% partial clinical response and angiographic stabilization in 60%. Tofacitinib appears to be particularly effective in TAK complicated by ulcerative colitis. The algorithm in treatment of TAK is described in Figure 9.4.4.

Supportive Measures in TAK

Aspirin has been recommended in the updated EULAR guidelines based on the observation that it decreases the risk of acute ischemic events. But aspirin use was not significantly associated with vascular complication-free survival. The recent studies on statins are contradictory in that one study showed a beneficial effect in reducing relapse rate after remission, while another study was not associated with a better relapse-free survival.

SURGERY

Delay in diagnosis and inadequate therapy lead to stenosis or occlusion of arteries which require interventions such as angioplasty or open surgery. Angioplasty is usually the initial approach, with stenting being reserved for post-angioplasty dissection or persisting stenosis despite intervention. The chances of restenosis are typically 15–30% at 5–20 years for open surgery and 30–50% at 5–10 years post angioplasty.

PROGNOSIS

Factors that contribute to significant morbidity in TAK include heart failure and ischemic events such as stroke and transient ischemic attacks and the leading cause of death is congestive heart failure.

LEARNING POINTS

- Takayasu arteritis is a granulomatous large vessel vasculitis with unknown etiology
- The diagnosis is mainly clinical
- There is no single marker available to assess disease activity with accuracy
- The treatment includes steroids with the addition of csDMARDs upfront
- The refractory cases need treatment with biologicals or JAK inhibitors to achieve remission which requires further randomised controlled studies for confirmation

FURTHER READING

1. Goel R, Danda D, Joseph G, et al. Long-term outcome of 251 patients with Takayasu arteritis on combination immunosuppressant therapy: Single centre experience from a large tertiary care teaching hospital in Southern India. Semin Arthritis Rheum. 2018;47:718–26.
2. Grayson PC, Alehashemi S, Bagheri AA, et al. 18 F-Fluorodeoxyglucose-Positron Emission Tomography As an Imaging Biomarker in a Prospective, Longitudinal Cohort of Patients With Large Vessel Vasculitis. Arthritis Rheumatol. 2018;70:439–49.
3. Ishikawa K. Diagnostic approach and proposed criteria for the clinical diagnosis of Takayasu's arteriopathy. J Am Coll Cardiol. 1988;12:964–72.
4. Keser G, Aksu K, Direskeneli H. Takayasu arteritis: an update. Turk J Med Sci. 2018;48:681–97.
5. Misra DP, Rathore U, Patro P, et al. Disease-modifying anti-rheumatic drugs for the management of Takayasu

arteritis-a systematic review and meta-analysis. Clin Rheumatol. 2021;40:4391–16.

6. Misra R, Danda D, Rajappa SM, et al.; Indian Rheumatology Vasculitis (IRAVAS) group. Development and initial validation of the Indian Takayasu Clinical Activity Score (ITAS2010). Rheumatology (Oxford). 2013;52:1795–801.

7. Nakaoka Y, Isobe M, Takei S, et al. Efficacy and safety of tocilizumab in patients with refractory Takayasu arteritis: results from a randomised, double-blind, placebo-controlled, phase 3 trial in Japan (the TAKT study). Ann Rheum Dis. 2018;77:348–54.

8. Perera AH, Youngstein T, Gibbs RG, et al. Optimizing the outcome of vascular intervention for Takayasu arteritis. Br J Surg. 2014;101:43–50.

9. Wen D, Feng L, Du X, et al. Biomarkers in Takayasu arteritis. Int J Cardiol. 2023;371:413–7.

Polyarteritis Nodosa

Benzeeta Pinto, Aman Sharma

INTRODUCTION

Polyarteritis Nodosa (PAN) is a systemic necrotizing vasculitis of medium vessels, first described by Kussmaul and Maier in 1866. Older reports of polyarteritis nodosa included patients with microscopic polyangiitis (MPA) also and the two were identified as distinct entities only after the introduction of ANCA testing. The nosology of primary vasculitis is based on the size of the vessel that is predominantly involved. The Chapel Hill Consensus Conference (CHCC) convened in 1994 defined MPA for the first time and differentiated it from PAN. PAN is defined by CHCC 2012 as a necrotizing arteritis of medium or small arteries without glomerulonephritis or vasculitis in arterioles, capillaries, or venules; and not associated with ANCA.

PAN is a rare disease with population prevalence varying from 2 to 33 per million. Infection with hepatitis B virus is a known etiological agent in PAN and the decrease in the occurrence of hepatitis B due to vaccination is another factor contributing to declining incidence. Untreated disease has a dismal prognosis with a five-year survival of 13%. PAN most commonly affects middle-aged or older adults with a slight male preponderance (1.5:1), although the disease can also be seen in children. A monogenic variant of PAN due to deficiency of ADA2 (DADA2) initially reported in children is being increasingly recognized in adults.

ETIOPATHOGENESIS

The etiopathogenesis of polyarteritis nodosa is not clear. Classical PAN is idiopathic. It can also be associated with hepatitis B virus (HBV) infection, hepatitis C virus (HCV) infection, and hairy cell leukemia. Recessive loss of function mutations in the adenosine deaminase 2 gene were described in 2014 to cause a monogenic vasculitis syndrome with a phenotype resembling classical PAN. The onset of disease in DADA2 PAN is usually in childhood or early adulthood with several differing clinical features. A more recently described adult-onset inflammatory disorder referred to as VEXAS (vacuoles, E1 enzyme, X-linked, autoinflammatory, somatic) syndrome may also present with a PAN like illness. Cutaneous PAN is a distinct entity that only involves the skin (Fig. 9.5.1) without systemic involvement

The pathogenetic mechanisms in PAN are poorly understood. Immune complex mediated disease may play a role in certain subsets like those associated with hepatitis B. The disease is characterized by necrotising inflammation of medium sized vessel

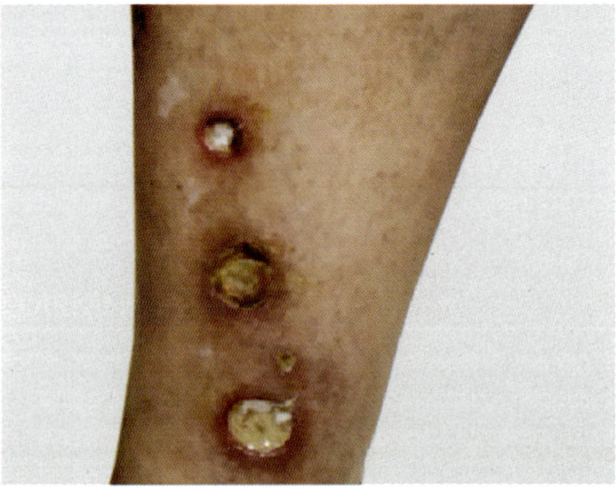

Fig. 9.5.1: Pyoderma gangrenosum like skin lesions in a patient with cutaneous PAN

wall and intimal proliferation leading to luminal narrowing, reducing blood flow and thrombosis leading to infarction of the end organ. This may also cause weakening of the vessel wall that leads to aneurysm formation and rupture resulting in life-threatening bleeding.

CLINICAL FEATURES

The clinical features of PAN are summarized in Table 9.5.1. Deficiency of adenosine deaminase 2 (DADA2) was first described in the context of PAN-like vasculitis. The clinical and histopathological manifestations can be just like classical PAN

Table 9.5.1: Clinical manifestations of polyarteritis nodosa

Clinical feature	*Frequency*
General symptoms Fever and weight loss Arthralgias and myalgias	93%
Neurological manifestations Mononeuritis multiplex Peripheral neuropathy Stroke Intracranial bleed	79%
Gastrointestinal manifestations Mesenteric ischemia Bleeding Perforation Cholecystitis Gastrointestinal microaneurysms and/ or stenoses	37.9%
Cutaneous manifestations Livedoid rash Palpable purpura Nodules Ulcers	49.7%
Renal and urological manifestations Hematuria New onset hypertension Renal dysfunction Testicular involvement Renal microaneurysm and stenoses	50.6%
Cardiac and vascular manifestations Myocarditis/cardiomyopathy Digital gangrene Limb claudication	22.4%

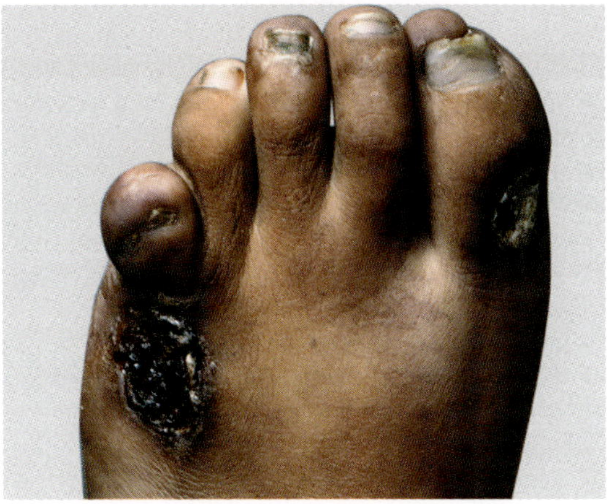

Fig. 9.5.2: Ulcerations with hemorrhagic crusting in a patient with DADA2

(Fig. 9.5.2). The age of presentation is usually in the first decade of life, however, presentation in adulthood has been reported. Livedoid reticularis/ racemosa like skin rash and central nervous system involvement in the form of ischemic or haemorrhagic stroke are dominant vascular manifestations.

DIAGNOSIS

The diagnosis of PAN is based on history and characteristic clinical features. The patient should be tested for hepatitis B, hepatitis C and HIV. Since ANCA vasculitis and vasculitis associated with connective tissue diseases are close differentials, antinuclear antibodies (ANA) and ANCA should also be tested. The diagnosis should ideally be based on histopathology of the involved organ. In case of skin biopsy deep incisional biopsy including the subcutaneous tissue has better yield compared to punch biopsies. Combined nerve muscle biopsies rather than nerve biopsy alone have a higher yield for vasculitis.

In patients in whom biopsy is not feasible classical angiographic manifestations on CT such as renal or gastroduodenal artery microaneurysms or vessel stenosis or end organ changes in the form of organ infarcts(renal/splenic/hepatic) are helpful in making the diagnosis.

The diagnosis of DADA2 PAN should be considered in patients presenting with PAN like vasculitis in the first decade, relapsing disease, recurrent strokes and extensive livedoid rash in the presence of family history and non-response to usual immunosuppressive drugs like azathioprine

Table 9.5.2: American College of Rheumatology (ACR) classification criteria for polyarteritis nodosa

- Otherwise unexplained weight loss greater than 4 kg
- Livedo reticularis
- Testicular pain or tenderness
- Myalgias (excluding that of the shoulder and hip girdle), weakness of muscles, tenderness of leg muscles, or polyneuropathy
- Mononeuropathy or polyneuropathy
- New-onset diastolic blood pressure greater than 90 mm Hg
- Elevated levels of serum blood urea nitrogen (>40 mg/dL or 14.3 mmol/L) or creatinine (>1.5 mg/dL or 132 μmol/L)
- Evidence of hepatitis B virus infection via serum antibody or antigen serology
- Characteristic arteriographic abnormalities not resulting from noninflammatory disease processes
- A biopsy of small- or medium-sized artery containing polymorphonuclear cells

The presence of 3 or more of these 10 criteria was associated with a sensitivity of 82.2% and specificity of 86.6% for classification of PAN

and cyclophosphamide, etc. Classification criteria for PAN were proposed in 1990 by ACR, however they are not meant for diagnosis and exclusion of mimics is essential for diagnosis (Table 9.5.2).

TREATMENT

Treatment of PAN depends on the severity of disease and organ involvement. As PAN is a rare disease there are no randomised controlled trials on treatment. Steroids along with a steroid sparing immunosuppressive is used in all. In mild to moderate disease azathioprine may be used, in severe disease cyclophosphamide IV monthly for 6 months as per the NIH regimen is used. In hepatitis B associated PAN steroids and plasma exchange along with antivirals are shown to be effective. DADA2 associated PAN is treated with tumour necrosis factor inhibitors which are effective for most vascular and inflammatory manifestations of the disease including prevention of stroke.

PROGNOSIS

The outcome of PAN has improved in patients receiving treatment; five-year survival is approximately 80%. Hepatitis B virus (HBV)-associated PAN has a lower survival rate than non-HBV-associated disease. The Five-Factor Score (FFS) introduced in 1996 and revised in 2011 is a simple prognostic tool for PAN. The revised score includes four factors associated with increased mortality:

i. Age >65 years,
ii. Cardiac symptoms,
iii. Gastrointestinal involvement, and
iv. Renal insufficiency (plasma creatinine >1.7 mg/dL [150 micromol/L]). Although PAN has a lower relapse rate compared to ANCA vasculitis, a 24% five-year relapse rate was found in the largest series of PAN.

LEARNING POINTS

- Polyarteritis nodosa is a systemic necrotizing vasculitis of medium vessels with varied manifestations.
- DADA2 PAN needs to be suspected in patients presenting with PAN like vasculitis in the first decade, relapsing disease, recurrent strokes and extensive livedoid rash, and non-response to usual immunosuppressive agents.
- The prognosis of classical PAN has improved with early diagnosis and use of immunosuppresive agents.
- Of note HBV-related PAN has a lower survival rate compared to non-HBV related PAN.

FURTHER READING

1. Naidu G, Kopp CR, Sharma V, et al. Validation of the provisional seven-item criteria for the diagnosis of polyarteritis nodosa. Rheumatol Int. 2021;41:1651–5.
2. Pagnoux C, Seror R, Henegar C, et al. French Vasculitis Study Group. Clinical features and outcomes in 348 patients with polyarteritis nodosa: a systematic retrospective study of patients diagnosed between 1963 and 2005 and entered into the French Vasculitis Study Group Database. Arthritis Rheum. 2010;62:616.
3. Sharma A, Naidu G, Sharma V, Jha S, Dhooria A, Dhir V, et al. Deficiency of Adenosine Deaminase 2 in Adults and Children: Experience From India. Arthritis Rheumatol. 2021;73:276–85.
4. Sharma A, Pinto B, Dhooria A, et al. Polyarteritis nodosa in north India: clinical manifestations and outcomes. Int J Rheum Dis. 2017;20:390–7.
5. Sharma A, Sharma K. Hepatotropic viral infection associated systemic vasculitides-hepatitis B virus associated polyarteritis nodosa and hepatitis C virus associated cryoglobulinemic vasculitis. J Clin Exp Hepatol. 2013;3:204–12.
6. Singhal M, Gupta P, Sharma A. Imaging in small and medium vessel vasculitis. Int J Rheum Dis. 2019;22 Suppl 1:78-85.

Granulomatosis with Polyangiitis

GSRSNK Naidu, Aman Sharma

INTRODUCTION

Granulomatosis with polyangiitis (GPA) is categorized under the anti-neutrophil cytoplasmic antibody (ANCA) associated small vessel vasculitis as per the Chapel Hill Consensus Conference nomenclature. Clinically, it is characterized by upper respiratory tract involvement, cavitary lung lesions, pauci-immune crescentic glomerulonephritis and sensorineural hearing loss.

CLINICAL FEATURES

The clinical manifestations of GPA are very diverse ranging from non-life-threatening manifestations like constitutional symptoms, nasal crusting, epistaxis, sensorineural hearing loss and scleritis to organ or life-threatening manifestations like diffuse alveolar hemorrhage, rapidly progressive renal failure due to pauci-immune crescentic glomerulonephritis, mononeuritis multiplex, scleromalacia and gastrointestinal vasculitis. Organ-wise clinical manifestations are shown in Table 9.6.1.

With such diverse clinical features of GPA, certain clinical manifestations should alert the physician to consider GPA in the differential diagnosis. These clinical features include nasal crusting, epistaxis, nasal septal perforation, the collapse of the nasal bridge with saddle nose deformity (Fig 9.6.1), chronic sinusitis not responding to usual medications, sensorineural hearing loss, strawberry gingivitis, lung nodules without cavitation along with the absence of significant lymphadenopathy (Fig. 9.6.2), scleromalacia perforans (Fig 9.6.3), mononeuritis multiplex and pachymeningitis.

Table 9.6.1: Clinical features of granulomatosis with polyangiitis

Organ	*Prevalence (%)*	*Manifestations*
Constitutional symptoms	50–60	Fever, weight loss, malaise, myalgia
Upper respiratory tract	79–98	Nasal congestion, nasal obstruction, nasal discharge, nasal crusting, epistaxis, nasal ulcers, septal perforation, saddle nose deformity, laryngeal or tracheal ulcerations, subglottic stenosis
Lungs	55–85	Nodules, cavities, infiltrates, mass like consolidations, hemoptysis, diffuse alveolar hemorrhage
Kidneys	33–77	Proteinuria, microscopic hematuria, oliguria, rapidly progressive renal failure
Eyes	31–52	Scleritis, episcleritis, conjunctivitis, scleromalacia perforans, corneal melts, uveitis, retinal vasculitis, orbital pseudotumor
Ears	18–20	Sensorineural hearing loss, tympanic membrane perforation

(Contd.)

Table 9.6.1: Clinical features of granulomatosis with polyangiitis *(Contd.)*

Organ	*Prevalence (%)*	*Manifestations*
Skin	21–46	Nodules, palpable purpura, skin ulcers, haemorrhagic bullae, digital infarcts, pyoderma gangrenosum
Peripheral nervous system	11–28	Mononeuritis multiplex, sensorimotor polyneuropathy
Central nervous system	5–27	Headache, cranial neuropathies, pachymeningitis, pituitary involvement
Oral cavity	5–10	Oral ulcers, Strawberry gingivitis, oroantral fistula, parotid or submandibular sialadenitis
Joints	42–81	Arthralgia, inflammatory oligoor polyarthritis
Heart	4–13	Pericarditis, myocarditis, conduction abnormalities
Gastrointestinal tract	3–12	Postprandial pain, upper or lower gastrointestinal bleed, bowel ischemia, bowel gangrene
Others	–	Prostatic vasculitis, mass lesions in muscles and breasts

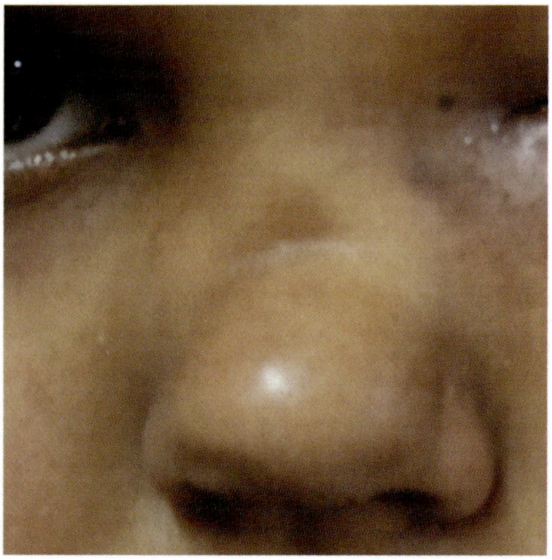

Fig. 9.6.1: Saddle nose deformity in a patient with GPA

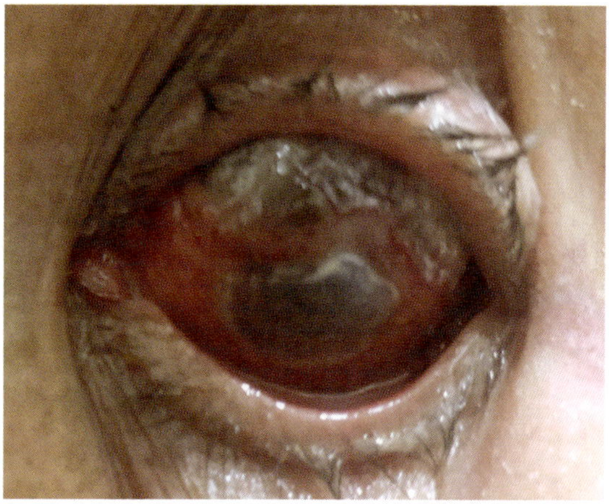

Fig. 9.6.3: Severe scleromalacia perforans in a patient with GPA

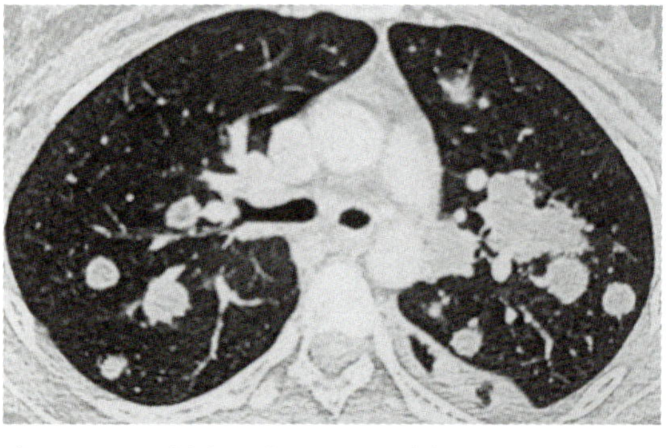

Fig. 9.6.2: Multiple pulmonary nodules in a patient with GPA

CLASSIFICATION

There are no diagnostic criteria for GPA while the 1990 American College of Rheumatology (ACR) criteria and the recent diagnostic and classification criteria in vasculitis (DCVAS) criteria can be used for classifying patients as GPA for epidemiological purposes. As per the ACR criteria, the patient can be classified as GPA if there is the presence of 2 out of the following 4 criteria: nasal or oral inflammation, abnormal chest radiograph, active urinary sediment and granulomatous inflammation on biopsy. The DCVAS criteria are weight-based and contain three clinical and seven laboratory criteria each with a separate weight and a total score of ≥5 is needed for classifying as GPA.

INVESTIGATIONS

There is no single diagnostic test for making a diagnosis of GPA and the diagnosis is made clinically. The various investigations that a patient with GPA should undergo depend on the clinical presentation and the organs that are involved (Table 9.6.2). Histopathology not only helps in establishing a diagnosis but also helps in determining the treatment response and prognosis of the patients; hence, every attempt should be made to obtain tissue samples. Renal biopsy is characterized by pauci-immune glomerulonephritis. Other commonly obtained tissues include nerves, skin and lungs. The presence of active or healed vasculitis and granulomas are consistent with a diagnosis of GPA.

Table 9.6.2: List of investigations and the expected findings in GPA

Investigation	*Findings to note*	*Timing of test*
Hemogram	Anemia, leukocytosis, thrombocytosis	Baseline, every visit during induction phase, every three months if in remission
Renal function tests	Serum creatinine	Baseline, every visit during induction phase, every three months if in remission
Liver function tests	Serum albumin, liver enzymes	Baseline, every visit during induction phase, every three months if in remission
Inflammatory markers	ESR, CRP	Baseline, at relapse
Urine analysis	Proteinuria, hematuria, granular casts 24-hour protein quantification	Baseline, every visit during induction phase, every three months if in remission, at relapse
ANCA by ELISA	PR3 and MPO ANCA	Baseline, at relapse
ANCA by IIF	c-ANCA or p-ANCA	Can be done if ELISA is not available
RF and ANA	RF may be positive in up to 50%	Not indicated
Chest X-ray	Infiltrates, consolidations, cavities	Baseline, at relapse
HRCT or CECT chest	Infiltrates, nodules, consolidations, cavities, masses	As clinically indicated
X-ray PNS	Opacities of sinuses	Baseline, at relapse
CECT PNS	Mucosal thickening, bone destruction	As clinically indicated
CECT abdomen	Bowel wall edema and enhancement (target sign), increased mesenteric vascularity (comb sign), pneumatosis intestinalis, bowel gangrene, perforation	As clinically indicated
CT or MRI brain	Infarcts, hemorrhages	As clinically indicated
PET/CT	Increased FDG uptake at sites of active inflammation, better characterization of tracheal involvement	As clinically indicated
Echocardiography	Pericardial effusion, myocarditis	As clinically indicated
Nerve conduction studies	Axonal or demyelination pattern	As clinically indicated
Pure tone audiometry	Conductive or sensorineural hearing loss	As clinically indicated

Assessment of Disease Activity

At baseline and every follow-up visit, the disease activity needs to be assessed. Birmingham vasculitis activity score (BVAS-version3) is used widely. BVAS-v3 consists of 51 items divided into 9 organ systems and each item should be scored if there is new onset involvement or worsening of preexisting involvement in the last 4 weeks. The scores can range from 0 to 63, with higher scores indicating a highly active disease. The persisting active disease has less weightage and the scores can range from 0 to 33. Damage related to vasculitis is measured using the vasculitis damage index (VDI) on follow-up.

MANAGEMENT

Timely initiation of appropriate immunosuppressants helps in attaining remission and improves the morbidity and mortality associated with this relapsing and life-threatening disease. The treatment decision is mainly based on the severity and extent of the disease. The European Vasculitis Study group (EUVAS) categorises them into five categories based on the extent and severity of the disease, as shown in Table 9.6.3.

Localized or Early Systemic Disease

In patients with localized or nonorgan threatening early systemic disease, a combination of oral glucocorticoids (GC) and methotrexate or mycophenolate mofetil (MMF) are recommended. One has to carefully remember that patients with nose and paranasal sinus disease with bony involvement, cartilage collapse, olfactory dysfunction, or deafness; skin involvement with ulceration; non-cavitating pulmonary nodules with hemoptysis, meningeal involvement, retro-orbital disease, cardiac involvement, mesenteric ischemia, acute mononeuritis multiplex or pulmonary hemorrhage of any severity are contraindications to remission induction with these drugs. Thus the indications of such treatment in real-life clinical practice are very limited and most of the time, on careful review the patients will have one or other feature necessitating the use of either cyclophosphamide (CYC) or rituximab (RTX) as detailed below. Even though many patients attain remission with this regimen, on long-term follow-up, many patients may have relapses and might require CYC induction. Hence, the patients should be kept under regular follow up and the physician should have a high index of suspicion for detecting relapses early.

Generalized and Severe Disease

In patients with generalized and organ or life-threatening disease, high-dose oral GC with or without intravenous methylprednisolone (IVMP) should be combined with either CYC or RTX. Depending on the response, GC is tapered over 3–6

Table 9.6.3: EUVAS categories for extent and severity of GPA

Category	*Definition*	*Example*
Localized	Upper and or lower respiratory tract disease without constitutional symptoms or any other organ involvement	Isolated nasal crusting, epistaxis. Asymptomatic lung nodules or cavities
Early systemic	Any other organ involvement without organ or life-threatening disease	Symptomatic lung nodules, cavities but not requiring oxygen or ventilator support. Proteinuria, hematuria without renal failure. Scleritis, episcleritis without vision loss. Constitutional symptoms.
Generalized	Organ threatening disease	Renal failure with serum creatinine <5.6 mg/dL. Diffuse alveolar hemorhage without requirement of ventilatory support. Uveitis, scleromalacia peforans, corneal melts. Mononeuritis multiplex
Severe	Vital organ failure	Renal failure with creatinine >5.6 mg/dL or requiring dialysis support. Lung involvement requiring ventilatory support. Severe myocarditis
Refractory	Progressive disease not responding to glucocorticoids and cyclophosphamide	–

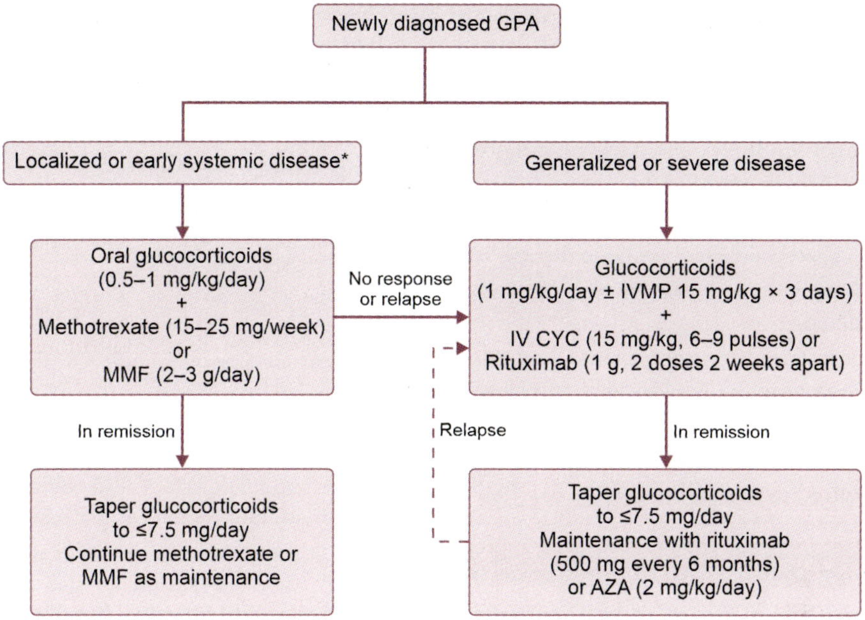

Fig. 9.6.4: Management algorithm for GPA

Nose and paranasal sinus disease with bony involvement, cartilage collapse, olfactory dysfunction, or deafness; skin Involvement with ulceration; non cavitating pulmonary nodules with hemoptysis, meningeal involvement, retro orbital disease, cardiac involvement, mesenteric ischemia, acute mono-neuritis multiplex or pulmonary hemorrhage of any severity would necessitate treatment like generalized or severe disease

months to a target dose of <10 mg/day. Intravenous CYC is preferred over oral CYC and administered every two weeks for the first three pulses, then every 3–4 weekly for another 3–6 pulses. In presence of renal failure, a dose of CYC should be reduced by 25% (Fig. 9.6.4). *Total IgG levels should be measured before administering RTX as patients with baseline hypogammaglobulinemia are at increased risk of infections with RTX.*

Remission Maintenance

GPA is a relapsing disease and hence, adequate and prolonged maintenance therapy is essential to prevent life-threatening relapses in these patients. The recommended drugs for remission maintenance are low-dose GC along with RTX or AZA. MAINRITSAN studies have shown that relapses are less common with RTX compared to azathioprine (AZA) and hence RTX is preferred over other drugs as maintenance therapy. Other drugs that can be used for remission maintenance are methotrexate and MMF. There is no data on the duration of maintenance therapy but it is usual practice to give for at least 2–3 years but needs to be continued for long in patients who had multiple relapses in the past.

Relapses

Minor relapses can be managed by increasing the dose of GC and if required the dose of maintenance drugs like AZA or methotrexate. In patients with major relapse, high dose GCs along with reinduction with RTX or intravenous CYC needs to be given. For patients who relapse while receiving CYC, a shift to RTX should be made and vice-versa. If a patient relapses on follow-up after having sustained remission or due to discontinuation of immunosuppressants, the same drug, CYC or RTX, which was used to induce remission previously can be used.

LEARNING POINTS

- GPA is characterized by upper respiratory tract, lung and renal involvement and the presence of ANCA.
- About 10–20% of patients with GPA can be ANCA negative.
- ANCA testing by ELISA for PR3 and MPO ANCA is preferred over the IIF method.

- Always think of GPA in patients with unexplained nasal crusting and epistaxis, saddle nose deformity, sensorineural hearing loss, cavitating lung nodules without accompanying lymphadenopathy, mononeuritis multiplex and pachymeningitis.
- Glucocorticoids along with immunosuppressants are the mainstay of therapy:
  - For localized and early systemic disease, oral GC along with methotrexate or MMF can be considered.
  - For generalized and severe disease, high- dose oral or intravenous GC along with intravenous CYC or rituximab is recommended.
  - For remission maintenance therapy, rituximab is preferred over azathioprine.

FURTHER READING

1. Aman Sharma, Pradeep Bambery. (2014) 'Granulomatosis with Polyangiitis (Wegener's Granulomatosis)'. Aman Sharma (ed.) *Textbook of Systemic Vasculitis.* New Delhi: Jaypee Brothers Medical Publishers (P) Ltd. 289–99.
2. Grygiel-Górniak B, Limphaibool N, Perkowska K et al. Clinical manifestations of granulomatosis with polyangiitis: key considerations and major features. Postgrad Med. 2018; 130:581–96.
3. Hoffman G, Kerr G, Leavitt R et al. Wegener's granulomatosis: an analysis of 158 patients. Ann Intern Med.1992;116:488–98.
4. Holle JU, Gross WL, Latza U et al. Improved outcome in 445 patients with Wegener's granulomatosis in a German vasculitis centre over four decades. Arthritis Rheum. 2011;63,257–66.
5. Sharma A, Naidu GSRSNK, Rathi M, et al. Clinical features and long-term outcomes of 105 granulomatosis with polyangiitis patients: A single centre experience from north India. Int J Rheum Dis. 2018;21:278–84.
6. Yates M, Watts RA, Bajema IM, et al. EULAR/ERA-EDTA recommendations for the management of ANCA-associated vasculitis. Ann Rheum Dis. 2016; 75:1583–94.

Chapter 9.7

IgA Vasculitis and Other Cutaneous Vasculitides

Siddharth Jain, Varun Dhir

INTRODUCTION

Purpura refers to bleeding in the skin, with petechiae specifically referring to <2 mm size of these lesions. The phenotypic correlate of cutaneous small-vessel vasculitis is palpable purpura (and petechiae). However, this is somewhat of a misnomer as all purpura due to small vessel vasculitis are not palpable. Indeed, some dermatologists refer to the color of the purpura—bright red being associated with vasculitis. There are a variety of causes of purpura, with probably the most common ones seen by rheumatologists being iatrogenic (due to steroid use) (Table 9.7.1).

Table 9.7.1: Causes of purpura	
Causes	*Etiologies*
Non-palpable = non-inflammatory = Blue	
Thrombocy-topenia	Disseminated intravascular coagulation Idiopathic thrombocytopenic purpura
Vessel wall weakness	Scurvy, steroid use
Palpable = Inflammatory = Red*	
Vasculitis	Immune complex–IgA vasculitis, Secondary–Connective tissue disease, rheumatoid arthritis, hypersensitivity vasculitis (drugs, infections, paraneoplastic) Pauci-immune–ANCA vasculitis
Embolism	Atheroembolism, infective embolism–rickettsia, *Meningococcus*

*Can be associated with cutaneous infarcts

Thus, it is important to bear in mind that all purpura (or petechiae) is not vasculitis. Once, one is sure there is no thrombocytopenia, and the 'red color' and 'palpable' nature suggest vasculitic etiology, it is important to consider what is the extent of the vasculitis (whether it is a systemic vasculitis) apart from what is its etiology (Fig. 9.7.1).

Finally, it is important to emphasize that cutaneous vasculitis comes in other shapes and sizes as well. Especially, small vessel vasculitis can also present as infarcts, bullae or urticaria. Medium vessel involvement of the skin can present as ulcers and nodules.

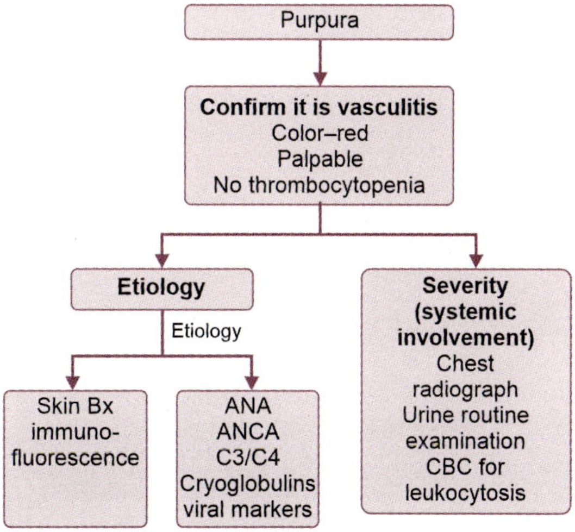

Fig. 9.7.1: An approach to a patient with purpura suggestive of cutaneous vasculitis

Nomenclature

Earlier known as Henoch–Schoenlein purpura or anaphylactoid purpura.

Epidemiology

IgA vasculitis is typically a childhood disease, with an incidence of 10–22 per 100,000 compared to 1 per 100, 000 in adults. More than 90% of the patients are children younger than 10 years of age, with a peak incidence at 6 years. In adults, the typical mean age is 50 years, and it is thought to be more chronic and has more renal involvement.

Clinical Features

The triad of IgA vasculitis consists of arthritis, purpura and gastrointestinal involvement; in some patients, it is a tetrad, with additional renal involvement which occurs in a subset of the patients.

The typical presentation is an abrupt onset of palpable inflammatory purpura over the legs and buttocks but can involve other parts as well, typically on the extensor surface (Figs. 9.7.2 and 9.7.3), which occurs in a small child following 1–2 weeks of an upper respiratory tract infection. The rash may start as erythematous papules (or urticaria) before transforming into purpura. There are accompanying mild constitutional features like fever and fatigue. Arthritis is transient and typically involves the knees and ankles, occurring in 3/4th of the patients. Abdominal pain starts 1 week after rash, is often the highest in intensity after meals, is colicky in character and may be accompanied by vomiting and hematochezia or melena. It must be noted that the onset of purpura, arthritis and gastrointestinal manifestations can be in any sequence, although typically the latter follow purpura.

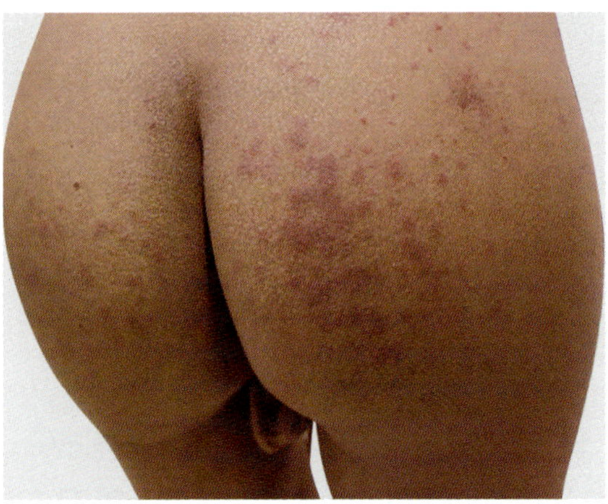

Fig. 9.7.2: A child with palpable purpura over the buttocks due to IgA vasculitis (*Courtesy:* Dr Deepti Suri, Pediatric Allergy and immunology Unit, Department of Pediatrics, PGIMER, Chandigarh)

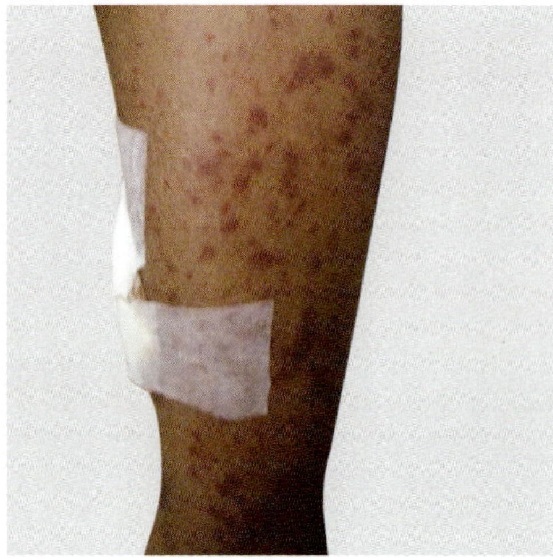

Fig. 9.7.3: A child with palpable purpura over the legs due to IgA vasculitis (*Courtesy:* Dr Deepti Suri, Pediatric Allergy and immunology Unit, Department of Pediatrics, PGIMER, Chandigarh)

Renal involvement occurs in 20–40%, more in adults, and is manifested by frothuria or generalized edema. It usually occurs 2–4 weeks after the rash but can ccur later as well. It is generally self-limiting; however, in a small subset of patients, it can lead to renal failure in the long-term (5%). The risk of renal disease is more in adults, those with persistent purpura, severe abdominal pain or multiple relapses. Thus, it is recommended that patients of IgA vasculitis undergo routine urine routine examinations and blood pressure recordings for the first 6 months.

Rarer manifestations include subcutaneous edema over the legs, hands or scrotum, diffuse alveolar hemorrhage, rapidly progressive renal failure (RPRF) and CNS abnormalities. The typical episode follows the rule of three—1/3rd last <2 week, one-third lasts 2–4 weeks and 1/3rd more than 4 weeks. Episodes can be recurrent.

Laboratory Features

Typical laboratory features include leukocytosis (mild), eosinophilia, increased IgA in 50% and increased acute phase reactants. In a typical child with typical features (and absence of any systemic involvement), the diagnosis can be presumed clinically. However, in all other cases, a skin biopsy with immunofluorescence for IgA can clinch the diagnosis.

In the case of abdominal pain or malena/ hematochezia, imaging of the bowel reveals some typical findings. Computed tomography of the abdomen reveals circumferential and symmetric bowel wall thickening which is typically multifocal with multiple skip areas of no involvement. It typically involves the small intestine–jejunum and ileum, but may also involve the stomach as well as the large intestine. The bowel loops may show a 'target sign' which is due to enhancement of the outer and inner walls, with a hypodense area in between them. (Fig. 9.7.4) In addition, mesenteric lymphadenopathy and vessel engorgement is also noted.

In case of renal involvement, there can be isolated proteinuria or active sediment.

Pathogenesis

Given that it often occurs post upper respiratory tract infection (URTI) in children and has a seasonal occurrence, a post-infectious 'reactive' process where the pathogen leads to IgA production which then deposits in the small vessels is considered likely. However, the exact infection remains to be conclusively defined. There have been reports of group A *Streptococcus*, as well as other organisms like Parvovirus B19, *Haemophilus, Helicobacter pylori,* etc.

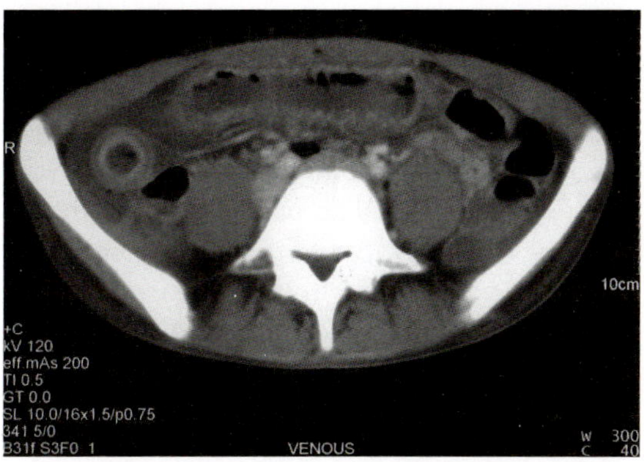

Fig. 9.7.4: A 16-year old boy with IgA vasculitis who presented with abdominal pain and underwent a CECT of the abdomen showing 'target sign'

Classification Criteria

Apart from the Chapel Hill Consensus Conference definition, two classification criteria exist for IgA vasculitis (Table 9.7.2). Since these are classification criteria, they are to be used primarily for research purposes, and preferably not for the diagnosis of individual patients. The ACR criteria were devised using 85 IgA vasculitis patients and adult patients with non-IgA systemic vasculitis were used as comparators, while the EULAR/PRINTO/PRES endorsed ankara 2008 criteria were based on larger international patient registry data and have been validated specifically for use in the pediatric setting . Recent studies have demonstrated better sensitivity and specificity of the latter even in adult IgA vasculitis. Thus, the European consensus-based SHARE initiative recommendations of 2019 endorse the EULAR/PRINTO/PRES criteria for the classification of IgA vasculitis.

Diagnosis

The diagnosis is usually clinical when straight-forward, especially in the pediatric population; however, in patients with incomplete or unusual presentations, histopathology of the affected organ (usually skin or kidney) is needed. Findings of small vessel leukocytoclastic vasculitis or proliferative glomerulonephritis with predominant IgA deposits on immunofluorescence are characteristic of IgA vasculitis. It is important to note, however, that absence of IgA staining does not exclude the diagnosis of IgA vasculitis.

No specific laboratory assay exists for the diagnosis of IgA vasculitis. Variable degrees of anemia, leukocytosis and elevated acute-phase reactants may be seen. Renal function tests including urinalysis, and abdominal imaging (ultrasonography) with fecal frank or occult blood testing should be done to look for renal and gastrointestinal involvement, respectively. Renal biopsy is indicated in cases of impaired eGFR, severe proteinuria (>250 mg/ mmol) or persistent proteinuria (severe proteinuria for 4 weeks, moderate proteinuria for 3 months or mild proteinuria for 6 months) as per the 2019 SHARE initiative consensus recommendations. Elevation in serum IgA levels is seen only in ~50% of cases and should not be relied upon for diagnosis. Autoantibodies (including ANA,

Table 9.7.2: Classification criteria for IgA vasculitis

ACR 1990	*EULAR/PRINTO/PRES 2008 Ankara*
Two or more of: i. Palpable purpura ii. Age at onset <20 years iii. Bowel angina iv. Histologic changes showing granulocytes in the walls of arterioles and/or venules	Purpura or petechiae with lower limb predominance without thrombocytopenia or coagulopathy (mandatory criterion) *plus* One or more of: i. Abdominal pain ii. Arthritis or arthralgia iii. Renal involvement iv. Histopathologic evidence of leucocytoclastic vasculitis or proliferative glomerulonephritis with predominant IgA deposition
Sensitivity 87.1%	Sensitivity 100%
Specificity 87.7%	Specificity 87%

ANCA, RF) and cryoglobulins are typically negative, and complements are usually normal.

Differential Diagnosis

Skin dominant Clinical Presentations (With Low Platelet or Coagulation Disorder)

- Disseminated intravascular coagulation
- Sepsis
- Immune-mediated thrombocytopenic purpura
- HUS/TTP
- Leukemia

With Normal Platelets and Normal Coagulation Profile

- ANCA-associated vasculitis
- Cryoglobulinemic vasculitis
- Connective tissue disease-related vasculitis
- Infection
- Drug-induced vasculitis
- Acute hemorrhagic edema of infancy.

In an arthritis-first presentation (~15% cases), standard evaluation for joint pain should be undertaken. In a GI-dominant presentation, medical and surgical causes of acute abdomen need to be considered and evaluated. IgA nephropathy is clinically, immunologically and histopathologically similar to renal involvement in IgA vasculitis and may in fact represent a renal-limited form of the disease.

Treatment

All cases of IgA vasculitis do not require immunosuppressive therapy since the disease process is self-limited. Management comprises symptom alleviation and prevention of the emergence of complications.

Symptomatic Therapy

Symptomatic treatment includes the use of analgesics (paracetamol or NSAIDs) for arthralgias, abdominal pain or painful skin lesions. Although rare in children, caution should be exercised against the GI and renal side effects of NSAIDs. Antihistaminics can be added for pruritus. Topical glucocorticoids may alleviate local skin symptoms but do not prevent the appearance of new lesions.

Immunosuppressive Therapy

Although there is some evidence that glucocorticoids reduce symptom intensity and duration in IgA vasculitis, whether they prevent the emergence of long-term complications is uncertain. The self-limited nature of the disease makes an assessment of treatment response even more difficult. Nonetheless, glucocorticoids are recommended in patients with orchitis, cerebral vasculitis, pulmonary hemorrhage, nephritis (see below), severe GI involvement, and other severe organ or life-threatening involvement. Dosage and route are usually oral (1–2 mg/kg/d for 1–2 weeks with subsequent weaning over the next 2 weeks); pulsed intravenous glucocorticoids (10–30 mg/kg up to 1 g/day) may be used for initial 3–5 days in severe cases. Glucocorticoids as preventive therapy for the development of nephritis are not indicated.

Table 9.7.3: Criteria for severity of nephritis in IgA vasculitis and its treatment		
Severity of nephritis in IgA vasculitis	*Definition*	*Management*
Mild	Normal eGFR* and mild^ or moderate$ proteinuria	1st line: oral pred 2nd Line: AZA/MMF/ pulsed MP
Moderate	<50% crescents and impaired** GFR or severe persistent proteinuria^^	1st line: Oral pred and/or pulsed MP 1st or 2nd line: AZA/MMF/IV CYC
Severe	>50% crescents and impaired GFR or severe persistent proteinuria	1st line IV CYC + pulsed MP and oral pred 2nd line: AZA/MMF + oral pred

*>80 mL/min/1.73 m^2

^spot (early morning) urine protein-creatinine ratio <100 mg/mmol in early morning urine sample (corresponds to <100 mg/mg creatinine or approximately <1 gram proteinuria in 24 hours)

$spot (early morning) urine protein-creatinine ratio 100–250 mg/mmol in early morning urine sample (corresponds to 100–250 mg/mg creatinine or approximately 1–2.5 grams proteinuria in 24 hours)

**<80 mL/min/1.73 m^2

^^spot (early morning) urine protein-creatinine ratio >250 mg/mmol for >4 weeks (corresponds to >2.5 mg/mg creatinine or approximately >2.5 grams per 24 hours)

Pred: Prednisolone; *MP:* Methylprednisolone; *AZA:* Azathioprine; *MMF:* Mycophenolate mofetil; *IV CYC:* Intravenous cyclophosphamide, *eGFR:* estimated glomerular filtration rate

Treatment of Nephritis in IgA Vasculitis

Treatment of IgA vasculitis-related nephritis is guided by its severity, which is determined by the renal function, amount and duration of proteinuria and histopathological findings (Table 9.7.3). The guidelines for management (based on currently available, low-quality evidence) as suggested by the European consensus-based SHARE initiative of 2019 have been summarized in Table 9.7.3. Although these share similarities with the KDIGO guidelines in the treatment of severe crescentic nephritis, there are differences between the two in the management of mild-moderate disease. The SHARE recommendations advocate earlier or upfront use of glucocorticoids in addition to ACE inhibitors or ARBs, even in patients with mild disease. Nonetheless, both recommendations emphasize the urgent need for RCTs to guide therapeutic decisions. Apart from the treatment options mentioned in the table, some adjunctive role of plasma exchange and rituximab in resistant cases has also been demonstrated.

Follow-up, Outcome and Prognosis

The disease is usually self-limited especially in children, and in the absence of significant renal involvement, outcomes are generally good. GI involvement is the major contributor to early morbidity, while renal involvement contributes majorly to long-term morbidity. Recurrence is seen in about one-third cases, more commonly in those with a severe initial disease course. The recurrences are usually milder in intensity, and/or of shorter duration compared to the initial episode.

Follow-up is important since there is risk of late renal damage in IgA vasculitis. Patients with normal urinalysis and blood pressure need to be periodically followed up for 6–12 months, while those with nephritis need to be closely followed up for at least 5 years.

OTHER CUTANEOUS VASCULITIS

As per the 2018 dermatologic addendum to the 2012 CHCC nomenclature, cutaneous vasculitis can exist in three forms:

i. Cutaneous component of systemic vasculitis.
ii. Skin-dominant or skin-limited phenotype of systemic vasculitis.
iii. Cutaneous single organ vasculitis. The existing vasculitis categories in the 2012 CHCC nomenclature can have a cutaneous component which is classifiable under the former two headings, while the third category of cutaneous single organ vasculitis was elaborated upon in the 2018 addendum.

Table 9.7.4: Cutaneous component (vasculitic) of systemic vasculitides (excluding IgA vasculitis)

Vasculitis category (2012 CHCC) and name	*Cutaneous component*
Large vessel vasculitis	
Takayasu arteritis	–
Giant cell arteritis	Rare (cutaneous infarcts)
Medium vessel vasculitis	
Polyarteritis nodosa	Infarcts, gangrene, livedo reticularis, dermal nodules, deep ulcers, purpura
Kawasaki disease	–
Small vessel vasculitis	
ANCA-associated vasculitis	Palpable purpura (most common). Papules, nodules, vesicles and necro-ulcerative lesions may also be seen
Cryoglobulinemic vasculitis	Palpable purpura (most common). Infarcts, hemorrhagic crusts and ulcers may also be seen.
Hypocomplementemic urticarial vasculitis	Urticarial plaques (most common). Angioedema, purpura and livedo reticularis may also be seen
Variable vessel vasculitis	
Behçet's disease	EN-like lesions, palpable purpura, papulopustular lesions, extragenital ulcerations, hemorrhagic blisters
Cogan's syndrome	Rare
Vasculitis associated with systemic disease	
Rheumatoid arthritis Systemic lupus erythematosusg Sjögren's syndrome	Palpable purpura, maculopapular erythema, hemorrhagic blisters, subcutaneous nodules, livedo reticularis, deep ulcers, gangrene

Cutaneous involvement (vasculitic) in different categories of systemic vasculitis is summarized in Table 9.7.4.

Cutaneous single organ vasculitides include:

i. IgM/IgG immune complex vasculitis,
ii, Erythema induratum of Bazin (nodular cutaneous vasculitis)
iii. Erythema elevatum et diutinum
iv, Recurrent macular vasculitis in hypergamma-globulinemia (hypergamma-globulinemic purpura of Waldenstrom)
v. Normocomplementemic urticarial vasculitis.

CONNECTIVE TISSUE DISEASE-ASSOCIATED CUTANEOUS VASCULITIS

Cutaneous vasculitis is the dominant presentation of RA vasculitis, which by itself occurs in <1% cases (those with severe and long-standing disease). It is characterized by small or medium vessel involvement, and manifests clinically as erythematous maculopapular rash, nailfold infarcts, digital ischemia or cutaneous ulcers.

A 19–28% of SLE patients have cutaneous vasculitis, which accounts for ~85% of lupus-associated vasculitis. Small vessel vasculitis (80–85%) is more common than medium vessel vasculitis (10–15%). The former can present either as leucocytoclastic vasculitis (~60%) or cryoglobulinemic vasculitis (~30%), while the latter has a cutaneous polyarteritis nodosa-like presentation.

Cutaneous vasculitis in Sjogren's syndrome is variably reported and usually takes the form of hypergammaglobulinemic purpura of Waldenstrom or cryoglobulinemic vasculitis, manifesting clinically with palpable purpura. A medium vessel PAN-like presentation is seldom reported.

Management Approach

Most cases of cutaneous vasculitis are self-limited, and do not need systemic therapy.

Systemic therapy is indicated only in severe, or chronic and recurrent cases; however the evidence to guide it is low-quality.

General Measures

Identifying the inciting trigger (if any) and removing it is alone effective in a number of cases. Removal of potential precipitants of disease flare, such as prolonged standing or sitting, heat, exhaustion or URTI are also beneficial. Conservative measures like limb elevation and compression stockings may be helpful for lower extremity lesions.

Application of emollients and topical steroids can reduce pruritus and other local skin symptoms. NSAIDs may be needed for skin discomfort.

Immunosuppression

Oral glucocorticoids (0.5–1 mg/kg/day prednisone equivalent) help in faster resolution of painful or ulcerative lesions or otherwise severe disease and retard the formation of new lesions. A taper over subsequent 3–6 weeks should be attempted. Patients who are poorly responsive to glucocorticoids, those who relapse on steroid taper, or those in whom symptoms last >4 weeks are candidates for steroid-sparing therapy. Colchicine (0.6 mg BD), dapsone (50–150 mg/day) and azathioprine (2 mg/kg/day) are commonly employed as first-line agents in view of their safety and tolerability, however hydroxychloroquine, methotrexate, sulfasalazine, mycophenolate mofetil, leflunomide or danazol are also beneficial. The duration of steroid-sparing therapy is unclear and needs to be individualized based on disease severity and treatment toxicity-attempting taper after sustained remission for 3–6 months may be reasonable.

Management of Recalcitrant Disease

Rare cases refractory to above agents may need more aggressive treatment with cyclosporine, cyclophosphamide, rituximab, infliximab or intravenous immunoglobulin.

LEARNING POINTS

- IgA vasculitis is the commonest cause of cutaneous vasculitis seen in children and young adults, with skin with or without joints , GI and renal involvement.
- Usually follows an upper respiratory tract infection.
- Diagnosis is straightforward and clinical, rarely needs skin biopsy to see for IgA depositis.
- Course is benign in the majority only needling assurance.
- Cutaneous vasculitis can be secondary due to underlying connective tissue disease such as SLE, RA, MCTD and rarely other systemic vasculitides.
- Needs to be differentiated from thrombocytopenic conditions.

FURTHER READING

1. Jennette JC, Falk RJ, Bacon PA, et al. 2012 Revised International Chapel Hill Consensus Conference Nomenclature of Vasculitides. Arthritis Rheum. 2013; 65:1–11.
2. Mills JA, Michel BA, Bloch DA, et al. The American College of Rheumatology 1990 criteria for the classification of henoch-schönlein purpura. Arthritis Rheum. 2010;17;33:1114–21.
3. Namgoong M. Management of IgA vasculitis nephritis (Henoch-Schonlein purpura nephritis) in Children. Child Kidney Dis. 2020;24:1–13.
4. Ozen S, Marks SD, Brogan P, et al. European consensus-based recommendations for diagnosis and treatment of immunoglobulin A vasculitis—the SHARE initiative. Rheumatology. 2019;58:1607–16.
5. Ozen S, Pistorio A, Iusan SM, et al. EULAR/PRINTO/PRES criteria for Henoch-Schonlein purpura, childhood polyarteritis nodosa, childhood Wegener granulomatosis and childhood Takayasu arteritis: Ankara 2008. Part II: Final classification criteria. Ann Rheum Dis. 2010;69:798–806.
6. Sharma A, Dhooria A, Aggarwal A. Connective Tissue Disorder-Associated Vasculitis. Curr Rheumatol Rep [Internet]. Jun [cited 2021 Jul 5]; c18. Available from: http://link.springer.com/10.1007/s11926-016-0584.
7. Sunderkötter CH, Zelger B, Chen K-R, et al. Nomenclature of Cutaneous Vasculitis: Dermatologic Addendum to the 2012 Revised International Chapel Hill Consensus Conference Nomenclature of Vasculitides. Arthritis Rheumatol. 2018;70:171–84.

Chapter 9.8

Behçet's Disease

Rajendra Varaprasad, G Narsimulu

INTRODUCTION

Behcet's disease (BD) manifesting with oro-genital, cutaneous, and ocular inflammation is a vasculitis that affects arteries and veins of all sizes. It is classified as a variable vessel vasculitis. The rarity of the disease, intermittent and incomplete manifestations and absence of a diagnostic test make BD a challenge to diagnose and manage.

EPIDEMIOLOGY AND PATHOGENESIS

Though BD is now reported internationally, the highest prevalence of BD lies in countries situated along the ancient silk route extending from Japan in the Far East to the Middle East and Mediterranean countries. The highest prevalence of BD is in Turkey. It is slightly more common in males, aged 20–40 years of age. Indian data shows that BD has a slight male predominance, it is a mild disease, with mucocutaneous and musculoskeletal manifestations being common presenting manifestations. Pan uveitis is a common form of eye involvement. Pathergy test is positive only in one-third of the patients.

The pathogenesis is unknown. It has a strong association with HLA B51. Various environmental triggers like bacterial (Streptococcus sanguinis) and viral (HSV) infections, and altered microbiomes have been implicated in the pathogenesis. Immunological perturbation leads to endothelial dysfunction, reduced vasodilatation and increased thrombogenicity. Unique histological features of BD are neutrophil-driven vasculitis involving arteries and veins of all sizes with the tendency towards thrombosis. Mucosal lesions show complex aphthosis, which features ulceration and granulation tissue with an underlying inflammatory infiltrate with occasional thrombi within vessels.

CLASSIFICATION CRITERIA

The International Study Group criteria are the most commonly used criteria for BD, they are less sensitive but more specific (Table 9.8.1).

Table 9.8.1: The International Study Group criteria (1990)

Recurrent oral ulcerations	Minor aphthous, major aphthous, or herpetiform ulceration observed by physician or patient, which recurred at least three times in one 12 month period
Plus, any two of the following:	
Recurrent genital ulceration	Aphthous ulceration or scarring observed by physician or patient
Eye lesion	Anterior uveitis, posterior uveitis or cells in vitreous on slit lamp examination or retinal vasculitis observed by ophthalmologist
Skin lesions	Erythema nodosum observed by physician or patient, pseudofolliculitis or papulopustular lesions, or acneiform nodules observed by physician
Positive pathergy test	Read by a physician at 24–48 hours

CLINICAL MANIFESTATIONS

Clinical features are variable (Table 9.8.2) with predilection of certain organs like the mouth, skin, eyes, gastrointestinal tract, brain, lungs, genitals, and joints.

Symptoms of vascular BD are usually seen in the first 5 years of disease onset. Arterial lesions resulting from inflammation cause aneurysms, stenosis with or without thrombosis; inflammation of veins presents as superficial or deep vein thrombosis. Lower limb DVT, superficial thrombophlebitis. Diarrhea, bleeding, and abdominal pain is presenting manifestations of GI involvement. In severe cases, fistula and perforations could be complications.

DIAGNOSIS

A meticulous history and systemic examination are essential to the diagnosis. It is essential to rule out other etiologies which could explain given symptoms in a patient. Most importantly infections including STDs, and other systemic autoimmune diseases have to be ruled out. The classic symptoms are often the only clues for diagnosis as there are no specific diagnostic tests. Raised inflammatory markers are usually associated with active disease. A positive pathergy test may aid in diagnosis. Imaging of large vessels and histopathological examination of mucus membranes and skin aid in the diagnosis.

TREATMENT

Treatment aims to reduce inflammatory exacerbations and recurrences. The treatment differs depending on the current illness presentation due to clinical heterogeneity.

Oro-genital ulcers: Topical corticosteroids are employed to treat isolated oral and vaginal aphthae. In addition to or instead of topical corticosteroids, topical sucralfate can be used. Systemic glucocorticoids should be utilized when topical corticosteroids, colchicine, or apremilast are ineffective.

In divided doses, colchicine can prevent recurring oral and vaginal ulcers. Apremilast has also been proven to be efficacious in the prevention of recurrent oral ulcers.

Arthritis: Colchicine, at split dosages of 1 to 2 mg per day, is effective for arthritis. Nonsteroidal anti-inflammatorydrugs (NSAIDs) can be used for symptomatic relief. Low-dose systemic glucocorticoids can be used to treat arthritis not controlled by colchicine.

Azathioprine and/or tumour necrosis factor (TNF)-alpha inhibitors can be used instead of colchicine for refractory or chronic arthritis. Other immunosuppressive drugs, such as interferon alfa or methotrexate, can be given in patients whose arthritis is resistant.

Anterior uveitis: Topical corticosteroids are typically used to treat anterior uveitis. Patients with anterior uveitis refractory to topical corticosteroids may need short-term systemic glucocorticoids.

Posterior uveitis: High-dose glucocorticoids combined with a second immunosuppressive

Table 9.8.2: Clinical features of behçet's

Oral ulcers	Painful and non-scarring
Genital Ulcers	Scrotal or vulval scarring
Cutaneous	Erythema nodosum, papulopustular lesions, pyoderma gangrenosum, superficial thrombophlebitis
Gastrointestinal	Ulcers involving the mouth, esophagus, ileocaecal and ascending colon, similar to IBD
Neuro-Behçet's disease	Parenchymal disease Non-Parenchymal disease Vascular BD
Eye disease	The spectrum of eye manifestations are episcleritis, scleritis, anterior uveitis, posterior uveitis, pars planitis, retinal vasculitis. Other ocular manifestations are thrombosis of retinal artery and vein and optic neuritis.
Musculoskeletal	Arthralgias, arthritis, and enthesitis
Vascular Involvement	Lower limb DVT, superficial thrombophlebitis, Budd Chiari syndrome Pulmonary arterial hypertension, Pulmonary arterial thrombosis

medication are the initial treatments. The prednisone dose is commonly 1 mg/kg per day. Pulse treatment with intravenous methylprednisolone (1 g/day for three days) is given for sight-threatening conditions. As the first line of treatment for posterior uveitis, azathioprine is used with steroids. A combination of azathioprine with a monoclonal TNF-alpha inhibitor can be used for individuals with refractory uveitis or sight-threatening disease. Cyclosporine, interferon alfa, cyclophosphamide, methotrexate, mycophenolate mofetil, or rituximab are the other choices.

Gastrointestinal (GI) illness: Systemic glucocorticoids combined with azathioprine is used for GI vasculitis. TNF-alpha inhibitors are often used in individuals who have failed therapy with glucocorticoids and azathioprine.

Vascular disease: High-dose glucocorticoids with an immunosuppressive drug, usually cyclophosphamide, are used as treatment of vascular disease. The cause of venous thrombotic events in Behçet syndrome is due to vascular inflammation rather than underlying coagulation abnormalities. Hence, anticoagulation is not required.

Neurologic disease: For individuals with a severe neurologic parenchymal illness, treatment depends on the severity. Mycophenolate, methotrexate, and cyclophosphamide are amongst other medications apart from azathioprine which is frequently used as the first-line treatment. Encephalitis, focal parenchymal lesions, and medium-vessel vasculitis are all potentially fatal disease presentations that should be treated with large doses of glucocorticoids combined with an immunosuppressive drug like cyclophosphamide.

PROGNOSIS

Male gender, early onset of disease, heavy disease burden, disease duration, and organ-specific prognostic factors predict the prognosis. Diagnosis is often delayed because of variable presentations, the relapsing and remitting nature of the disease, and the lack of specific diagnostic tests. Pregnant BD patients with active disease and on colchicine have an increased risk of preterm delivery and low birth weight. Morbidity is predominantly due to ocular and neurological manifestations. The cause of death is usually vasculitis and CNS involvement.

LEARNING POINTS

- Behçet's Disease is a unique inflammatory disease characterized by oro-genital ulcers and other systemic manifestations
- Morbidity is predominantly due to ocular and neurological manifestations.
- Treatment depends upon organ involvement: Corticosteroids, immunosuppressive and biological agents have been shown to benefit.
- Prognosis depends on the type of organ involved.

FURTHER READING

1. Ahn CS, Strowd LC, Jorizzo JL.. Behcet's Disease. In: Firestein GS, Budd RC, Gabriel SE, Koretzky GA, McInnes IB, O'Dell JR, editors. Firestein and Kelley's Textbook of Rheumatology. Philadelphia: Elsevier; 2021. pp. 1666–75.
2. Pande I, Uppal SS, Kailash S, et al. Behcet's disease in India: a clinical, immunological, immunogenetic and outcome study. Br J Rheumatol. 1995;34:825–30.
3. Sachdev N, Kapali N, Singh R, et al. Spectrum of Behçet's disease in the Indian population. International Ophthalmol. 2009;29:495–501.
4. Singal A, Chhabra N, Pandhi D, et al. Behcet's disease in India: A dermatological perspective. Indian J Dermatol Venereol Leprology. 2013;79:199-204.
5. Karadag O, Bolek EC. Management of Behçet's syndrome. Rheumatology (Oxford). 2020;59(Supplement_3): iii108–17.
6. Yazici H, Seyahi E, Hatemi G, et al. Behçet syndrome: a contemporary view. Nature Rev Rheumatol. 2018; 14:107–119.

IgG4-related Disease

Rashmi Roongta, Ritambra Nada, Arghya Chattopadhya

INTRODUCTION

IgG4-related disease (IgG4-RD) is an immune-mediated fibroinflammatory condition first described in 2003. It can involve multiple organs producing sclerotic or tumefactive masses, and has an insidiously progressive course. Response to immunosuppression suggests an autoimmune etiology; however, definite evidence of autoimmunity is lacking. The disease is most commonly seen between the 5th and 7th decade with a male predominance (60–80%). It has been mostly reported from Japan.

CLINICAL FEATURES

IgG4-RD can cause symptoms and signs for years before diagnosis. A long latency period is responsible for irreversible organ dysfunction in 60% of the patients at the time of diagnosis. Around 60–90% of patients have multi-organ involvement. Fever is uncommon and its presence warrants consideration of an alternative diagnosis. Weight loss can occur due to malabsorption caused by pancreatic failure. Four distinct subtypes of IgG4-RD have been identified:

a. Pancreaticohepatobiliary
b. Retroperitoneum and aorta
c. Head and neck—limited
d. Mikulicz and systemic

The clinical features of IgG4-RD can be divided broadly into the fibrotic and proliferative subtypes as depicted in Figure 9.9.1.

LABORATORY AND IMAGING FINDINGS

Serum IgG4 is elevated in 55–97% of patients (Table 9.9.1). ESR and CRP are only modestly elevated. Autoantibodies are negative, except for low titers ANA and RF. Imaging can reveal characteristic findings (Table 9.9.2), namely orbital pseudotumor, pancreatic masses, enlarged kidneys, etc.

DIAGNOSIS

Diagnosis can be challenging due to the difficulty in obtaining biopsy samples, especially from the pancreas or retroperitoneum. Organ-specific criteria can be used when a biopsy is unobtainable or when serum IgG4 levels are expected to be low, e.g in retroperitoneal fibrosis. Isolated lymph nodal involvement does not classify as IgG4 RD.

The 2012 revised comprehensive diagnostic criteria consist of three major items:

1. Organ involvement such as diffuse/localized swelling.
2. Serum IgG4 concentrations >135 mg/dL and
3. Marked plasmacytic infiltration defined as >10 IgG4+ cells per high-powered field (HPF) and IgG4+/ IgG+cells >40%, accompanied by fibrosis on histopathology (Fig. 9.9.2). Fulfilment of all three criteria makes a diagnosis of definite IgG4-RD.

Difficulty in obtaining biopsy samples, poor sensitivity and specificity of IgG4 level, difficulty in IgG4 staining, and uniqueness of storiform fibrosis and obliterative phlebitis for IgG4-RD, led to the proposition of the 2020 criteria which requires 3 items for a definitive diagnosis of IgG4 RD. Items 1 and 2 remain unchanged. Item 3 requires positivity of 2 out of the following-1. "dense lymphocyte and plasma cell infiltration with fibrosis", 2. "IgG4+/ IgG+ >40% and >10 IgG4+ plasma cells/ HPF",

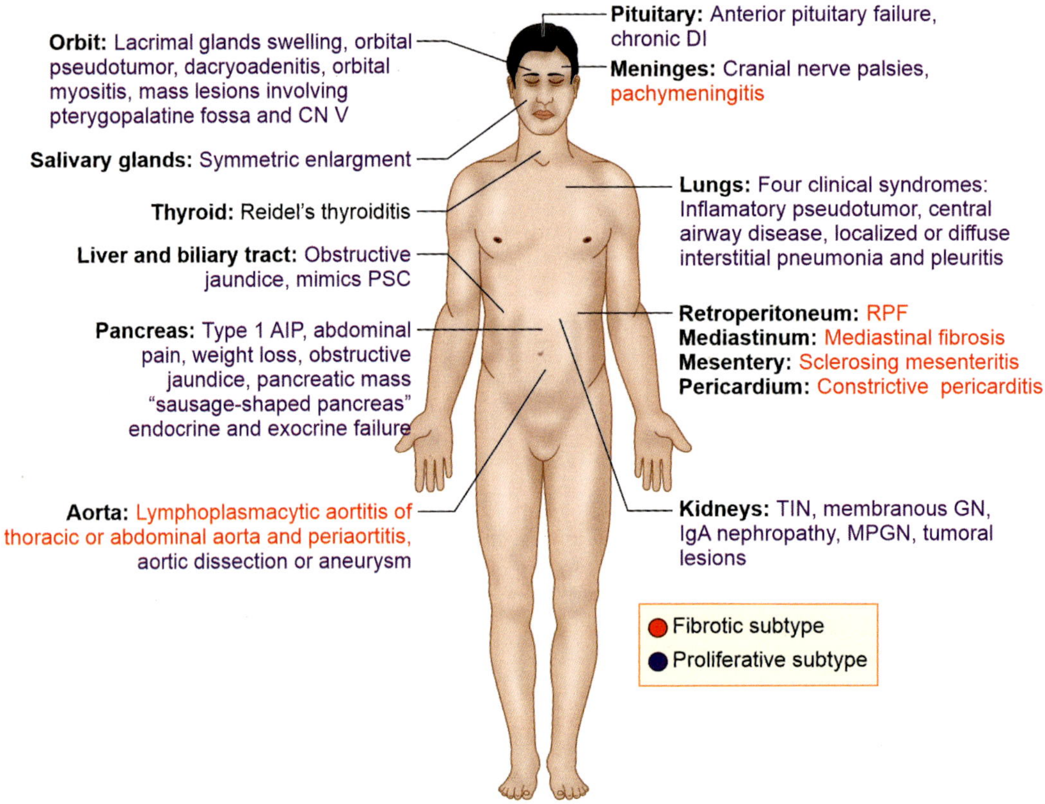

Fig. 9.9.1: Clinical manifestations of IgG4-related disease

CN: Cranial nerve; *PSC:* Primary sclerosing cholangitis; *DI:* Diabetes insipidus; *GN:* Glomerulonephritis; *MPGN:* Membranoproliferative GN; *RPF:* Retroperitoneal fibrosis

Table 9.9.1: Laboratory parameters in IgG4-RD

Laboratory parameters	*Comments*
ESR	Can be modestly elevated
CRP	Typically normal, slight increase can be seen in RPF and aortic involvement
Eosinophilia, elevated serum IgE	Seen in 30% of patients, levels reduce with treatment, higher baseline values predict relapse
Serum IgG4	Elevated in 55–97% of patients, correlates with disease severity and number of organs involved, levels reduce with treatment, higher baseline values predict relapse
Serum IgG1, IgG2, IgG3	May be elevated
C3, C4	Low in 25%, might indicate concurrent TIN
ANCA, SSA, SSB, dsDNA, RNP, Sm	Autoantibodies are absent, if present should prompt an alternate diagnosis of autoimmune disease
ANA, RF	May be present in low titers
Anti-galectin-3, laminin 511, annexin A11, prohibitin antibodies	Novel biomarkers present in <30% of patients

RPF: Retroperitoneal fibrosis; *ANCA:* Anti-neutrophilic cytoplasmic antibody; *TIN:* Tubulointestinal nephritis

Table 9.9.2: Imaging characteristics of different organs in IgG4-RD

Organ	*Imaging features*
Salivary and lacrimal gland	**CT:** Homogeneous attenuation and enhancement **MRI:** Low signal intensity on T1 and T2 weighted images
Orbital pseudotumors	**CT:** Soft-tissue attenuation and homogeneous enhancement **MRI:** Low signal intensity relative to brain on T2-weighted images, hyperintense on DWI because of fibrosis
Pancreas	**CT:** Diffuse type: Enlarged, sausage like pancreas, loss of lobulation, irregular pancreatic duct, hypodense rim/halo sign (edema surrounding the organ in the form of halo) and minimal peripancreatic fat stranding **Focal type:** enlargement of pancreatic head, body or tail-mass like (hypoattenuating), duct penetrating sign, ice pick sign
Sclerosing cholangitis	**ERCP, MRCP:** Multiple focused strictures, >2.5 mm thickening in bladder wall, and long segment narrowing, upstream dilatation, intrapancreatic segment of CBD most commonly affected **CT/MRI:** circular and symmetric rind of tissue encasing the bile duct wall, with relatively smooth margins and homogeneous enhancement in the delayed phase
Retroperitoneal fibrosis	Medial displacement of ureter, soft tissue mass lesion involving surroundings of aorta and inferior vena cava
Kidneys	Enlarged kidneys and hypoattenuating lesions on arterial phase, isoattenuating on later phase **MRI:** Low signal intensity on T1 and T2 images
Lungs	Interstitial or nodular opacities, ground glass opacities, hilar lymphadenopathy
Aorta and branches	Heterogeneous soft tissue densities surrounding aorta, 'mistletoe sign in CT angiography

CT: Computed tomography; *ERCP:* Endoscopic retrograde cholangiopancreatography; *MRCP:* Magnetic resonance cholangiopancreatography; *CBD:* Common bile duct

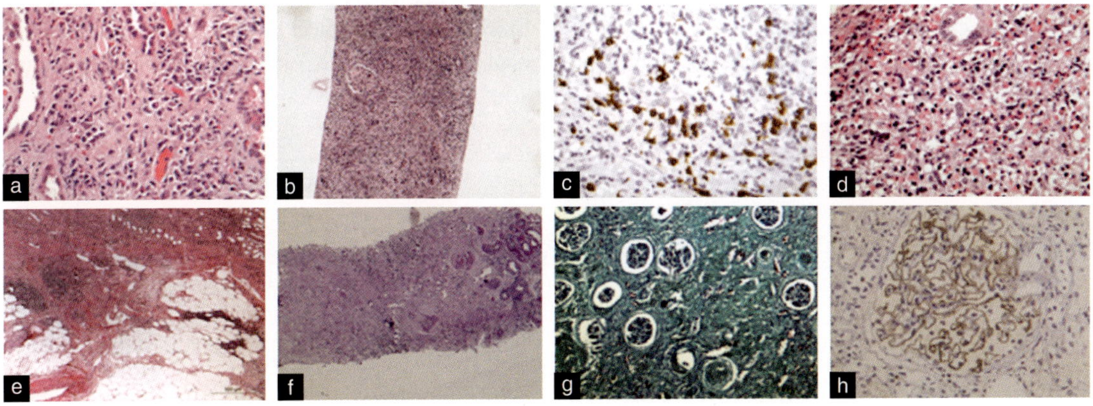

Fig. 9.9.2: Histopathology of IgG4-RD depends upon whether the infiltrate is tumoral or diffuse and the stage at which we biopsy the patients-cellular or fibrotic. Classic morphology consists of plasma rich infiltrate which has an insinuating pattern of infiltrate (a), storiform fibrosis (b) and IgG4+plasma cells (c). Eosinophils can be variably present (d). Obliterative venulitis (e) is generally not emphasized in IgG4-RD, though it can be seen in resected specimens. Accompanying granular IgG deposition along tubular basement membrane on immunofluorescence may be seen.

Tumoral lesions can be identified by sharp demarcation of the lesions even in the fibrotic stage. Different looking scar with sharp cut off (f) was the clue to diagnosis of IgG4-RD in a patient who had a history of pancreatic resection 17 years back which did not show tumor on histopathology.

Glomeruli are normal most often but all patterns of glomerular injury are seen. Secondary glomerular sclerosis can be seen in areas with chronic interstitial fibroses (g). Membranous GN with isolated IgG4 (h) staining can be seen. MPGN pattern and pauci-immune disease with ANCA have also been documented.

and 3. "Typical tissue fibrosis, particularly storiform fibrosis, or obliterative phlebitis". The presence of items 1+ 3 leads to a probable and 1+2 leads to a possible diagnosis of IgG4RD. [The reader is referred to the 2019 ACR/EULAR classification criteria for IgG4-RD for further reading].

Many diseases are associated with high serum IgG4 levels including respiratory diseases such as bronchiectasis, and rhinosinusitis; biliary tract diseases like primary sclerosing cholangitis (PSC), and cholangiocarcinoma; pancreatic diseases like non-IgG4 related pancreatitis, pancreatic cancer; cirrhosis;Systemic vasculitis, lupus, and atopic dermatitis. Hence IgG4-RD should not be diagnosed based solely on raised serum IgG4 levels.

When considering IgG4-RD rule out solid tumors of the pancreas, prostate, cholangiocarcinoma, lymphoma, and autoimmune diseases (Sjögren's syndrome, ANCA-associated vasculitis, large vessel vasculitis, Erdheim-Chester disease, sarcoidosis).

TREATMENT

Guidelines for management are lacking due to the rarity of the disease and the lack of trials. A possible window of therapeutic opportunity exists when intervention can prevent the transformation from the inflammatory to the fibrotic phase. Six monthly follow up can be considered for patients with asymptomatic lymphadenopathy, slight salivary gland enlargement, and incidentally detected lung nodules.

The ACR recommends glucocorticoids as the first-line agents for induction of remission. Improvement occurs within days to weeks. Steroid-sparing agents are used in the maintenance phase or in refractory/relapsing disease. Rituximab has been used for induction of remission with good results but is not recommended as a first-line agent currently due to the higher risk of relapse. The duration of therapy is not defined but a commonly accepted strategy is to discontinue maintenance therapy after 3 years with biochemical and radiological follow-up. Debulking surgery should be considered in single organ disease/obstructive lesions (ureters, bile duct). Novel therapies involving B and T cell inhibition, plasma cell depletion, complement, and cytokine blockade are being studied. Treatment strategies for IgG4-RD are given in Table 9.9.3.

Outcomes of Treatment

Although nearly all patients respond to glucocorticoids, 40% fail to show complete remission or relapse within 1 year despite 5 mg prednisolone per day. The IgG4- Responder Index is a tool that has been developed to assess response to treatment. Higher IgG4 level, number of organs involved at baseline, head and neck involvement, and cessation of glucocorticoids are risk factors for relapsing disease.

Table 9.9.3: Treatment strategies for IgG4-RD

Drug	*Induction*	*Maintenance*
Glucocorticoids (Prednisolone)	0.5–1 mg/kg/day for 2–4 weeks followed by tapering at 5 mg every 1–2 weeks	2.5–10 mg/day (6–36 months) Maintenance therapy considered in high-risk patients—high serum IgG4, IgE, eosinophilia at onset, multiple organ involvement, previous history of relapse
Azathioprine	0.5–2.5 mg/kg/day	0.5–2.5 mg/kg/day
Methotrexate	15–20 mg/week	15–20 mg/week
Leflunomide	10–20 mg/day	10–20 mg/day
Mycofenolate mofetil	1–1.5 g/day	0.5–1 g/day
Cyclophosphamide	50–100 mg/day	50–100 mg/day
Cyclosporine	100 mg/day	100 mg/day
Tacrolimus	1–2.5 mg/day	1–2.5 mg/day
Rituximab	1 g 2 infusions 15 days apart	1 g 2 infusions 15 days apart or single infusion every 6 months

LEARNING POINTS

- IgG4-RD is a slowly progressive disease that can present with tumefactive or sclerotic lesions.
- Pancreatobiliary system, retroperitoneum, aorta, head and neck, and salivary gland are the most frequently involved organs.
- IgG4RD can mimic malignancy and infective conditions.
- Fever is uncommon and its presence warrants consideration of an alternative diagnosis.
- Diagnosis of IgG4-RD must not be made solely based on raised IgG4 levels in the absence of appropriate clinical, histopathological, and radiological evidence.
- Due to the lack of any specific biomarker, histopathology is the mainstay of diagnosis.
- Glucocorticoids are the mainstay of treatment and recently rituximab has also shown excellent results.

FURTHER READING

1. Khosroshahi A, Wallace ZS, Crowe JL, et al. International Consensus Guidance Statement on the Management and Treatment of IgG4-Related Disease. Arthritis Rheumatol. 2015;67:1688–99.
2. Lanzillotta M, Mancuso G, Della-Torre E. Advances in the diagnosis and management of IgG4 related disease. BMJ. 2020;369:m1067. doi: 10.1136/bmj.m1067.
3. Maritati F, Peyronel F, Vaglio A. IgG4-related disease: a clinical perspective. Rheumatology (Oxford). 2020; 59(Suppl 3): iii123-iii131. doi: 10.1093/rheumatology/kez667.
4. Perugino CA, Stone JH. IgG4-related disease: an update on pathophysiology and implications for clinical care. Nat Rev Rheumatol. 2020;16:702–14.
5. Wallace ZS, Naden RP, Chari S, et al. The 2019 American College of Rheumatology/European League Against Rheumatism Classification Criteria for IgG4-Related Disease. Arthritis Rheumatol. 2020;72:7–19.
6. Zhang W, Stone JH. Management of IgG4-related disease. Lancet Rheumatol 2019;1:e55–e65.

Section

X

CRYSTAL ARTHRITIDES, SARCOIDOSIS, OSTEOARTHRITIS, OSTEOPOROSIS, JIA, AOSD, MACROPHAGE ACTIVATION SYNDROME, AND SEPTIC ARTHRITIS

Chapter 10.1

Gout

Binoy J Paul, Reeta James

INTRODUCTION

Gout result from the deposition of monosodium urate (MSU) crystals in the joint or soft tissues. Serum levels of uric acid vary from 2 to 7 mg/dL (0.12–0.42 mmol/L) in health. In normal men taking purine-free diets, the daily urinary excretion of uric acid is 350–500 mg. Uric acid is formed as a result of the metabolism of purines which are derived partly from the diet and partly from the endogenous pathway. Hyperuricemia may result either from underexcretion (85–90% cases) or overproduction (10–15% cases) (Table 10.1.1). Though uric acid levels in the serum above the saturation threshold of urate (>7 mg/dL) may predispose to gout, neither does everyone with high urate levels develop gout nor are high urate levels (>7 mg/dL in men and >6 mg/dL in females) found in all patients with gout.

Gout is now considered to be more of a *transportpathy* with a genetic basis- SLC2A9, ABCG2, SLC17A1 and gene encoding the anion exchanger URAT1 (SLC22A12) being the major genes involved. GLUT 9 (Glucose transporter) transports uric acid along with glucose and fructose and thus explains the pivotal role of dietary glucose and fructose in hyperuricemia.

Table 10.1.1: Causes of hyperuricemia

Increased urate production	*Decreased renal clearance*
Inherited enzyme defects HGPRT deficiency (Lesch–Nyhan syndrome) Glucose-6-phosphatase deficiency (G6PD) Phosphoribosyl pyrophosphate synthetase overactivity Myeloproliferative disorders Psoriasis Hemolytic diseases Malignancies Tumor lysis syndrome High-purine diet Alcohol	**Renal** Primary gout (90%), chronic kidney disease, polycystic kidney disease, lead nephropathy **Endocrine** Hyperparathyroidism, hypothyroidism, diabetes insipidus **Metabolic** Lactic acidosis, starvation, ketoacidosis, severe dehydration **Metabolic syndrome** Obesity, dyslipidemia, hypertension **Drugs** Diuretics, Low-dose aspirin, pyrazinamide, cyclosporin, ethambutol **Miscellaneous** Sarcoidosis, toxemia of pregnancy, Down syndrome

PATHOGENESIS

The pathological hallmark of a gout attack is neutrophil influx into the synovium and joint fluid triggered by the interaction between MSU crystals with synovial lining cells. This leads to activation of inflammasome leading to caspase activation that produces IL-1 causing the release of inflammatory mediators (Fig. 10.1.1)

CLINICAL FEATURES

Gout occurs mainly in men, postmenopausal women, and any condition that causes hyperuricemia. It progresses through phases of asymptomatic hyperuricemia, acute attacks, intercritical period, and chronic stage. Typically attack of gout is acute onset of pain, swelling and erythema of the 1st metatarsophalangeal joint ('podagra', Fig. 10.1.2) though it may involve the midtarsal joint, ankle, knee, wrist, or elbow. The pain and swelling build up in 24 hours with fever and constitutional features and subside within 5–7 days with desquamation of the skin. In 3–14% it may have a polyarticular presentation, though shoulders, hips, spine and sacroiliac joints are rarely involved. The course is typical of recurrent episode if serum uric acid is not maintained below 7 mg/dL.

Intercritical Phase

During the interval between 2 episodes of acute arthritis, the patient is usually free of pain but uric acid crystals can be demonstrated from the joint fluid. Gradual and progressive destruction of the joints can occur during this period.

Chronic Tophaceous Gout

Uncontrolled persistent or fluctuant hyperuricemia leads to repeated attacks of gout in the same joint or progresses to involve other joints. At one point the acute attacks do not remit completely and the joints become painful and swollen over a prolonged period leading to osteoarthritic changes, ankylosis of joints and tissue destruction. Tophi develop around the joints and on tendons (Fig. 10.1.3). Persistently high uric acid levels can lead to urolithiasis and urate nephropathy and chronic renal impairment.

DIAGNOSIS

Gout should be considered in all cases of acute or subacute mono/oligoarticular joint pain and swelling in an individual with predisposition factors. The presence of positive family history, hyperuricemia, and imaging abnormalities suggestive of gout will further support the diagnosis.

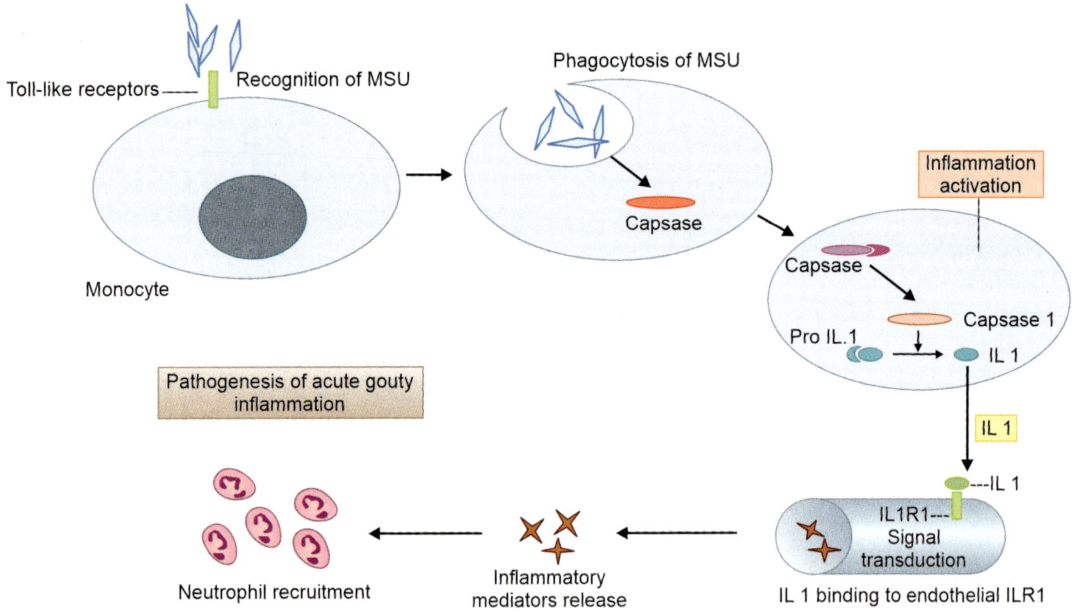

Fig. 10.1.1: Pathogenesis of gout. Steps leading to inflammasome activation and production of IL-1, a key inflammatory cytokine

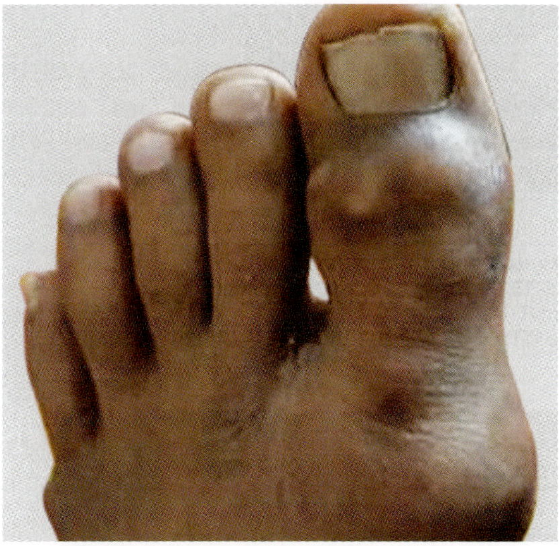

Fig. 10.1.2: Acute gouty arthritis of the metatarsophalangeal and interphalangeal joint of the great toe

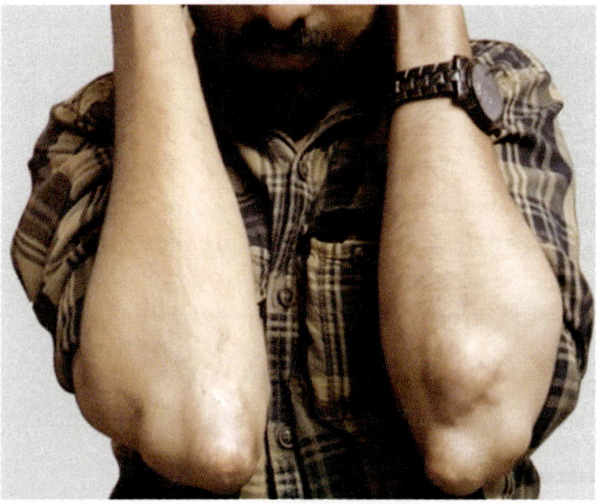

Fig. 10.1.3: Large tophi over both elbows in chronic tophaceous gout

Serum uric level is not useful in the diagnosis of acute gout as during acute attacks serum uric acid levels are normal or low in 30%, because of the uricosuric effect of stress induced ACTH and cortisol. Chronic gout is usually associated with hyperuricemia.

Synovial Fluid Examination

Demonstration of MSU crystals in synovial fluid (SF) is the gold standard for the diagnosis of gout. In real life, aspirating an inflamed joint such as MTP is difficult, however, the physician should make every effort to draw even a few drops of fluid. It is easier with the ankle and knees. Diagnostic arthrocentesis during acute gout is a safe procedure with a low frequency of adverse events. SF should not be taken in formalin as it dissolves the MSU crystals. In light microscopy, urate crystals are seen as needle-shaped crystals (Fig. 10.1.4a), and under a polarised microscope, crystals are identified intracellularly or outside the cells as negatively birefringent crystals (Fig. 10.1.4b).

Radiological Changes

It is not essential to order radiographs in the acute or first attack, as changes are seldom seen. In long-standing chronic gout, **plain radiograph** shows periarticular small punched-out erosions with overhanging margins (Fig. 10.1.5). In the late phases, there will be osteoarthritic changes and destruction and subluxation of joints.

Fig. 10.1.4a: Light microscopy shows needle-shaped monosodium urate monohydrate crystals

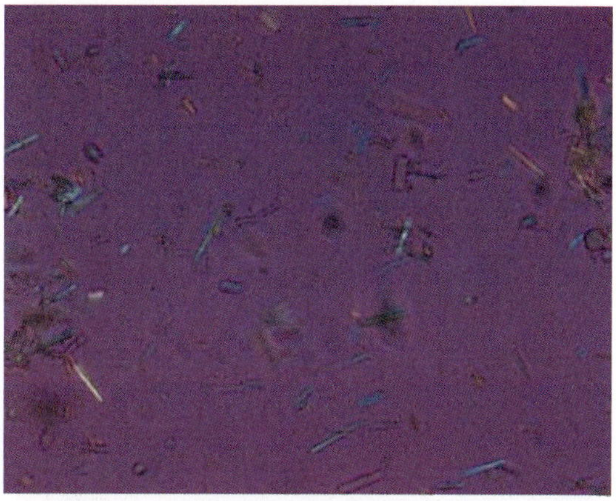

Fig. 10.1.4b: Polarized microscopy demonstrating negatively birefringent needle-shaped monosodium urate monohydrate crystals

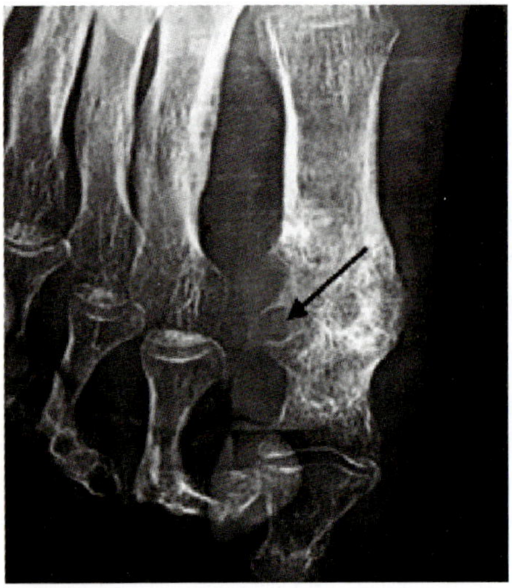

Fig. 10.1.5: Plain radiograph of the foot showing punched out lytic lesion with overhanging margin (arrow) involving the first metatarsophalangeal joint

Ultrasonography (USG)

MSU crystals within the synovial fluid give a 'snow storm appearance' and those deposited on the superficial articular cartilage cause hyperechoic band- '**double contour sign**' (Fig. 10.1.6). Deposition of MSU on tendons and ligaments are also commonly seen in USG. Tophi are seen as hypoechoic, hyperechoic, or mixed echogenicity nodules.

Dual Energy Computed Tomography (DECT)

DECT is a new technique, which can demonstrate MSU crystal deposition even at rare locations. It uses two different energies at orthogonal angles to each other and the software assigns different color codes to materials with different spectral profiles. This enables differentiation of low-density urate deposition from other denser materials like calcium (Fig. 10.1.7)

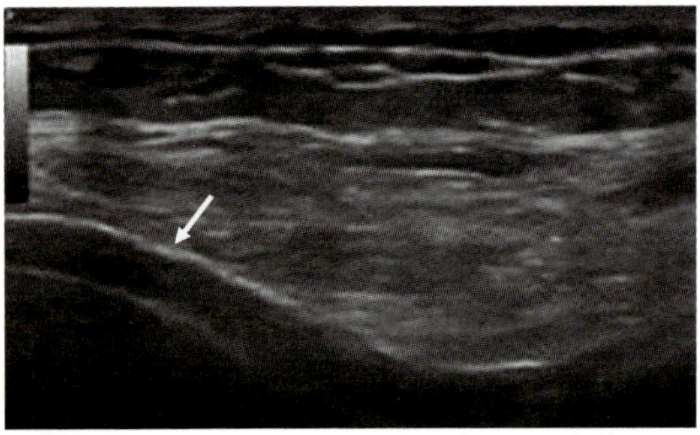

Fig. 10.1.6: Double contour sign (arrow head) on ultrasonography

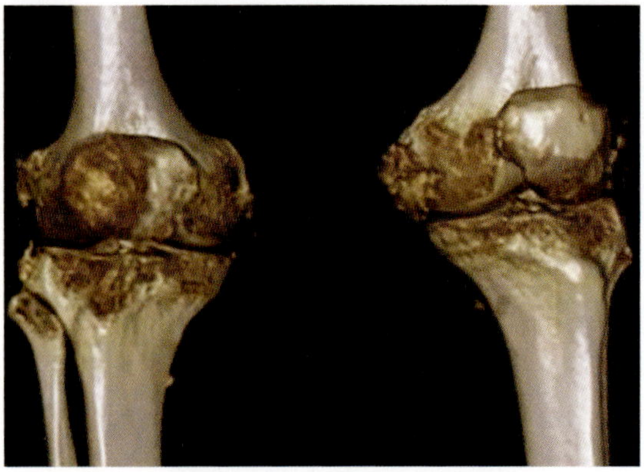

Fig. 10.1.7: Dual Energy CT (DECT) scan showing heavy deposits of uric acid around the knee joint

TREATMENT

Therapy of gout depends upon the phase of the disease.

Asymptomatic Hyperuricemia

Currently, there is no evidence of benefit from treating sustained asymptomatic hyperuricemia unless there is inherited enzyme defects, tophus, uric acid stones, urate nephropathy or persistently elevated serum uric acid above 9 mg/mL.

Acute Attacks of Gout

NSAIDS or oral colchicine are first line therapy and when contraindicated corticosteroids either intramuscular or oral effectively relieves the severe pain of acute gouty arthritis (Table 10.1.2). Urate lowering therapy (ULT) with allopurinol or febuxostat is not started during an acute attack for fear of further worsening the pain. These drugs are started after 1–2 weeks of subsidence of the acute phase. If the patient is already on urate lowering agents, it may be continued in the same dosage throughout the acute phase.

Chronic Gout

The aim of treatment is sustained reduction of serum uric acid to <6 mg/dL in non-tophaceous gout and <5 mg/dL in presence of tophi, in order to eliminate acute gouty attacks, reduce tophi and prevent ongoing joint or organ damage. Diet and lifestyle changes such as weight reduction, optimal control of hypertension and dyslipidemia

Drug	Indications	Dosage
NSAIDs	First choice if the diagnosis is fairly certain	Indomethacin 25–50 mg thrice daily initially and then reduced to a maintenance dose or Naproxen (750–1500 mg) daily
Colchicine	Preferred when the diagnosis is uncertain	An initial dose of 1mg orally followed by 0.5 mg after 1 hour and an additional 0.5 mg after 12 hours if required. Then continued at 0.5 mg thrice a day until acute attack resolves
Glucocorticoids	Used when NSAIDs and colchicine are contraindicated (such as chronic renal insufficiency, established peptic ulcer disease with a history of GI bleed on NSAIDs use)	Oral prednisolone 30–40 mg daily or equivalent parenteral preparations tapered over 7–10 days Intra-articular steroids
Corticotropin (ACTH)	In post-surgical and post-transplant patients	Single injection of 60 IU IM Can be repeated after 24 –48 hours, if needed

Table 10.1.2: Drugs used for the treatment of acute gout

and reducing purine-rich diet (such as meat, sea foods, and alcohol) are essential along with drugs to lower serum uric acid level.

There are 3 classes of drugs: Uricostatics (allopurinol or febuxostat), uricosurics (probenecid, benzbromazone, sulfinpyrazone) and uricolytics (rasburicase or pegloticase). Commonly used drugs available in India are allopurinol and febuxostat. Both are equally effective. Severe drug allergies including Steven Johnson syndrome are unusual with febuxostat which made the drug more popular in Asian countries, as the drug hypersensitivity to allopurinol is more common in Asian populations compared to Caucasians. Probenecid and Topiroxostat have limited availability in our country (Table 10.1.3).

Many new drugs are in the pipeline or available abroad (Table 10.1.4). Of the new drugs only Topiroxostat and Canagliflozin are available in India.

Table 10.1.3: Urate-lowering drugs

Drug	Mechanism of action	Daily dose	Adverse effects
Allopurinol	Xanthine oxidase inhibitor	100–800 mg	Hypersensitivity, Steven–Johnson syndrome, cytopenias
Probenecid	Uricosuric	500–2000 mg	Nephrolithiasis, aplastic anemia, nephrotic syndrome
Febuxostat	Xanthine oxidase inhibitor	40–240 mg	Rash, hepatitis, cytopenias
Topiroxostat	Xanthine oxidase inhibitor	20–160 mg	Nasopharyngitis, elevated transaminases, leucopenia

Table 10.1.4: Newer drugs for hyperuricemia

Urate transporter (URAT1) inhibitors	Lesinurad, verinurad, arhalofenate, tranilast, levotofisopam, canagliflozin
Purine nucleotide phosphorylase inhibitors	Ulodesine
Xanthine oxidase inhibitors	Topiroxostat
Melanocortin 3 receptor agonists	γ-MSH
Selective inflammasome inhibitor	Dapansutrile
Capsase inhibitors	Pralnacasan, emricasan
Uricases	Pegsiticase, SEL-212
Urate transporters to intestinal lumen	ABCG2 activators

Box 10.1.1: Treatment options for refractory gout

Lifestyle modifications
- Low purine diet
- Avoidance of nonessential drugs

Dose escalation of conventional ULT
- Allopurinol to 800 mg daily
- Febuxostat to 240 mg daily
- Probenecid to 2000 mg daily

Combination therapy
- Xanthine oxidase inhibitor + Uricosuric agent

Biologic therapy
- Uricase
- IL-1 antagonists

ULT: Urate-lowering therapy

Refractory Gout

This is symptomatic gout in which maximum dose of ULT does not control hyperuricemia or optimal ULT cannot be achieved because of adverse effects, contraindications or drug interactions. Treatment options available for refractory gout is given in Box 10.1.1.

LEARNING POINTS

- Diagnosis of gout is often clinical.
- Demonstration of urate crystals in the joints is the gold standard for diagnosis. The aspirated synovial fluid should not be taken in formalin as it dissolves the MSU crystals.
- Newer imaging modalities include joint ultrasound and DECT.
- Treatment with urate-lowering therapy is lifelong.

FURTHER READING

1. Paul BJ, James R. Gout-an Asia Pacific update; Int J Rheum Dis 2017;20:407–16.
2. Paul BJ. Crystal arthritis- Past, present and future. JK Science 2006;8;232–4.
3. Paul BJ, Anoopkumar K, Krishnan V. Asymptomatic hyperuricemia: is it time to intervene? Clin Rheumatol. 2017;36:2637–44.
4. Zell M, Zhang D, FitzGerald J. Diagnostic advances in synovial fluid analysis and radiographic identification for crystalline arthritis. Curr Opin Rheumatol. 2019; 31:134–43.

Chapter 10.2

Crystal Arthritis other than Gout

V Krishnamurthy

INTRODUCTION

Crystal arthritis other than gout are usually due to calcium pyrophosphate dihydrate crystal and basic calcium phosphate (BCP) crystal deposition. They are uncommon and mimic several musculoskeletal disorders.

CPPD DISEASE

Crystal arthritis induced by calcium pyrophosphate deposition (CPPD) and BCP deposition manifests in several clinical forms (Table 10.2.1). Pseudogout is the term that denotes acute calcium pyrophosphate (CPP) crystal arthritis simulating acute gout. The term chondrocalcinosis is a radiological term and is not a synonym of CPPD; several other crystals can cause it.

Pathophysiology

The pathophysiology of CPP crystal deposition in the articular and hyaline cartilage is not well known. Aging and damaged chondrocytes result in an increase in anionic inorganic pyrophosphate and a decrease in pyrophosphatases. Pyrophosphates interact with the calcium cations in the cartilage matrix, causing the deposition of CPP crystals. ATP is the source of pyrophosphate, which is hydrolyzed by increased activity of ATP pyrophosphohydrolase and 5'-nucleotidase. Phagocytosis of these crystals by monocyte-macrophages and neutrophils induces inflammation through the NLRP3 inflammasome complex and cytokine IL-1b. Cartilage glycosaminoglycans inhibit crystal formation. Conditions that predispose to crystal deposition include:

- Hemochromatosis
- Hyperparathyroidism
- Hypophosphatasia
- Hypomagnesemia
- CKD
- ANKH gene mutations

CPPD is a disease of the elderly and chondrocalcinosis is seen only in 40% of patients. Trauma and acute systemic illness also can predispose to CPPD, and there is no dietary association.

Table 10.2.1: Clinical presentations of CPPD disease and BCP deposition disease

CPPD	*BCP*
Asymptomatic	Asymptomatic
Acute CPPD arthritis	Acute BCP periarthritis
Chronic CPPD arthritis	Destructive arthropathy of BCP
OA with CPPD	OA with BCP

CPPD: Calcium pyrophosphate deposition; *BCP:* Basic calcium phosphate; *OA:* Osteoarthritis

Clinical Presentation

Four types of presentations are seen asymptomatic, acute CPPD arthritis, chronic CPPD arthritis, and OA with CPPD.

Asymptomatic Disease

Incidentally discovered without signs or symptoms.

Acute Arthritis

This manifests as acute inflammatory monoarthritis mimicking gout and affects larger joints like knees, wrists, and elbows. They differ from gout, by lasting for several days to weeks. They also can present as oligoarthritis or polyarthritis mimicking rheumatoid arthritis by involving metacarpal (MCP) joints. False-positive rheumatoid factor in the elderly, elevated CRP may add to the confusion. Sometimes, arthritis can be migratory or additive in presentation. Fever, malaise, leukocytosis, and elevated ESR and CRP can mimic septic arthritis.

Axial Disease

CPPD in the atlantoaxial joint, facet joints, intervertebral joints and discs can occur causing pain in these areas. Acute attacks cause severe neck pain, and rigidity and can mimic meningitis, polymyalgia rheumatica or giant cell arteritis. Cervical instability and crowned dens syndrome have been described.

CPPD as Osteoarthritis

CPPD simulates osteoarthritis (OA) but differs by affecting the shoulder glenohumeral joint, MCP, wrist and elbow joints, with acute flares.

Diagnosis

A high index of suspicion in acute inflammatory arthritis of the elderly is the key to diagnosis. Blood tests include serum calcium, phosphorous, alkaline phosphatase, PTH, uric acid magnesium, ferritin, TSH and liver function tests to find associated metabolic derangement. The diagnosis is achieved by demonstraton of rhomboid-shaped positively birefringent CPP crystals in the synovial fluid aspirate (Fig. 10.2.1). During an acute attack the synovial fluid is inflammatory with high leukocyte

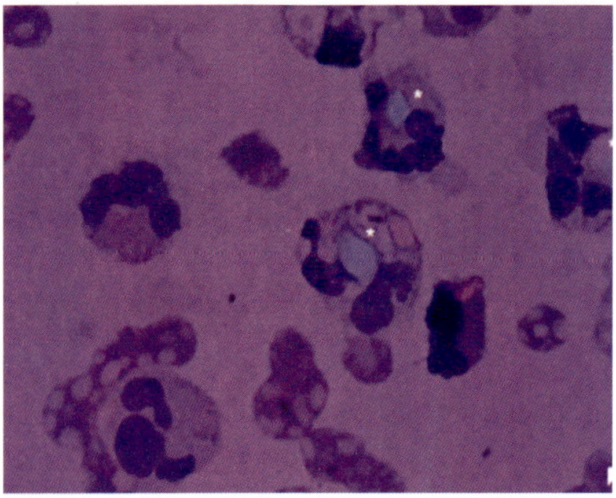

Fig. 10.2.1: CPP crystals: Positively birefringent rhomboids within neutrophils (*Courtesy*: Sidari and Jordan M Hall)

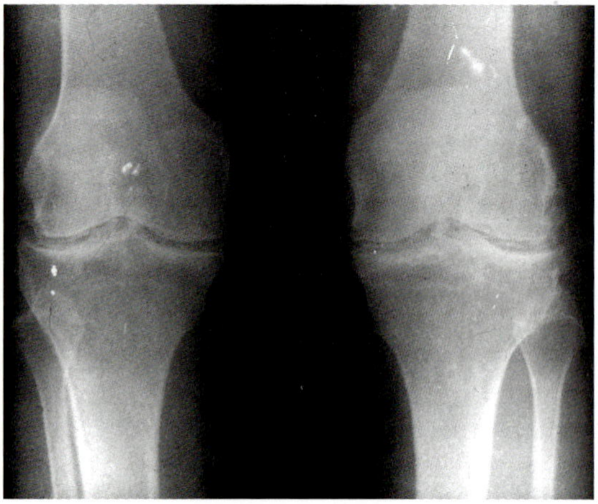

Fig. 10.2.2: Linear calcification of CPPD in X-ray of the knee joints. CPPD is associated with OA

counts. An X-ray of the knee reveals linear or rounded calcification along the meniscus and triangular in the wrist due to fibrocartilage calcification (Fig. 10.2.2) Ultrasonogram reveals hyperechoic rounded deposits differing from the linear pattern of gout. DECT is an advanced imaging technique for detection of CPP crystal deposition.

Treatment

An acute inflammatory attack is treated with oral or intra-articular steroids, NSAIDs and colchicine as in acute gouty arthritis. There is no crystal dissolution therapy.

In chronic disease, the treatment is not very satisfying, and one must combat comorbid conditions also. Colchicine, IL-1 inhibitors, and hydroxychloroquine have been studied. Low-dose methotrexate is not useful.

BCP CRYSTAL DEPOSITION

BCP crystals are of several types: calcium carbonate, hydroxyapatite, octa calcium and tricalcium phosphates and whitlockite. Hydroxyapatite is common. The BCP gets deposited in both intra-articular and periarticular areas.

Pathogenesis

Deposition occurs in areas of tissue damage. Hypercalcemia, hyperparathyroidism, and hyper-phosphatemia seen in chronic kidney disease aid apatite deposition. BCP crystals often coexist with CPP crystals in osteoarthritis (OA).

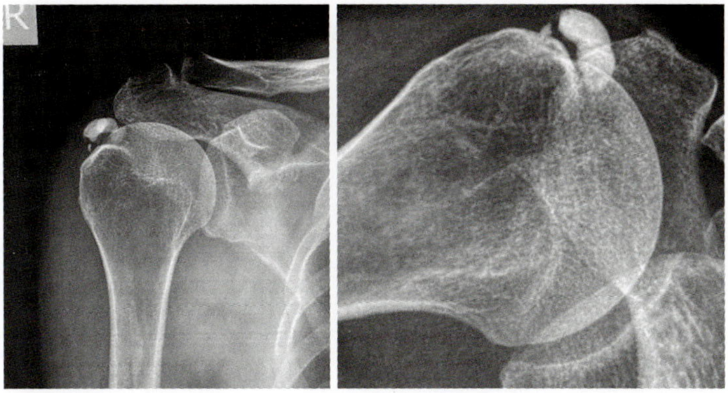

Fig. 10.2.3: Periarticular intensive BCP deposition of bicipital tendon joint at insertion

Clinical Features

Like CPPD, 4 types of clinical presentations occur:

- Asymptomatic
- Acute BCP arthritis
- Destructive arthropathy
- OA wth BCP

Periarticular joint capsule, bursae, tendons, and articular areas are affected (Fig. 10.2.3). It can manifest either as acute inflammatory or chronic destruction.

Periarticular calcification can occur in both sexes and all age groups, including children. It can be seen in younger women. Shoulder calcifications can be asymptomatic and are associated with diabetes mellitus, hypomagnesemia, dyslipidemia, CTD, and trauma.

Apatite-associated destructive arthropathy (AADA) is a different BCP disorder and is known as the Milwaukee shoulder, common in elderly women. Apart from shoulders, it can affect knees, hips, elbows, and ankles. Trauma, overuse, dialysis, and neurological disorders have been associated with this condition.

Diagnosis

BCP crystals are not visible in polarizing light and need a special staining technique (Alizarin red). They can be identified only by electron microscopy and X-ray diffraction. Intra- and periarticular calcifications with or without destruction are the characteristic radiographic findings.

Treatment

Symptomatic treatment with NSAIDs, colchicine for 2 weeks, intra- or periarticular steroid injection after aspiration of effusion are effective. Diffuse calcinosis has been treated with IVIG, rituximab, calcium channel blockers and bisphosphonates. Hemodialysis is effective in renal failure with hyperphosphatemia.

CALCIUM OXALATE

These crystals can cause arthritis, periarthritis, visceral and bone deposits. It is common in chronic kidney disease and certain hereditary metabolic disorders. Hemodialysis, reduction in intake of ascorbic acid and avoiding a diet rich in oxalates help.

LEARNING POINTS

- The most common crystal arthritis other than gout is due to calcium pyrophosphate crystal deposition (CPPD) disease.
- The radiological findings are characteristic and the demonstration of CPP crystals in synovial fluid is diagnostic.
- Acute attacks are treated with oral or intraarticular steroids, NSAIDs and colchicine.

FURTHER READING

1. Abhishek A, Doherty M. Epidemiology of calcium pyrophosphate crystal arthritis and basic calcium phosphate crystal arthropathy. Rheum Dis Clin North Am. 2014;40:177–91.
2. El-Zawawy H, Mandell BF. Crystal-Induced Arthritides in the Elderly: An Update. Rheum Dis Clin North Am. 2018;44:489–99.
3. Schumacher HR, Chen XL. Gout and other Crystal-Associated Arthropathies. In: Jameson JL, Fauci AS, Kasper DL, Hauser SL, Longo DL, Loscalzo J, editors. Harrison's Principles of Internal Medicine (20th Ed) New York: McGraw Hill; 2018. p. 2633–5.
4. Sidari A, Hill E. Diagnosis and Treatment of Gout and Pseudogout for Everyday Practice. Prim Care. 2018;45:213–36.

Chapter 10.3

Sarcoidosis

Durga Prasanna Misra, Vikas Agarwal

INTRODUCTION

Sarcoidosis is a chronic granulomatous disease of unknown etiology. The epidemiology, pathophysiology, clinical features, differential diagnosis and management of sarcoidosis, including specific features of particular relevance are presented.

EPIDEMIOLOGY

Sarcoidosis is a rare disease. Although epidemiological data from India is unavailable, studies from the West have reported an incidence of 2.3–11.5 and a prevalence of 2.17–160 per 100,000 persons per year. Sarcoidosis most commonly starts in the 5th to 6th decade of life. Sarcoidosis is associated with greater mortality risk, with estimated all-cause mortality at 1 year of 2%. Risk factors for sarcoidosis include obesity, exposure to crystalline silica (increased risk) and smoking (decreased risk).

PATHOGENESIS

Non-caseating granulomas are the characteristic histopathologic feature of sarcoidosis (Fig. 10.3.1), resulting from aberrant activation of CD4+ T lymphocytes in response to an unknown antigenic stimulus. The dominance of Th1 lymphocytes results in granuloma formation followed by its resolution, whereas Th2 lymphocytes drive a phenotype of fibrosis following granulomatous inflammation. In patients with sarcoid arthritis, increased proportions of circulating Th1, Th2 and Th17 cells (ratio versus T regulatory cells) and higher CD8+ cytotoxic T cells in peripheral blood have been detected when compared with those without articular sarcoidosis.

CLINICAL FEATURES

Various organ systems can be affected by sarcoidosis. Table 10.3.1 summarizes different organ systems

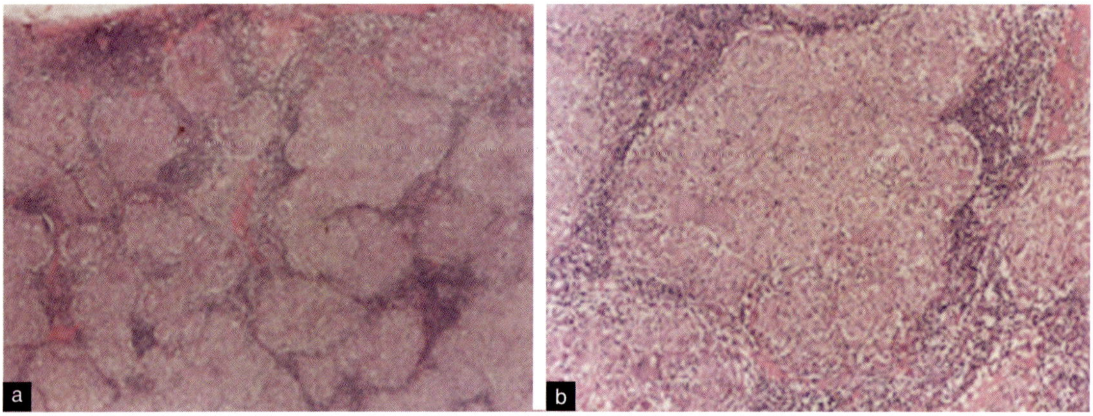

Fig. 10.3.1: Non-caseating granulomas on lymph node biopsy in a patient with sarcoidosis

Table 10.3.1: Major organ systems involved in sarcoidosis

• Lungs are the most common organ involved. – Hilar adenopathy and mediastinal adenopathy – Interstitial lung disease – Peribronchovascular nodules
• Lymphoreticular system – Lymph nodes and spleen enlargement
• Eyes – Uveitis is commonly chronic, most often anterior uveitis or panuveitis – Rarely optic neuritis, scleritis or episcleritis
• Liver – Hepatomegaly, raised alkaline phosphatase
• Skin – Erythema nodosum, papuloplaque lesions
• Musculoskeletal system – Arthritis, myositis, bone cysts–(further detailed in Table 10.3.2)
• Cardiac sarcoidosis – Conduction abnormalities, less commonly restrictive cardiomyopathy
• Kidneys – Interstitial nephritis, hypercalcemia causing acute tubular necrosis
• Brain – Neurosarcoidosis commonly involves brainstem and posterior fossa – Cranial nerve palsies
• Peripheral nervous system – Pure sensory or sensorimotor peripheral neuropathy are more common
• Bone marrow infiltration causing cytopenias

commonly involved in sarcoidosis. Fever, weight loss and other constitutional symptoms might be presenting features in sarcoidosis. Sarcoidosis presenting with fever, hilar adenopathy (Fig. 10.3.2), erythema nodosum and ankle arthritis is also called Lofgren's syndrome. Heerfordt syndrome comprises the triad of uveitis, parotitis and fever in a patient with sarcoidosis. It is important to note that pleural effusion is distinctly unusual in sarcoidosis.

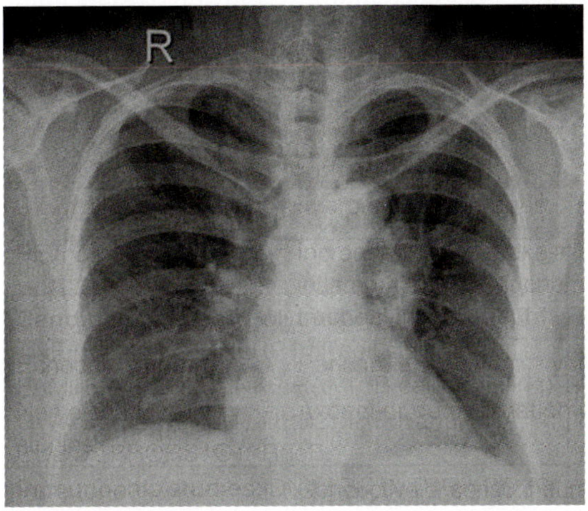

Fig. 10.3.2: Hilar adenopathy on chest radiograph

Sarcoidosis for the Rheumatologist

Patients with sarcoidosis might present to the rheumatologist with sarcoid arthritis. The features of arthritis in sarcoidosis are detailed in Table 10.3.2. Focal myositis is rarely associated with sarcoidosis. Bone lesions commonly include bone cysts (Fig. 10.3.3) and lytic lesions, more common in the phalanges. A common presentation is erythema nodosum (Fig. 10.3.4) and ankle arthritis. In this instance, differential diagnoses to be considered are sarcoidosis, tuberculosis, and erythema-nodosum associated arthritis. Cross-consultations from ophthalmology (for uveitis), cardiology (for cardiac sarcoidosis) and pulmonary medicine (for sarcoid

Table 10.3.2: Salient features of arthritis in sarcoidosis

- Age of onset: 3rd to 4th decade
- Characteristics of arthritis:
  - Both acute or chronic arthritis (duration >3 months).
  - Monoarthritis is unusual.
  - Arthritis with tenosynovitis is typical.
  - Oligoarthritis more common in acute stage.
  - Both oligoarthritis and polyarthritis have similar prevalence in chronic sarcoid arthritis.
- Joints involved:
  - Ankle is the most commonly affected joint in both oligoarthritis and polyarthritis.
  - Wrists, metacarpophalangeal, proximal interphalangeal joints of hands, shoulder and knee are more commonly affected with sarcoid polyarthritis than with oligoarthritis.
- Extra-articular manifestation:
  - Commonest associated extra-articular manifestations in both oligoarthritis and polyarthritis are hilar adenopathy and erythema nodosum.
- Serology:
  - Generally seronegative for RF
- Response to treatment:
  - There is a favorable response to corticosteroids and non-steroidal anti-inflammatory drugs.
  - Few patients with polyarthritis might require further immunosuppressant therapy for steroid-sparing effect.

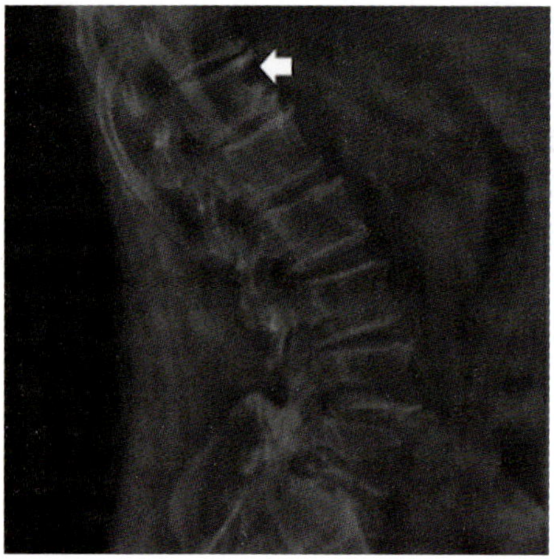

Fig. 10.3.3: Bone cyst in the spine of a patient with sarcoidosis

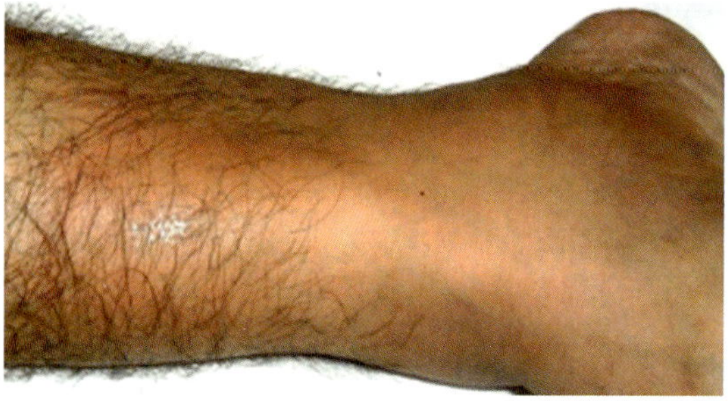

Fig. 10.3.4: Erythema nodosum in a patient with sarcoidosis

lymphadenopathy or interstitial lung disease) might also bring a patient with sarcoidosis to the rheumatologist.

DIFFERENTIAL DIAGNOSIS

Tuberculosis is an important differential diagnosis for sarcoidosis, particularly in regions where it is endemic such as India. Past tuberculosis infection has been proposed as one of the antigenic triggers driving sarcoidosis. It is imperative to document a negative tuberculin test and interferon-gamma release assay before concluding a diagnosis of sarcoidosis. Table 10.3.3 summarizes the differences between tuberculosis and sarcoidosis.

MANAGEMENT

Investigations in an individual with sarcoidosis are summarized in Table 10.3.4. Hilar adenopathy is a characteristic finding on chest radiography (Fig. 10.3.2).

After ascertaining a diagnosis of corticosteroids, the first line of therapy, generally prednisolone started at a dose of 0.5–1 mg/kg/day (higher doses preferred in those with neurological, renal or cardiac involvement), tapered over 6 months to 1 year.

Table 10.3.3: Features that help to distinguish tuberculosis from sarcoidosis		
Feature	*Favors tuberculosis*	*Favors sarcoidosis*
Caseating granulomas	Yes	No
Positive tuberculin test or interferon gamma release assay	Yes	No
Choroid tubercles	Yes	No
Peripheral arthritis	Less common: Poncet's arthritis	Yes
Myositis	Uncommon	Focal myositis is well described but still rare
Cavitary lung lesions	Yes	No
Pleural effusion	Yes	No
Bone cysts	No	Yes
Osteomyelitis	Yes	No

Table 10.3.4: Investigations in sarcoidosis	
Test	*Expected findings*
Serum calcium	Elevated
Serum ACE	Elevated
CBC	Cytopenias involving all three lineages less commonly seen in individuals with bone marrow infiltration
Liver function tests	Raised alkaline phosphatase
1,25 dihydroxy vitamin D	Elevated
Serum creatinine	May be raised in the presence of interstitial nephritis. Associated with hypercalciuria but not with active urinary sediments
Chest X-ray	Mediastinal and hilar adenopathy Pulmonary infiltrates
CT thorax	Mediastinal and hilar adenopathy Lung nodules in a peribronchovascular distribution Interstitial lung disease
Neuroimaging	In neurosarcoidosis–white matter lesions more common in the posterior fossa may be seen on MRI
Nerve conduction studies	Axonal sensory or sensorimotor neuropathy are more common

ACE: Angiotensin converting enzyme; *CBC:* Complete blood counts

Major organ involvement (brain, kidneys, heart) or relapses while tapering corticosteroids may require the addition of maintenance immunosuppressants such as azathioprine, mycophenolate mofetil, cyclophosphamide or anti-tumor necrosis factor alpha agents. Cardiac arrhythmias might require the insertion of an implantable cardioverter and defibrillator.

CONCLUSION

Sarcoidosis is a great mimic of different diseases. Differentiation from tuberculosis is essential although not always simple. When in doubt, it is better to provide a therapeutic trial of anti-tubercular therapy. Sarcoid arthritis can behave just like rheumatoid arthritis, although often seronegative, and often associated with a good response to therapy.

LEARNING POINTS

- Sarcoidosis most commonly affects lungs, lymph nodes, skin and joints.
- Cardiac, renal and nervous system involvement is associated with greater morbidity.
- Histopathological demonstration of non-caseating granulomas is characteristic.
- Renal failure due to interstitial nephritis or hypercalciuria causing polydipsia and acute tubular necrosis, neurosarcoidosis, and cardiac sarcoidosis causing ventricular arrhythmias are manifestations of sarcoidosis requiring urgent medical attention.
- Treatment of sarcoidosis is with corticosteroids, with or without other immunosuppressants.

FURTHER READING

1. Agarwal V, Agrawal V, Aggarwal A, et al. Arthritis in sarcoidosis: A multicentric study from India. Int J Rheum Dis 2018; 21:1728–33.
2. Arkema EV, Cozier YC. Epidemiology of sarcoidosis: current findings and future directions. Ther Adv Chronic Dis. 2018; 9:227–40.
3. Govindarajan V, Agarwal V, Aggarwal A, Misra R. Arthritis in sarcoidosis. J Assoc Physicians India. 2001; 49:1145–7.
4. Sève P, Pacheco Y, Durupt F, et al. Sarcoidosis: A Clinical Overview from Symptoms to Diagnosis. Cells. 2021; 10:766.
5. Tana C, Mantini C, Donatiello I, et al. Clinical Features and Diagnosis of Cardiac Sarcoidosis. J Clin Med. 2021; 10:1941.

Osteoarthritis

Pooja Dhaon, Siddharth Kumar Das, Ghan Shyam Pangtey

INTRODUCTION

Osteoarthritis (OA) results from primary age-related degeneration of the cartilage compounded by mechanical stress such as obesity or secondary to inflammatory arthritis. The initial changes include bone marrow edema, meniscal damage and sometimes inflammation of the synovium (visualized by MRI). Subsequently, there is focal cartilage loss along with subchondral bone formation, which appears as bony overgrowths called osteophytes on radiographs. The central component of OA is destruction of cartilage, but subsequently, the entire joint (organ) is affected as a whole.

Hip and knee OA accounts for 1.12% of all years lived with disability. In India the prevalence of OA in rural Pune is 5.78%, while our data from Lucknow shows a prevalence of 4.2% in rural and 11.5% in urban areas.

Risk Factors and the Role of Inflammation in OA

The risk factors for OA are extrinsic, intrinsic, and systemic (Fig. 10.4.1). OA is considered to be a mechanical-driven, non-inflammatory and degenerative disease. However, there is data that shows the presence of synovial inflammation, and activation of the inflammatory complement system in the pathogenesis of knee OA. The major risk factors for knee OA namely obesity, local knee trauma are associated with local articular cartilage and systemic production of inflammatory mediators. Obesity and excessive abnormal loading of joints

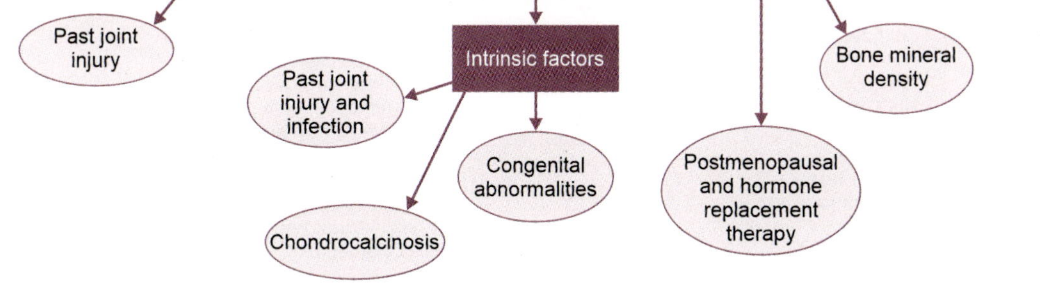

Fig. 10.4.1: Extrinsic, intrinsic, and systemic risk factors for osteoarthritis

also stimulate protease enzymes that are responsible for the degradation of cartilage proteoglycan and collagens leading to irreversible damage.

CLINICAL FEATURES

OA is classified as primary and secondary based on whether there is an underlying cause of degeneration of cartilage (Fig. 10.4.2). The most common joint affected in primary OA is the knee, hand joints: distal interphalangeal (DIP), first carpometacarpal, proximal interphalangeal (PIP) joints, and the hip. Other joints are less frequently involved. In primary OA symptoms usually occur in one or two large joints typically in a middle-aged to an elderly person. Symptoms are joint pain, stiffness, and reduced mobility of the joint (Table 10.4.1). Pain occurs during activity or weight bearing with or without non-inflammatory swelling, that is progressive over the years and with disability. OA has a more severe course in women, extensive involvement along with the increased prevalence of knee and hand involvement. On the contrary, men have more hip involvement.

Hand OA or nodal OA: This subset is characterized by pain and bony swelling over the DIP and to a lesser extent the PIP joints, with familial clustering. On examination, we can find Heberden's nodes: bony enlargement of DIP joint, Bouchard's nodes: bony enlargement at PIP joints. Usually non-erosive on plain radiographs. Primary OA of the base of the thumb (first carpometacarpal joint) is the second most common OA of the hand.

Table 10.4.1: Symptoms and signs of osteoarthritis

Symptoms	*Signs*
Pain	Altered gait
Stiffness	Tenderness
Gelling	Bony swelling over the joint **Heberden's nodes:** over the DIPs **Bouchard's nodes:** over the PIPs
Weakness	Effusion of the joint
Grinding or clicking	Crepitus of the joint
Instability or buckling	Limitation of motion
	Deformity
	Ligamentous instability

Erosive hand OA (EOA): This is a subset of hand OA, manifesting with an inflammatory picture. The clinical features are pain, swelling, warmth, redness, and limited function of the hand joints. Heberden and Bouchard's nodes may be present or absent. Plain radiographs of the hands show cartilage loss and joint space narrowing, subchondral erosions, and bony proliferation involving the first CMC, DIP, and PIP joint giving the typical "gull-wing" appearance. It leads to deformities and ankylosis. Rheumatoid factor, anticitrullinated peptide

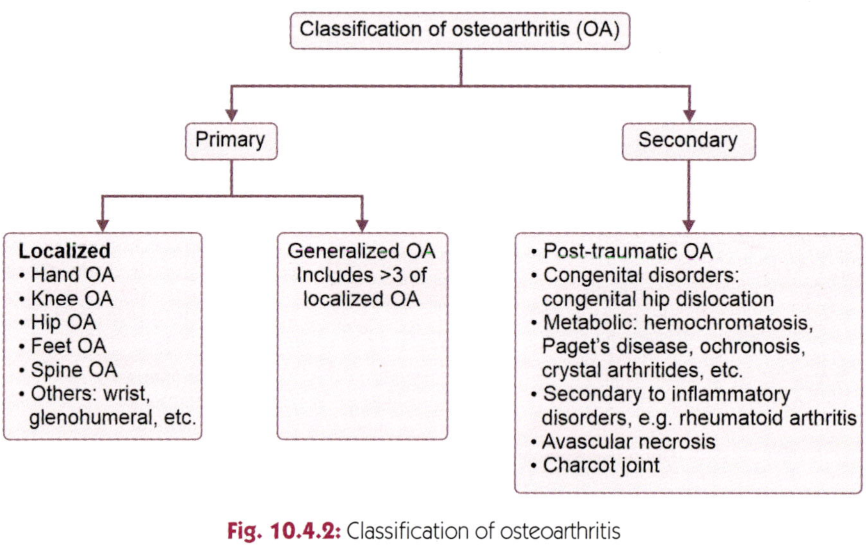

Fig. 10.4.2: Classification of osteoarthritis

antibodies, and CRP are negative. EOA mimics rheumatoid arthritis and psoriatic arthritis.

Isolated knee OA: It is the most common form of OA. The knee joint may be the only joint involved. It usually starts unilaterally in the beginning but becomes bilateral over a period of time. Obesity, female sex, and knee bending are important risk factors. It may involve predominantly medial femorotibial, lateral femorotibial or patellofemoral compartment.

Spinal OA: Apophyseal joint involvement is the only true form of OA of the spine. Back pain on bending backwards is the typical physical sign of such involvement. Intervertebral disc degeneration with osteophyte formation is considered an integral part of OA. It is common in the lumbar and cervical spondylitis regions, the sites of maximum spinal motion. It gives rise to local pain and/or radicular pain. Diffuse idiopathic skeletal hyperostosis (DISH) and ossification of posterior longitudinal ligament (OPLL) are considered to be variant forms of OA.

INVESTIGATIONS AND DIAGNOSIS

Plain radiographs are the most common method of imaging in clinical practice for diagnosis and grading severity although there is discordance between radiographic severity and clinical symptoms. The advantage of radiographs is that they are inexpensive and widely available. The most reliable method for radiographs is the standing semi-flexed view. The Kellgren–Lawrence (KL) system is used to grade radiographs on a scale of 0–4 (Fig. 10.4.3). The typical radiographic findings in OA are summarized in Table 10.4.2.

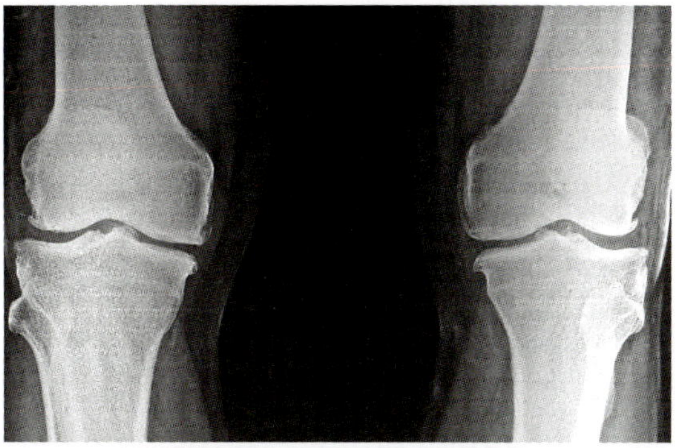

Fig. 10.4.3: Radiograph of both knees. Anteroposterior view showing medical compartment joint space narrowing, loss of tibial spike, multiple osteophytes and subchondral sclerosis

Table 10.4.2: Radiographic findings in osteoarthritis (OA)

Finding	*Description*
Joint space narrowing (JSN)	It is the earliest finding, indicating cartilage thinning, meniscus degeneration. It is focal and not uniform that helps to differentiate from rheumatoid arthritis. JSN is used to monitor progression of disease.
Osteophytes	Osteophytes are bony outgrowths at sites where mechanical stress is less. Hallmark of OA, their presence is considered important for diagnosis.
Subchondral sclerosis	Sclerosis of the subchondral bone is one of the earliest changes to appear, and it correlates with disease progression
Bone remodeling and attrition	There is flattening and increased congruity between articular surfaces. With increase in cartilage loss the bone is further flattened and ultimately the surfaces become deformed.
Calcification	Linear calcification can be seen due to CPPD deposition, while spotty calcification is due to hydroxyapatite deposition.

The synovial fluid shows mild leukocytosis with mononuclear predominance. There may be the presence of crystals in about 30–70% of patients. The most commonly found crystals are CPPD, however, sometimes hydroxyapatite (HA) or basic calcium phosphate crystals (BCP) may also be detectable.

The diagnosis of OA is clinicoradiological using the American College of Rheumatology (ACR) criteria. As it is known there is clinicoradiological discordance in OA using radiographs, an early diagnosis of OA using MRI must be attempted. Additional imaging or laboratory test may be required in a case of OA if the patient is young, have atypical symptoms (unusual joint involvement, joint synovitis, nocturnal or resting pain, and constitutional symptoms) and in patients who have joint locking history, suggestive of additional mechanical derangement.

Recent guidelines published by the ACR and OARSI (Osteoarthritis Research Society International) for the management of osteoarthritis, a holistic approach must be followed for these patients. Treatment must be individualized considering the patient's medical status and patient preference. Before starting the treatment, every patient must be assessed as shown in Table 10.4.3. The management can be divided into non-pharmacological, pharmacological, surgical, and experimental therapies.

Table 10.4.3: Assessment of a patient with osteoarthritis before commencing treatment

The following points need to be considered
1. Confirm diagnosis and site of osteoarthritis
2. Identify comorbidities
3. Clinical status
a. Pain, stiffness, and function using WOMAC
b. Joint effusion, instability, and malalignment
4. Assess emotional and environment
a. Health belief and expectations
b. Mood
c. Sleep quality
d. Depression
e. Financial status
f. Social network

WOMAC: The Western Ontario and Mcmaster Universities osteoarthritis index

Non-pharmacologic Treatment

This includes weight loss, exercise, and psychosocial interventions among others (Table 10.4.4).

Physical Medical Rehabilitation (PMR)

The PMR specialist consultation should be sought for optimal management of OA. Appropriate footwear with shoe orthotics can reduce pain. Unloading the joint by using an assisted device and realignment of joints (splint, brace), is appropriate for individuals who have problems with activities of daily living.

Pharmacological Therapy

It must be initiated for all patients having mild to moderate disease (Table 10.4.5). Most studies have been published for knee OA and very few trials have been published regarding pharmacological management of hip OA. There are as yet no effective disease modifying agents for OA though clinical trials are underway.

Experimental Therapies

The most promising ones are tanezumab (Anti nerve growth factor), sprifermin (A recombinant human fibroblast growth factor) and canakinumab (monoclonal targeting IL-1β molecule). Other experimental treatments include the development of regenerative medicine and tissue engineering

Table 10.4.4: Nonpharmacological therapy of osteoarthritis

1. Weight loss
a. All obese and overweight patients should be advised for weight loss.
b. Modest weight loss decreases the risk of the development of OA, as well as pain in established disease.
2. Exercise
a. General aerobic fitness, and range of motion exercises, and strength training programs incorporating resistance-based lower limb and quadriceps strengthening exercises, are effective in reducing pain and improving physical function.
3. Nutraceuticals
a. According to ACR and OARSI, considering the lack of evidence, glucosamine or chondroitin sulfate are not recommended, but European guidelines suggest they can be used for disease modification.
b. Similarly, acupuncture therapy for pain management should not be offered to patients with OA.
4. Thermotherapy and electrotherapy
a. Heat or cold application, stretching, and electrotherapy with transcutaneous electric nerve stimulation (TENS) may be beneficial as adjunctive therapy over.

Table 10.4.5: Pharmacological therapy of osteoarthritis

1. **Topical NSAIDs**
   a. For knee and hand OA, excellent safety profile.
   b. Topical rubefacients should be avoided in treating OA.
2. **Oral acetaminophen and NSAIDs**
   a. High-dose acetaminophen (paracetamol) was considered the drug of choice for OA, however recent OARSI recommendations advice to limit its use due to its hepatotoxicity potential and less efficacy.
   b. NSAIDs are currently the drug of choice for pain relief.
   c. Co-oxygenase 2 (COX-2) inhibitors are GI safe
   d. Use the lowest effective dose for the shortest duration of time
3. **Opioid analgesics**
   a. Highly efficacious, but has excess risk of chemical dependency
   b. Tramadol can be tried
4. **Intra-articular glucocorticoid**
   a. Useful for short-term relief in flares of OA in the hip and knee, which is not controlled by oral drugs or where NSAIDs are contraindicated.
   b. Conditionally recommended in hand osteoarthritis
5. **Intra-articular hyaluronans**
   a. Improve the viscosity of synovial fluid, reduce pain, and reduce proinflammatory cytokines and matrix metalloproteinases. However, they do not modify disease progression and are not recommended in OA.
6. **Cochicine**
   a. Small studies favor its usefulness in osteoarthritis, though the ACR does not recommend its use.
   b. Specifically useful to reduce pain and inflammation in patients with associated chondrocalcinosis.
7. **Duloxetine: selective serotonin and norepinephrine reuptake inhibitor.**
   a. Approved for use in OA.
   b. Used at a higher dose (120 mg/day) compared to its use in fibromyalgia.

Table 10.4.6: Experimental therapies in osteoarthritis

- Nerve growth factor inhibitors: Tanezumab (phase 3 trials)
- Interleukin 1 β inhibitors
- Tumor necrosis factor α inhibitors
- Matrix metalloproteinase inhibitors
- Mitogen-activated protein kinase inhibitors
- Inducible nitric oxide inhibition
- Bradykinin B2 receptor antagonist
- Intra-articular bone morphogenic protein 7
- Intra-articular recombinant human fibroblast growth factor
- Calcitonin, bisphosphonates and strontium

approaches to restore damaged articular cartilage (Table 10.4.6).

Surgical therapy is the most definitive, and effective. It can be minimally invasive procedures (arthroscopic), related procedures including bone grafting, and total joint replacement surgery.

LEARNING POINTS

- Osteoarthritis is the most common rheumatological disease affecting the whole joint.
- Knee is the most common joint involved in osteoarthritis.
- Plain radiographs of the joints are the most common and the lowest cost modality for assessment of the joints involved.
- Management of patients includes a combination of non-pharmacological and pharmacological modalities.
- Associated comorbidities like depression, osteoporosis must be diagnosed and treated simultaneously.

FURTHER READING

1. Berenbaum F. Osteoarthritis is an inflammatory disease (osteoarthritis is notosteoarthrosis). Osteoarthritis and Cartilage. 2013; 21:16–21.

2. Bannuru RR, Osani MC, Vaysbrot EE, et al. OARSI guidelines for the non-surgical management of knee, hip, and polyarticular osteoarthritis. Osteoarthritis Cartilage. 2019; 27:1578–89.
3. Deveza LA, Hunter DJ, Unraveling osteoarthritis pathogenesis: New insights into pre-radiographic disease and patient phenotypes. Arthritis Rheumatology 2015; 67:3097–100.
4. Favero M, Belluzzi E, Ortolan A, et al. Erosive hand osteoarthritis: latest findings and outlook. Nat Rev Rheumatol. 2022; 18:171–83.
5. Kolasinski SL, Neogi T, Hochberg MC, et al. 2019 American College of Rheumatology/Arthritis Foundation Guideline for the Management of Osteoarthritis of the Hand, Hip, and Knee [published correction appears in Arthritis Care Res (Hoboken). 2021 May;73(5):764]. Arthritis Care Res (Hoboken). 2020; 72:149–62.
6. Loeser RF, Goldring SR, Scanzello CR, et al. Osteoarthritis: a disease of the joint as an organ. Arthritis Rheum. 2012; 64:1697–707.
7. Mandl LA. Osteoarthritis year in review 2018: clinical. Osteoarthritis Cartilage. 2019; 27:359–64.

Osteoporosis

Sanjiv Kapoor, Pankti Mehta

DEFINITION AND DIAGNOSIS

The WHO defines osteoporosis as a "progressive systemic skeletal disease characterized by low bone mass and microarchitectural deterioration of bone tissue, with a consequent increase in bone fragility and susceptibility to fracture." The American Association of Clinical Endocrinology has defined the diagnostic criteria for osteoporosis as described in Table 10.5.1. Common sites for major osteoporotic fractures include the hip, spine (thoracolumbar junction, T12–L1 is the most common site), distal radius and proximal humerus. In contrast, minor osteoporotic fractures commonly involve the pelvis, sacrum, ribs, distal humerus, distal femur, and ankle.

Table 10.5.1: Diagnosis of osteoporosis

Clinical	*BMD*	*FRAX*
Fragility fractures* in absence of other metabolic bone disorders and even with a normal BMD	• T score of –2.5 or lower in the lumbar spine, femoral neck, total hip or 1/3rd radius • T score between –1.0 and –2.5 and a fragility fracture of proximal humerus, pelvis or distal forearm	T score between –1.0 and –2.5 with increased fracture risk based on FRAX[#]

*Fractures secondary to trivial trauma such as fall from a standing height; [#]10-year major osteoporotic fracture risk ≥3% for hip fractures or ≥20% for other major osteoporotic fractures; *BMD:* Bone mineral density; FRAX: Fracture risk assessment tool

Clinical Assessment

A medical history and clinical examination are desirable in all women >50 years to look for:

- History of prior fragility fracture.
- Clinical risk factors for osteoporosis: age >65 years, low body weight <57.6 kg, smoking, early menopause, family history of fragility fractures, alcohol intake >3 drinks per day, secondary osteoporosis (type 1 diabetes mellitus, hypercortisolism, hyperparathyroidism, malabsorption syndromes, chronic liver disease, glucocorticoid use, rheumatoid arthritis, chronic obstructive lung disease, malignancies, thalassemia).
- Height loss or kyphosis.
- High risk of falls due to impaired vision, neurologic diseases, sedative use, or poor lighting/slippery floors/wet floors.

Osteoporosis is a painless condition and are asymptomatic. Patients develop pain and height loss once they develop fragility fractures. Therefore, a high index of suspicion in an appropriate clinical scenario is required.

INVESTIGATIONS

Bone Mineral Density (BMD)

Indications for BMD assessment with dual energy X-ray absorptiometry (DXA) include:

- Women aged ≥65 years and men aged ≥70 years
- Postmenopausal women <65 year and men <70 years old with clinical risk factors for fracture (patients on corticosteroids >3 months, rheumatoid arthritis, h/o fractures, low BMI,

smoking other medical conditions and drugs associated with decrease in BMD.)

- Women during menopausal transition with clinical fracture risk factors (low body weight, prior fracture or high-risk medication use)
- Adults with a fragility fracture
- Adults with a disease or condition associated with low bone mass or bone loss
- Adults taking medications associated with low bone mass or bone loss

Other indications are as listed by the International Society for Clinical Densitometry 2019.

Utility of BMD

BMD helps in screening, establishing severity, determining fracture risk (for every 1-standard deviation decline in BMD, the relative fracture risk increases by 1.6–2.6-fold), and monitoring response to therapy.

Site of Measurement

A dual-energy X-ray absorptiometry (DXA) of the lumbar spine (L1–L4) and bilateral proximal femur accurately measures the BMD. The distal 1/3 radius is a valuable alternative site when the former two sites cannot be used.

Pitfalls of BMD Assessment by DXA

Inaccuracies can result from:

- Improper positioning of the patient
- Fractured vertebrae
- Osteophytes in cases with osteoarthritis, syndesmophytes in spondyloarthritis, extra-articular calcifications leads to overestimation of BMD.
- Use of different machines for follow-up
- Vertebral fracture assessment: lateral spinal radiographs or vertebral fracture assessment can supplant BMD (T score < –1.0) measurement to look for vertebral fractures in patients with unexplained height loss >4 cm, women ≥70 years and men ≥80 years, self-reported spinal fractures or glucocorticoid therapy (≥5 mg per day for ≥3 months)

Other Laboratory Tests

Other laboratory tests are needed to look for causes of secondary osteoporosis.

- Complete blood count
- Serum chemistry (calcium, phosphate, total protein, albumin, liver enzymes, alkaline phosphatase, creatinine, electrolytes)
- 25-hydroxy vitamin D
- Additional tests like parathormone levels for hyperparathyroidism, T3, T4, TSH, anti-tissue transglutaminase antibodies for celiac disease, serum protein electrophoresis for multiple myeloma, etc. can be done as clinically indicated.

Bone turnover markers like C-terminal telopeptide type-1 collagen (CTX) and serum carboxy-terminal propeptide of type-I collagen (PINP) are not indicated in all patients. They may be tested in certain situations, like assessing rapid response to therapy or during drug holidays.

MANAGEMENT

The therapy aims to prevent fractures. Treatment failure is defined as a significant decline in BMD or recurrent fractures after ruling out non-compliance to treatment (Fig. 10.5.1).

Nonpharmacologic

These include:

- Physical therapy to improve strength and balance.
- Fall prevention: Modification of drugs (sedatives, antihypertensives), a transformation of the environment (anti-slip mats, railings, walking aids, etc.), correction of visual impairment, and control of other comorbidities.
- Smoking cessation.
- Restrict alcohol intake to 2 drinks per day.
- Adequate dietary/supplemental calcium intake (1000–1200 mg/day).

Pharmacologic

A summary of the drugs approved for the treatment of osteoporosis and their fracture risk reduction are described in Table 10.5.2. The choice of medication depends on the severity of osteoporosis, cost of therapy, comorbidities, and adverse effect profile.

Antiresorptive Agents

Oral or intravenous bisphosphonates and denosumab are preferred for patients diagnosed with osteoporosis without any prior fragility fractures. Amongst the former, alendronate and risedronate are preferred as they prevent vertebral and hip fractures, unlike ibandronate. Alendronate is given for five years

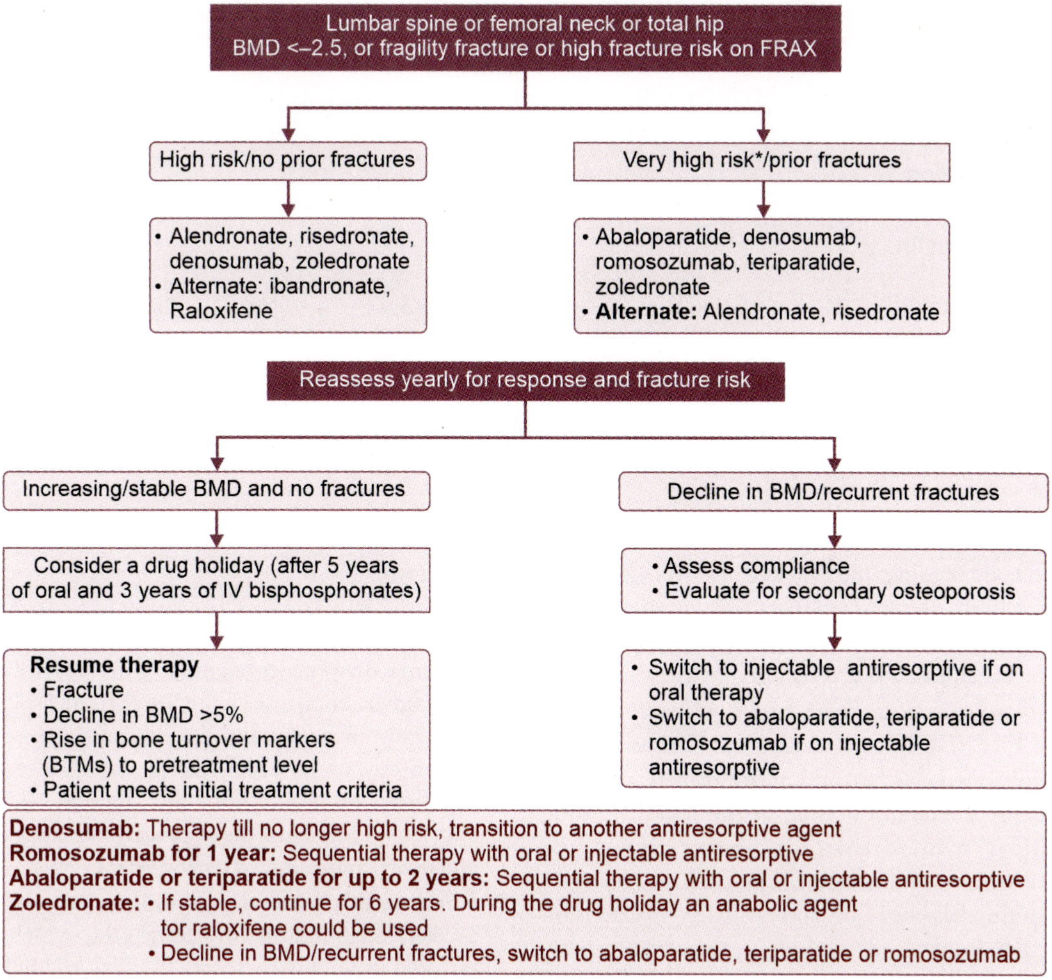

Fig. 10.5.1: Management strategy of osteoporosis; *BMD:* Bone mineral density. *Advanced age, frailty, high risk of fall, very low BMD, glucocorticoid use

Table 10.5.2: Drugs used for the treatment of osteoporosis

Drugs	*Dose*	*Fracture risk reduction*			*Special adverse effects*
		Vertebral fracture	*Nonvertebral fracture*	*Hip fracture*	
Bisphosphonates					
Alendronate	10 mg/day or 70 mg/week	Yes	Yes	Yes	ONJ, atypical femur fractures
Risedronate	5 mg/day or 35 mg/week	Yes	Yes	Yes	
Ibandronate	2.5 mg/day or 150 mg/month	Yes	No*	No*	
Zoledronate acid	5 mg IV yearly	Yes	Yes	Yes	
Anti-RANKL antibody					
Denosumab	60 mg sc 6 monthly	Yes	Yes	No*	High fracture risk after stopping the drug

(Contd.)

Table 10.5.2: Drugs used for the treatment of osteoporosis (*Contd.*)

Drugs	*Dose*	*Fracture risk reduction*			*Special adverse effects*
		Vertebral fracture	*Nonvertebral fracture*	*Hip fracture*	
PTHrP analog					
Abaloparatide	80 mg sc/day	Yes	Yes	No*	—
Anti-sclerostin antibody					
Romosozumab	210 mg sc/month	Yes	Yes	No*	Cardiovascular risk
Others					
Calcitonin	200 IU intranasally/day	Yes	No*	No*	
Raloxifene	60 mg/day	Yes	No*	No*	

*Study may not powered adequately

PTH: Parathormone; *rP:* related peptide; *sc:* subcutaneous; *RANKL;* Receptor activator of nuclear factor kappa-B ligand

and zoledronate for three years, followed by a drug-free holiday as per the FIT and HORIZON trials, respectively. Response to therapy is monitored with a yearly BMD to look for a response. Compliance of 80% for at least a year is required to assess response.

Denosumab is given for 5–10 years as per the FREEDOM trial extension. Denosumab is transitioned over to oral antiresorptive drugs to prevent a rebound decline in the BMD. A drug holiday reduced risks for adverse effects like osteonecrosis of the jaw and atypical femur fractures because trials like FLEX and HORIZON extension for alendronate and zoledronate, respectively, show a nonsignificant decline in BMD during this period despite withholding therapy. The period of drug holiday is monitored for the occurrence of fractures or a decrease in BMD. The patient can be switched to zoledronate or denosumab in case of intolerance or non-response to oral therapy (Fig. 10.5.1).

Anabolic Agents

In very high-risk cases or prior fragility fractures, anabolic agents are preferred as the first line. Teriparatide and abalopartaide are given for 18–24 months and romosozumab for 12 months, followed by antiresorptive therapy. Romosozumab should be avoided in patients with high cardiovascular risk. Zoledronate is also an alternative and can be given for six years, followed by a drug holiday (Fig. 10.5.1).

PREVENTION

Adequate calcium and vitamin D intake, regular weight-bearing, balance exercises, and avoidance of tobacco and alcohol is the key to preventing osteoporosis.

Special Populations

1. **Patients on glucocorticoids:** Glucocorticoid-induced osteoporosis is an important aspect, especially in rheumatology. It translates into a high risk of vertebral fractures due to more significant trabecular bone loss. Figures 10.5.2 and 10.5.3 highlight the approach to managing glucocorticoid-induced osteoporosis.
2. **Rheumatoid arthritis:** These patients have accelerated inflammatory bone loss, which is factored in the FRAX score.

CONCLUSION

Rheumatologists have an essential role in carefully evaluating the risk, therapy, monitoring, and prevention of osteoporosis, especially in patients with glucocorticoid use.

LEARNING POINTS

- Osteoporosis is a risk factor for fracture. Bone strength = bone mineral density (60%) + bone quality/architecture (40%).
- Defining osteoporosis-BMD–T score < –2.5 SD, clinical–fragility fracture, FRAX based–10 years risk fracture >20% major osteoporotic fracture risk or hip fracture risk >3%.
- Most fractures occur in the osteopenic range, clinical assessment FRAX, comorbidities, and the patient profile should be taken into account for management.

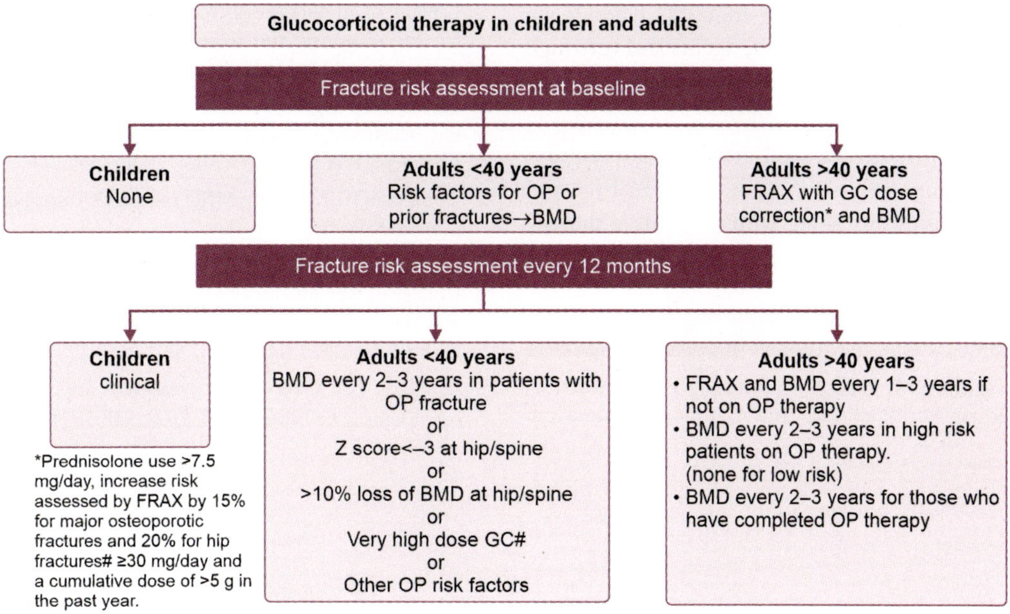

Fig. 10.5.2: Evaluation of a patient on glucocorticoids (GC) for osteoporosis (OP). *Prednisolone use >7.5 mg/day, increase risk assessed by FRAX by 15% for major osteoporotic fractures and 20% for hip fractures #>30 mg/day and a cumulative dose of >5 g in the past year.

Adapted from: Buckley L, et al. Arthritis Care Res (Hoboken). 2017; 69:1095–110.

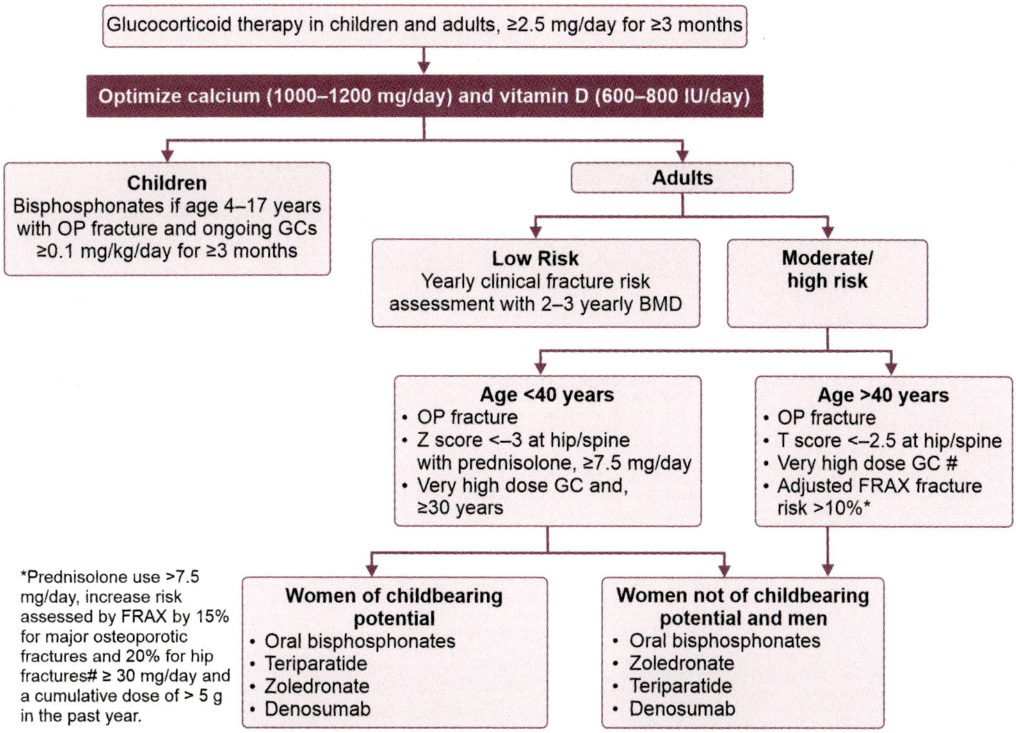

Fig. 10.5.3: Treatment of glucocorticoid (GC)-induced osteoporosis (OP). *Prednisolone use >7.5 mg/day, increase risk assessed by FRAX by 15% for major osteoporotic fractures and 20% for hip fractures #>30 mg/day and a cumulative dose of >5 g in the past year.

Adapted from: Buckley L, et al. Arthritis Care Res (Hoboken). 2017;69:1095–110.

- Patient risk stratification–high-risk patients are treated with anti-resorptive agents and very high risk with anabolic followed by antiresorptive drugs (sequential therapy).
- Glucocorticoid-induced osteoporosis requires assessment for osteoporosis at baseline and regular intervals along with preventive therapy in high-risk cases.

FURTHER READING

1. Camacho PM, Petak SM, Binkley N, et al. American Association of clinical endocrinologists/American College of Endocrinology Clinical Practice guidelines for the diagnosis and treatment of postmenopausal osteoporosis-2020 Update. Endocr Pract. 2020;26:1–46.
2. Chotiyarnwong P, McCloskey EV. Pathogenesis of glucocorticoid-induced osteoporosis and options for treatment. Nat Rev Endocrinol. 2020;16:437–47.
3. Compston JE, McClung MR, Leslie WD. Osteoporosis. *Lancet.* 2019; 393:364–76.
4. Buckley L, Guyatt G, Fink HA, et al. 2017 American College of Rheumatology Guideline for the Prevention and Treatment of Glucocorticoid-Induced Osteoporosis. Arthritis Care Res (Hoboken). 2017;69:1095–110.
5. Langdahl BL. Overview of treatment approaches to osteoporosis. Br J Pharmacol. 2021;178:1891–906.

Chapter 10.6

Juvenile Idiopathic Arthritis

Anu Punnen, Sathish Kumar

INTRODUCTION

Juvenile idiopathic arthritis (JIA) is the most common cause for chronic arthritis in childhood. According to International League of Associations for Rheumatology (ILAR) JIA is defined as a chronic arthritis that occurs before the 16th birthday and persists for at least 6 weeks with other known etiology is excluded. The 2001 ILAR classification of JIA is accepted by clinicians worldwide and is based upon clinical features and certain laboratory parameters namely rheumatoid factor (RF), anti-nuclear antibody (ANA), and HLA B27. In this classification there are eight distinct clinical types of JIA. These are: Systemic onset, oligoarthritis, polyarthritis RF+, polyarthritis RF-, psoriatic arthritis, enthesitis-related arthritis (ERA), and others. This classification of JIA into relatively homogeneous subset by the ILAR is mainly for research purposes and management.

SUBTYPES

Classification of JIA as per ILAR requires the presence of certain features and exclusion criteria during the first 6 months of presentation.

To classify a child as oligoarthritis the number of joints involved is <4, it can remain 'persistent' or 'extended' if >4 joints get involved after the six months of illness.

Polyarthritis is involvement of >5 joints and can be with or without RF.

Systemic onset JIA (SoJIA) is typified by the fever of at least >2 weeks duration. The fever is quotidian in pattern (at least once a day goes up to >39°C and falls down to 37°C) and must be present for at least 3 days. One other feature must be present either an evanescent rash, lymphadenopathy, hepatomegaly and/or splenomegaly, or serositis to classify a child as SoJIA.

Psoriatic arthritis is arthritis and psoriasis OR arthritis with two of: psoriasis in a blood first degree relative, dactylitis, and nail pitting.

ERA is classified based on arthritis and enthesitis. Or the child should have arthritis/enthesitis with two of the following: sacroilitis, HLA-B27+, arthritis in a male child older than 6 years old, acute anterior uveitis, positive family history (1st degree relative) of HLA B27 related disease.

TREATMENT

Goals of therapy are as follows:

1. Stop ongoing inflammation
2. Prevent joint damage in long-term
3. Enhance normal growth and development in child with JIA
4. To reduce medication side effects especially with corticosteroids

Multidisciplinary team with pediatric rheumatologist, paediatrician, occupational therapist and physiotherapist are required for successful management of child with JIA.

Oligoarthritis and Polyarthritis

Consider oligo JIA when a young girl presents with <4 large joint arthritis with positive ANA. Large joints like knees, ankles, wrists, or elbows are involved. Unusually hip joint can be involved very late in disease course. ANA is positive in 60–80% of children with oligo JIA. ANA positivity is associated with a higher risk of asymptomatic chronic anterior uveitis. Hence regular eye examination is advised. The frequency of eye examination depends on the age of the child, and the duration of the disease, and the status of ANA (Table 10.6.1). In children where the onset of disease was at younger than 6 years, and where the duration of disease is <4 years, and are ANA positive need more frequent eye examination preferable every three months. Whereas those older than 6 years, longer disease duration, and ANA negative fall in the moderate to low risk of uveitis and can have eye examination between 6 monthly to one yearly (Tables 10.6.1 and 10.6.2). The frequency of eye examination in systemic JIA is annual, irrespective of ANA status and disease duration. The steps to management of oligoarticular JIA is illustrated in Figure 10.6.1.

RF positive polyarthritis is usually seen in adolescent girls and they present with symmetrical polyarthritis of large and small joints. They may develop rheumatoid nodules and joint erosions. This subtype is equivalent to adult rheumatoid arthritis. In the management (Fig. 10.6.2) apart

Table 10.6.1: Eye examination in ANA positive children with oligoarthritis/polyarthritis

Risk for uveitis	*Age at onset, years*	*Duration of JIA*	*Frequency of eye examination*
High	≤6	≤4 years	Every 3 months
Moderate	≤6 >6	>4 years ≤4 years	Every 6 months
Low	≤6 >6	>7 years >4 years	Every 12 months

Table 10.6.2: Eye examination in ANA negative children with oligoarthritis/polyarthritis

Risk for uveitis	*Age at onset, years*	*Duration of JIA*	*Frequency of eye examination*
Moderate	≤6	≤4 years	6 months
Low	≤6	>4 years	12 months
Low	>6	Any duration	12 months

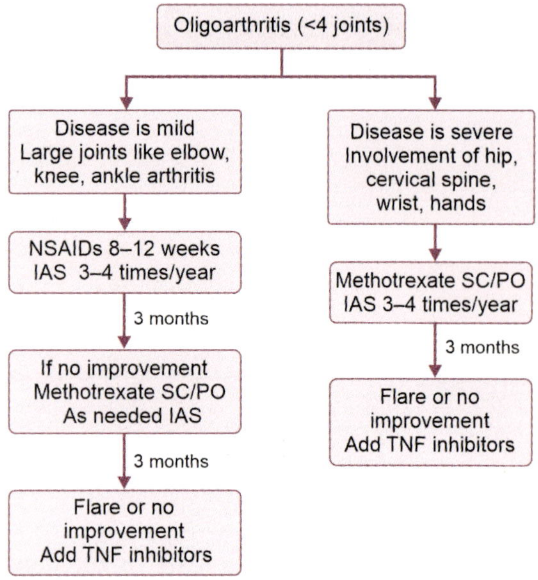

Fig. 10.6.1: Management algorithm for oligoarticular JIA
NSAIDs: Nonsteroidal anti-inflammatory drugs; *IAS:* Intra-articular steroids; *PO:* Per orally; *SC:* Subcutaneous

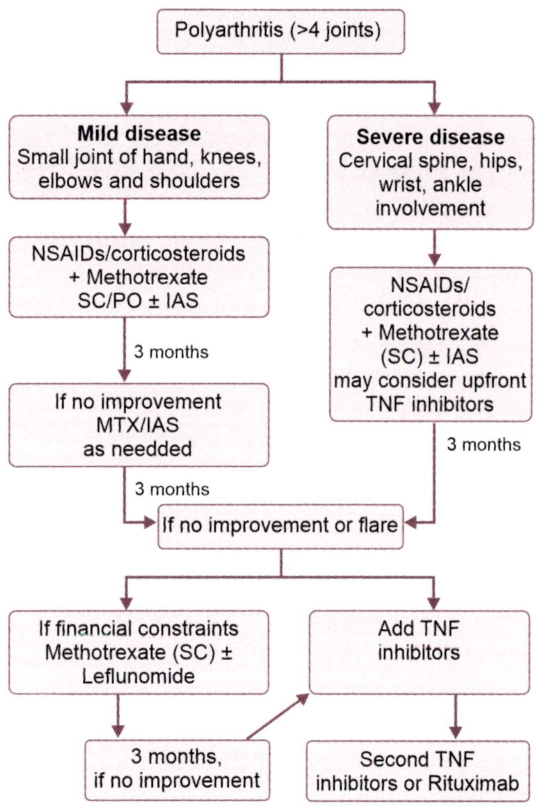

Fig. 10.6.2: Management algorithm for polyarticular JIA
NSAIDs: Non steroidal anti-inflammatory drugs; *IAS:* Intra-articular steroids; *PO:* Per orally; *SC:* Subcutaneous

Table 10.6.3: Dosage and monitoring of commonly used DMARDs

DMARD dose and route of administration	*Monitoring*
Methotrexate Dose is 10–15 mg/m² once a week, by oral or subcutaneous administration. The maximum dose is 25 mg/day. Folic acid twice a week.	CBC, LFT, and serum creatinine at baseline and every 3 months once
Sulfasalazine This drug is given by mouth. Start with 10–15 mg/kg daily (maximum 500 mg) in divided doses. Increase every week up to 30–50 mg/kg daily (maximum 2 g).	CBC, LFT, creatinine at baseline and every 2 weeks till you reach full dose and then every 3 months
Leflunomide It is given by mouth. The dose of Leflunomide is as per weight of the child <20 kg: 10 mg on alternate days Between 20–40 the dose is 10 mg once a day If weight >40 kg, then the dose is 20 mg once a day	CBC, LFT, creatinine at baseline and then every 3 months

DMARDs: Disease modifying antirheumtic drugs; *CBC:* Complete blood counts; *LFT:* Liver function test

from NSAIDs, corticosteroids and methotrexate, upfront TNF inhibitors can be considered in case of severe disease. The dose of conventional DMARDs in children is summarized in Table 10.6.3.

Systemic Arthritis

As the name indicates, systemic JIA have both systemic symptoms and arthritis:

- Classical quotidian fever: Fever spikes >38.5°C, which return to baseline or below and occurs once or twice daily fever. Children appear unwell during fever episodes and well during afebrile periods.
- Evanescent, salmon-colored rash over trunk and extremities which occurs with fever and occasionally pruritic
- Hepatosplenomegaly
- Generalized lymphadenopathy
- Serositis (pleuritis, pericarditis, ascites)
- Arthritis can occur at presentation or develop later. Arthritis can be oligoarticular, affecting knees, wrists and ankles or polyarticular involving small and large joints. Cervical spine and hip joints can be also involved

While managing systemic disease it is useful to categorize them as 'active systemic and articular' dominant or 'articular' dominant (Fig. 10.6.3). Those with predominantly active systemic will need corticosteroids and methotrexate upfront with pulse dose corticosteroids in severe disease (Fig. 10.6.3). Further this group if not having adequate response to such treatment is best managed with IL-1 or IL-6 blocking agents, in contradistinction to articular dominant where TNFi are preferred (Table 10.6.4). Leflunomide (Table 10.6.3) is an option for arthritis dominant disease when TNFi are unavailable due to financial constraints.

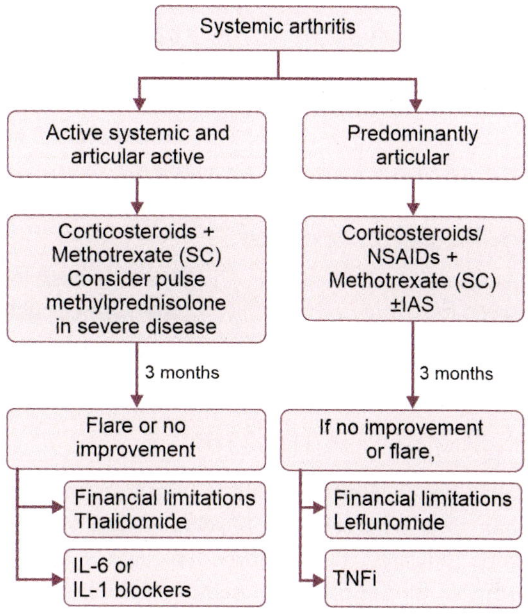

Fig. 10.6.3: Management algorithm for systemic JIA

NSAIDs: Non steroidal anti-inflammatory drugs; *IAS:* Intra-articular steroids; *PO:* Per orally; *SC:* Subcutaneous; *IL-6 blocker:* Interleukin-6 inhibition; *TNFi:* Tumor necrosis factor-α inhibitor

Table 10.6.4: Biological agents used in treatment of JIA

Biologic	*Dosage*
Etanercept is a TNFi given by subcutaneous (SC) route	Dose is 0.8 mg/kg given once a week or 0.4 mg/kg every two weeks. Maximum 50 mg/week.
Adalimumab is also a TNFi given by SC	Dose is based on weight of the child. Weight between 15–30 kg, dose is 20 mg every two weeks Weight >40 kg, dose is 40 mg every two weeks.
Infliximab is a TNFi given intravenously (IV)	The dose is 5 mg/kg at week 0, 2, 6 weeks, then every 8 weeks.
Tocilizumab is an IL-6 blocker, given either IV or SC	**IV Tocilizumab preparation** In polyarticular JIA, IV tocilizumab is administered every 4 weeks. 10 mg/kg if child's weight <30 kg 8 mg/kg if weight is >30 kg. Systemic arthritis 12 mg/kg every 2 weeks for those <30 kg 8 mg/kg every 2 weeks if weight >30 kg **SC tocilizumab preparation** Polyarticular JIA 162 mg every 3 weeks if the child is <30 kg; 162 mg every 2 weeks if child is >30 kg. Systemic arthritis 162 mg every 2 weeks if weight <30 kg 162 mg every week if weight is >30 kg
Rituximab targets CD20+ B cells is given by IV infusion	It is given 500 mg/m^2 × 2 doses at 15 days apart
Anakinra is a IL-1 blocker given SC	Maximum dose is 100 mg/day Otherwise calculated as 1–4 mg/kg/day

TNFi: Tumor necrosis factor-α inhibitor; *IL-6:* Interleukin-6; *IL-1:* Interleukin-1

ENTHESITIS-RELATED ARTHRITIS

Enthesitis-related arthritis is common in boys than girls who are over 6 years of age. As the name indicates, these children have enthesitis and arthritis. Enthesitis (inflammation of the insertion sites of tendons, ligaments and fascia to bone) is pathognomonic of this subtype. Examine for enthesitis at the insertion sites of the achilles tendon, plantar fascia and quadriceps tendon. Lower limb joints like knees, ankles and hips are commonly affected. Spine involvement typically develops after second decade. Other manifestations of ERA include tarsitis and Dactylitis. Acute symptomatic anterior uveitis presenting with eye pain and redness (unilateral/bilateral) occurs in children with ERA.

Children with ERA with active sacroiliitis and/or enthesitis are first managed with NSAIDs, if there is inadequate response or no improvement the next step is TNFi (Table 10.6.3). Those with hip or tarsal joint disease are given both NSAIDs and methotrexate/or sulfasalazine failing which TNFi is indicated. Those with only peripheral arthritis will benefit from intra-articular steroid injections and NSAIDs, failing which methotrexate and sulfasalazine are indicated (Fig. 10.6.4).

LEARNING POINTS

- JIA is clinical diagnosis.
- Consider/Suspect JIA in children with persistent arthritis >6 weeks when other causes of arthritis are excluded.
- Use investigations like RF, ANA and HLA-B27 to distinguish different clinical subtypes.
- Treatment is based on clinical phenotype

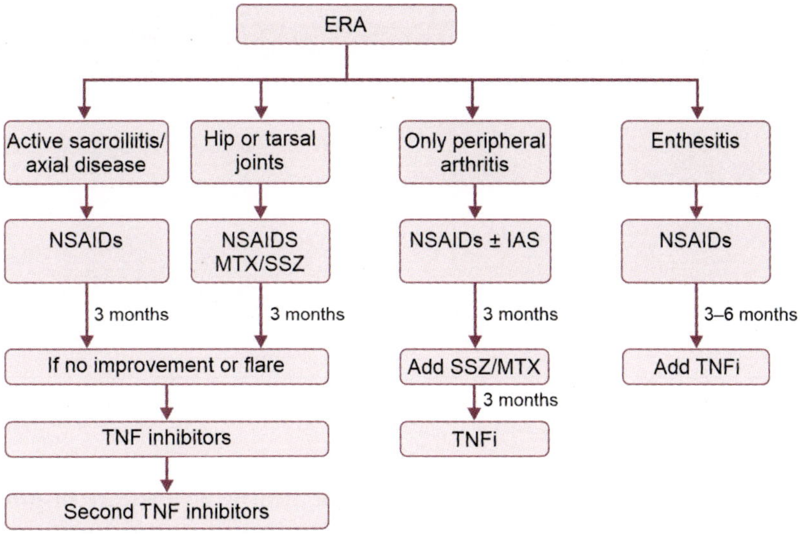

Fig. 10.6.4: Management algorithm for enthesitis-related arthritis (ERA)

NSAIDs: Nonsteroidal anti-inflammatory drugs; *IAS:* Intra-articular steroids; *MTX:* Methotrexate; *SSZ:* Sulphasalazine; *TNFi:* Tumor necrosis factor-α inhibitor

- Start conventional DMARDs followed by biological DMARDs if there is no response or inadequate response.

FURTHER READING

1. Heiligenhaus A, Niewerth M, Ganser G, et al.; German Uveitis in Childhood Study Group. Prevalence and complications of uveitis in juvenile idiopathic arthritis in a population-based nation-wide study in Germany: suggested modification of the current screening guidelines. Rheumatology (Oxford). 2007;46:1015–9.
2. McCurdy D, Parsa MF. Updates in Juvenile Idiopathic Arthritis. Adv Pediatr. 2021; 68:143–70.
3. Momah T, Ray L. Juvenile idiopathic arthritis: Old disease, new tactics. J Fam Pract. 2019; 68:E8-E13.
4. Onel K, Rumsey DG, Shenoi S. Juvenile Idiopathic Arthritis Treatment Updates. Rheumatic Disease Clinics. 2021;47:545–63.
5. Petty RE, Southwood TR, Manners P, et al.; International League of Associations for Rheumatology. International League of Associations for Rheumatology classification of juvenile idiopathic arthritis: second revision, Edmonton, 2001. J Rheumatol. 2004;31):390–2.
6. Vanoni F, Minoia F, Malattia C. Biologics in juvenile idiopathic arthritis: a narrative review. Eur J Pediatr. 2017;176:1147–153.

Adult-onset Still's Disease

Kavitha Mohanasundaram, Molly Mary Thabah

INTRODUCTION

Adult-onset Still's disease (AOSD) is characterized by a symptom complex of fever, evanescent rash, arthritis, and elevated acute phase response. It shares many clinical features with systemic onset juvenile idiopathic arthritis (SoJIA). It is a disease of young adults, though older people can also be involved. The presentation of AOSD with high-grade fever, rash, and arthritis often mimics infections, malignancy and systemic autoimmune diseases. Thus, it cannot be overemphasized that all these conditions need to be ruled out before establishing a diagnosis of AOSD.

PATHOGENESIS

AOSD considered to be a nonfamilial, polygenic, autoinflammatory syndrome has several features of monogenic autoinflammatory syndromes, namely fever, polyserositis, polymorphonuclear leukocytosis, markedly elevated acute phase reactants, absence of autoantibodies, and a good response to interleukin 1 (IL-1) blockade. Typically, the onset of autoinflammatory syndromes is abrupt and settles down spontaneously most of the time, only to recur. However, the characteristic pattern of fever of AOSD, the absence of a single gene defect, and the presence of destructive arthritis argue against it being an autoinflammatory syndrome. Various viral or bacterial agents such as Epstein Barr virus, measles, mumps, *Chlamydia*, and *Campylobacter jejuni* are implicated as triggers of an attack that initiates an inflammatory cascade (Fig. 10.7.1). Amplification of the inflammatory cascade is contributed by an increase in proinflammatory activity and defective regulatory cytokines.

CLINICAL FEATURES

The classical features of AOSD are fever, arthritis or arthralgia, and rash. Sore throat, myalgia, weight loss and lymphadenopathy can be accompanying features.

Fever: It is a universal feature, with >90% of affected individuals presenting with fever. Fever is usually high grade (>39°C), accompanied by chills and rigors, with a quotidian or double quotidian pattern; typical spiking is observed in the evenings. Fever is present during the active phase of the disease and is associated with rapid weight loss.

Arthritis/arthralgia: It is present in >70% of AOSD patients, most times accompanying spiking fever. The usual pattern is polyarthritis, with symmetrical involvement of the wrists, knee and ankle. Interphalangeal joints of the hand, elbow, hip, sacroiliac, metacarpophalangeal, metatarsophalangeal joints and temporomandibular joints can also be involved. Synovial fluid is inflammatory, can be thick and purulent due to neutrophilic predominance often mimicking septic arthritis. Arthritis if left untreated result in destructive symmetrical arthritis. Isolated carpal ankylosis in the absence of erosions in metacarpophalangeal joints and proximal interphalangeal joints is a hallmark feature of AOSD.

Skin rash: It is present in more than 2/3rd of affected individuals. It is typically described as a salmon-colored, evanescent, maculopapular rash (Fig. 10.7.2), occurs during fever spikes, involves

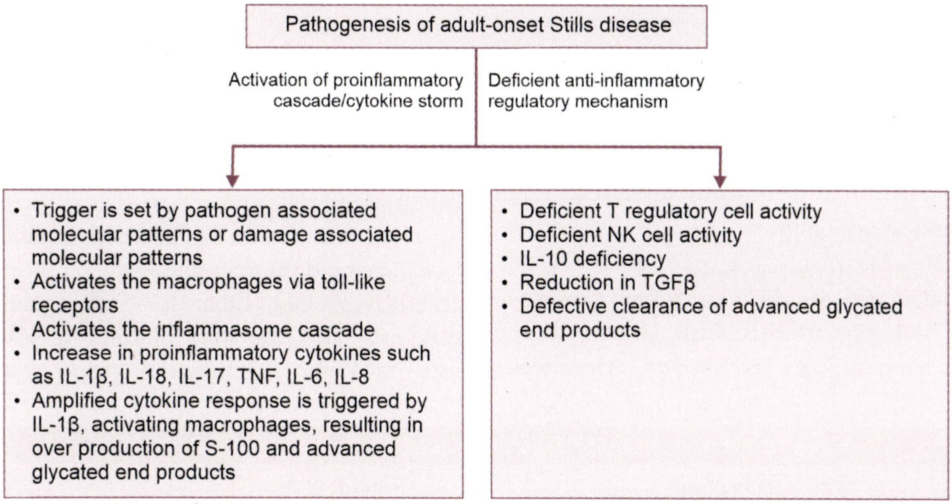

Fig. 10.7.1: Laboratory and clinical studies indicate that an important pathophysiological mechanisms of adult-onset Still's disease is an inappropriate activation of the innate immune system, with hypersecretion of the proinflammatory cytokines, namely IL-1 and IL-6, and a defective anti-inflammatory regulatory mechanism

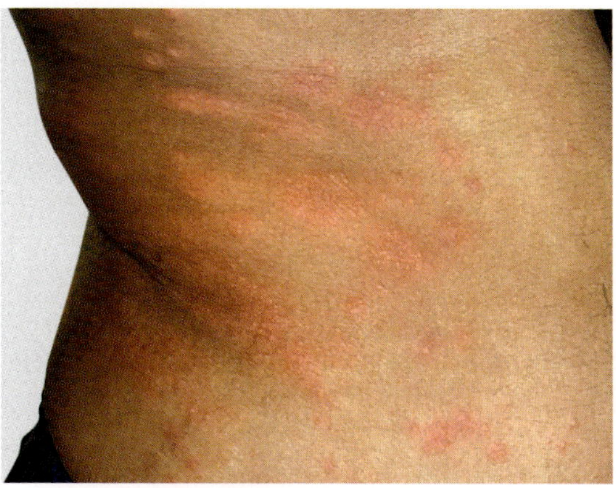

Fig. 10.7.2: Maculopapular erythematous rash over the trunk in a patient with adult onset Still's disease

the trunk and proximal limbs and typically spares the face, palms and sole. They are pruritic at times, and exhibit dermographism and Koebner's phenomenon. Purpura is uncommon, if present patients will need to be evaluated for hemophagocytic lymphohistiocytosis and disseminated intravascular coagulation (DIC), both of which are known complications of AOSD (Table 10.7.1).

Other clinical features: They are sore throat associated with odynophagia (due to inflammation of cricoarytenoid joints), myalgia, serositis (pleuritis and pericarditis), lymphadenopathy, hepatomegaly, splenomegaly, weight loss and abdominal pain. Involvement of lung (12.5%) is associated with

Table 10.7.1: Complications of adult-onset Still's disease (AOSD)

Life-threatening complications
1. Macrophage activation syndrome
2. Disseminated intravascular coagulation
3. Pulmonary arterial hypertension
4. Fulminant hepatitis
5. Acute respiratory distress syndrome
6. Myocarditis
7. Thrombotic microangiopathy
8. Diffuse alveolar hemorrhage
9. Cardiac tamponade
Long-term complications
systemic AA amyloidosis

high ferritin levels, and is associated with increased mortality.

PRESENTATION AND COURSE

The presentation may be predominantly systemic with fever and weight loss (60%), or predominant chronic polyarthritis (40%). The further course of systemic form is either **monocyclic with a single episode** which can go through for months but does not recur. Or it follows a polycyclic **course where** there are frequent systemic flares, the duration between each flare can range anywhere from months to years. Arthritis symptoms may or may not be present and the patient is in complete remission between flares. Patients who present with **predominant chronic polyarthritis** have a chronic course resulting in destructive arthropathy and a poor response to treatment. AOSD can result in complications, some of them life-threatening (Table 10.7.1).

In Indian patients, the most common course of AOSD is chronic arthritis. Rash, sore throat and lymphadenopathy are uncommon. Most series report macrophage activation syndrome as a major complication and one series suggested sulphasalazine as a trigger.

DIAGNOSIS

Investigations must be carried out to rule out infectious diseases, malignancies (lymphoma and leukemias) and autoimmune diseases. Classification criteria for AOSD (Table 10.7.2) may guide in the diagnosis. The laboratory findings in AOSD are listed in Table 10.7.3. Serum ferritin apart from

Table 10.7.2: Classification criteria for adult-onset Still's disease (AOSD)

	Yamaguchi et al.	*Fautrel et al.*
Major criteria	1. Fever 2. Arthralgia 3. Typical rash 4. Leukocytosis	1. Spiking fever ≥39°C 2. Arthralgia 3. Transient erythema 4. Pharyngitis 5. Polymorphonuclear leukocytes ≥80% 6. Glycosylated ferritin ≤20%
Minor criteria	1. Sore throat 2. Lymphadenopathy and/ or splenomegaly 3. Transaminitis 4. Negative RF and Negative ANA	1. Maculopapular rash 2. Leukocytes >10,000 cells/mm^3
Exclusion criteria	Malignancy, infections, autoimmune connective tissue diseases	None
Classification	Requires five criteria, two of which should be major. The exclusion criteria should be applied.	Requires four or more major criteria OR three major and two minor criteria
Comment	Yamaguchi criteria is widely used in the classification of AOSD. The sensitivity and specificity are 96% and 98%, respectively	Fautrel criteria differ from Yamaguchi in that glycosylated ferritin is included, while doing away with the exclusion criteria. It has a sensitivity of 87% and a specificity of 97%.

Table 10.7.3: Laboratory features of adult-onset Still's disease (AOSD)

- Neutrophilic leukocytosis is a major feature of AOSD with polymorphonuclear leukocytes contributing to >80% of WBCs.
- C-reactive protein and erythrocyte sedimentation rate are markedly elevated
- Mild transaminitis is a common feature
- Rheumatoid factor is negative
- Antinuclear antibodies are typically negative
- Serum ferritin >5 times of the normal limit (typically >1,000 µg/L)
- Glycosylated ferritin <20% of the total ferritin level
- Lymph node histopathology often shows reactive lymphoid hyperplasia

being an acute phase reactant in AOSD has been hypothesized to contribute towards pathogenesis too, by activating NF-κB resulting in excess IL-1β production. Serum ferritin >5 times of the normal limit (typically >1,000 μg/L) has a sensitivity and specificity of 40% and 80% respectively for the diagnosis of AOSD. When combined with values of glycosylated ferritin that are <20% of the total ferritin level, sensitivity further increases to 70% and specificity to 93%. Normally glycosylated ferritin is >50% of total serum ferritin.

Fluorodeoxyglucose Positron Emission Tomography (FDG-PET)

The usefulness of FDG-PET lies in ruling out infections and malignancy before attributing a fever of unknown origin to AOSD. The findings on FDG-PET scan in AOSD *per se* is a diffuse uptake in the spleen, bone marrow and symmetrical involvement of lymph nodes, with joint involvement. But a biopsy of lymph nodes is needed to rule out neoplastic lesions. Lymph node biopsy findings in AOSD are nonspecific with reactive lymphoid hyperplasia.

MANAGEMENT

NSAIDs: They are used for symptomatic relief of arthritis. Often there is a prompt response to naproxen for fever; which may be a clue to the diagnosis. Once the diagnosis is established definitive treatment is commenced (Fig. 10.7.3).

Prednisolone: A 0.5–1 mg/kg forms the first-line treatment. Fever and rash respond well to glucocorticoids, and responses to glucocorticoids is often quick. Tapering of glucocorticoids is initiated once systemic and articular symptoms are controlled, usually after a month. However, close to 40% of patients flare while tapering glucocorticoids resulting in steroid dependence and consequent increase in side effects.

Methotrexate: Up to 25 mg/week by the oral route is effective in controlling systemic and articular symptoms in 40–70% of patients who fail monotherapy with glucocorticoids or in patients who are steroid dependent.

Cyclosporine a and leflunomide: They are second-line agents when glucocorticoids are ineffective or steroid-dependent.

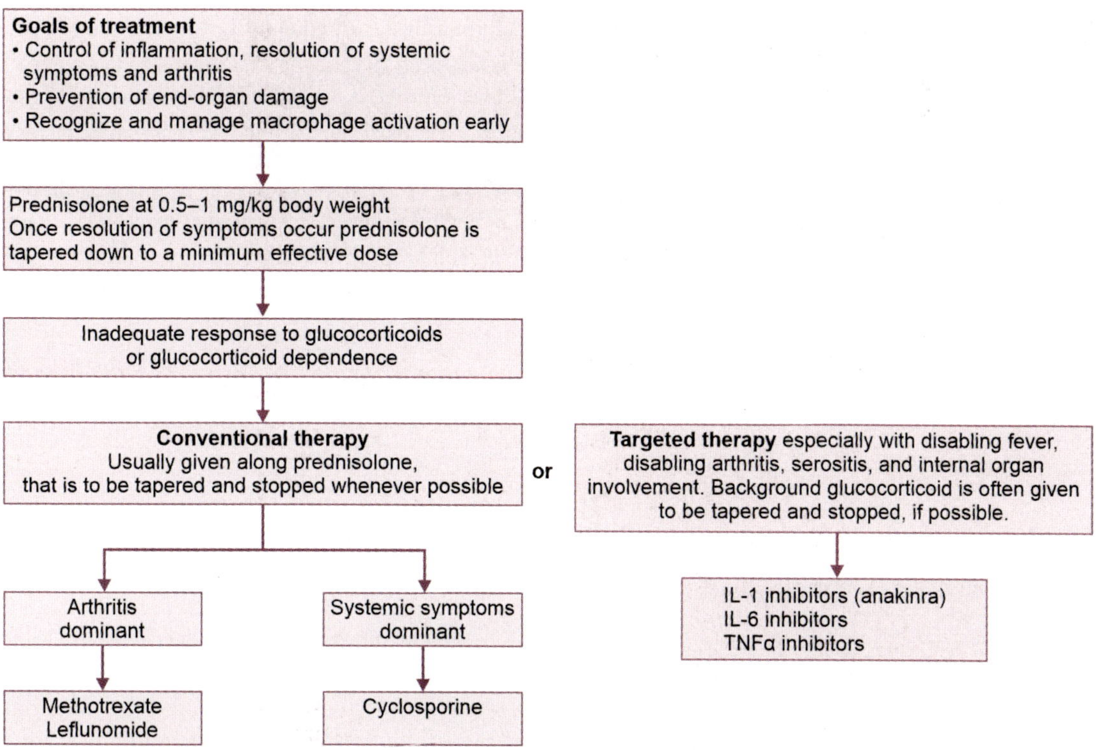

Fig. 10.7.3: An approach to the treatment of adult-onset Still's disease (Indian scenario)

Biological DMARDs: About 30% do not respond to the conventional lines of management. These refractory AOSD patients will require targeted therapy.

Interleukin 1 (IL-1) blockers: Anakinra, an IL-1 receptor antagonist is approved for the treatment of AOSD. It results in rapid resolution of systemic and articular symptoms with normalization of inflammatory markers. It also has a steroid-sparing effect. Other IL-1 blockers used in AOSD are rilonacept and canakinumab. Anakinra is indicated in AOSD when there are active systemic features and moderate to high disease activity, or in patients with continued disease activity after treatment with NSAIDs or glucocorticoids. For patients weighing >50 kg the dose is 100 mg/day by subcutaneous injection or 1–2 mg/kg/day if body weight <50 kg. It is approved as monotherapy or with other DMARD. Currently, none of the IL-1 blockers are available in India.

Tumor necrosis factor α inhibitors (TNFi): Infliximab, etanercept, and adalimumab are sometimes employed in arthritis-dominant disease when glucocorticoids and methotrexate fail. Systemic dominant AOSD responds poorly to TNFi.

Interleukin 6 (IL-6) inhibitors: Tocilizumab gives a good improvement in both articular and systemic symptoms in patients where methotrexate, anakinra, or TNFi have failed. Systemic symptoms respond much better, articular symptoms might persist. Tocilizumab is given either subcutaneously 162.5 mg once a week or intravenously (IV) at 8 mg/kg once in 4 weeks. The duration of treatment in most series is 12–24 months. About 75% of patients achieve remission on tocilizumab.

Other drugs: B cell and T cell-targeted therapies like rituximab and abatacept have been tried in AOSD with variable success. IL-18 inhibition by tadekinig alfa, a human recombinant IL-18 binding protein proved to be safe and efficacious in phase II trials for the treatment of AOSD refractory to conventional therapy. Role of JAK inhibitors are under evaluation for the treatment of AOSD.

LEARNING POINTS

1. AOSD is a rare disease presenting with fever, arthritis and rash.
2. Infections, malignancy, and other autoimmune diseases need to be ruled out before making a diagnosis of AOSD.
3. Anakinra and Tocilizumab are the most effective for the treatment of AOSD.

FURTHER READING

1. Fautrel B, Zing E, Golmard JL, Le Moel G, Bissery A, Rioux C, et al. Proposal for a new set of classification criteria for adult-onset still disease. Medicine (Baltimore). 2002;81:194–200.
2. Feist E, Mitrovic S, Fautrel B. Mechanisms, biomarkers and targets for adult-onset Still's disease. Nat Rev Rheumatol 2018;14:603–18.
3. Yamaguchi M, Ohta A, Tsunematsu T, Kasukawa R, Mizushima Y, Kashiwagi H, et al. Preliminary criteria for the classification of adult Still's the disease. J Rheumatol. 1992;19:424–30.
4. Zhou S, Qiao J, Bai J, Wu Y, Fang H. Biological therapy of traditional therapy-resistant adult-onset Still's disease: an evidence-based review. Ther Clin Risk Manag. 2018; 14:167–71.

Macrophage Activation Syndrome

Rutviz Mistry

INTRODUCTION

Hemophagocytic lymphangiohistiocytosis (HLH) seen in the context of autoimmune rheumatic diseases is called macrophage activation syndrome (MAS). It is caused by inappropriate activation and survival of cytotoxic T cells and histiocytosis leading to systemic hyperinflammation. It is characterized by fever, pancytopenia, high C-reactive protein (CRP), liver insufficiency, coagulopathy, and neurologic symptoms. If undiagnosed, macrophage activation syndrome has mortality ranging from 5 to 39%.

MAS is commonly seen in systemic onset juvenile idiopathic arthritis (sJIA), its adult variant adult onset still's disease (AOSD). Its incidence is around 10% in longitudinal series of sJIA depending on the definition used for diagnosis. However, it is being increasingly acknowledged that it is underdiagnosed, especially in adult rheumatic conditions like SLE, dermatomyositis, and Sjogren's disease, highlighting a need for increased education and index of suspicion. Early diagnosis and timely treatment can be lifesaving.

CLINICAL PRESENTATION

Fever is the cardinal feature of MAS seen in almost all pediatric and adult patients. The transition of fever pattern from intermittent to continuous suggests the onset of MAS in the setting of sJIA/AOSD. It mimics sepsis with progressive worsening cytopenia, multiorgan failure, and inadequate response to treatment. Certain clinical features help in early recognition of MAS (Table 10.8.1).

Table 10.8.1: Clinical features that helps early recognition of MAS
• Change in the pattern of fever from intermittent to non-remitting
• Deterioration of hepatosplenomegaly and lymphadenopathy
• Presence of central nervous system symptoms: irritability, lethargy, coma
• Hemorrhagic manifestations
• Fall in ESR
• Fall in platelet counts

Cytopenia, especially thrombocytopenia and leukopenia are seen in >80% of patients with MAS. Normal leukocyte and platelet count in the setting of sJIA/AOSD should raise the suspicion of MAS. Cytopenia may occur late in a small subset of patients making diagnosis difficult.

Very high serum ferritin level is one of the cardinal laboratory features of MAS. In the HLH-94 study, ferritin greater than 500, 5000, and 10,000 ng/mL were seen in 93, 42, 25% of the patients respectively. In a retrospective study, ferritin of more than 10,000 ng/mL was found to have 90% sensitivity and 96% specificity for the diagnosis of HLH/MAS. Furthermore, ferritin levels have prognostic value. A fall in Serum ferritin levels of less than 50% after 48 hours portends a poor prognosis and increased mortality.

Liver dysfunction is seen in almost all patients of MAS. Transaminitis (>3 times upper limit normal), lactate dehydrogenase (LDH), and increased bilirubin are seen in 50–90%, 85% and

Table 10.8.2: Classification Criteria for MAS in systemic onset JIA: The 2016 EULAR/ACR/PRINTO criteria

1. Fever
2. Serum Ferritin >684 ng/mL
• AND any two of the following:
• Platelets ≤181 × 10^9/L
• AST >48 U/L
• Fibrinogen ≤360 mg/dL
• Serum triglycerides >156 mg/dL
The lab abnormalities should not be otherwise explained by any other conditions such as immune thrombocytopenia, infectious hepatitis, etc.

EULAR/ACR/PRINTO: European league against rheumatism/american college of rheumatology/paediatric rheumatology international trials organisation.

80% respectively. Hypertriglyceridemia, seen in 68% of patients, is associated with significant liver involvement.

Other features: Neurologic involvement, although reported in 25% of patients with primary HLH, is less common in patients with MAS associated with rheumatic diseases. Respiratory involvement (42%), renal dysfunction (16%) and skin rashes (25%) have been reported. Hypotension and bleeding due to coagulopathy might warrant extensive supportive care.

Various classification criteria exist for the diagnosis of MAS in different clinical settings. Pediatric Rheumatology International Trials Organization (PRINTO) criteria for diagnosis of sJIA associated MAS (Table 10.8.2). The HScore calculator is useful to calculate the percentage probability of secondary (reactive) HLH.

TREATMENT

HLH is a disease of unchecked inflammation and if untreated, is fatal due to multiple organ failure. The treatment of MAS is traditionally based on guidelines and protocols of familial HLH devised in 1994 and 2004. The 2004 HLH management protocol consists of glucocorticoids, etoposide and cyclosporine. However, it is increasingly believed that HLH-specific therapy is not routinely required in patients with MAS associated with rheumatic diseases and they can be controlled with the treatment of the underlying condition.

Parenteral high-dose glucocorticoids (methylprednisolone 30 mg/kg, maximum 1 g) form the cornerstone of treatment with MAS. After 3–5 days of IV glucocorticoids, 1 mg/kg oral prednisolone is started and tapered over the next 2–3 months. Along with glucocorticoids, increased immunosuppression of the underlying rheumatic condition is sufficient.

However, a significant proportion of patients are steroid-resistant. Acutely ill patient, persistent fever, cytopenia, absence of rapid reduction of serum ferritin (>50% fall in 48 hours), relapse of fever/cytopenia on tapering steroid suggest aggressive disease. Cyclosporine or other immunosuppressants are likely to be needed in such cases. Cyclosporine-A (CsA) use in MAS is based on its successful use in familial HLH. Some authors advocate its use as a first-line treatment for MAS associated with sJIA. The dramatic response has been achieved with CsA in combination with glucocorticoids, using a dose of 2–7 mg/kg/day.

Evidence and recent guidelines support the use of the anakinra (IL-1) blockade in MAS. It has been shown to be effective in patients where glucocorticoids, cyclosporine and other biologics have failed. Although IL-6 receptor inhibitor tocilizumab is effective in sJIA, patients treated with tocilizumab remain at risk of MAS. Intravenous immunoglobulin (IVIg) has been used in the treatment of MAS anecdotally. Rituximab has a special role in the treatment of Ebstein Bar virus (EBV) associated with MAS.

Apart from sJIA, MAS is commonly seen in the setting of systemic lupus erythematosis (SLE) and autoinflammatory syndromes. MAS is one of the life-threatening complications of uncontrolled SLE. Infections are the most common trigger of MAS. Viral infections and intracellular bacteria like salmonella and tuberculosis are more likely to cause MAS.

Autoinflammatory syndromes are dysregulation in the innate arm of the immune system. Reports of MAS in cryopyrin-associated periodic syndrome (CAPS), mevalonate kinase deficiency (MKD), familial Mediterranean fever (FMF), and tumour necrosis factor receptor-associated periodic syndrome (TRAPS). Corticosteroids along with IL1 inhibition (anakinra) form the first line of therapy in this group of diseases.

Current strategy of glucocorticoids, cyclosporine, cytokine specific therapies seem to be effective in reducing mortality and morbidity of MAS associated with rheumatic diseases. However, further studies and larger trials are required to delineate their exact clinical role.

CONCLUSION

MAS/secondary HLH can be triggered by a broad range of triggers, including infection, autoimmunity, and malignancy. A lower threshold for diagnosis of MAS can enable earlier diagnosis and aggressive treatment thereby can be lifesaving. MAS should be considered as a differential in patients with pyrexia of unknown origin in "at risk" patients of sJIA, AOSD, systemic lupus erythematosus and other connective tissue diseases.

LEARNING POINTS

- Secondary HLH seen in autoimmune diseases is known as macrophage activation syndrome.
- It is characterized by fever, pancytopenia, high C-reactive protein, liver dysfunction, coagulopathy.
- Ferritin levels are useful for diagnosis and monitoring therapy in MAS.
- Early diagnosis and aggressive treatment are important for a favorable outcome.

FURTHER READING

1. Carter SJ, Tattersall RS, Ramanan AV. Macrophage activation syndrome in adults: recent advances in pathophysiology, diagnosis and treatment. Rheumatology (Oxford). 2019;58:5–17.
2. HScore for Reactive Hemophagocytic Syndrome-MDCalc." HScore for Reactive Hemophagocytic Syndrome-MDCalc, ww.mdcalc.com/calc/10089/hscore-reactive-hemophagocytic-syndrome. Accessed 28 Sept. 2022.
3. Ramos-Casals M, Brito-Zerón P, López-Guillermo A, et al. Adult haemophagocytic syndrome. Lancet. 2014;383: 1503-1516. Erratum in: Lancet. 2014;383:1464.
4. Ravelli A, Minoia F, Davì S, et al. Paediatric Rheumatology International Trials Organisation; Childhood Arthritis and Rheumatology Research Alliance; Pediatric Rheumatology Collaborative Study Group; Histiocyte Society. 2016 Classification Criteria for Macrophage Activation Syndrome Complicating Systemic Juvenile Idiopathic Arthritis: A European League Against Rheumatism/American College of Rheumatology/Paediatric Rheumatology International Trials Organisation Collaborative Initiative. Arthritis Rheumatol. 2016;68:566–76.
5. Trottestam H, Horne A, Aricò M, et al.; Histiocyte Society. Chemoimmunotherapy for hemophagocytic lymphohistiocytosis: long-term results of the HLH-94 treatment protocol. Blood. 2011;118:4577–84.

Septic Arthritis

Gautam Dhar Choudhury

INTRODUCTION

Septic arthritis is usually a monoarthritis of acute onset due to antecedent infection with a pyogenic bacteria. It involves large joints like the knee and hip in most cases. The hematogeneous route is the most common mode of infection. It is a medical emergency in rheumatology because if not diagnosed early or adequately treated it lead to rapid joint destruction and impairment of function.

Septic arthritis is nowadays rarely seen due to over the counter use of antibiotics for any infection. Still the incidence is 6 cases per 10,0000 population per year in industrialized nations, the incidence increases to 70 per 10,0000 in patients with preexisting joint pathologies like rheumatoid arthritis (RA) or in prosthetic joints (Table 10.9.1).

ETIOLOGICAL AGENTS

The most common microorganisms in both adults and children is *Staphylococcus aureus.* The etiological agent also depends on the predisposing factor (Table 10.9.1). Studies have shown that it is the

Table 10.9.1: Predisposing factors and microbiological agents for septic arthritis

Predisposing factors

- Extremes of age, <15 years and >80 years
- Prosthetic joint
- Recent joint surgery
- Gout and pseudogout
- Rheumatoid arthritis
- Diabetes mellitus
- Local skin infection

Microbiological agents	Comment
Staphylococcus aureus *Streptococcus pneumonia* *Neisseria gonorrhoeae*	*Staphylococcus aureus* is the most common cause of septic arthritis, mainly attributed to its arthritogenic virulence factors. *Neisseria gonorrhoeae* remains an important cause of septic arthritis in the US, though rare in Europe.
Hemophilus influenzae	More common in immunocompromised conditions like hypogammaglobulinemia, asplenia, and systemic lupus erythematosus. In young children, septic arthritis due to *H. influenzae* is less common now due to widespread vaccination policy.
Gram-negative organisms *Escherichia coli, Pseudomonas aeruginosa, Klebsiella pneumoniae,* and *Proteus mirabilis*	Gram-negative organisms are important causes of septic arthritis in the elderly, IV drug abuse, or immunocompromised individuals.
Escherichia coli	The most common gram-negative organism causing septic arthritis.

(Contd.)

Table 10.9.1: Predisposing factors and microbiological agents for septic arthritis (*Contd.*)	
Burkholderia pseudomallei	Melioidosis is an important differential of septic arthritis in diabetes mellitus patients
Anaerobes	Traumatic conditions and penetrating wounds
Listeria monocytogenes, Streptobacillus moniliformis, and *Pasteurella multocida*	Rare
Polymicrobial	Uncommon, but if so it is in cases due to penetrating trauma involving the joint space or small joint septic arthritis

primary cause of bacterial arthritis in 40% cases from England and Wales, 56% from France, and 37% from Australia. The predominance of *Staphylococcus aureus* is mainly attributed to its arthritogenic virulence factors.

Other organisms are *Streptococcus pneumoniae,* and *Neisseria gonorrhoeae* etc. Gram-negative organisms also cause septic arthritis and are more common in the elderly. Anaerobic infection is commonly seen in traumatic conditions and penetrating wounds.

MECHANISM OF INFECTION

Septic arthritis is generally considered a secondary infection that is spread of bacteria through the bloodstream from a primary site. Mechanisms that allow the infectious agents to disseminate from blood to the joint are endothelial attachment, transcytosis, and bacteria transportation by professional phagocytes.

Common modes of infection are:

- Bacterial infection from distant sites, e.g. infective endocarditis, meningitis.
- Direct inoculation during surgery or joint injection.
- Complications of procedures like sternoclavicular joint infection in case of subclavian vein catheterization.
- Septic arthritis of the hip from femoral venipuncture.

CLINICAL FEATURES

Septic arthritis classically presents with acute onset fever, joint pain, swelling and limited range of motion. Usually occurs in a single joint, most commonly in the lower extremity. Knee is the most common joint involving around 50 % followed by the hip and then ankle. Polyarticular septic arthritis accounts for <10% of cases, is more common in older people, immunosuppressed, RA, and is associated with sepsis.

Injection drug users have a predilection to develop septic arthritis of axial joints, such as the sternoclavicular or manubriosternal joint.

DIAGNOSIS

Clinical Evaluation

- Acute onset monoarthritis of the lower limb, especially the knee joint, should always raise the suspicion of joint infection (Fig. 10.9.1).
- In addition to pain there will be a limitation in range of motion.
- Systemic response like fever will be present in immunocompetent patient.

Laboratory Evaluation

- Complete blood count (CBC) will show polymorphonuclear leukocytosis.

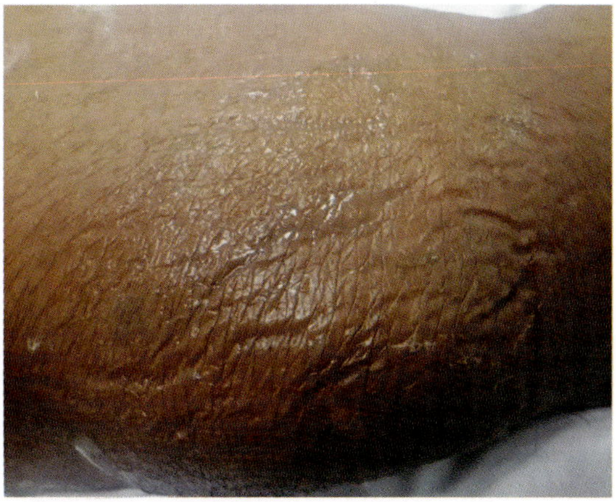

Fig. 10.9.1: Septic arthritis right knee with peau-d'orange appearance of overlying skin

- Erythrocyte sedimentation rate (ESR) and C-reactive protein (CRP) levels are raised and help in ascertaining response to treatment.
- Blood culture should be advised in patients with a profound systemic response and is positive in around 30% of cases.
- Polymerase chain reaction and other advanced diagnostic methods such as MALDI-TOF [Matrix Assisted Laser Desorption Ionization-Time Of Light] mass spectrometry may be useful when routine cultures are negative and the suspicion of infection remains high.
- Measurement of serum or synovial procalcitonin level is not a good marker to diagnose or rule out septic arthritis.

Synovial Fluid Analysis

Should be performed as soon as possible when bacterial arthritis is suspected. The identification of organisms in synovial fluid is the primary criterion for the diagnosis of septic arthritis. Fluid should be examined for crystals also to rule out gout or pseudogout. Typically the fluid is purulent with a high leukocyte count of more than 50000–150,000/dL. Gram stain and culture should be done in all cases. In special cases acid-fast bacilli stain and culture polymerase chain reactions are also undertaken.

Imaging

- Plain radiograph is an important adjunct to the physical examination. It is imperative to compare the involved extremity with the opposite healthy side. Widening of joint space, increased opacity within the joint, subluxation, erosion of subchondral bone are a few important findings. It helps in ruling out osteomyelitis, erosions due to gout and fracture if any.
- Ultrasonography is useful in identifying and quantifying joint effusions which are located deep like the hip joint, sacroiliac joints.
- Magnetic resonance imaging is not advised frequently in septic arthritis. Its use is mainly to evaluate possible concomitant osteomyelitis.
- FDG-PET is not indicated in diagnosing septic arthritis.

Septic Arthritis in Children

Septic arthritis in children is common in those under 4 years of age. In young infants, it may manifest primarily as septicemia, cellulitis, or fever without any localising sign of infection. Malaise, poor appetite, irritability, tachycardia may be presenting symptoms. The signs and symptoms can be subtle. At times the patient may awake at night contrary to juvenile idiopathic arthritis where there is early morning stiffness. More than one joint may be involved.

Causative organisms are mainly *S. aureus*, Group A *Streptococcus*, gram-negative bacilli (enterobacter), and *Hemophilus influenzae B* in the unvaccinated. The most common route of infection is hematogenous, although bacterial arthritis at times may represent a complication of osteomyelitis, especially if the metaphysis is within the joint capsule. Septic arthritis may be suspected case of juvenile idiopathic arthritis with a recent injection of a joint or on chronic immunosuppression. Vaso-occlusive disease like sickle cell anemia can develop septic arthritis as a complication

MANAGEMENT

Septic arthritis should be managed on the following principles:

- Antibiotic therapy
- Joint lavage or arthrocentesis
- Rapid mobilization of the affected joint.

Antibiotic Therapy

Diagnostic and therapeutic joint aspiration is the keystone in the management of septic arthritis. However one need not wait to initiate antibiotic therapy. The initial choice of antimicrobial regimens is generally based on coverage of the most likely organisms to cause infection. Regimens may be streamlined to a single agent once antimicrobial susceptibility data are available. There is no role for intra-articular antibiotics. Choice of antibiotics is given in Table 10.9.2.

Joint Drainage

There is a requirement of joint drainage in the setting of septic arthritis to drain out the pus from the affected joint. Options for drainage include needle aspiration, arthroscopic drainage, or arthrotomy (open surgical drainage). Knee joint can be drained by a large bore needle. Decrease in joint temperature, reduction in leukocyte count and amelioration of pain with increased mobility

Table 10.9.2: Antibiotics in septic arthritis		
Organisms	*Antibiotics*	*Duration of therapy*
Gram positive cocci	Vancomycin	2 weeks followed by switch over to oral antibiotics for another 2 weeks
Gram negative bacilli	Ceftriaxone, cefotaxime, or ceftazidime	Same
Pseudomonas aeruginosa	Ceftazidime plus aminoglycoside	Same
Methicillin-resistant *S. aureus* (MRSA)	Vancomycin Daptomycin Linezolid Clindamycin	Same
Cephalosporin allergic patients	Ciprofloxacin plus aminoglycoside	Same

signifies adequate drainage. Drainage of bigger joints like the hip and shoulder should be done by arthroscopy or arthrotomy. A few studies have shown that arthroscopy with large volume irrigation is better than arthrotomy.

LEARNING POINTS

- Septic arthritis is a common cause of acute onset monoarthritis due to bacterial infection.
- Bacteremia is more likely to localize in a joint with preexisting arthritis.
- Organisms such as *S. aureus* and streptococci are the commonest to cause joint infections. Infection due to gram-negative bacilli is generally seen following trauma or in patients with severe underlying immunosuppression.
- The most common joint involved is the knee joint followed by wrists, ankles and hip joint respectively.
- Isolation of bacteria in the synovial fluid is the definitive diagnostic test. Crystals need to be ruled out.
- Treatment consists of antibiotic therapy and joint drainage. The duration of therapy is around 3–4 weeks.

FURTHER READING

1. Lieber SB, Fowler ML, Zhu C, et al. Clinical characteristics and outcomes in polyarticular septic arthritis. Joint Bone Spine. 2018;85:469–473.
2. Mathews CJ, Weston VC, Jones A, et al. Bacterial septic arthritis in adults. Lancet. 2010;375:846–55.
3. Petty RE. Septic arthritis and osteomyelitis in children Curr Opinion Rheumatol. 1990;616–621.
4. Ross JJ. Septic Arthritis of Native Joints. Infect Dis Clin North Am. 2017;31:203–218.
5. Wall C, Donnan L. Septic arthritis in children. Aust Fam Physician. 2015;44:213–5.

Section

XI

ARTHRITIS IN SYSTEMIC DISEASES AND INFECTIONS, RELAPSING POLYCHONDRITIS, OPTICOSPINAL SYNDROME, IPAF, AND PAH IN CTDs

Musculoskeletal Tuberculosis

Kodali Ramya, Benzeeta Pinto

INTRODUCTION

Tuberculosis (TB) continues to be a major public health problem despite remarkable advancements in the diagnosis and treatment of TB in the past century. India with one-sixth of the global population accounts for about one-fourth of the global TB burden. Extrapulmonary tuberculosis (EPTB) accounts for about one-fifth of all tuberculosis cases. TB is equally relevant in rheumatology practice and it can closely mimic several rheumatic diseases as well. The use of immunosuppression and biologicals, especially tumour necrosis factor inhibitors, puts this group of patients at increased risk of opportunistic infections. Tuberculosis may also be associated with drug-induced rheumatic syndromes. Thus, the tuberculous infection may manifest with musculoskeletal features by virtue of direct infection, hypersensitivity or as a result of drug-related adverse effects (Table 11.1.1).

PATHOGENESIS

Musculoskeletal tuberculosis results from hematogenous spread, most commonly from a pulmonary, genitourinary, or from lymphatic dissemination from a lymph node focus. The rich arterial plexus in the subchondral region of the vertebral body as well as the metaphysis of bones account for the predilection of these sites for tuberculous bacilli dissemination. In case of tuberculosis of diarthrodial joints, the bacilli enters by invasion from adjacent osteomyelitis or by hematogenous dissemination to the synovial tissue. Arthritis may also be a hypersensitive response to visceral tuberculosis.

CLINICAL PRESENTATIONS

Musculoskeletal tuberculosis accounts for 10–50% of all extrapulmonary cases. They often occur concurrently with a pulmonary or extrapulmonary focus (Table 11.1.2).

Table 11.1.1: Rheumatic syndromes caused by tuberculosis

Direct infection	*Indirect effects*
Osteoarticular tuberculosis TB spine TB of peripheral joints TB osteomyelitis TB dactylitis	Para-infectious/reactive syndromes Poncet's disease Erythema nodosum Tubercular uveitis
TB soft tissue rheumatism Myositis Bursitis Tenosynovitis	Iatrogenic rheumatism Drug-induced polyarthralgia Isoniazid-induced lupus Hyperuricemia and gout associated with pyrazinamide

Table 11.1.2: Clinical features of musculoskeletal tuberculosis (TB)

Type of disease	*Involved region*	*Clinical presentation*
TB of spine	Lower thoracic, lumbar vertebrae	Chronic low back ache May present with red flag signs of back pain
TB arthritis	Knee, hip, shoulder	Chronic monoarthritis of weight bearing joints
TB osteomyelitis	Any bone can be affected. Long tubular bones are rarely involved.	Painful swelling of shaft of the bones Multifocal osteomyelitis is seen in children and immunocompromised patients
TB dactylitis	Metacarpals, metatarsals, phalanges	Fusiform 'spindle like' painful swelling
TB tenosynovitis	Tendons of hand	Exposure to cattle predisposing to *M. bovis* Formation of cold abscess and skin ulceration at the site
TB bursitis	Greater trochanteric bursa Subdeltoid bursa Pes anserine bursa	Localized swelling with mild pain

Spinal Tuberculosis

Spinal tuberculosis is the most common site of musculoskeletal involvement and accounts for 1–2% of tuberculous infections. The common presentation is axial pain of variable intensity. A neurological deficit can be seen in up to 75% of cases as a result of vertebral kyphosis or paradiscal abscess and compression of the spinal cord. The disease is characterized by paradiscal vertebral involvement with late involvement of the disc. The dorsal spine is most commonly affected; however, both the cervical as well as the lumbar spine can also be involved. It is not rare to see noncontiguous involvement of the spine. A cold abscess may track along the skin and produce a sinus.

Tuberculosis Arthritis

This is the second most common form of osteoarticular tuberculosis. In 85% of cases the manifestation is as chronic monoarthritis, while in immunosuppressed persons, involvement of two or more joints may be seen. Tuberculous arthritis occurs commonly in weight-bearing joints such as the hip and knee joints. Rarely, upper extremity joints and small joints of hands and feet may be involved. Sacroiliac involvement can be confused with axial spondyloarthritis, especially psoriatic arthritis which may also produce unilateral sacroiliitis. Joints affected by inflammatory arthritis as well as osteoarthritis are also predisposed to tuberculous infection. Patients usually present with swelling, pain, stiffness and limitation of movement. Joint swelling is often not accompanied by warmth or tenderness. Systemic symptoms may or may not be there. Monoarticular disease with periarticular destruction should raise the suspicion of infectious arthritis like tuberculosis. Radiologically joint space narrowing due to cartilage erosions and soft tissue swelling are other radiological features (Figs. 11.1.1 and 11.1.2).

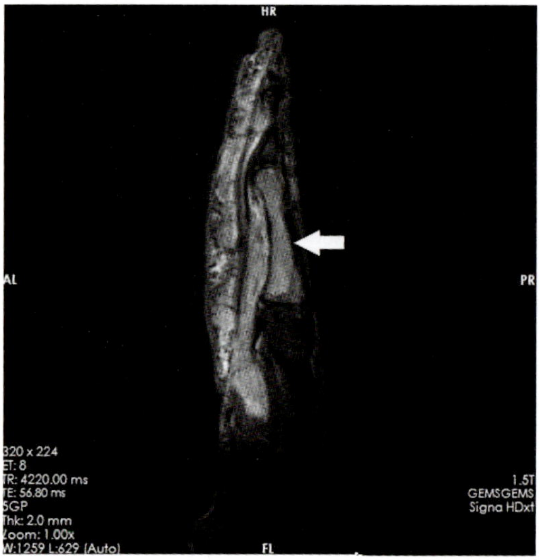

Fig. 11.1.1: A 24-year-old male presented with constitutional symptoms, chronic pain and swelling of the left 3rd digit. An MRI of the left hand oblique STIR sequence shows hyperintensities in the middle phalynx of left 3rd digit (arrow) with surrounding soft tissue inflammatory changes with sparing of PIP, DIP. Tissue biopsy showed caseous necrosis with granulomas suggestive of tuberculosis (TB). The final diagnosis was TB dactylitis.

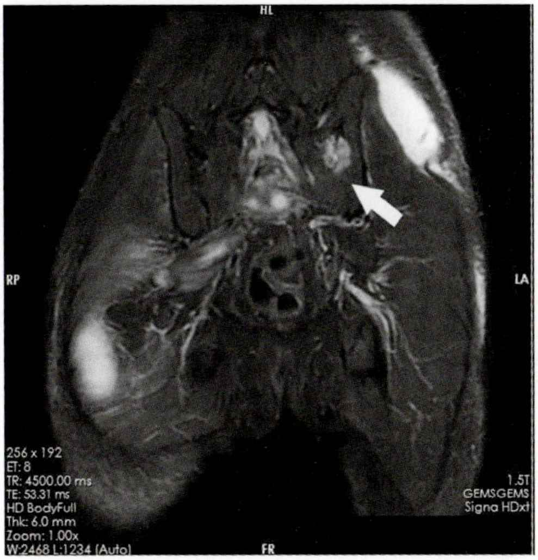

Fig. 11.1.2: A 31-year-old male, presented with chronic inflammatory back pain with tenderness over left buttock region, and significant constitutional changes. MRI hip joint coronal STIR sequence showed hyperintensity involving articular portion of sacral and iliac bone with joint space narrowing (arrow) noted on the left side suggestive of sacroiliitis. Percutaneous CT-guided aspiration from SI joint was positive for acid fast bacilli.

Tuberculous Osteomyelitis

The common bones affected by osteomyelitis include the short bones of hands and feet. The diaphysis is affected. Prominent periosteal reaction is a common feature. Involvement of the phalanges may produce a fusiform swelling of the digit. This swelling can be confused with dactylitis associated with rheumatological diseases like psoriatic arthritis and reactive arthritis. Multifocal osteomyelitis may be common in children.

Poncet's Arthritis

Poncet's arthritis is a form of reactive arthritis seen in patients with active tuberculosis without mycobacterial infection of the joint. The arthritis is different from reactive arthritis in that it is non-erosive and nondeforming; hence, this has also been described as parainfectious arthritis by some commentators. It often involves the large joints of the lower limb. The pattern of involvement is commonly oligo- or polyarthritis, with monoarthritis occurring less frequently. Poncet's arthritis may present as long-standing arthritis or rarely as an acute explosive polyarthritis of fewer than 4 weeks duration. It may predate or coincide with the diagnosis of tuberculosis and is characterised by a prompt improvement once antituberculous therapy is started. A classification criteria has been recently developed for Poncet's arthritis to enable uniformity in reporting of this disease (Table 11.1.3).

Tuberculous Myositis

Tuberculous infection of the muscles is rare. Immunosuppressed states such as chronic kidney disease and immunosuppressive medications are risk factors for infectious myositis. Patients with inflammatory myositis are also at increased risk. The thigh is the most commonly affected site. Multifocal involvement may also be seen with some case series describing it to be present in nearly half the cases. Similar to osteoarticular tissue, muscle tissue is also paucibacillary, hence the presence of caseous necrosis and identification of a pulmonary or another extrapulmonary focus that could be responsible for the hematogenous dissemination is important. However, tuberculous infection of the muscle may also develop from contiguous spread from the underlying bone.

Other less commonly seen musculoskeletal manifestations include tuberculous tenosynovitis, bursitis and fasciitis.

Table 11.1.3: Sharma and Pinto's diagnostic criteria for Poncet's arthritis

Essential criteria	Inflammatory, non-erosive, nondeforming arthritis Exclusion of other causes of inflammatory arthritis
Major criteria	Concurrent diagnosis of extra-articular tuberculosis Complete response to antitubercular therapy
Minor criteria	1. Mantoux positivity 2. Associated hypersensitivity phenomenon, such as erythema nodosum, tuberculids or phlyctenular keratoconjuctivitis 3. Absence of sacroiliac and axial involvement

For diagnosis: Definite – Essential + two major Probable – Essential + one major + three minor Possible – Essential + one major + two minor, or Essential + three minor

Nontuberculous mycobacterial infections may occur rarely. They often affect the synovial sheath rather than osteal tissue. HIV infection is the predominant risk factor, but they may also occur in healthy individuals.

DIAGNOSIS

Musculoskeletal tuberculosis runs an indolent course and may or may not be accompanied by constitutional symptoms. Mycobacterial culture remains the gold standard for diagnosis. It comes with the added advantage of assessing drug sensitivity. Tissue specimens have a higher yield than pus. Microscopic assessment for acid-fast bacilli is a less sensitive test as osteoarticular and muscle tissue are generally paucibacterial. Polymerase chain reactions for genetic components of tubercle bacilli have enhanced diagnostic capabilities. Apart from sensitivity and specificity of >80%, they have added benefits of providing a quick diagnosis and also provide information on drug resistance. Radiological features add to the armamentarium of diagnostic tests. Peripheral joints classically show cartilage destruction and joint space narrowing along with often large erosions, soft tissue swelling and even calcification. In spinal tuberculosis, peridiscal involvement with relative sparing of the disc space is seen. Osteomyelitis of phalanges produces a marked periosteal reaction. Computed tomography and magnetic resonance imaging have increased the sensitivity and specificity for the diagnosis of musculoskeletal tuberculosis (Table 11.1.4).

Table 11.1.4: Diagnostic tools for musculoskeletal tuberulosis

Diagnostic test	*Advantages*	*Disadvantages*
Histopathological diagnosis: synovial/tissue biopsy (Arthroscopy/fine needle aspiration)	'Gold standard' for diagnosis Achieves more than 90% of yield Indicated in chronic inflammatory monoarthritis	Technical difficulty in obtaining the sample Invasive procedure
Microbiological diagnosis 1. Culture	Also considered as gold standard • Low cost, highly specific • Assessment of drug resistance	Poor culture yield (10%–30%) is reported due to initiation of empirical ATT, paucibacillary state, deep seated lesions. Delayed results
2. Molecular diagnostic methods (Polymerase chain reaction) • GeneXpert • Gene Xpert MTB/RIF	Results obtained within 2 hours Highly specific (>90%)	Sensitivity depending on the tissue tested
3. Synovial fluid smear	Low cost, easily accessible	Less sensitive for biological fluids (5–20%)
X-ray joint	Low cost, feasible Gradual narrowing of joint space Peripherally placed osseous erosions suggestive of TB	Limited use in early stages of disease. Lesions take 3–6 months to appear
MRI	Detailed anatomical evaluation (fibrous tissue, abscess, spinal cord) Extent of soft tissue involvement in soft tissue TB	Less details on bony lesions
CT	Superior in depicting the degree of bony destruction and facilitating image-guided biopsy for spinal TB	Lack of imagining facilities and high-cost burden Less details on bony lesions

MANAGEMENT

The treatment of musculoskeletal tuberculosis involves mainly antituberculous therapy with surgical intervention in certain situations.

The WHO recommends 2 months of intensive phase comprising a four-drug regimen of isoniazid (H), rifampicin (R), pyrazinamide (Z), and ethambutol (E) followed by 7 months continuation phase including HR.

The American Thoracic Society recommends 6 months of ATT in adults and 12 months in children. In India the recent Index TB guidelines suggest a 3 month intensive phase of HRZE followed by 10–16 month continuation phase of HRE.

Surgical treatment may be required in case of paraspinal abscesses. A costotransversectomy is often done for drainage of the abscess. In case of kyphosis, resection of the anterior compartment followed by reconstruction using allograft humeral shaft and fixation is the most commonly done procedure.

LEARNING POINTS

- Spinal tuberculosis is the most common type of musculoskeletal tuberculosis.
- Tuberculous arthritis most commonly affects the hip and knee and is mostly monoarticular.
- Poncet's disease is a form of reactive arthritis in the presence of extra-articular TB presenting either as oligoarthritis or polyarthritis.
- Diagnosing osteoarticular tuberculosis is challenging. Microbiological diagnosis from tissue specimens remains the 'gold standard'.
- Musculoskeletal tuberculosis may mimic rheumatic diseases.
- Early diagnosis and management can reduce morbidity, social and economic burden of tuberculosis in our country.

FURTHER READING

1. Dunn RN, Ben Husien M. Spinal tuberculosis: review of current management. Bone Joint J. 2018; 100–B:425–31.
2. Malaviya AN, Kotwal PP. Arthritis associated with tuberculosis. Best Pract Res Clin Rheumatol. 2003; 17:319–43.
3. Sharma A, Pinto B, Dogra S, et al. A case series and review of Poncet's disease, and the utility of current diagnostic criteria. Int J Rheum Dis 2016; 19:1010–7.
4. Sharma SK, Mohan A. Extrapulmonary tuberculosis. Indian J Med Res 2004; 120:316–53.
5. Sharma SK, Ryan H, Khaparde S, et al. Index-TB guidelines: Guidelines on extrapulmonary tuberculosis for India. Indian J Med Res. 2017; 145:448–63.

Arthritis in Leprosy

Latika Gupta, Anupam Wakhlu, Vikas Agarwal

INTRODUCTION

Leprosy is a chronic granulomatous infectious disease caused by *Mycobacterium leprae* with skin and nerves being predominantly affected. In India, the states of Uttar Pradesh and Bihar have the highest number of leprosy cases (Fig. 11.2.1).

EPIDEMIOLOGY

The frequency of arthritis in leprosy is difficult to estimate because the prevalence varies from 1 to 78%. Rheumatic symptoms occur in as many as 75% of leprosy patients and are the third most common reason for hospital admission. Rheumatologic manifestations can occur in all types of leprosy, but are more common in the lepromatous variety.

CLINICAL FEATURES

The classical clinical presentation of leprosy is in form of hypo- or anesthetic and anhidrotic macules, patches or plaques or widespread papulonodular lesions, with or without paresthesias or loss of nerve function in the distribution of mononeuropathy or mononeuritis multiplex/polyneuropathy and blindness.

Rheumatological manifestations of leprosy are less commonly recognized. Rheumatological manifestations can be divided into three broad categories: (a) due to infiltration of synovium by *M. leprae,* (b) Reactional states, (c) complications such as peripheral neuropathy (neuropathic joints). Though neuropathic joints and septic arthritis

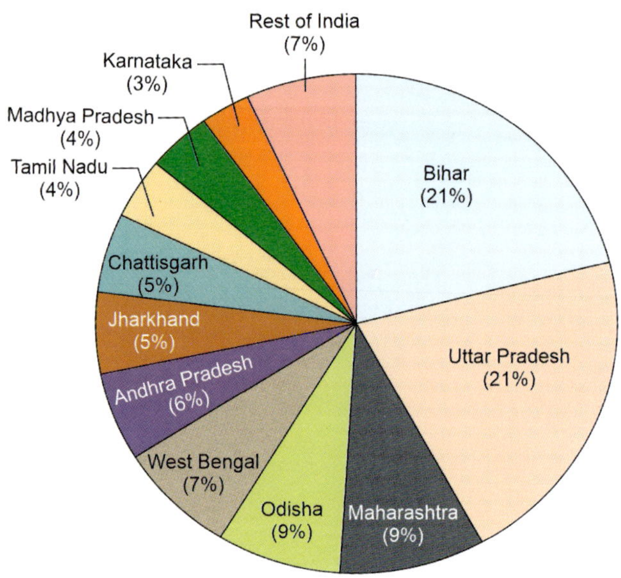

Fig. 11.2.1: Registered prevalence per state of India

are well known types of articular involvement in leprosy, inflammatory arthritis is much more common during the reactional states. The pattern of arthritis may vary from monoarticular involvement to symmetric polyarticular disease mimicking rheumatoid arthritis (RA) and or oligoarticular involvement with/without sacroiliitis or enthesitis mimicking seronegative spondyloarthropathy.

Charcot's arthropathy is usually seen in long-standing cases with neuropathy. Characteristically, these patients have severely damaged joints with little pain. Ankle and knee are most commonly involved. Findings may range from subluxation, dislocation or pathologic fractures to complete joint destruction.

Inflammatory arthritis is the characteristic presentation of leprosy during reactional states, both type 1 and type 2 lepra reactions. It may present as acute painful symmetric polyarthritis involving hand joints mimicking RA. It usually begins abruptly and is associated with constitutional symptoms: fever, weight loss, new/worsening of cutaneous lesions or paresthesias. It may last for a few weeks to months. Patients may have repeated episodes of such type of arthritis (Box 11.2.1). Synovial biopsy may show granulomatous reactions without evidence of *M. leprae* infiltration, nonspecific inflammation, or demonstrate *M. leprae* (Table 11.2.1).

Another presentation reported during reactional states is **swollen hand and feet syndrome (HFS)**. Patients present with acute onset painful edema over the dorsum of the hands with marked restriction of the movements and nodules along the extensor tendons (Fig. 11.2.2). Biopsy of the nodules may show granulomatous reaction with positivity for *M. leprae*.

Erythema nodosum leprosum (ENL) is type 2 reaction marked by the sudden appearance of numerous painful nodules and polyarthritis. Some of these lesions can ulcerate and exude pus. The patients with ENL may have high fever, lymphadenopathy, orchitis, iridocyclitis, muscle tenderness and arthritis. The natural course of the condition is 1–2 weeks, but recurrences are common.

Reaction independent **chronic RA-like arthritis** has also been reported (Box 11.2.2). Chronic RA-like presentations are most likely to be misdiagnosed. Boutonnière and swan neck deformities may occur.

Box 11.2.1: Characteristics of arthritis in reactional states

- May precede, accompany or follow the reaction
- Acute in onset
- Severe pain, morning stiffness and disability
- Parallels the duration and course of reaction
- Responds to antileprosy and anti-inflammatory therapy especially glucocorticoids
- Mostly resolve without sequelae
- Synovial biopsies do not show *M. leprae*
- Radiographs do not show erosions

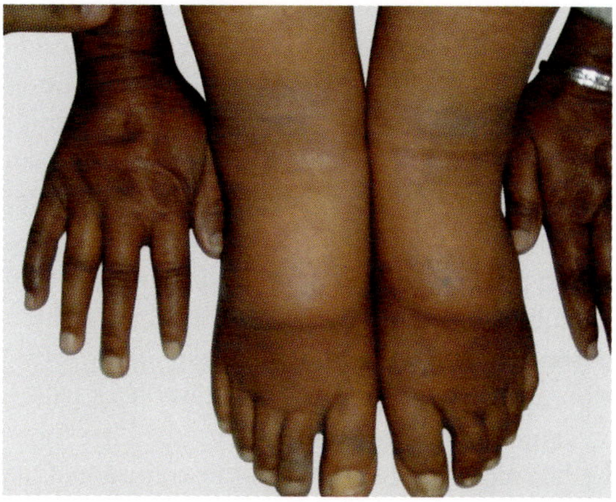

Fig. 11.2.2: Swollen hand and feet syndrome

Table 11.2.1: Reaction associated acute arthritis

Author, year	*No. of patients*	*Type of arthritis*	*Joints involved*	*Synovial histology*
Lele et al. 1965	13	Acute symmetric polyarthritis	Wrists, PIP, knee	Granuloma + No AFB
Modi et al. 1969	27		Wrists, PIP, ankle	AFB +
Chandrasekaran et al. 1993	7		MCP, PIP, ankle, knee	ND
Gibson et al. 1994	20		Wrist, MCP, PIP, ankle, MTP	AFB –

MCP: Metacarpophalangeal; *PIP:* Proximal interphalangeal; *ND:* Not done

Box 11.2.2: Characteristics of chronic arthritis in leprosy

- Insidious onset
- Seen in all forms of leprosy
- Usually polyarticular and symmetric
- May be asymmetric and oligoarticular
- Spontaneous exacerbations and remissions
- Responds to antileprosy therapy but rarely resolves completely
- Radiographs may show erosions
- Synovial biopsy may show *M. leprae*/granuloma

Though these patients may have considerable relief with antileprosy therapy, their arthritis never resolves completely. Few of the patients had erosive arthritis just like RA (Table 11.2.2). Some of them respond to disease modifying antirheumatic drugs such as hydroxychloroquine and sulfasalazine.

Asymmetric lower limb oligoarthritis and sacroiliitis akin to spondyloarthropathy has been described in lepromatous leprosy. Sacroiliitis, although, did not correlate with lower back pain.

Leprosy can sometimes mimic vasculitis (non-healing ulcers) leading to diagnostic confusion. One such extremely severe presentation is "lucio leprosy". This happens in cases with high bacillary load and bacilli infiltrating the vascular endothelium. This variety is rare in Asia, most cases being described from Mexico and Costa Rica. Rarely, cryoglobulinemia can be another cause for vasculitis in a leprosy patient without lucio phenomenon. The cryoglobulins in these cases are polyclonal IgG and IgM.

Leprosy is a great masquerader; cases of leprosy with heliotrope rash, muscle weakness and elevated muscle enzymes; oral ulcers, malar rash and photosensitivity, or mimicking scleroderma with Raynaud's, pitting scars and skin thickening have been described. Isolated enthesitis and tenosynovitis (Fig. 11.2.3) have been reported.

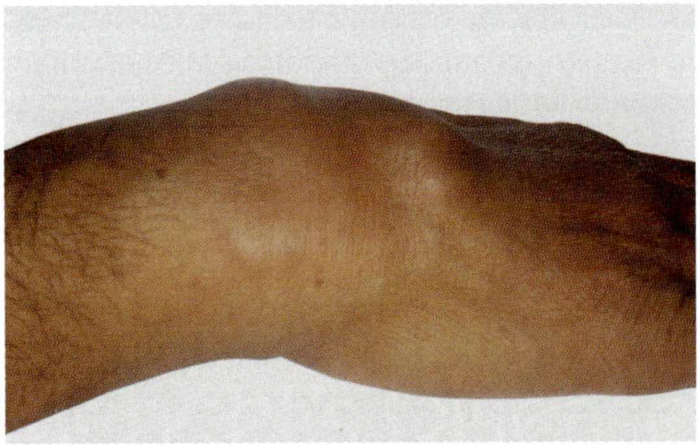

Fig. 11.2.3: Isolated tenosynovitis of extensor tendons of the hand

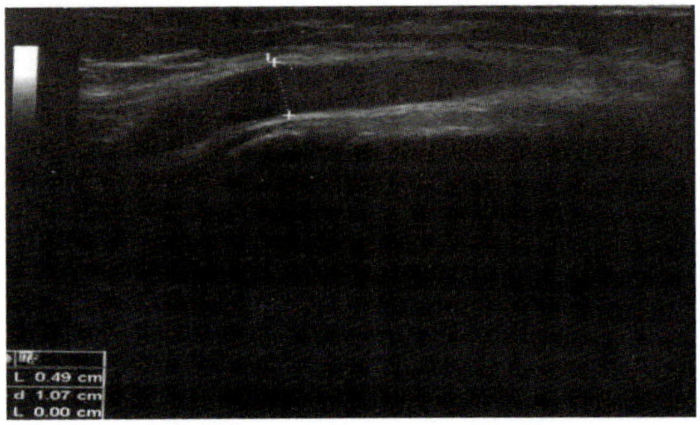

Fig. 11.2.4: Markedly thickened ulnar nerve mimicking localized collection

Recently, pure neuritic subtypes of leprosy cases with arthritis, tenosynovitis with/without paresthesias and thickened nerves have been reported. Nerve biopsy is confirmatory. Arthritis in such cases may mimic RA, or swollen hands and feet syndrome (HFS). Presence of thickened (Fig. 11.2.4) or tender nerves can clinch the diagnosis.

DIAGNOSIS

Clinical clues: Hypo/anesthetic macules or patches or erythematous macules, nodules (Fig. 11.2.5), with history of paresthesias, thickened and tender peripheral nerves and or sensory and motor neuropathy. Nerves that should be examined

Table 11.2.2: Reaction independent chronic arthritis

Author, year	*No. of patients*	*Type of arthritis*	*Joints involved*	*Radiology*
Atkins et al. 1987	31	Symmetrical polyarthritis	Wrists, MCP, PIP, Knee, MTP	ND
Atkins et al. 1989	20			Erosive disease ($n = 12$)
Cossermelli et al. 1998	39			Erosive disease

MCP: Metacarpophalangeal; *PIP:* Proximal interphalangeal; *MTP:* Metatarsophalangeal; *ND:* Not done

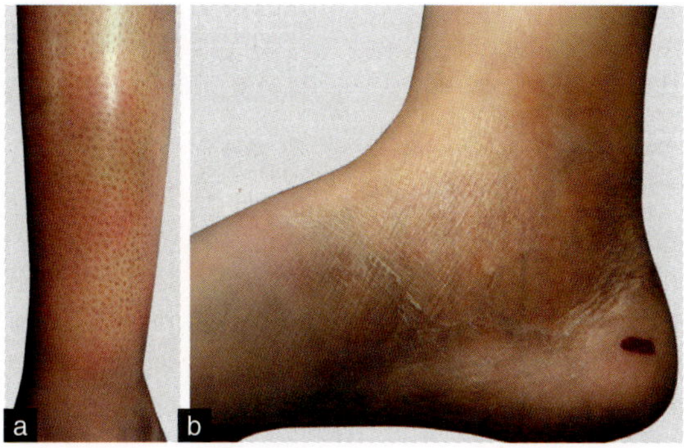

Fig. 11.2.5: (a) Erythema nodosum lesions with (b) ankle arthritis mimicking sarcoidosis

are ulnar, common peroneal nerve, radial, supraclavicular, greater auricular (Fig. 11.2.6), and facial. Careful attention to dystrophic nails (Fig. 11.2.7) and cutaneous infarcts/gangrene (Fig. 11.2.8) may suggest leprosy. Radiologically, juxta-articular erosions, periostitis, bone resorption, sacroiliitis and deformed joints have been reported. Histopathologically, synovium demonstrating granuloma, epithelioid cells and *Mycobacterium leprae* (Wade fite positive). Synovial fluid may demonstrate *Mycobacterium leprae*. Serological test, phenolic glycolipid 1 (PGL-1) for detection of antibodies to the *M. leprae* may help in appropriate clinical scenarios. These antibodies are present in 90% of patients with untreated lepromatous disease, but only 40–50% of patients with paucibacillary disease, and 1–5% of healthy controls. Skin smears have high specificity, but low sensitivity, as up to 70% of all leprosy patients may be smear negative.

TREATMENT

All patients should receive multidrug therapy (MDT): Rifampicin, clofazimine, and dapsone. For paucibacillary disease: Rifampicin 600 mg along with clofazimine 300 mg once monthly and dapsone 100 mg plus clofazimine 50 mg daily for 6 months

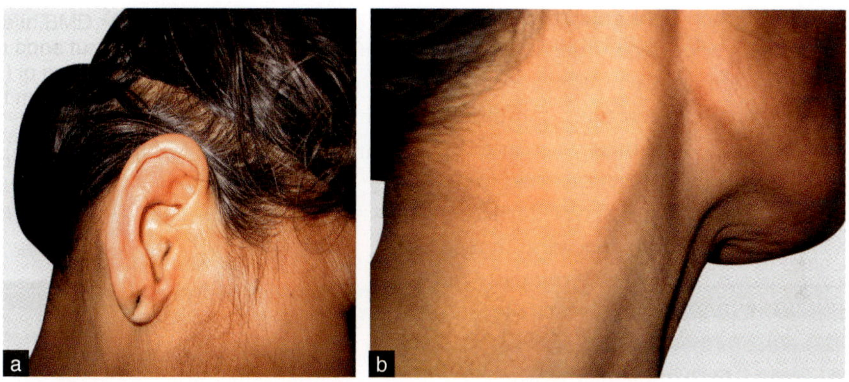

Fig. 11.2.6: Auricular chondritis with thickened right greater auricular nerve mimicking relapsing polychondritis

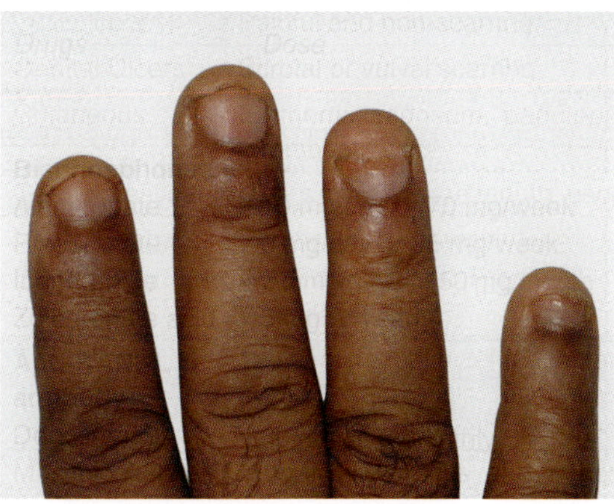

Fig. 11.2.7: Dystrophic nails

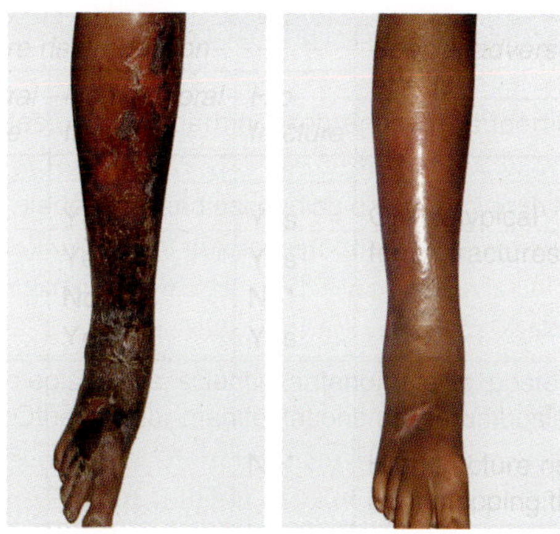

Fig. 11.2.8: Lucio phenomenon mimicking necrotizing vasculitis (before and after MDT)

Table 11.2.3: Characteristics of different forms of arthritis in leprosy

	Onset	*Symmetric*	*Oligo/ polyarthritis*	*Antimicrobial*	*Glucocorticoid*	*Joint erosions*	*M.leprae in synovium*
Lepra reaction	Acute	Yes	Yes	Poor	Good	No	No
Chronic arthritis	Insidious	Yes	Yes	Good	Not much	Yes	Yes
Swollen hand	Acute	Yes	Yes	Poor	Good	No	No
Pure* neuritic	Acute to insidious	Yes	Yes	Yes	Yes	No	No

**M. leprae* can only be demonstrated in the nerve biopsy. May present with tenosynovitis alone.

and for multibacillary leprosy, for 24 months. For paucibacillary single lesions, rifampicin 600 mg, ofloxacin 400 mg, and minocycline 100 mg single dose is enough.

The treatment of reaction-associated arthritis include glucocorticoids along with MDT. Prednisolone administration should be started at the dose of 1mg/kg/day and gradually tapered by 5 mg every 2–4 weeks depending upon the improvement in the signs and symptoms. Patients with borderline-tuberculoid reactions commonly need corticosteroids for 3–4 months, whereas those with borderline-lepromatous reactions may need treatment for 6 months. Sometimes, type 2 reaction may not respond to MDT and prednisolone; in such cases, clofazimine can be used at 300 mg daily for several months or thalidomide (TNF-α blocker) (100–400 mg daily) is better than steroids and is the drug of choice for young men with severe ENL. Monoclonal antibodies targeting the TNF-α molecule seem logical choice for therapy of severe refractory ENL in exceptional cases.

CONCLUSION

Leprosy may mimic various rheumatological disorders. A high index of suspicion and careful attention to cutaneous lesions and thickened peripheral nerves may help in clinching the diagnosis (Table 11.2.3).

LEARNING POINTS

- Rheumatological manifestations of leprosy are due to infiltration of synovium by *M. leprae*, reactional states, and complications such as peripheral neuropathy (neuropathic joints).
- During the acute reaction states patients may present with acute inflammatory arthritis, or acute onset painful edema over the dorsum of the hands (swollen hand and feet syndrome), or erythema nodosum leprosum.
- Chronic arthritis mimicking RA can occur independent of reaction states.
- It is a great mimicker and can mimic vasculitis and myositis also.
- Pure neuritic subtypes of leprosy cases with arthritis, tenosynovitis with/without paresthesias and thickened nerves have been reported.

FURTHER READING

1. Albert DA, Weisman MH, Kaplan R. The rheumatic manifestations of leprosy (Hansen disease). Medicine 1980;59:442–8.
2. Agarwal V, Wakhlu A, Aggarwal A, et al. Tenosynovitis as the presenting manifestation of Leprosy. J Indian Rheumatol Assoc 2002;10:69–70.
3. Chandrasekaran A. Infection and arthritis, our experience, a retrospective and prospective study. J Indian Rheumatol Assoc 1993;1:7–20.
4. Cossermelli-Messina W, Festa Neto C, Cossermelli W. Articular inflammatory manifestations in patients with different forms of leprosy. J Rheumatol 1998;25:111–9.
5. Gibson T, Ahsan Q, Hussein K. Arthritis of leprosy. British Journal of Rheumatology 1994;33:963–6.
6. Modi TH, Lele RD. Acute joint manifestations in leprosy. J Assoc Physicians India 1969;17:247–54.
7. Prasad S, Misra R, Aggarwal A, et al. Leprosy revealed in Rheumatology clinic: a case series. Int J Rheum Dis 2013;16:129–33.
8. Haroon N, Agarwal V, Aggarwal A, et al. Arthritis as presenting manifestation of pure neuritic leprosy—a rheumatologist's dilemma. Rheumatology (Oxford). 2007;46:653–6.

Chikungunya Arthritis and Rheumatism

Arvind Chopra, Anuradha Venugopalan, Sanat Phatak

INTRODUCTION

Following the epidemic that swept across central and southern India in 2006, post-chikungunya arthritis and rheumatism (PCAR) emerged as an important disease entity in rheumatology practice.

EPIDEMIOLOGY

Chikungunya virus (CHIKV) is an alphavirus and a member of the Togaviridae family. Three viral genotypes are recognized-West African genotype, East Central South African (ECSA) genotype, and Asian genotype. The 2006 India epidemic had roots in the African variant but is known to have undergone mutations and express unique characteristics. Though the intense devastation of the 2006 abated within few years, several local outbreaks (often endemic) are reported every year in India. A rapid surge was reported in 2016 and 2017 by the Government of India's surveillance system.

MICROBIOLOGY AND PATHOGENESIS

CHIKV is a single-stranded positive-sense RNA virus. The virus bears a spike appearance which facilitates penetration into susceptible cells. The surface viral envelope (E) proteins E1 and E2 bind to the host cells (membrane fusion and surface receptor binding) and are critical antigenic determinants. Virus RNA and/or viral remnants have been demonstrated in the synovium and synovial fluid of chikungunya arthritis.

NATURAL HISTORY

CHIKV disease ustually follows the following natural history:

Acute Illness

The initial 24 hours of illness in over 90% of adult patients is characterized by high fever and often preceded by chills and rigors, severe myalgia and stiffness in the back legs and peripheral joints. One-third have erythematous maculopapular/morbilliform skin rash (Fig. 11.3.1). The illness is generally more severe in the elderly, while it is mild in children.

Fever lasts for 2–3 days and most patients recover completely within 3 weeks.

CHIKV disease is reported uncommonly to affect other systems—gastrointestinal (21%), cardiac (5%) and neurological (12%). Other complications reported include encephalitis, myelitis, neuropathy (Guillain –Barre syndrome), diarrhea, vomiting, hepatitis, flaccid paralysis, myopericarditis, pericarditis, iridocyclitis, severe thrombocytopenia and associated hemorrhage. A maternal-fetal viral transmission was described in a neonate with CHIKV infection (especially skin features) at birth.

Subacute and Chronic Arthritis

About 40% of cases persisted with PCAR after 30 days of acute illness and more than 10% have it after 1 year. Patients with a known connective tissue disease often have a flare. The diagnosis of acute illness and PCAR is often clinical.

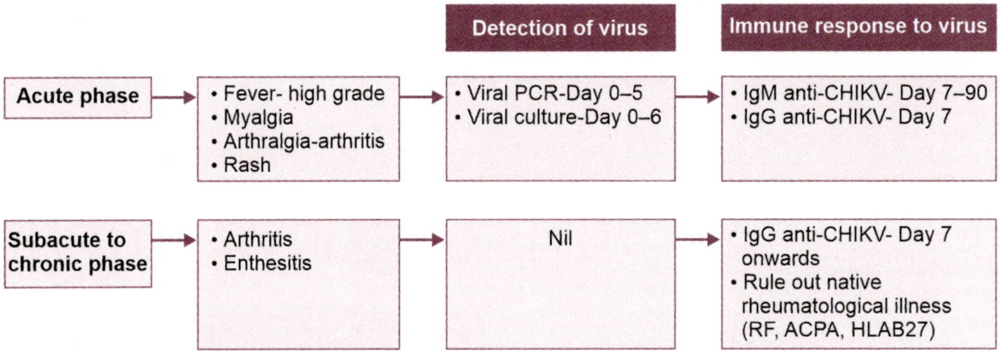

Fig. 11.3.1: Detection of Chikungunya virus (CHIKV) and immune response

Clinical Features

Disease patterns of rheumatic MSK sequelae are as follows:

i. **Inflammatory arthritis (PCAR-IA):** Sero-negative, non-erosive polyarthritis that mimics RA. With associated tenosynovitis of wrist and ankle joint. Infrequently, erosive arthritis and oligoarticular pattern in ankle or wrist are reported.

ii. **Spondyloarthritis (PCAR-SpA):** Presents with enthesitis and tenosynovitis in the foot ankle region, resembling peripheral spondyloarthritis. HLA B27 may be positive.

iii. **Soft tissue pain and inflammation (PCAR-STP):** Common sites are feet, ankle, knee, shoulder, wrist and back, accompanied by disproportionate fatigue.

iv. **Knee pains (PCAR-KP):** A large proportion of PCAR is chronic painful knees features of osteoarthritis (OA) that may progress in time. The association of Chik with OA knee is speculated.

v. **Nonspecific arthralgias (PCAR-NSA):** Poly- or monoarticular, episodic or persistent, usually involving large joints with ill-defined sensory symptoms in limbs.

DIAGNOSIS

The diagnosis of CHIKV disease is confirmed by:

- Demonstration of the virus RNA by reverse transcriptase-polymerase chain reaction (RT-PCR) assay, for 6 days after acute illness, or viral cultures.

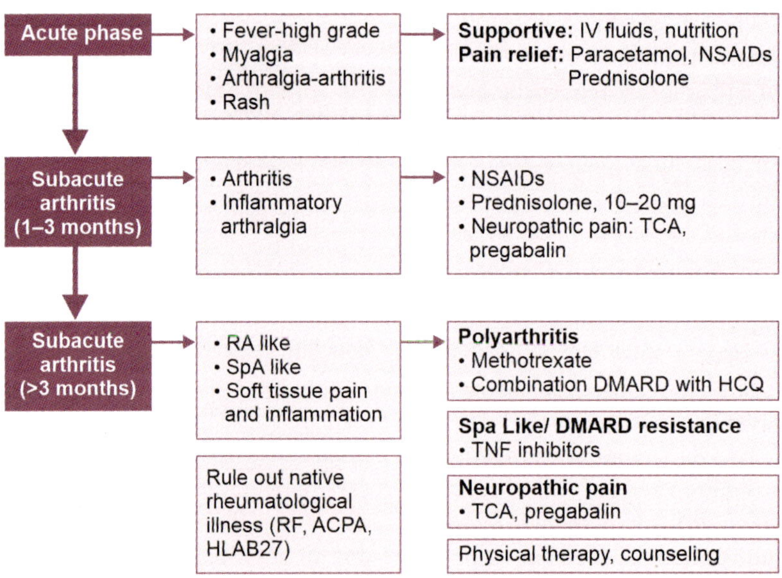

Fig. 11.3.2: Management of CHIKV disease

- Serological tests for specific IgM and/or IgG antibodies. IgM response is reported for up to last 3 months in several reports, IgG response may be evident for several years and may be protective.

MANAGEMENT

There are no specific drugs or vaccines available for acute CHIK illness and PCAR. Management depends on the duration of symptoms and manifestations (Fig. 11.3.2). Principles of management include:

Acute CHIKV

1. Pain management: NSAIDs
2. Supportive therapy—will require adequate oral hydration and nutrition. The elderly and the debilitated and those with prior severe chronic medical illnesses (such as uncontrolled diabetes or hypertension) may require intensive care and close watch. Opioid analgesia can be used where NSAID is contraindicated.
3. An oral steroid may be added in acute therapy for pain. A trial showed greater pain relief in patients receiving prednisolone (10 mg) than those who did not receive it.
4. Though experimental studies did show the antiviral effect of oral chloroquine and hydroxychloroquine, there is no clinical evidence for its use in acute illness.
5. Reassurance and counseling to allay anxiety and apprehension.

Subacute-chronic Rheumatic Sequelae

Acute Arthritis (1–3 Months)

1. Continuation of modalities used during acute febrile phase—including paracetamol and NSAIDs.
2. Systemic or intra-articular glucocorticoids are used in patients with raised inflammatory markers, demonstrable synovitis and those not responding to NSAID alone.
3. It is important to recognise the added burden of neuropathic pain and agents such as pregabalin may be useful.

Chronic Arthritis (>3 months)

The principles of usage of DMARD is similar to treatment for other inflammatory arthritis:

1. PCAR 1a: For chronic peripheral arthritis (resembling RA), methotrexate can be used. In a trial of 160 patients, a dose of 15 mg per week showed a positive therapeutic response and most patients did not require change or dose escalation. An Indian trial showed that combination therapy (Methotrexate, sulfasalazine and HCQ) was superior to HCQ alone.
   HCQ monotherapy seems to be ineffective in this situation.
2. PCAR-SpA: NSAIDs and TNF inhibitors have been used. There is no separate evidence to support the use of any one particular DMARD in this subgroup.
3. Several small molecules (such as Bindaret and oligonucleotides, and biologic agents have been researched but none were evaluated in Phase III clinical studies

Since an acute infection can lead to chronic, debilitating disease, CHIKV prevention is important to consider. Since it is a vector-borne disease, public health strategies for prevention revolve around vector control. Vaccine development holds promise in endemic areas. A measles vector vaccine and a CHIK virus-like particle (VLP) have undergone phase 2 trials, while an mRNA-based vaccine has undergone a phase 1 trial.

LEARNING POINTS

- MSK complaints are seen in up to 40% of cases in the subacute or chronic phase of the disease.
- Chronic arthritis can manifest like RA, spndyloarthropathy, fibromyalgia, knee pain or non specific arthralgia.
- Diagnosis is based on IgG or IgM antibodies to CHIKV.
- Treatment depends upon the type of arthritis.
- Methotrexate therapy has shown benefit in chronic arthritis of RA like.

FURTHER READING

1. Chopra A, Anuradha V, Ghorpade R, Saluja M. Acute chikungunya and persistent musculoskeletal pain following the 2006 Indian epidemic: a 2-year prospective rural community study. Epidemiol Infect 2012;140:842–50.
2. Chopra A, Anuradha V, Lagoo-Joshi V et al. Chikungunya virus aches and pains: an emerging challenge. Arthritis Rheum 2008;58:2921–2.

3. Chopra A, Saluja M, Venugopalan A. Chloroquine effectiveness and inflammatory cytokine response in early persistent post chikungunya musculoskeletal pain and arthritis. Arthritis Rheum 2014;66:319–26.
4. Marks M, Marks JL. Viral arthritis. Clin Med (Lond). 2016;16:129–34.
5. Miner JJ, Aw-Yeang HX, Fox JM et al. Chikungunya viral arthritis in the United States: A mimic of seronegative rheumatoid arthritis (Brief Report). Arthritis Rheumatol. 2015;67:1214–20.
6. Ravindran V, Alias G. Efficacy of combination DMARD therapy vs. hydroxychloroquine monotherapy in chronic persistent chikungunya arthritis: a 24-week randomized controlled open label study. Clin Rheumatol. 2017;36:1335–40.

Chapter 11.4

Rheumatic Manifestations of Human Immunodeficiency Virus Infection

Ajay Wanchu, Paul T Antony, Harikrishnan V

INTRODUCTION

Musculoskeletal (MSK) disorders are common with human immunodeficiency virus (HIV) infection and the prevalence increases in the late stages of the disease. These disorders can result in significant morbidity and may impair the patient's quality of life. MSK manifestations of HIV may be subdivided based on their uniqueness, association or rarity with the HIV infection (Table 11.4.1).

Table 11.4.1: Classification of rheumatic disorders in HIV-infected patients

Manifestations unique to HIV infection
• HIV-associated arthralgias and arthritis including crystal induced arthritis
• Diffuse infiltrative lymphocytic syndrome (DILS)
Manifestations commonly seen in HIV infection
• HIV-associated seronegative arthritides, including reactive, psoriatic and undifferentiated spondyloarthritis
• Vasculitis
• Myopathy
• Bone disorders
Infections associated with HIV infection
• Septic arthritis
• Osteomyelitis
• Pyomyositis
Manifestations associated with HIV treatment
• Osteoporosis
• Avascular necrosis (AVN)
• Zidovudine-associated myopathy
Manifestations associated with immune reconstitution syndrome (IRIS)
• Rheumatoid arthritis (RA)
• Systemic lupus erythematosus (SLE)
• Sarcoidosis

ARTICULAR AND BONE DISEASE ASSOCIATED WITH HIV

HIV-associated Arthralgia

It is seen in 25% of HIV-positive cases usually as a part of seroconversion illness. Treatment is usually symptomatic and spontaneous resolution is the norm.

HIV-associated Arthritis

An aseptic predominantly oligoarthritis involving the lower limbs is seen in HIV individuals. Arthritis is usually non-erosive and self-limiting and usually last for <6 weeks. There is a good response to NSAIDS and DMARDS like hydroxychloroquine and sulfasalazine.

Painful Articular Syndrome

It is an HIV-specific MSK feature characterized by episodes of acute bone and joint pain that is acute in onset, ans lasts for <24 hours. It usually occurs in advanced HIV. Large joints like knees and elbows are generally involved. Treatment is usually symptomatic; however, severe pain can be disabling.

HIV-associated Reactive Arthritis

Reactive arthritis is frequently encountered in HIV patients presenting with lower limb peripheral arthritis along with enthesitis and dactylitis. The main distinguishing features between HIV-associated arthritis and HIV-associated reactive arthritis are presented in Table 11.4.2. Treatment includes NSAIDs, sulfasalazine, hydroxychloroquine and methotrexate based on severity and chronicity. Anti-TNF blockers may be needed in refractory cases.

Table 11.4.2: Contrasting features of HIV-associated arthritis and HIV-associated reactive arthritis

Feature	HIV-associated arthritis	HIV-associated reactive arthritis
Joint involvement	Variable	Asymmetric oligoarthritis
Enthesopathy	Absent	Present
Mucocutaneous involvement	Absent	Present like keratoderma blenorrhagicum and circinate balanitis
Synovial fluid white blood cells	500–2000/μL	2000–10,000/ μL
Organisms in synovium	? HIV	*Chlamydia*
HLA–B27	Absent	Present
Course	Self-limited	Chronic/relapsing

HIV-associated Psoriatic Arthritis

The prevalence of psoriasis and psoriatic arthritis is increased among HIV positive patients. Usually, the arthritis is lower limb predominant and polyarticular. The skin lesions are of the guttate-plaque type. The treatment options include methotrexate, cyclosporine, apremilast, anti-TNF blockers and anti IL17 receptor blockers.

Avascular Necrosis of Bone (AVN)

Highly active antiretroviral therapy (HAART) especially the protease inhibitors along with or without corticosteroids has been associated with AVN in HIV patients.

Osteopenia and Osteoporosis

HIV-positive patients have a threefold prevalence of osteoporosis and osteopenia. Risk factors include protease inhibitors, poor nutrition, low body mass, advanced HIV, high viral load, smoking and alcohol abuse. Adequate calcium and vitamin D supplementation along with bisphosphonates may prevent fractures.

Hypertrophic Pulmonary Osteoarthropathy

This has been reported to occur in HIV patients with *Pneumocystis jiroveci* pneumonia.

MUSCLE DISEASE ASSOCIATED WITH HIV

Myopathy

Skeletal muscle disease may be due to:

1. HIV-associated myopathies
2. Complications of antiretroviral therapy
3. Opportunistic infections
4. Tumor infiltrations of skeletal muscle, and
5. Rhabdomyolysis (Table 11.4.3):

Involvement of skeletal muscle can happen at any stage of HIV disease.

HIV-associated polymyositis typically occurs early in HIV infection. The presentation is a subacute onset, proximal muscle weakness, with high creatine kinase enzyme levels. Auto-antibodies are typically absent. Muscle biopsies reveal interstitial inflammatory infiltrates similar to polymyositis. The treatment is similar to that for other inflammatory myopathies. Both muscle weakness and creatine

Table 11.4.3: Myopathies associated with human immunodeficiency virus (HIV) infection

HIV-associated myopathies	*Myopathies secondary to antiretrovirals*	*Others*
Vasculitic processes, HIV wasting syndrome, diffuse infiltrative lymphocytosis syndrome, nemaline myopathy, inclusion body myositis, HIV polymyositis, myasthenia gravis and other myasthenic syndromes, chronic fatigue syndrome and fibromyalgia.	Zidovudine myopathy, toxic mitochondrial myopathies related to other NRTIs, immune reconstitution syndrome related to HAART, HIV-associated lipodystrophy syndrome.	Opportunistic infections involving muscles, tumor infiltrations of skeletal muscle, rhabdomyolysis.

kinase respond well to glucocorticoids. Refractory cases may require methotrexate or azathioprine.

Rhabdomyolysis can be caused by HIV infection itself, as a consequence of the interaction between protease inhibitors and statins, or as an adverse effect of integrase inhibitors (raltegravir) or abacavir.

HIV wasting syndrome should be distinguished from other causes of generalized weight loss in HIV like infections, lactic acidosis, etc. Muscle biopsy may show diffuse atrophy without much inflammation.

A reversible mitochondrial myopathy characterized by myalgia and muscle weakness was observed among patients on zidovudine and didanosine. This myopathy related to HAART is characterized by the presence of ragged red fibers in the muscle biopsy histopathology. Thus, this condition should be suspected in individual with HIV who presents with an elevated CK with or without myalgia/muscle weakness. Offending drug/drugs should be discontinued for 4 weeks before further tests with EMG or muscle biopsies are contemplated.

Diffuse Infiltrative Lymphocytosis Syndrome (DILS)

DILS is an HIV-specific syndrome characterized by painless salivary gland swelling (mainly parotid), sicca symptoms and some extraglandular features (Table 11.4.4). It mimics primary Sjogren's syndrome with a few dissimilarities (Table 11.4.5). The incidence has reduced with the advent of HAART therapy. HIV patients who develop DILS

Table 11.4.4: Extraglandular manifestations of HIV patients with diffuse infiltrative lymphocytosis syndrome (DILS)

Neurological
- 7th cranial nerve palsy
- Aseptic lymphocytic meningitis
- Peripheral neuropathy

Pulmonary
- Lymphocytic interstitial pneumonitis (LIP)

Gastrointestinal
- Lymphocytic hepatitis

Renal
- Renal tubular acidosis
- Interstitial nephritis

Hematological
- Lymphoma

Musculoskeletal
- Peripheral arthritis
- Polymyositis

Table 11.4.5: Differences between diffuse infiltrative lymphocytosis syndrome (DILS) and Sjogren's syndrome (SS)

Variables	*Sjogren'syndrome*	*DILS*	*Hepatitis C*
Sicca	Present	Present	Present
Glandular manifestations	Moderate parotid enlargement	Moderate-to-severe parotid enlargement	Mild-to-moderate parotid enlargement
Extraglandular manifestations	Mainly pulmonary, gastrointestinal, renal, and neurologic involvement	Mainly musculoskeletal, pulmonary, gastrointestinal, and neurologic involvement	Mainly gastrointestinal and musculoskeletal involvement
Infiltrating lymphocytic phenotype	CD4	CD8	CD4
Autoantibodies	High frequency of rheumatoid factor (RF), ANA, anti-Ro/SSA and anti-La/SSB	Low frequency of RF. ANA and anti-Ro mostly absent	High frequency of RF and ANA, anti-Ro/SSA present, though less frequently than primary SS
HLA	B8, DR2, DR3 and DR4	B45, –B49, –B50 DR11 (DRS) and DRw6(DRBI*130 1*1302)	DR11 (DRS)

Table 11.4.6: Treatment of diffuse infiltrative lymphocytosis syndrome
• Reassurance and education
• Regular dental care
• No specific treatment for asymptomatic individuals
• Effective antiretroviral treatment
• Pilocarpine or cevimeline for sicca symptoms
• Systemic glucocorticoids
• Drainage and instillation of corticosteroids into parotid lymphoepithelial cysts
• Radiation of parotid cysts

progress less rapidly to AIDS as they demonstrate a robust CD8+ T cell response against the virus. Treatment of DILS is described in Table 11.4.6.

VASCULITIS

All types of vasculitis have been described in patients with HIV infection. All patients presenting with suspected vasculitis should be routinely tested for chronic viral infections before planning any immunosuppressive therapy. In HIV the vasculitis may occur either due to the HIV virus, coinfection with other viruses or as a result of HIV treatment.

A type of aneurysmal large vessel vasculitis occurs in adult males who are untreated and in the advanced stage of HIV. They present with critical limb ischemia and aneurysms involving the aorta and its branches.

Pediatric HIV patients can present with aneurysmal disease involving cerebral vessels presenting as a stroke-like disease which can cause fatal cerebral haemorrhage. This usually occurs in the setting of advanced HIV disease and regresses with effective HAART therapy.

Polyarteritis nodosa (PAN) is the most common vasculitis seen in HIV-infected individuals. The differences between classical and HIV-associated PAN described in Table 11.4.7.

Cerebral vasculitis or primary angiitis of the central nervous system is the cause of stroke in about 13% of HIV with stroke. It can occur at any time during the course of HIV disease irrespective of CD4 count.

Prevalence of cryoglobulinemic vasculitis (mostly types II and III mixed cryoglobulins) in HIV-positive patients ranges from 1 to 27% but it is much more frequent with HIV and hepatitis C coinfection. Rituximab may be needed to be used with caution in the treatment of this vasculitis.

Infectious vasculitis due to cytomegalovirus (CMV) infection leads to gastrointestinal and cutaneous manifestations. The diagnosis is by demonstration of its inclusion bodies on GI or skin specimens. Management consists of ganciclovir or foscarnet and any concomitant immunosuppressive therapy reduced. Life-threatening complications affecting the lungs, kidneys or nervous system should be treated with steroids and immunosuppressants. Antiretroviral drugs may help.

INFECTIONS ASSOCIATED WITH HIV

Pyomyositis

There is a hematogenous origin of infection involving the muscles seen in HIV patients with a CD4+ count less than 200/μL. *Staphylococcus aureus* is the most common organism. Lower limb muscle groups are typically involved. Diagnosis is usually

Table 11.4.7: Differences between different forms of polyarteritis nodosa (PAN)

Feature	*Classical PAN*	*Non-classical PAN*	*Non-classical PAN*
Association	HBV	HIV	HCV
Symptoms	Waxing, waning	Acute	Acute
Organs involved	Renal, GI and CNS	Skin, joints	Skin and others like HBV
Response to therapy	Fair (steroids and cytotoxic)	Excellent (mostly steroids only; HAART)	Good (Rituximab); relapses common; Peg IFN+Ribavarin
Severity	Severe	Mild	Moderate
Relapses	Common	Uncommon	Very common
Prognosis	Poor (35% mortality)	Excellent	Fair (10% mortality)

made with imaging using ultrasonography or MRI. Treatment consists of appropriate antibiotics and drainage of the pus.

Bacterial Arthritis and Osteomyelitis

The most common cause is staphylococcus aureus and the sites involved include the wrist, tibia, femoral head and thorax. Appropriate antibiotics with or without drainage are the corner stone of therapy.

Musculoskeletal Tuberculosis

Skeletal tuberculosis in HIV patients is usually multicentric. The most common site is the thoracolumbar vertebrae. The other sites include peripheral arthritis, osteomyelitis, bursitis and tenosynovitis. Extended duration of multi-drug antituberculous therapy is usually effective.

Atypical Mycobacterial Infection

Common organisms causing septic arthritis and osteomyelitis are *Mycobacterium hemophilum* and *Mycobacterium kansasii.* Cutaneous ulcers, nodules, sinuses and draining tracts occur in 50% of cases. These infections occur in HIV patients with CD4 count <100/µL. Treatment includes ATT and clarithromycin.

Parasitic Infections

Muscle toxoplasmosis occurs in advanced HIV infection presenting as subacute myopathy. Treatment is a combination of pyrimethamine and sulfadiazine.

Fungal Infections

Oligoarticular or polyarticular infections and tenosynovitis with *Candida albicans* or *Sporothrix schenckii* occurs in HIV cases with low CD4 counts. Disseminated infections with histoplasmosis, cryptococcosis and blastomycosis can occur.

Response of other Rheumatic Diseases to HIV Infection

Owing to low CD4+ counts HIV patients with rheumatoid arthritis and systemic lupus erythematosus (SLE) usually goes into remission but not exclusively. HIV may mimic SLE in many ways (Table 11.4.8).

Table 11.4.8: Clinical and laboratory features common to SLE and HIV/AIDS

Organ involved	*Clinical feature*
General	Fever, weight loss, fatigue
Skin and nails	Alopecia, vasculitis, blue nails
Mucous membrane	Oral ulcers, candidiasis
Musculoskeletal	Arthralgia, arthritis, osteonecrosis, osteoporosis, myopathy
Cardiovascular	Pericardial effusion, myocarditis, accelerated atherosclerosis, noninfective verruccous endocarditis
Pulmonary	Pleural effusion, pulmonary infiltrates, pulmonary hypertension
Reticuloendothelial	Lymphadenopathy, hepatosplenomegaly
Nervous system	Aseptic meningitis, seizures, stroke, peripheral neuropathy, transverse myelitis
Renal	Proteinuria, urinary infection
Ocular	Optic neuritis, keratoconjuctivitis sicca
Hematology	Leukopenia, thrombocytopenia, Coombs positive hemolytic anemia, anemia of chronic disease
Autoantibodies	ANA, anti-dsDNA, anti ENA, antiplatelet, antiphospholipid

IMMUNE RECONSTITUTION SYNDROME

Immune reconstitution inflammatory syndrome (IRIS) is a paradoxical clinical deterioration that occurs in patients with HIV who receive HAART as a result of improvement in cellular immunity. This usually occurs within 6–9 months after initiation of HAART therapy. Organ specific autoimmune disease like Graves disease, alopecia, ileitis, hepatitis, Guillain–Barré syndrome are more common. There are reports of systemic rheumatic diseases like rheumatoid arthritis, SLE and sarcoidosis occurring as a part of IRIS. If there is a risk of organ damage or mortality, HAART may need to be discontinued and corticosteroids initiated.

SEROLOGICAL ABNORMALITIES IN HIV

Multiple autoantibodies are found in HIV sera. This is due to involvement of the humoral arm of the immune system and spontaneous B cell proliferation. Development of B cell lymphoma is well described in HIV. A partial list of B cell defects in HIV infection related to rheumatologic manifestations is shown in Table 11.4.9.

Treatment for HIV itself can result in some rheumatic complaints in the patients. HAART-associated rheumatic problems are enumerated in Table 11.4.10.

Thus an entire spectrum of rheumatic diseases occurs in HIV-positive individuals, with most of them being typical of what is seen in non-HIV populations. Others may be particular to the setting of HIV (DILS, HIV-associated arthritis). Treatment of the HIV infection is part of the management of many of these disorders. Antiretroviral agents improve the clinical symptoms of HIV-associated rheumatic diseases. Some drugs used in the treatment of the rheumatic diseases (indomethacin, hydroxychloroquine) have antiretroviral properties too. With the availability of highly active antiretroviral agents the effects that these agents have on the presentation, course, and outcome of the HIV-associated rheumatic diseases remain to be determined.

Table 11.4.9: Consequences of B cell defects related to HIV infection, resulting in production of various autoantibodies

Autoantibodies	*Prevalence (%) in HIV*
Polyclonal hypergammaglobulinemia	45
Circulating immune complexes	20
Antineutrophil cytoplasmic antibodies	18–43
Antinuclear antibodies	17–30
IgG and IgA rheumatoid factor	15–32
Antiphospholipids	40–90
Antiplatelet	<5
Anti-RBC	<5
Antilymphocyte surface antigen	<5
Antineuronal cells	<5
Antineurotransmitters	<5

Table 11.4.10: Rheumatic manifestations of anti-retroviral drugs

Medication	*Class*	*Manifestations*
Zidovudine, stavudine	NRTI	Myopathy, myalgia, rhabdomyolysis
Tenofovir	NRTI	Osteopenia
Lamivudine, emtricitabine	NRTI	Arthralgia, myalgia, rhabdomyolysis
Efavirenz	NNRTI	Arthralgia, myopathy, myalgia
Nevirapine	NNRTI	Arthralgias
Nelfinavir, lopinavir, atazanavir	PI	Osteopenia, osteoporosis, AVN
Saquinavir, ritonavir	PI	Myalgia, arthralgia, arthritis, osteopenia, osteoporosis
Indinavir	PI	Adhesive capsulitis shoulder, TM joint pain, osteopenia, osteoporosis, AVN

NRTI: Nucleotide reverse transcriptase inhibitors; *NNRTI:* Non-nucleotide reverse transcriptase inhibitors; *PI:* Protease inhibitors; *AVN:* Avascular necrosis of bone

LEARNING POINTS

- HIV can have myriad rheumatic manifestations as a result of the HIV virus itself, concomitant infections, treatments with HAART, and owing to the changes in the immune system induced by the HIV virus.
- Some manifestations are unique to HIV like DILS, HIV-associated arthritis and painful articular syndrome.
- Most of the rheumatic manifestations are unrelated to HIV like reactive arthritis, spondyloarthritis and psoriatic arthritis.
- As the HIV virus depletes CD4+T cells, rheumatic diseases like rheumatoid arthritis and systemic lupus erythematosus may go into remission with active HIV infection only to flare on treatment with HAART as what happens with IRIS.
- HAART has led to a reduction in some HIV-associated clinical manifestations like DILS but has its share of problems like drug-induced myopathy and osteonecrosis.

FURTHER READING

1. Dau J, Reveille JD. Rheumatic Manifestations of HIV Infection. In: Firestein GS, Budd RC, Gabriel SE, Koretsky GA, McInnes IB, O'Dell JR, editors. Firestein and Kelleys's Textbook of Rheumatology. Philadelphia: Elsevier; 2021. pp. 2033–47.
2. Fox C, Walker-Bone K. Evolving spectrum of HIV-associated rheumatic syndromes. Best Pract Res Clin Rheumatol. 2015;29:244–58.
3. Vassilopoulos D, Calabrese LH. Viral Infections. In: Hochberg MC, Gravallese EM, Smolen JS, van der Heijde, Weinblatt ME, Weisman MH, editors. Rheumatology. Philadelphia: Elsevier; 2023. pp. 982–7.

Relapsing Polychondritis

Sanat Phatak, Abhichandra Madineni

INTRODUCTION

Relapsing polychondritis (RP) is an autoimmune disease in which inflammation has predilection for cartilage tissue. Consequently, organs with cartilage: ears, nose, joints, respiratory tract are involved. RP is a rare disease, and most commonly affects Caucasians. However, all ethnic groups can be affected and is now increasingly being diagnosed in India with a higher awareness among physicians. Men and women are equally affected, and most patients present in the 5th or 6th decade of life.

CLINICAL FEATURES

RP is characterized by cartilage inflammation in anatomically independent sites: including the ear auricles, nasal cartilage, joint cartilage, large airways, and blood vessels. Inflammation of the external ear is the most common manifestation. Systemic manifestations of inflammation namely fatigue, weight loss, malaise are common, as is fever.

One-third of patients have an associated, recognized illness in addition, which may be present prior to diagnosis or may be diagnosed during evaluation for RP. Illnesses associated with RP include connective tissue diseases (SLE, rheumatoid arthritis), systemic vasculitides (polyarteritis nodosa, ANCA-associated vasculitis, large vessel vasculitis syndromes) and hematological malignancies or premalignant states such as myelodysplastic syndrome.

Ear involvement: The external ear is inflamed in nearly half patients at diagnosis and eventually in 90%. Involvement presents with pain and redness, which may be patchy or diffuse with characteristic sparing of the ear lobule. Repeated attacks or persistent untreated inflammation results in fibrosis of the cartilage producing a 'cauliflower' ear.

Nasal involvement: Patients present with pain over the nasal bridge with local redness or warmth, and may have accompanying nasal stuffiness, rhinorrhea and loss of smell. In late cases, the structural integrity of nasal cartilage is affected, rarely leading to a saddle nose.

Eye involvement: Most common manifestations include episcleritis (redness, asymptomatic) or scleritis (redness, pain, thinning). Rarer and more serious ocular manifestations include uveitis (both anterior and posterior uveitis have been described), peripheral ulcerative keratitis and proptosis.

Airway involvement: The larynx, trachea and proximal bronchial tree is most commonly affected. Initial inflammation produces laryngeal pain, hoarseness, secretions and cough. Luminal narrowing may occur, occasionally severe enough to hamper breathing. Long-standing inflammation leads to fibrotic contractures and tracheal collapse.

Articular involvement: Joint inflammation is seen in 50–70% patients through the disease course, and the pattern varies from monoarticular to polyarticular involvement. It is usually non-erosive and responds well to NSAIDs and steroids. Inflammation of the costochondral and other parasternal joints is characteristic of RP.

Blood vessel involvement: Variable vessel vasculitis, ranging from capillaritis to aortitis can be seen. Patients may present with palpable purpura, nodules, panniculitis, features suggestive of aortic involvement (pulseless disease) may be seen.

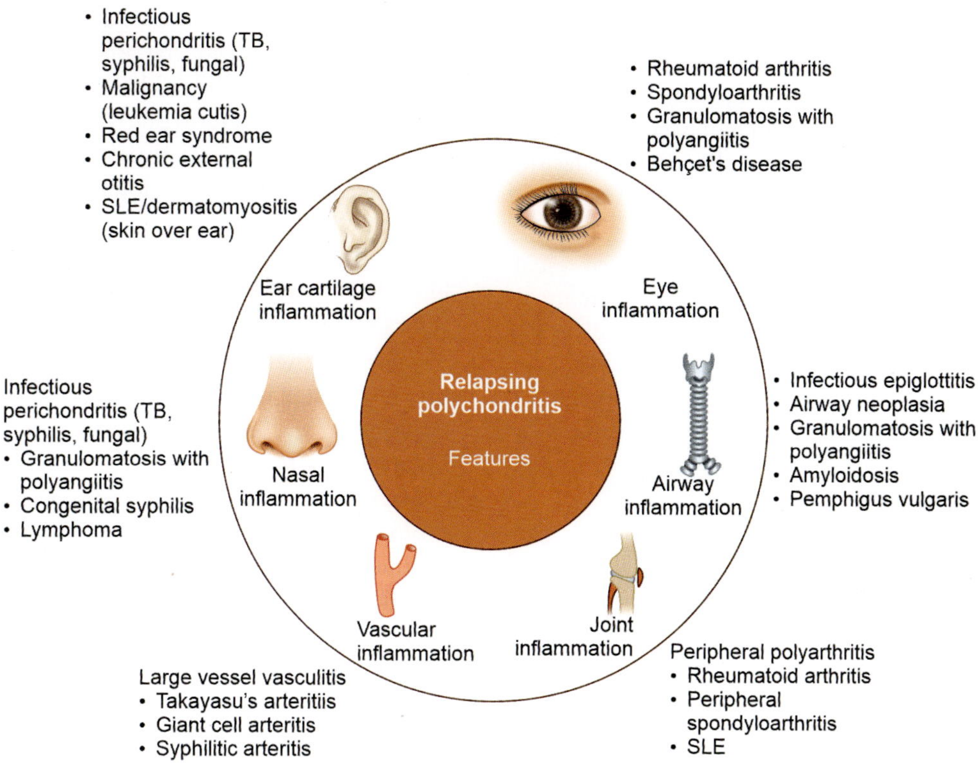

Fig. 11.5.1: Differential diagnosis of relapsing polychondritis, based on organs involved

Other rare presentations: One fourth of patients may have clinical involvement as evidenced by proteinuria and renal derangements. Many of these have an associated vasculitis. CNS involvement has been described, most commonly presenting as cranial neuritis. About 10% have cardiac involvement, mainly as regurgitant valvular lesions, pericarditis or myocarditis.

DIAGNOSIS AND DIFFERENTIAL DIAGNOSIS

Empirical diagnostic criteria are available for diagnosis of RP. These include McAdam's criteria or its modification (Damiani criteria). As a rule, these are based on the clinical features of noncontiguous cartilage inflammation. Biopsy is useful in patients not fulfilling criteria—as many patients may present with inflammation at one site alone—or in those who have atypical features, or a lack of steroid responsiveness. Biopsy is most commonly taken in an inflamed auricle, which demonstrates a pleomorphic perichondrial infiltrate in the early phases. A tissue biopsy is also useful in ruling out differentials like chronic infections. Late stages may show granulation tissue, tissue architecture loss and fibrosis.

Differential diagnoses (Fig. 11.5.1): Depend upon the patterns of organs involved. RP may resemble seronegative spondyloarthritis (arthritis, costochondritis, eye involvement); rheumatoid arthritis (arthritis, scleritis), Granulomatosis with polyangiitis (nasal bridge, scleritis, systemic). Infectious causes of auricular inflammation and epiglottitis need to be ruled out.

INVESTIGATIONS (FIG. 11.5.2)

The goals of investigations in RP include:

1. Ruling out other diagnoses, include blood or tissue culture for infections, biopsy for malignancy.
2. Ascertaining extent and severity of disease: This includes imaging for lung, renal functions, systemic inflammation markers
3. Coexistent disease: Since RP is often associated with other autoimmune diseases, ANCA and ANA serology is usually done. If hematological parameters are suggestive, a bone marrow biopsy is indicated for MDS.

Autoantibody Testing

Autoantibody testing is not necessary for diagnosis. ANA are present in up to half patients with RP, are usually speckled on immunofluorescence and target nonspecific nuclear antigens. Rheumatoid factor, anti phospholipid antibodies and ANCA have also been seen to be positive.

Antibodies to type II collagen have been tested in research settings and are positive in most patients with RP. However these are only seen in the early active phase, and do not add to the clinical diagnosis and thus not routinely tested. In addition, these are non-specific and have been seen in many other autoimmune diseases such as RA and spondyloarthritis.

MANAGEMENT AND PROGNOSIS (FIG. 11.5.2)

The general principles of treatment include the following considerations:

1. **Immunosuppression:** The degree of immune suppression depends on the severity and extent of disease involvement. Mild diseases or those restricted to ear or nose inflammation can be managed with NSAID alone, or glucocorticoids if NSAID resistant. Moderate-to-severe disease usually mandates the addition of steroid sparing agents. Methotrexate, azathioprine and leflunomide are often used for arthritis and moderate disease. Cyclophosphamide is usually preferred in induction of life threatening disease. Anecdotal reports of utility of biological DMARDs (tocilizumab, abatacept) exist; in contrast rituximab does not seem to be useful.
2. **Supportive therapy:** Surgical interventions may be required in chronic airway involvement (stenting for tracheal reconstruction) and nasal involvement (saddle nose repair). Patients are susceptible to infections and may require prolonged antibiotic therapies and abscess drainages. Patients have variable natural histories and prognosis depends upon the organ involvement and pattern of disease: despite being labeled 'relapsing' monocyclic illness, fulminant progressive, benign and indolent inflammatory disease courses have all been described. Those with associated MDS had the worst prognosis in a clustering analysis.

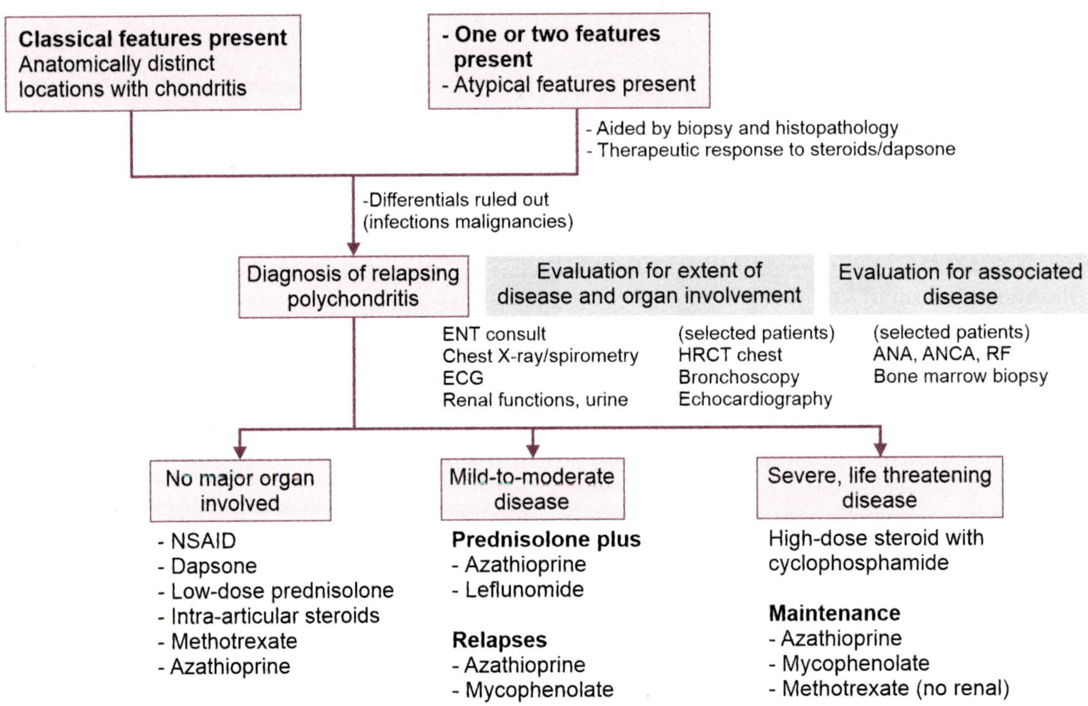

Fig. 11.5.2: Diagnosis and management of relapsing polychondritis

LEARNING POINTS

1. Relapsing polychondritis is characterized by inflammation of independent cartilaginous tissue.
2. One-third patients have an associated, well described autoimmune or hematological disease.
3. Diagnosis is clinical, biopsy is useful when features are early, atypical or treatment resistant.
4. Management and prognosis depends upon severity of organ involvement and associated illness.

FURTHER READING

1. Kingdon J, Roscamp J, Sangle S, D'Cruz D. Relapsing polychondritis: a clinical review for rheumatologists. *Rheumatology (Oxford)*. 2018; 57:1525–32.

Chapter 11.6

Opticospinal Syndrome

P Damodaram

INTRODUCTION

Neuromyelitis optica (NMO) also called Devic's disease is the prototype disease that manifests with optic neuritis and transverse myelitis (opticospinal syndrome). The other causes of the opticospinal syndrome are multiple sclerosis (MS), autoimmune diseases, and drugs (Table 11.6.1).

NMOSD

NMO is an inflammatory CNS syndrome characterized by optic neuritis, transverse myelitis, and antibodies to aquaporin 4 (AQP4-IgG). However, brain syndromes can also occur with or without optic neuritis and myelitis. So the NMO spectrum disorders (NMOSD) include limited forms of NMO and other brain syndromes. NMOSD can occur by itself or as a manifestation of autoimmune diseases namely Sjogren's syndrome, systemic lupus erythematosus (SLE), and antiphospholipid syndrome (APS).

Table 11.6.1: Causes of opticospinal syndrome

1. Inflammatory CNS disease
   - Neuromyelitis optica or Devic's disease
   - Acute encephalomyelitis
   - Multiple sclerosis
2. Autoimmune diseases
   - Systemic lupus erythematosus
   - Sjögren's syndrome
   - Antiphospholipid antibody syndrome
   - Sarcoidosis
3. Paraneoplastic syndromes
4. Drug-induced opticospinal syndrome

CLINICAL FEATURES

NMO and NMOSD are conditions more prevalent in Asians as compared to Caucasians, and more prevalent in women with a monophasic or relapsing course. Ocular pain is common (eye headache). Optic neuritis is commonly unilateral, symptoms may be preceded by a prodrome like an upper respiratory infection. Initially attacks are reversible and recover completely, but sometimes there is permanent visual loss.

Patients may also present with transverse myelitis: motor weakness, sensory involvement with a typical sensory level, and bladder and bowel disturbances. Symptoms may begin unilaterally, progressing to paraparesis or quadriparesis depending on the level of cord involvement.

Other symptoms of NMOSD are intractable vomiting and hiccups (due to inflammation of dorsal medulla). Whereas diplopia, dysarthria, and bulbar dysfunction indicate brainstem involvement. The first manifestation can also be encephalopathy with confusion, seizure, and coma. Hypothalamic involvement can also occur but is rare, and presents with hypotension/hypertension, narcolepsy, syndrome of inappropriate antidiuretic hormone secretion (SIADH), etc.

Aquaporin 4 (AQP4) antibodies

IgG to the water channel protein aquaporin-4 (AQP4) is observed in ~70% of patients. AQP4 is concentrated in the spinal cord gray matter, periaqueductal, periventricular regions, and astrocytic foot processes at the blood-brain barrier. Experimental studies show that AQP4 IgG is directly pathogenic and causes complement-mediated lysis of the astrocytes. The concentration of AQP4 is especially high in the area postrema leading to astrocyte dysfunction and the clinical manifestations of nausea and vomiting (area postrema syndrome). Certain differences exist between seronegative and seropositive cases (Table 11.6.2). One is seronegative NMOSD are more responsive to steroids and less likely to relapse.

Thirty percent of AQP4 negative patients have IgG to myelin oligodendrocyte glycoprotein (MOG-IgG). Generally, MOG+ affects both sexes equally, attacks are less severe, the prognosis is better.

IMAGING

On MRI the presence of edema of the optic nerve, and T2 hyperintense signals of the cord spanning more than three spinal cord segments, i.e. longitudinally extensive transverse myelitis (LETM) is the hallmark feature of NMOSD. Atrophy and central cavitation are seen in the later stages of the disease. Abnormalities of the brain on MRI imaging (Table 11.6.3) are present in a variable number of patients depending on serology status. These brain lesions can be symptomatic or asymptomatic.

DIAGNOSIS

The 2005 diagnostic criteria for NMO (Table 11.6.4) mandate the presence of optic neuritis and myelitis with no other CNS disease. Recent 2015 criteria are based on AQP4 status and include imaging findings as well.

Differential Diagnosis

In the patient presenting with opticospinal syndrome, one should consider autoimmune disorders as an underlying disease and investigations should proceed accordingly. Another diagnosis to consider is multiple sclerosis (MS).

Differentiating NMOSD from MS

The presence of AQP4-IgG distinguishes NMOSD from MS. In the early stages MS can present with the opticospinal syndrome in a small proportion of cases but LETM is rare. So optic neuritis and myelitis tend to be more severe in NMOSD, and the CSF is negative for oligoclonal bands.

In the Japanese population opticospinal MS (OSMS) clinically and immunologically similar to NMOSD, is reported in 15–40% of MS. It was

Table 11.6.2: Some clinical differences between AQP4 positive versus AQP4 negative NMOSD

Seropositive	*Seronegative*
• Predominantly women • Autoimmunity features • Severe clinical attacks • Motor symptoms more common • Higher spinal cord lesion load (higher vertebral segments or even entire spinal cord involvement)	• Bilateral optic neuritis • Simultaneous optic neuritis and myelitis at onset (thus time to diagnosis is shorter) • Higher frequency in children • Monophasic disease in majority • More responsive to steroids • Better prognosis

Table 11.6.3: Findings on brain MRI in NMOSD

• During an acute attack there is edema of the optic nerve enhanced with gadolinium.
• Periventricular areas are located immediately next to the lateral ventricle following the ependymal lining. Lesions are distributed in the medulla, supratentorial and infratentorial white matter, midbrain, cerebellum, thalamus, and hypothalamus. – In multiple sclerosis (MS) periventricular lesions are discrete, ovoid, perpendicular to the ventricles, and perivenular extended (e.g. Dawson's fingers).
• In Japanese patients lesions in the corpus callosum are multiple, large, and edematous with heterogeneous intensity "marbled pattern" during the acute phase, can appear like an arch bridge when there is the involvement of entire thickness of the corpus callosum including the splenium.
• Hypothalamic lesions (5%): The lesions can be there in MS too but they are small and triangular unlike NMO where they are extensive.

Table 11.6.4: Criteria to diagnose NMOSD

<table>
<tr><td colspan="2">Revised diagnostic criteria for neuromyelitis optica (NMO) 2006</td></tr>
<tr><td colspan="2">Definite NMO
Required: Optic neuritis and acute myelitis
At least two of three supportive criteria
1. Contiguous spinal cord MRI lesion extending over three vertebral segments
2. Brain MRI not meeting diagnostic criteria for multiple sclerosis
3. NMO-IgG seropositive status</td></tr>
<tr><td colspan="2">National MS Society 2008 task force criteria</td></tr>
<tr><td colspan="2">Required: Optic neuritis and Myelitis (cord MRI T2 lesion >3 vertebral segments and T1 hypointense during attack)
Sarcoidosis, vasculitis and lupus (clinically manifest) exclude diagnosis
Supportive: Initial brain MRI normal
Positive serology for NMO-IgG (AQP4 specific antibodies)</td></tr>
<tr><td colspan="2">International consensus diagnostic criteria 2015</td></tr>
<tr><td>NMOSD, AQP4-IgG positive</td><td>NMOSD, AQP4-IgG negative</td></tr>
<tr><td>At least one clinical manifestation of NMOSD</td><td>At least two different clinical manifestations of NMOSD
MRI in accordance with clinical manifestations</td></tr>
<tr><td colspan="2">Clinical manifestations:
1. Optic neuritis
2. Acute myelitis
3. Area postrema syndrome
4. Acute brainstem syndrome
5. Symptomatic narcolepsy
6. Symptomatic brain syndrome (ADEM/PRES) with MRI lesions</td></tr>
<tr><td colspan="2">These criteria should be applicable only in cases with better no clinical explanation
Recommendation for AQP4-IgG should be cell based assay</td></tr>
</table>

ADEM: Acute demyelinating encephalomyelitis; *PRES:* Posterior reversible encephalopathy

identified as a spectrum of conventional MS. But is now considered as part of NMOSD because it is associated with HLA-DPB1-0501 while MS is associated with the HLA-DRB1-1501 allele. Moreover, AQP4 +ve patients are HLA-DPB1 positive.

Autoimmune Diseases and NMOSD

NMOSD has a known association with systemic autoimmune disorders and organ-specific autoimmunity such as hypothyroidism, pernicious anemia, myasthenia gravis, thyroiditis, etc. Antinuclear autoantibodies (ANA) are present in about 50% of patients with NMOSD, while SSA/SSB in up to 17%. Apparently, the disease duration of NMOSD is shorter in ANA+ patients and can predict severe NMOSD.

Systemic Lupus Erythematosus and NMOSD

Myelitis is a devastating neurological feature of SLE and can present either as acute transverse myelitis or LETM. Myelitis can predate SLE. Two third myelitis cases occur in active lupus and one-third during inactive SLE. AQP4-IgG is present in almost 100% of cases of neurological SLE (NPSLE) with LETM. A population-based study from Denmark showed that AQP4 is present in just 2% of non-neurological SLE but positive in all cases who have LETM and antiphospholipid antibodies (aPLs). Though rare, patients with SLE can develop brain and brainstem syndrome. Thus patients with demyelinating NPSLE should be tested for AQP4-IgG and MOG to help identify NMOSD.

Sjögren's Syndrome and NMOSD

Neurological manifestations are common extraglandular manifestations of Sjögren's syndrome, of which sensorimotor polyneuropathy is most common. Others are cranial neuropathy, mononeuritis multiplex, progressive myelopathy, or transverse myelitis. In a review of Sjögren's syndrome ($n = 116$) who presented with NMOSD, the majority were females, AQP4+ in 83%, anti-SSA in 97%. NMOSD preceded Sjögren's syndrome by ~55%. Transverse myelitis was the most common presentation, followed by optic neuritis. NMOSD associated with Sjögren's syndrome has a more severe course compared to idiopathic NMOSD. The CSF in Sjogren's syndrome with myelopathy may show elevated protein, moderate pleocytosis, and negative oligoclonal bands.

It is probable that vasculopathy with breakage of blood–brain barrier in systemic autoimmune illnesses aids the transfer of AQP4-IgG to enter the CNS.

Antiphospholipid Antibody Syndrome (APS) and NMOSD

The prevalence of transverse myelopathy in APS according to data from the Euro-phospholipid project is 0.4%. Optic neuritis is even less frequent. The prevalence of aPLs in NMOSD is 45%. NMOSD patients with positive anticardiolipin (aCL) IgG and IgM have worse outcomes than the isolated presence of IgG or IgM. Also, SLE with transverse myelitis with high aPLs also has poor outcomes. Because aPLs are found in many inflammatory disorders and infections, it can be assumed that they indicate underlying inflammation rather than a pathogenic role. Pulse methylprednisolone and cyclophosphamide are used to treat transverse myelitis with APS. Anticoagulation decisions may be made based on clinical judgment.

Sarcoidosis and NMOSD

Sarcoid myelopathy is rare, predominantly subacute or chronic, and often occurs in males, and clinical courses may be monophasic, or progressive. Diagnosis of sarcoid myelopathy is difficult unless there is a high index of suspicion for possible underlying sarcoidosis in patients with LETM and or optic neuritis. A definitive diagnosis can only be made through tissue diagnosis and biopsy of an affected organ system. MRI of sarcoid myelopathy is predominantly central, involves cervical or thoracic regions, and is longitudinally extensive.

Paraneoplastic NMOSD and Drugs

AQP4 expression in tumor tissue has been reported, and NMOSD presenting as a paraneoplastic syndrome in association with carcinomas are also reported. The possibility of underlying malignancy should be considered in elderly patients with NMOSD. New therapeutic agents and biologics can trigger NMOSD (Table 11.6.5).

Table 11.6.5: Drug-induced NMO

Drug	*Remarks*
TNF inhibitors (TNFi) such as infliximab, etanercept, and adalimumab	TNFi have been associated with optic neuritis, NMO like picture the proposed mechanism is TNFi induced demyelination.
Immune checkpoint inhibitors **Ipilimumab** a human monoclonal antibody directed against CTLA-4, inhibits downregulation activation of T-cells and therefore leads to activation of the immune system, stimulating an immune response against cancer cells	Ipilimumab is associated with optic neuritis, NMO-like presentations are reported.
PD-1 and PDL-1 antibodies	NMOSD has been reported in association with nivolumab therapy. Also atypical neurological complications have been associated with PD-1 antibodies (pembrolizumab and nivolumab).
Interferon-alpha (IFN-α) treatment has been reported to induce NMOSD	IFN-α has also been detected significantly more often in the serum of NMO than in MS patients, and increase disease severity with increasing IFN-α level.

TREATMENT

For acute attacks IV methylprednisolone 1gm for 3 days, followed by oral prednisolone 1mg/kg with taper over the next 6 months. Plasma exchange is indicated in severe attacks when the patient has not responded even 5 days after IV pulse methylprednisolone.

Maintenance treatment is with low dose steroid and a steroid-sparing agent either azathioprine, or mycophenolate mofetil, or rituximab. Presence of a coexisting systemic autoimmune disease and the number of attacks prior are important factors that will help decide therapy.

Biologics in NMOSD

- Satralizumab a humanized IgG2 monoclonal antibody (Mab) that binds to soluble and membrane-bound human interleukin-6 (IL-6) receptors is effective to prevent relapses.
- Eculizumab, an inhibitor of the terminal complement protein (C5), is effective to prevent relapse. Eculizumab is associated with increased susceptibility to opportunistic meningococcal infection. It is an approved treatment for AQP4+ NMOSD.
- Inebilizumab is a humanized Mab that binds to CD19. In seropositive NMO it led to fewer attacks compared to placebo. It has been approved by the US FDA.

LEARNING POINTS

- NMOSD is the prototype disease that manifests with optic neuritis and transverse myelitis (opticospinal syndrome).
- Other causes of opticospinal syndrome are multiple sclerosis (MS), autoimmune diseases, and drugs.
- It is important to differentiate NMOSD from MS as treatments for MS often aggravates NMOSD.
- NMOSD has a known association with systemic autoimmune disorders, hence it is important to look for features of autoimmune diseases in opticospinal syndrome/NMOSD.

FURTHER READING

1. Dutra BG, da Rocha AJ, Nunes RH, et al. Neuromyelitis Optica Spectrum Disorders: Spectrum of MR Imaging Findings and Their Differential Diagnosis. Radiographics. 2018; 38:169–93.
2. Jarius S, Paul F, Weinshenker BG, et al. Neuromyelitis optica. Nat Rev Dis Primers. 2020;6:85.
3. Kira J. Neuromyelitis optica and opticospinal multiple sclerosis: Mechanisms and pathogenesis. Pathophysiology. 2011;18:69–79.
4. Shahmohammadi S, Doosti R, Shahmohammadi A, et al. Autoimmune diseases associated with Neuromyelitis Optica Spectrum Disorders: A literature review. Mult Scler Relat Disord. 2019;27:350–63.
5. Weinshenker BG, Wingerchuk DM. Neuromyelitis Spectrum Disorders. Mayo Clin Proc. 2017;92: 663–79.

Chapter 11.7

Interstitial Pneumonia with Autoimmune Features

Siddharth Jain, Uma Kumar

INTRODUCTION

Interstitial lung disease (ILD) is a heterogeneous group of diffuse lung parenchymal disorders with varied etiology both known and unknown (idiopathic interstitial pneumonias). ILDs have variable clinical, radiographic, and histopathological features. Connective tissue diseases (CTDs) are a prominent cause of ILD. The relationship of ILD with CTD is intricate, wherein ILD is associated with a definite well-established CTD in a majority of cases, with an undifferentiated CTD in about a quarter, while it predates the CTD in the remaining cases as the first, forme fruste manifestation of CTD. Determining that an ILD is CTD-associated is important therapeutically and prognostically.

In clinical practice it is found that some patients with idiopathic interstitial pneumonia (IIP) have serological, clinical, radiological or histopathological features that are suggestive of an underlying autoimmune etiology but do not fulfil all the criteria for a definite CTD. These patients are often grouped as having undifferentiated CTD (UCTD) ILD. Another term used is autoimmune ILD or lung-dominant CTD.

To remove the ambiguity associated with the usage of these non-standardized, overlapping terms and to bring them under a single unified umbrella, the term "interstitial pneumonia with autoimmune features" (IPAF) was proposed and defined by the European Respiratory Society/ American Thoracic Society task force in 2015 (Table 11.7.1). The development of a uniform IPAF cohort was intended to be the starting point for the conduct of prospective research studies aimed at better characterization of these patients, their management, and their similarities and differences vis-a-vis CTD-ILD.

Notably, the ATS/ERS criteria are classification criteria for research, rather than diagnostic criteria for clinical use.

EPIDEMIOLOGY

The prevalence estimates of IPAF vary from 7 to 34% of all ILDs. As per preliminary studies (low quality), IPAF demographics including age, gender (balanced male-to-female) and smoking prevalence seem to lie somewhere in-between CTD-ILD (predominantly younger age, women, nonsmokers) and idiopathic pulmonary fibrosis (predominantly older age, males, smokers). However, IPAF demographics are expected to vary considerably with the study design, eligibility criteria and sampled population characteristics.

DIAGNOSIS AND PROBLEMS IN ESTABLISHING IT

The first step to a diagnosis of a suspected IPAF is reliably excluding an underlying CTD-ILD. Rheumatologists thus occupy a central role in the evaluation of IPAF. It has been shown that a greater proportion of IIP are labeled as IPAF, and a large chunk of IPAF is relabeled as CTD-ILD with the involvement of a rheumatologist in the multidisciplinary team.

All patients with a presumed IIP should be screened for the presence of autoimmune features

Table 11.7.1: Classification criteria for IPAF

Interstitial pneumonia should be confirmed either by HRCT chest or by lung biopsy. Other causes of ILD must be ruled out. The patient must not have a well defined autoimmune rheumatic disease.
There must be at one feature from at least two of the domains detailed below:

Clinical	*Serologic*	*Morphologic*
1. Inflammatory arthritis 2. Raynaud's 3. Digital tip ulcers 4. Mechanic's hands 5. Gottron sign 6. Unexplained digital edema 7. Palmar telangiectasia	1. Rheumatoid factor ≥2 × upper limit of normal 2. Anti-citrullinated peptide antibodies 3. Positive ANA ≥1:320 titer, diffuse, speckled, homogeneous patterns or ANA nucleolar pattern (any titer) or ANA centromere pattern (any titer) 4. Anti-dsDNA 5. Anti-Smith 6. Anti-RNP 7. Anti-Ro 8. Anti-La 9. Anti-topoisomerase 10. Anti-tRNA synthetase 11. Anti-PM-Scl 12. Anti-MDA-5	1. HRCT pattern a. NSIP b. OP c. NSIP with OP overlap d. LIP 2. Lung biopsy histopathology patterns a. NSIP b. OP c. NSIP with OP overlap d. LIP e. Diffuse lymphoplasmacytic infiltration (with or without lymphoid follicles) f. Interstitial lymphoid aggregates with germinal centers 3. Multi-compartment involvement a. Unexplained pleural effusion or thickening b. Unexplained pericardial effusion or thickening c. Unexplained intrinsic airways disease d. Unexplained pulmonary vasculopathy

NSIP: Nonspecific interstitial pneumonia; *OP:* Organizing pneumonia; *LIP:* Lymphoid interstitial pneumonia (Fischer A, et a. Eur Respir J. 2015)

using a detailed review of systems (history and examination) and laboratory tests including tests for autoantibodies (Table 11.7.2). This review should not be limited to the parameters specified in the ATS/ERS classification criteria since important clinical parameters like rash, sicca, oesophagal dysmotility, gastroesophageal reflux disease (GERD), fever, proximal muscle weakness with or without myalgia, and autoantibodies including ANCA have been excluded from the criteria despite their relevance to diagnosis.

Other tests like nailfold capillaroscopy and salivary gland biopsy which fall under a rheumatologist's purview may be needed to include/exclude an underlying CTD. Ordering of necessary/sufficient autoantibody testing and interpretation of their results can be challenging, considering the ever-expanding pool of available autoantibodies and numerous false-positive and false-negative results. Finally, defining a multicompartment involvement on radiology may be challenging in the presence of significant smoking, concomitant emphysema, and advanced ILD (where significant pulmonary hypertension may set in secondarily).

MANAGEMENT

Patients with IPAF require multidisciplinary care. The importance of general measures like smoking cessation, vaccination, avoidance of environmental and occupational exposure to lung detrimental factors, treatment of GERD, pulmonary rehabilitation and management of comorbidities needs to be emphasized to all patients.

Table 11.7.2: Systems review and laboratory investigations for evaluating an underlying autoimmune etiology to ILD (IPAF or CTD-ILD)

Domain	*Characteristics*
History	• Arthralgia/arthritis • Raynaud's phenomenon • Skin tightening • Proximal muscle weakness +/– myalgia • Dysphagia • Skin rash • Puffiness of hands or feet • Sicca symptoms • Photosensitivity • Oral ulcers • Alopecia • Hemoptysis • Frothuria or oliguria • Constitutional symptoms
Clinical examination	• Skin rash (after disrobing): all skin signs of dermatomyositis and SLE • Mechanic's hands • Digital pits or ulcers • Microstomia • Sclerodactyly • Muscle power testing including neck, trunk, bulbar and respiratory muscles • Synovitis • Oral ulcers • Dental caries • Sublingual salivary pool • Schirmer's test (keep Schirmer's strips handy)
Laboratory tests	
Routine tests	• CBC, LFT, RFT, urinalysis
Inflammatory markers	• ESR • CRP
Muscle enzymes	• CK • LDH • AST, ALT • Aldolase (if available)
Autoantibodies	• RF • Anti-CCP • ANA by IIF (Hep-2) **Systemic sclerosis autoantibody panel:** • Anti–Scl70 or topoisomerase-1 • Anti-centromere • Anti-RNA polymerase III • Less commonly: Anti-Th/To, Anti-PM/Scl75 and 100, Anti-U3RNP, Anti-Ku **Inflammatory myopathy autoantibody panel:** • Anti-synthetase antibodies (Jo-1, PL-7, PL-12, EJ, OJ, etc.) • Anti–Mi-2 • Anti–MDA5 • Anti-SRP • Anti-HMGCR • Anti-NXP2 • Anti–TIF1-gamma • Anti-SAE • Anti-PM/Scl75 and anti-PM/Scl100 • Anti-Ku **Sjögren syndrome:** • Anti-Ro/SS-A • Anti-La/SS-B **SLE:** • Anti-dsDNA • Anti-Sm **MCTD:** • Anti-U1RNP **AAV (repeated remote covert DAH may manifest as ILD):** • PR-3-ANCA • MPO-ANCA

Since IPAF is a relatively new entity, data to guide evidence-based treatment is limited to a few observational (predominantly retrospective) studies and management principles are largely extrapolated from CTD-ILD (Fig. 11.7.1). Immunosuppressive therapy forms the cornerstone of therapy based on the premise of an underlying autoimmune/inflammatory pathophysiology. However, all patients of IPAF do not need treatment as emphasized in the algorithm (Fig. 11.7.1).

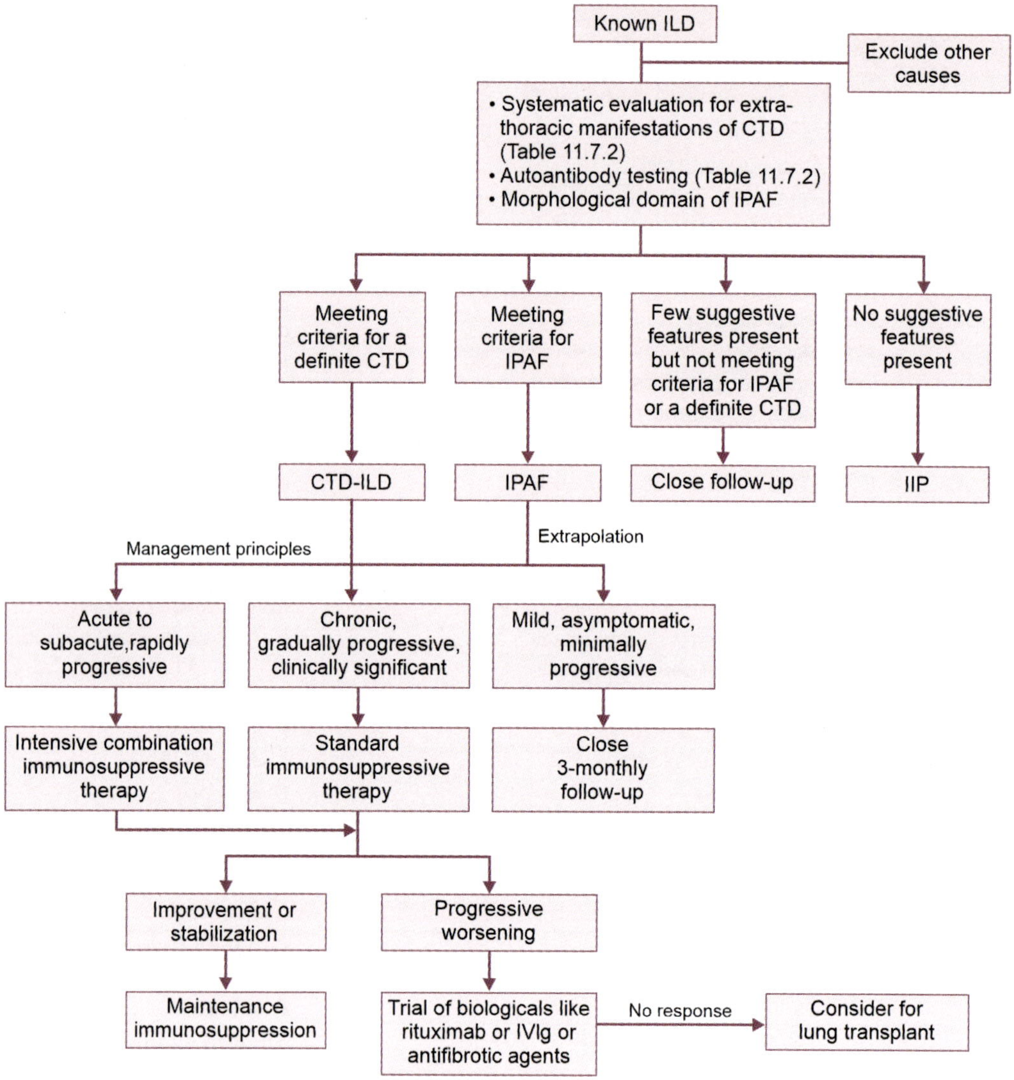

Fig. 11.7.1: Algorithm for diagnosis and management of IPAF

Cyclophosphamide or mycophenolate mofetil are most commonly used steroid-sparing immunosuppressive drugs in IPAF cohorts, based on evidence of efficacy in systemic sclerosis-ILD; other agents include azathioprine, cyclosporine, tacrolimus, etc. Biologics including rituximab and tocilizumab, and immunomodulators like intravenous immunoglobulins can also be used in select cases. However, which therapy is to be preferred in which set of patients is currently unknown.

Some patients of IPAF may benefit from antifibrotic therapy, especially the ones with a progressive fibrosing phenotype, although the exact position of antifibrotic therapy in IPAF treatment remains unclear. There is positive data on the role of nintedanib in chronic, progressive, fibrosing ILD (including the IPAF subgroup) from the INBUILD trial. Whether there is a role of concurrent or sequential immunosuppressive and antifibrotic therapy in IPAF needs to be explored.

Candidates for long-term oxygen therapy are decided the same way as IPF. Advanced cases with end-stage lung disease require referral for lung transplantation.

FOLLOW-UP AND PROGNOSIS

A small fraction (10–15%) of IPAF evolve into a definite CTD-ILD over time laying the credence to a "pre-CTD-ILD" hypothesis.

Since IPAF includes a heterogenous group of conditions, the prognosis as a group is variable but generally believed to be intermediate between CTD-ILD and IPF. The UIP subset of IPAF tends to have a worse prognosis similar to idiopathic pulmonary fibrosis (IPF), while the NSIP subset has a better prognosis and behaves closer to CTD-ILD. Based on data from prospective and retrospective observational cohorts, other factors favoring a good prognosis include presence of features from the clinical domain, and myositis specific antibodies especially anti-synthetase. On the other hand, older age, smoking, lower baseline pulmonary function, concomitant pulmonary hypertension, RNP antibodies, and MUC5B polymorphism seem to confer a worse prognosis.

FUTURE PERSPECTIVE AND CHALLENGES

Considering the heterogeneity of the IPAF group and limitations of the current criteria, a revision of the classification criteria is in the pipeline. The parameters incorporated in the clinical, serological and morphological domains need to be carefully chosen in order to maximize the sensitivity and specificity. Dedicated RCTs and large-scale prospective cohort studies are needed to frame evidence-based treatment strategies and identify factors reliably determining prognosis.

LEARNING POINTS

- IPAF is a group of diffuse parenchymal lung disorders characterized by clinical, serological, and/or morphological features suggestive of but not definitive for a CTD.
- A rheumatologist holds a central position in the recognition, monitoring and management of IPAF.
- Since IPAF is a relatively new entity, data on its epidemiology, appropriate treatment, prognosis and long-term follow-up is currently limited.

FURTHER READING

1. Fischer A, Antoniou KM, Brown KK, et al.; "ERS/ATS Task Force on Undifferentiated Forms of CTD-ILD". An official European Respiratory Society/American Thoracic Society research statement: interstitial pneumonia with autoimmune features. Eur Respir J. 2015; 46:976–87.
2. Joerns EK, Adams TN, Sparks JA, et al. Interstitial Pneumonia with Autoimmune Features: What the Rheumatologist Needs to Know. Curr Rheumatol Rep. 2022; 24:213–26.

Pulmonary Hypertension in Connective Tissue Diseases

Nilesh Nolkha

DEFINITION

Pulmonary Hypertension and Pulmonary Arterial Hypertension

Pulmonary hypertension (PH) is a broad umbrella term (Table 11.8.1) and as per 6th World Symposium on PH, PH is now defined as mean pulmonary arterial pressure (mPAP) >20 mm Hg versus the earlier definition of >25 mm Hg. Pulmonary arterial hypertension (PAH) is a subgroup of PH that is characterized by an elevated mPAP >20 mm Hg and elevated pulmonary vascular resistance (PVR) >3 Wood (W) units and a normal pulmonary artery wedge pressure (PAWP <15) on right heart catheterization (RHC). Connective tissue diseases (CTD)–PAH (CTD–PAH) comes under group 1 PH (Table 11.8.1).

Table 11.8.1: Clinical classification of pulmonary hypertension (PH)

Group 1:	Pulmonary arterial hypertension (PAH) (includes primary and CTD-PAH)
Group 2:	PH due to left heart disease (pulmonary artery wedge pressure > 15 mm Hg)
Group 3:	PH due to lung diseases and/or hypoxia
Group 4:	Chronic thromboembolic PH and other pulmonary artery obstructions
Group 5:	PH with unclear and/or multifactorial mechanisms

Adapted from: Simonneau, Gérald, et al. Haemodynamic definitions and updated clinical classification of pulmonary hypertension. European Respiratory Journal 53.1 (2019).

PREVALENCE AND CAUSES

Systemic sclerosis related PAH (SSc-PAH) accounts for almost 75% of all CTD-PAH, with 8–12% of SSc patients developing PAH. PAH occurs in 1–5% of patients with mixed connective tissue disease (MCTD) and systemic lupus erythematosus (SLE). It is rarely seen in other CTDs like rheumatoid arthritis, primary Sjogren syndrome and idiopathic inflammatory myositis (IIM).

PH in CTDs can be due to causes other than group 1 classified PAH. Group 3 PH can be seen in a significant number of patients with SSc-associated interstitial lung disease (ILD). Other causes could be left ventricular dysfunction (group 2), chronic thromboembolic PH (group 4), and pulmonary veno-occlusive disease. In a given patient usually, one predominant component is identifiable.

PATHOGENESIS

The pathogenesis of PAH in SSc can be oversimplified as the progressive remodeling of small and medium-sized pulmonary vasculature propagated by a combination of inflammation, hypoxia, endothelial injury, and tissue proliferation. In certain subsets of SLE and MCTD patients, response to immunosuppression suggests a predominance of immune-mediated inflammation.

CLINICAL FEATURES AND PHYSICAL FINDINGS

A high degree of suspicion is required as PAH in CTDs is clinically silent or may present with nonspecific symptoms like atypical chest pain, fatigue, dyspnoea or syncope. Certain features in SSc such as telangiectasias, limited cutaneous disease, anti-centromere antibody, longer disease duration (>4 years) and severe nail capillaroscopy changes are associated with increased risk of incident PAH. Specific physical examination is unrevealing for PAH until late and may later reveal signs of right sided heart failure (RHF).

SCREENING AND DIAGNOSIS

A combination of clinical parameters and relevant investigations (Table 11.8.2) help achieve the diagnosis in these patients (Fig. 11.8.1). Though right heart catheterization (RHC) is the gold standard for the diagnosis of PAH, in resource-poor settings like India, RHC is expensive and not widely practiced. Echocardiography forms the mainstay of PAH diagnosis in such settings and it is important to liaise with the reporting cardiologist (Table 11.8.2).

MANAGEMENT OF CTD-PAH

A. **General measures:** Patients should be educated, given advice on vaccinations, exercise tolerance and cardiopulmonary rehabilitation. PAH patients should avoid high altitudes and may need oxygen therapy for flight travel. Pregnancy is not advisable, especially if moderate-to-severe

Table 11.8.2: Screening and diagnostic evaluation for patients with suspected CTD-PAH

1. Baseline and annual screening for PAH is recommended in patients with SSc or CTDs with SSC like overlap features.
2. Electrocardiogram (ECG)—may reveal presence of P pulmonale and RV strain pattern.
3. Chest X-ray—enlarged pulmonary artery, obliteration of retrosternal space
4. Echocardiography—forms the mainstay of PAH diagnosis when RHC is not routinely done. The mean pulmonary artery pressure (mPAP) is calculated by formula mPAP = 0.6 × PASP + 2 mm Hg. Pulmonary artery systolic pressure (PASP) cut off of > 36 mm Hg is widely used to diagnose PAH. In view of variations in PASP calculations, direct mention of tricuspid regurgitation velocity (TRV) can be helpful to make clinical decisions.
   PASP = 4 × (TRV)2 + right atrial pressure (~5 mm Hg).

TRV	PH likelihood
<2.8 m /s	Less likely
2.8 m/s – 3.4 m/s	Intermediate
>3.4 m/s	Highly likely

   Echocardiography can also help with some other suggestive signs of PAH and ruling out other alternative possibilities.
5. Diffusion capacity of lung for carbon monoxide (DLCO)—parameters like isolated low DLCO (<60%) with normal lung function test, forced vital capacity (FVC)/DLCO ratio >1.6 or a 20% unexplained decline in DLCO can be strong predictors of underlying PAH.
6. Six-minute walk test distance (6MWD)—more useful in assessing risk status and response to therapy. A worsening value with desaturation may be indicative of underlying PAH.
7. Brain natriuretic peptide (BNP) and N-terminal pro-BNP—can help as a part of diagnostic algorithms (>2-fold elevation), predicting prognosis and assessing response to therapy.
8. DETECT 1 and ESC/ERS 2 (2015) algorithm can be helpful to categorize probability of PAH in patients with scleroderma and other CTDs, respectively.
9. Right heart catheterization (RHC)—gold standard for PH diagnosis, PAH is characterized by an elevated mPAP >20 mm Hg and PVR >3 Wood (W) units and a normal PAWP <15 mm Hg. Can be helpful for assessing severity and monitoring also.

Adapted from: [1]Coghlan JG, Denton CP, Grunig E et al. Evidence based detection of pulmonary arterial hypertension in systemic sclerosis: the DETECT study. Ann Rheum Dis. 2014;73:1340–9 and Rreference 1 in Further Reading section.

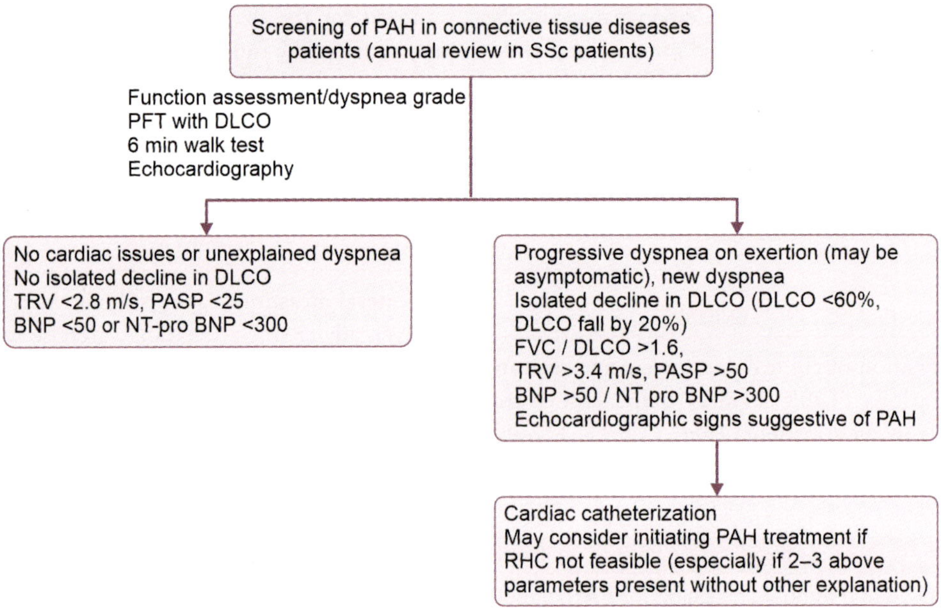

Fig. 11.8.1: Screening for PAH in CTD patients

PAH is present. Estrogen free contraception measures may be more appropriate. Supportive measures like oxygen therapy (especially if PO_2 <60 mm Hg), digoxin, and diuretics may also be needed. Oral anticoagulation should not be used as a routine in CTD-PAH unless indicated for CTEPH or other issues. Immunosuppressive therapy (steroids, cyclophosphamide, etc), though not helpful in SSc-PAH, can be helpful to control or reverse PAH in certain patients with SLE and MCTD.

B. **Medical management:** The drugs used in PAH are summarized in Table 11.8.3, and Figure 11.8.2 provides a treatment algorithm for PAH patients. Calcium channel blockers have very poor efficacy and are not recommended in CTD-PAH. PAH patients should be assessed at baseline and classified as low, intermediate, or high risk, depending on various hemodynamic parameters provided by ESC/ERS guidelines (Table 11.8.4). Generally, low-risk patients are patients who are stable with WHO functional class (WHO-FC) II or better. Therapy is initiated according to risk status or WHO-FC (Fig. 11.8.2) with considerations of local drug availability, possible side effects, tolerability, and costs. Monitoring is done every 3–6 months for symptomatic improvement and the goal is to achieve a low-risk status (Table 11.8.4). If the goal is not achieved, then sequential triple

Table 11.8.3: Drugs used in pulmonary arterial hypertension (PAH)

Class of drug	*Drug and dose (gradually titrated upwards in most cases as per efficacy and tolerability)*	*Remarks*
PDE5 inhibitors (PDE5i)	**Sildenafil:** 5–20 mg thrice daily	Class specific common side effects include hypotension, flushing, headache, sinus congestion. Other side effects include myalgia, priapism and paresthesia. Should not be combined with soluble guanylate cyclase stimulators (GCs) such as riociguat in view of risk of hypotension. Preferred class for initial combination therapy with ERA in WHO FC II–III patients.
	Tadalafil: 5–40 mg once or twice daily in divided doses	
	Vardenafil: 5 mg once or twice daily	

(Contd.)

Table 11.8.3: Drugs used in pulmonary arterial hypertension (PAH) *(Contd.)*

Class of drug	*Drug and dose (gradually titrated upwards in most cases as per efficacy and tolerability)*	*Remarks*
Endothelin receptor antagonists (ERA)	**Bosentan:** 62.5 mg to 125 mg twice a day **Ambrisentan:** 5–10 mg once daily **Macitentan:** 10 mg once daily	Side effects include transaminitis, flushing, headache, sinus congestion, peripheral edema, hematologic changes (anemia), decreased sperm counts and urinary tract infections. Metabolized by the CYP450 system and drug interactions to be checked (bosentan especially). Preferred class for initial combination therapy with ERA in WHO FC II–III patients.
Prostacyclin analogs (PC)[1]	**IV Epoprostenol:** 2–40 ng/kg/min–very slowly titrated through a device/central venous catheter) (very short half life of 2–3 minutes)	Needs a specialized device. Class specific side effects include headache, myalgia, anxiety, jaw pain, flushing, dizziness, pruritus, edema, flu like symptoms, hypotension, gastrointestinal/liver issues. Additional side effect includes line infection. Sudden stoppage may lead to rebound PH or death. Preferred initiation with parenteral PC in WHO-FC III/IV patients or as add on to sequential combination therapy. Only drug to show survival benefit.
	IV or SC treprostinil: 2–40 ng/kg/min	Class specific side effects.
	Inhaled treprostinil: 18–54 μg, 3–9 breathes per dose	Special oral inhalation system.
	Inhaled Iloprost 2.5–5 μg/dose using special aerosolization, may use up to 9 times per day (max 45 μg/day)	Class specific side effects. Additional side effects include transaminitis, congestive heart failure and pneumonia.
	Oral treprostinil: 0.125 mg thrice a day or 0.25 mg twice a day with slow escalation by 0.125/0.25 mg in each dose	Class specific side effects. Parenteral/inhaled have better evidence in WHO FC III/IV.
	Oral beraprost: 20–40 μg 3–4 times per day	Available only in some countries. Class specific side effects.
Prostacyclin receptor agonist (PRA)[1]	**Oral selexipag:** 200 μg twice a day–1600 μg twice a day	Class specific side effect like prostacyclin analog. Can used as a part of sequential combination therapy.
Soluble guanylate cyclase stimulators	**Riociguat:** 1 mg thrice daily, orally. Decrease to 0.5 mg if patient do not tolerate due to hypotension	Riociguat has good safety profile. Most adverse effects are mild-moderate intensity and include nausea, vomiting, headache, dyspepsia, dizziness, diarrhea, and hypotension. It should be discontinued 24 hours prior to initiating PDE5i.

CYP: Cytochrome P enzyme system.

combination therapy should be tried to achieve the same (Fig. 11.8.2).

C. **Surgery:** In patients who fail medical management heart-lung or double lung transplantation may have to be considered. Balloon atrial septostomy (BAS) may help as a bridge to transplantation in patients without severe hypoxemia. In carefully selected patients, without significant

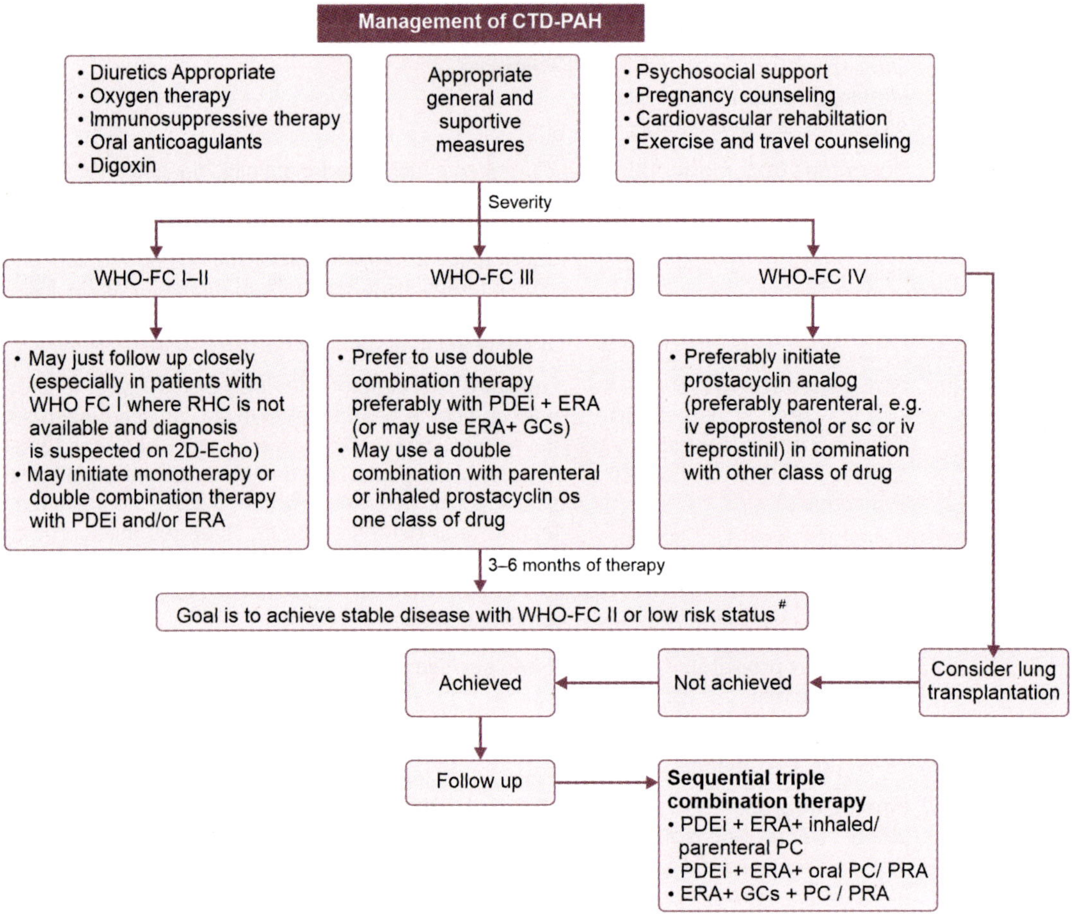

Fig. 11.8.2: Management algorithm for PAH patients.

Severity can be assessed as per risk status suggested by ECS/ERS guideline (Table 11.8.4). *FC:* Functional capacity; *PDE5i:* Phosphodiesterase inhibitors; *ERA:* Endothelin receptor antagonists; *GCs:* Soluble guanylate cyclate stimulators; *PC:* Prostacyclin analog; *PRA:* Prostacyclin receptor agonist; Based on: Galiè N, Channick RN, Frantz RP, et al. Risk stratification and medical therapy of pulmonary arterial hypertension. Eur Respir J. 2019 Jan 1;53(1)1801889.

Table 11.8.4: Intermediate or high risk PAH patients (based on ERS/ESC guidelines 2015*)

1.	Presence of right heart failure signs
2.	World health organization function class III/IV
3.	Rapid progression of symptoms
4.	Plasma BNP level >50 ng/L or NT-pro BNP >300 ng/L
5.	Six minute walk distance (6MWD) <380–440 m
6.	Right atrium area >18–26 cm^2 or presence of pericardial effusion on echocardiography
7.	Right atrial pressure >8–14 mm Hg, Cardiac index <2.5 L/min/m^2

Goal is to achieve consistent low risk status with WHO FC-II or better class, with minimal symptoms, with better exercise capabilities, with normalization or decrease in BNP/NT-pro-BNP levels and improvement in 6MWD. *See Further Reading#1

RV dysfunction, a modified unidirectional valve Potts shunt procedure (anastomosis of main pulmonary artery and descending aorta) can be offered. These are high risk procedures which are individualised and not a part of routine PAH treatment guidelines.

SUMMARY

CTD-PAH needs a higher degree of suspicion and carries a poorer prognosis than idiopathic PAH. Early diagnosis and intervention can improve quality of life and may have survival benefits. Recent drug advances have improved PAH therapy, though five-year mortality remains significantly high (25–50%).

LEARNING POINTS

1. PH is now defined as mean pulmonary arterial pressure (mPAP) >20 mm Hg.
2. CTD-PAH requires a high degree of suspicion and regular screening is recommended to diagnose it early.
3. There can be significant variations in echocardiographic reporting of PAH with significant under and overdiagnosis.
4. If RHC is not available, a combination of echocardiography findings and other parameters may be used to arrive at a treatment decision.
5. Early intervention, sequential combination & goal based therapies are recommended and can have major survival benefits in CTD-PAH patients.

FURTHER READING

1. Condon DF, Nickel NP, Anderson R, et al. The 6th World Symposium on Pulmonary Hypertension: what's old is new. F1000Res. 2019;8:F1000 Faculty Rev-888. doi:10.12688/f1000research.18811.1.
2. Galiè N, Channick RN, Frantz RP, et al. Risk stratification and medical therapy of pulmonary arterial hypertension. Eur Respir J. 2019;53:1801889. doi:10.1183/13993003.01889–2018.
3. Galiè N, Humbert M, Vachiery JL, et al. 2015 ESC/ERS Guidelines for the diagnosis and treatment of pulmonary hypertension: The Joint Task Force for the Diagnosis and Treatment of Pulmonary Hypertension of the European Society of Cardiology (ESC) and the European Respiratory Society (ERS): Endorsed by: Association for European Paediatric and Congenital Cardiology (AEPC), International Society for Heart and Lung Transplantation (ISHLT) [published correction appears in Eur Respir J. 2015 Dec;46(6):1855–6]. Eur Respir J. 2015;46:903–75.
4. Galiè N, McLaughlin VV, Rubin LJ, et al. An overview of the 6th World Symposium on Pulmonary Hypertension. Eur Respir J. 2019; 53:1802148.

Rheumatic Manifestations of Endocrine Disorders

Sanjeeb Kakati, Vishal Agarwal

INTRODUCTION

Endocrine disorders often show symptoms related to musculoskeletal system. In this chapter we give an overview of the rheumatic manifestations seen in commonly encountered endocrine disorders.

DIABETES MELLITUS

Diabetes is commonly linked to rheumatic syndromes. Rheumatic manifestions in diabetes commonly include Charcot joints, diffuse idiopathic skeletal hyperostosis (DISH), osteopenia and diabetic muscle infarction (Table 11.9.1). Involvement of hands frequently occurs in diabetics and can present in various forms, including Dupuytren's contracture, flexor tenosynovitis, carpal tunnel syndrome, and diabetic sclerodactyly.

Hand and Shoulder Syndrome

This syndrome occurs in patients with long-standing diabetes. This includes:

- Limited joint mobility (diabetic cheiroarthropathy) is characterized by skin thickening involving dorsal surface of hands leading to restricted mobility of multiple joints of fingers (Fig. 11.9.1).

Table 11.9.1: Rhematological manifestations in Diabetes

Condition	*Comments*
1. Limited Joint Mobility (Diabetic cheiroarthropathy)	Thickening of skin over the dorsum of the hands and restricted mobility of multiple joints of fingers.
2. Dupuytren contracture	Palmar fascia thickening : flexion contraction of involved joints.
3. Flexor tenosynovitis (Trigger finger)	Proliferation of fibrous tissue in tendon sheaths; painful
4. Carpel tunnel syndrome	Involves median nerve distribution.
5. Diabetic sclerodactyly	Thickening of skin. Usually involves distal fingers, may gradually progress to involve entire hand.
6. Diabetic neuropathy	Distal symmetrical sensorimotor polyneuropathy (most common), diabetic amyotrophy, mononeuropathy and autonomic neuropathy.
7. Shoulder capsulitis (adhesive capsulitis or frozen shoulder)	Joint capsule of shoulder joint gets thickened and adheres to the humeral head, causes pain and stiffness in the involved joint.
8. Charcot joints	Painless joint swelling, laxity, subluxation, and bone resorption.
9. Diffuse idiopathic skeletal hyperostosis (DISH)	Osteophytes along anterolateral surface of vertebral bodies, may lead to stiffness and back pain.
10. Diabetic muscle infarction	Swelling and pain usually affecting the lower extremities. Can spontaneously resolve but tends to recur.

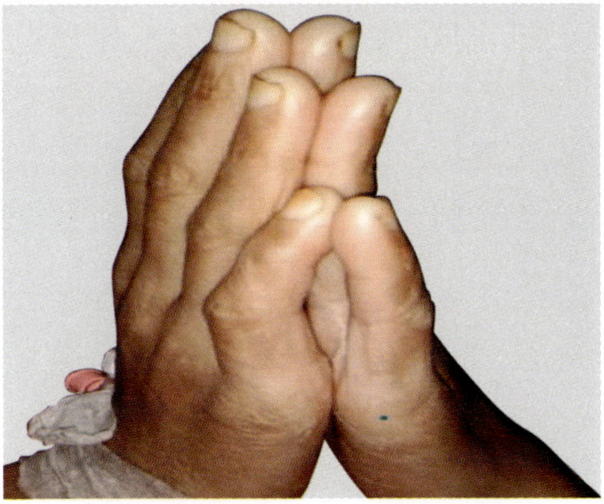

Fig. 11.9.1: Diabetic cheiroarthropathy

- Dupuytren contracture is characterized by focal flexion deformity of fingers due to fibrosis of palmar fascia. The fingers are involved in following order of decreasing frequency: 4th finger, followed by 5th, 3rd, and 2nd finger.
- Shoulder capsulitis (Adhesive capsulitis or Frozen shoulder) has prevalence in the range of 4–29%. Its prevalence is 5–6 times higher in diabetes patients. It is characterized by three distinct clinical phases:
  - **Initial phase or freezing phase (2–4 months):** Characterized by pain, stiffness and restriction of range of motion.
  - **Adhesive phase (4–12 months):** Pain gradually subsides but stiffness persists.
  - **Resolution phase (12–42 months):** During this phase, the range of motion gradually improves.
- Flexor tenosynovitis is characterized by inability to carry out active flexion and extension of fingers smoothly, with or without pain.

DIABETIC MUSCLE INFARCTION

This occurs especially in type 1 diabetes patients. It commonly involves thigh muscles and is associated with sudden onset of pain and swelling in the involved group of muscles. Calf muscles are less commonly involved.

DIFFUSE IDIOPATHIC SKELETAL HYPEROSTOSIS

Metabolic derangements of type 2 diabetes are associated with DISH. Its pathogenesis is complex. IGF-1 stimulates osteoblast proliferation, whose production is increased by increase in insulin levels and growth hormone.

THYROID DISEASE

In thyroid disorders, musculoskeletal manifestations are common.

- Musculoskeletal manifestations of hypothyroidism includes muscular pain and stiffness of extremities, pain and paresthesia in the fingers, carpel tunnel syndrome and tenosynovitis.
- Hyperthyroidism is associated with increased bone resorption, osteoporosis and increased risk of fracture.

PARATHYROID DISEASE

Hyperparathyroidism

Hyperparathyroidism leads to excessive bone resorption and turnover. Patients usually complains of muscle weakness, arthralgia and bone pain. Osteitis fibrosa cystica occurs in long-standing disease.

Hypoparathyroidism

Hypoparathyroidism can present clinically with spondyloarticular features. These features along with biochemical parameters of hypocalcemia and low PTH suggest the possibility of hypoparathyroidism. Pseudohypoparathyroidism is a rare disorder resulting from resistance to parathyroid hormone (Fig. 11.9.2).

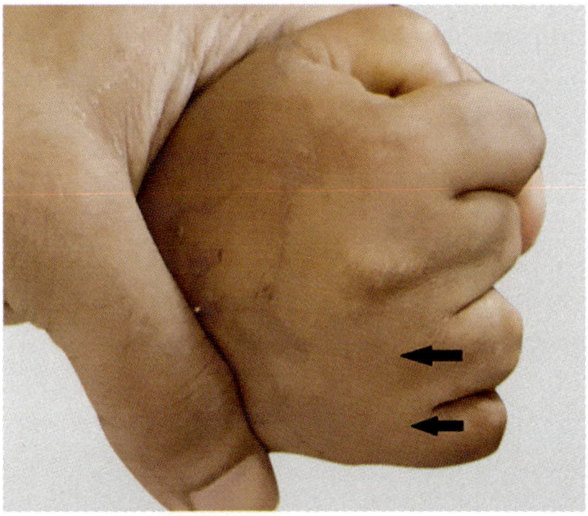

Fig. 11.9.2: Pseudohypoparathyroidism. (Arrows: Shortened metacarpals causing absence of knuckles at 4th and 5th digits resulting in classic "knuckle, knuckle, dimple, dimple" sign)

Acromegaly

Patients of acromegaly may experience arthralgia, joint stiffness, swelling, and hypermobility. In advanced and long-standing cases, restricted joint mobility and carpal tunnel syndrome can also occur. On contrary, fracture risk is shown to be decreased in patients with acromegaly in some studies and according to the researchers, this is likely due to the anabolic effects of growth hormone on bone.

Cushing's Syndrome

Musculoskeletal manifestations of hypercortisolism differ in adults than that of children. Adult Cushing's syndrome patients usually have muscle atrophy and about half of these patients are osteoporotic. In contrast, children with Cushing's syndrome frequently show growth retardation, muscle weakness, reduced bone mineral density and increase in long term risk of osteoporosis.

Addison's Disease

Painful flexion contractures at hip and knee joints are common during adrenal crisis, which resolves on administration of intravenous fluids and corticosteroids. Hyperpigmentation of skin and mucous membranes occurs commonly (Fig. 11.9.3).

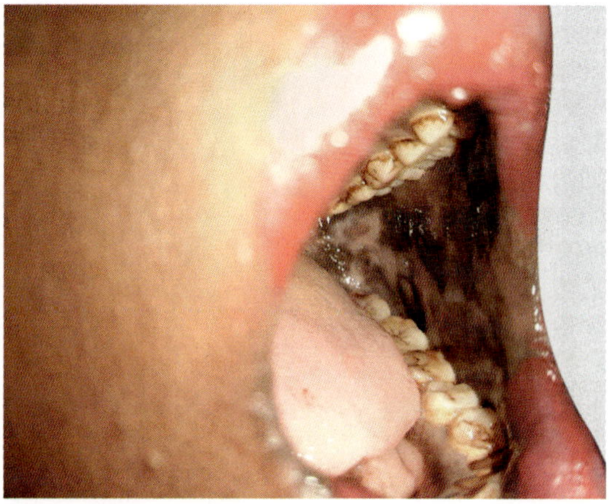

Fig. 11.9.3: Hyperpigmentation of oral mucosa in Addison's disease

CONCLUSION

The evaluation and workup of endocrine disorders is important in patients presenting with musculoskeletal symptoms. Early consideration and evaluation of an endocrine cause may improve management in such patients.

LEARNING POINTS

- Diseases of the endocrine system often cause musculoskeletal symptoms.
- Diabetic cheiroarthropathy, Carpal tunnel syndrome, Dupuytren's contracture commonly occur in Diabetics.
- Hypothyroidism and Cushing's disease can present with proximal myopathy.

FURTHER READING

1. Leatherwood C, Hoffgott SE. RheumatIc manifestations of endocrine and lipid disease. In: Hochberg MC, Gravallese EM, silman AJ, Smolen JS, Weinblatt, Weisman MH, editors. Rheumatology. 7th Edition. Philadelphia: Elsevier; 2019. pp. 1735–41

Rheumatic Manifestations of Malignancies

Prasanta Padhan

INTRODUCTION

Malignancy associated rheumatic diseases pose a special challenge to clinicians in view of their varied clinical manifestations. Malignancies can cause rheumatic manifestations either by direct spread or invasion, treatment related, e.g. check point inhibitors or by paraneoplastic rheumatism. The aim of this chapter is to give an overview of various paraneoplastic rheumatic conditions and their possible mechanisms and treatment.

Paraneoplastic syndromes related to malignancies are mediated by cytokines or hormones; due to abnormal immune activation by tumor cells. Hence the clinical manifestations occur at a distant site which can involve joints, muscles, fasciae, ligaments, bones or vessels. The musculoskeletal manifestations are considered as paraneoplastic if the symptoms appear simultaneously or within one year of detection of neoplasia; but no later than 2 years.

Common paraneoplastic rheumatic conditions include carcinomatous arthritis(CA), hypertrophic osteoarthropathy (HOA), palmar fasciitis with polyarthritis syndrome(PFPAS), remitting seronegative symmetrical synovitis with pitting edema (RS3PE), pancreatic panniculitis and polyarthritis (PPP), cancer associated myositis (CAM), paraneoplastic vasculitis and tumor induced-osteomalacia (TIO).

CARCINOMATOUS ARTHRITIS (CA)

It is commonly seen with breast cancer in females and lung cancer in males. Features include late onset arthritis (>60 years), rapid onset, lower limb arthritis, asymmetrical and seronegative. Arthritis correlates well with cancer regression or recurrence and symptomatic therapy include low dose glucocorticoids or NSAIDs.

HYPERTROPHIC OSTEOARTHROPATHY (HOA)

It is often seen with intra-thoracic especially lung malignancies and the clinical features include digital clubbing, bone pain (often in tibia or fibula), arthralgia or arthritis involving knee or ankle joints. Mechanisms include periosteal proliferation due to growth factors produced by tumor cells like VEGF , PDGF. Resolution of symptoms occurs with tumor resection and NSAIDs can provide symptomatic relief.

PALMAR FASCIITIS WITH POLYARTHRITIS SYNDROME (PFPAS)

It is characterized by progressive digital contractures, inflammatory fasciitis and polyarthritis; with a characteristic "woody hands" appearance (Fig. 11.10.1). This syndrome often precedes

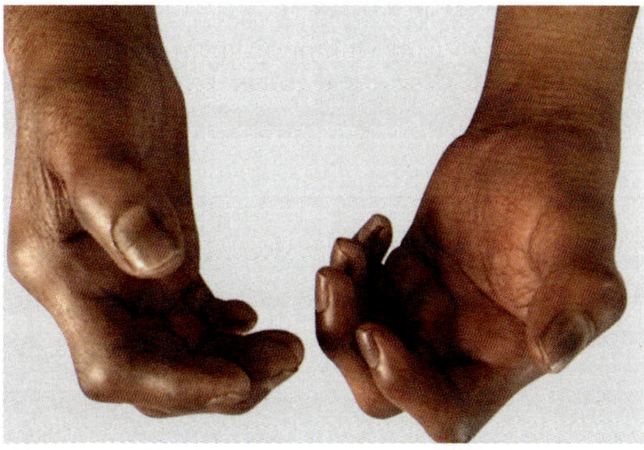

Fig. 11.10.1: "Woody hands" in a case of palmar fasciitis and polyarthritis syndrome (PFPAS) in breast carcinoma

onset of malignancies; commonly seen with ovarian, rarely gastric, uterine, breast, prostate and pancreatic cancer. Treatment includes that of underlying cancer, along with steroids or NSAIDS for symptomatic relief.

REMITTING SERONEGATIVE SYMMETRICAL SYNOVITIS WITH PITTING EDEMA (RS3PE)

Often seen in elderly, it commonly affects bilateral hands and feet with raised acute phase reactants without erosions in X-rays and a negative rheumatoid factor. This condition is often associated with edema of dorsum of hands and feet which responds well to steroids. Both solid and hematological malignancies have been associated with RS3PE.

PANCREATIC PANNICULITIS AND POLYARTHRITIS (PPP)

It is associated with acinar cell pancreatic cancer along with pancreatitis and high lipase levels bearing a dismal prognosis. Clinical features include polyarthritis with erythema nodosum involving legs.

CANCER-ASSOCIATED MYOSITIS (CAM)

Inflammatory myositis (dermatomyositis~30% and polymyostis~15%) are known to be associated with malignancies; mostly within one year of diagnosis of myositis. Risk of malignancy is higher with older age, male gender, rapid onset of symptoms, skin necrosis, periungual erythema and presence of antibodies to transcription intermediary factor TIF-1γ. The most common associated malignancies are ovarian, lung, pancreatic, stomach, bladder, colorectal cancer and non Hodgkin's lymphoma. Appropriate cancer screening is recommended with tumor markers; PET–CT may be indicated for detection of occult neoplasia.

PARANEOPLASTIC VASCULITIS

Commonly seen with hematological magnancines, the findings include those of cutaneous leukocytoclstic vasculitis. The histology include immune complexes with tumor antigens and IgA, hence all adult patients with a diagnosis of HSP, a malignancy search should be obtained.

TUMOR-INDUCED OSTEOMALACIA (TIO)

This condition is seen with mesenchymal tumors, there is bone pain, muscle weakness and spontaneous fracture; due to high levels of circulating fibroblast growth factor 23(FGF 23) resulting in increased renal phosphate wasting. Biochemical abnormalities include hypophosphatemia, normal serum calcium, PTH and raised alkaline phosphatase level. Often whole body PET scan is required for tumor localization and tumor removal is curative.

LEARNING POINTS

Identification of an underlying malignancy in the background of a rheumatic disease could be challenging. The following are a few clues which suggest the presence of occult neoplasia.

- Positive family history of malignancy.
- History of exposure to carcinogen/radiation
- Explosive onset arthritis in elderly.
- Out of proportion constitutional symptoms.
- Inadequate response to conventional therapy.
- Presence of tumor markers.
- Presence of other paraneoplastic features.

FURTHER READING

1. Manger B, Schett G. Paraneoplastic syndromes in rheumatology. Nat Rev Rheumatol. 2014;10:662–70.
2. Naschitz JE, Rosner I. Musculoskeletal syndromes associated with malignancy (excluding hypertrophic osteoarthropathy). Curr Opin Rheumatol. 2008; 20:100–5.
3. Scalapino KJ, Thomas CR Jr. Paraneoplastic and cancer treatment-related rheumatic disorders. Rheum Dis Clin North Am. 2011;37:ix-x.

Section

XII

KAWASAKI DISEASE, PRIMARY IMMUNODEFICIENCY DISEASES, AUTOINFLAMMATORY SYNDROMES, AMYLOIDOSIS, PANNICULITIS, AND SOFT TISSUE RHEUMATISM

Kawasaki Disease

Surjit Singh, Nutan Kamath, Rakesh Kumar Pilania

INTRODUCTION

Kawasaki disease (KD) is an acute, systemic inflammatory, medium vessel vasculitis of childhood. It is not only the most common vasculitis in childhood but is perhaps more common than all the other vasculitides combined. Etiopathogenesis of KD remains an enigma. It has been hypothesized that various environmental and infectious triggers are responsible for the pathogenesis of KD in a genetically predisposed individual. KD has special predilection for coronary arteries and is associated with significant long-term morbidity and mortality in these patients. Timely diagnosis and prompt treatment is essential to reduce cardiovascular complications.

EPIDEMIOLOGY

KD is usually seen in children below 5 years. Annual incidence of KD is ~10–25/100,000 children below 5 years of age in North America and Europe. The annual incidence in children of Japanese ancestry is 353/100,000 children below the age of 5. It has been estimated that, in Japan approximately 1% children develop KD by 10 years of their age. There is a paucity of nationwide incidence figures of KD from developing world including India. Based on extrapolations of hospital data at Chandigarh, incidence of KD in North India is at least 9-10/100,000 children below the age of 5.

CLINICAL FEATURES AND DIAGNOSIS

The course of the disease in KD can be divided into 3 phases (Table 12.1.1). It is important to note that diagnosis of KD remains clinical and there are no pathognomonic laboratory tests for confirmation of clinical suspicion. There are a set of clinical criteria meant to help the clinician arrive at a diagnosis (Table 12.1.2). Diagnosis of KD is based on recognition of a temporal sequence of various clinical features, although none of these have any diagnostic significance individually. Clinical manifestations in a given patient evolve over several days and all the features may not be seen at a given point of time. However, it is essential to make the diagnosis during the acute phase of disease as appropriate treatment in this phase results in a significant reduction in coronary artery complications. These criteria for diagnosis have virtually remained unchanged over 55 years since the initial description of this enigmatic disorder. Furthermore, as many as half of all children diagnosed with KD may never actually fulfill the criteria for KD and have an 'incomplete' presentation.

Important differential diagnoses to consider include viral infections, amongst others (Table 12.1.3). The following characteristic features may help distinguish KD from its mimics:

- Infants and young children with KD typically have extreme irritability.
- Fever in children with KD is usually high spiking with peak temperatures >39°C.
- Presence of a conjunctival discharge, and especially a purulent discharge, corneal ulceration, and conjunctival edema are strong pointers toward an alternative diagnosis.
- Pharyngeal erythema is usually diffuse. Discrete oral ulcers or tonsillar exudates are pointers against a diagnosis of KD.

Table 12.1.1: Disease course of Kawasaki disease

Kawasaki disease phase	*Approximate time period*	*Characteristics*
Acute (febrile) phase	1–14 days	• Fever is typically high grade and remittent, with peak temperatures usually >39°C. • After the onset of fever in the first week of illness, usually the child develops cervical lymphadenitis, nonexudative conjunctival injection, oral cavity changes, pleomorphic rash, edema and erythema of hands and feet.
Subacute phase	2–4 weeks	• Periungual desquamation and thrombocytosis are characteristic of this phase.
Convalescent or recovery period	May last for several months or even years	• Beau's lines (transverse furrows across fingernails) may be seen during the convalescent phase of KD. These are present for several days and tend to grow out with the nail. • If coronary artery abnormalities have developed in a given patient, the affected vessels would undergo healing, remodeling and ultimately, scarring during this phase. Coronary aneurysmal dilatation due to KD may end up as coronary stenosis later in life.

KD: Kawasaki disease

Table 12.1.2: Definition for diagnosis of Kawasaki disease

1. **Fever more than 5 days**
2. **At least 4 of the following 5 clinical findings**
   i. Bilateral conjunctival injection.
   ii. Changes in the oropharyngeal mucous membranes: including one or more of: cracked lips (Fig. 12.1.1), strawberry red tongue (Fig. 12.1.2), pharyngeal erythema.
   iii. Changes in the peripheral extremities, including erythema and/or edema of the hands and feet (acute phase) or periungual desquamation (convalescent phase) (Fig. 12.1.3).
   iv. Polymorphous rash, primarily truncal; nonbullous and nonvesicular.
   v. Cervical adenopathy with at least one node >1.5 cm.
3. **Illness not explained by any other disease process**

Table 12.1.3: Differential diagnosis of Kawasaki disease

Differential diagnosis	*Comments*
Viral diseases (e.g. measles, adenoviral infection, and Epstein–Barr virus infection)	• Children with viral exanthemata usually do not have evidence of systemic inflammation. • Nasal catarrh and cough are predominant in measles and adenoviral infections but not in KD. • Viral infections do not manifest the typical extremity changes seen in KD.
Scarlet fever	• Children with scarlet fever do not have ocular, lip, and articular changes. • Scarlet fever is unusual before 2 years of age. • Pastia lines are typically seen in children with scarlet fever. These are faint erythematous lines seen in various skin folds.
Stevens–Johnson syndrome or serum sickness	• Oral ulceration, exudative conjunctivitis, pseudomembrane formation, and targetoid skin lesions are prominent clinical features in children with drug reactions.
Systemic juvenile idiopathic arthritis (systemic JIA)	• Persistent, prolonged febrile illness along with generalized lymphadenopathy, hepatosplenomegaly, and characteristic evanescent rash are suggestive of systemic JIA. • Overlap of KD and systemic JIA has been reported.

KD: Kawasaki disease

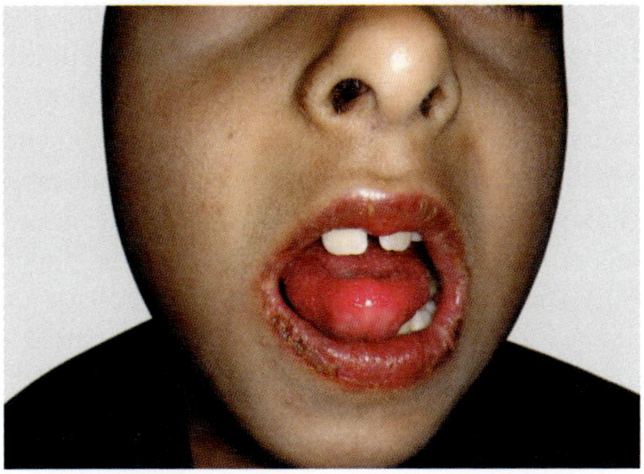

Fig. 12.1.1: Injected and fissured lips

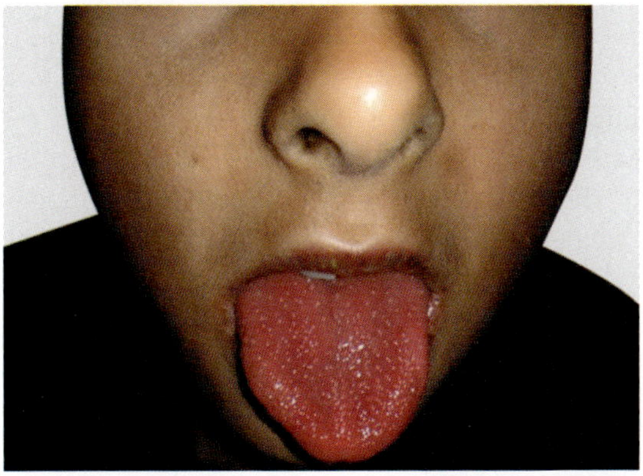

Fig. 12.1.2: Strawberry tongue

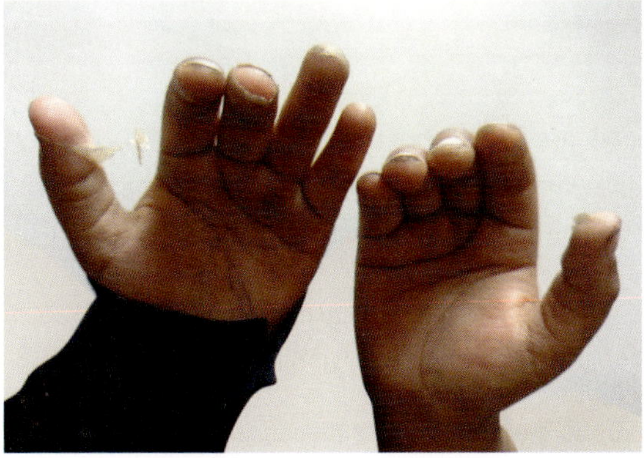

Fig. 12.1.3: Periungual desquamation

- Diffuse lymphadenopathy especially with axillary and inguinal node involvement, or the presence of splenomegaly would be unusual for KD.
- Bullous or vesicular rash are almost never seen in children with KD. Unlike measles, the rash of KD usually fades without residue.

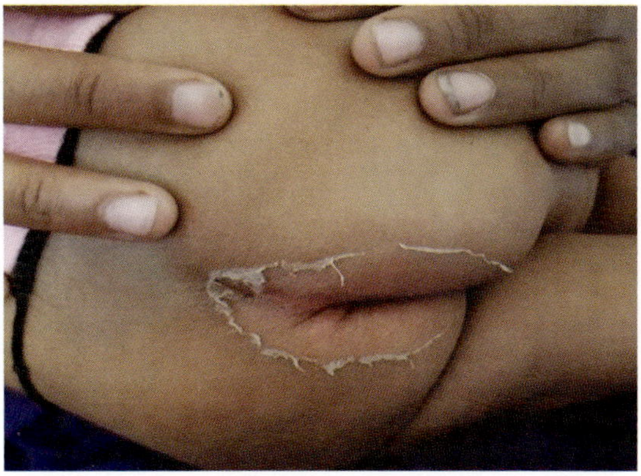

Fig. 12.1.4: Perineal desquamation

- Perineal desquamation (especially when perianal in localization) is characteristically seen in the first few days of fever and points towards a diagnosis of KD (Fig. 12.1.4).
- Periungual desquamation occurs during the subacute phase of illness (during second week of illness) and is typically seen at the tips of fingers and toes just short of the distal edge of the nails (Fig. 12.1.3).

KD is a systemic childhood vasculitis and may involve several other organ systems. Other clinical features that are often seen include arthralgia/arthritis, myositis, aseptic meningitis, facial nerve palsy, sensorineural hearing loss, peripheral aneurysms, and macrophage activation syndrome (MAS). MAS may present as thrombocytopenia. KD is also known to present with pulmonary infiltrates, pleural effusion, diarrhea, vomiting, pain abdomen, gallbladder hydrops, acute surgical abdomen, hepatomegaly, testicular swelling, redness, and crusting at the site of BCG inoculation. Beau's lines may be seen during the convalescent phase of KD. It is important to be aware of these varied clinical features lest the condition be confused with an entirely unrelated disease. In fact, it is the presence of these additional (and apparently misleading) clinical features which makes the diagnosis of this condition so challenging.

KD and Cardiac Complications

Cardiovascular complications remain important manifestations of KD and are associated with significant morbidity and mortality in children with KD. Coronary artery abnormalities (CAAs) are seen in 15–25% of patients with KD if left undiagnosed and untreated. However, it is often not appreciated that 3–5% patients can develop CAAs even after treatment with intravenous immunoglobulin (IVIg). Although CAAs remain a defining cardiovascular complication of KD, other cardiac manifestations can also occur during the acute phase of disease. These include myocarditis, valvular regurgitation and pericardial effusion. Myocarditis in children with KD has been considered as almost universal; however, symptomatic myocarditis is uncommon. Myocarditis usually manifest during first week of illness and may present as tachycardia out of proportion of fever or signs of congestive heart failure. Children with KD can also develop aneurysms of systemic arteries—these are, however, almost always seen only in children who also have large coronary aneurysms. Risk factors for increased chances of development of CAAs include persistent fever, IVIg resistant KD (persistence or recurrence of fever after more than 36–48 hours of IVIg infusion), delays in diagnosis and treatment (IVIg treatment beyond day 10 of the onset of symptoms), infants, male gender and macrophage activation syndrome.

Incomplete/atypical Kawasaki Disease

KD can sometimes present with "incomplete" and "atypical" features. Children presenting with fever and <4 of principal clinical features are classified as "incomplete" KD. A child is said to have "atypical" KD when the clinical presentation is unusual (e.g. with nephritis, seizures, stroke, or hepatitis). Infants with KD often have incomplete forms of the disease. "Incomplete" and "atypical" KD do not connote milder forms of the disease. KD should be under consideration in all infants and young children with fever >7 days in whom the cause of fever remains unclear especially when this is associated with elevated acute phase reactants. KD can occasionally be present in adolescents and adults. The diagnosis is often delayed in such cases because of the rarity of this presentation.

LABORATORY FINDINGS

Diagnosis of KD is clinical and there are no pathognomonic laboratory tests for confirmation of clinical suspicion. However, certain laboratory findings may help the pediatrician with arriving at a diagnosis (Table 12.1.4).

Imaging in KD for Cardiovascular Assessment

2D-echocardiography is used to detect CAAs and assess other cardiovascular abnormalities and in experienced hands, can provide useful information. Other imaging modalities such as Dual Source

Table 12.1.4: Laboratory findings in KD

Laboratory abnormalities	*Comments*
Neutrophilic leukocytosis	• Leukopenia and lymphopenia are usually not seen.
Anemia	• Anemia is usually normocytic normochromic. Post intravenous immunoglobulin infusion drop in hemoglobin can be seen in several children.
Elevated erythrocyte sedimentation rate	• Not reliable for monitoring post IVIg infusion.
Elevated C-reactive Protein (CRP)	• Persistence of elevated CRP levels despite IVIg therapy warrants consideration for second lien therapy.
Elevated serum transaminases	• Elevated transaminases can be a sign of severe disease.
Hyponatremia	• Markers of severe disease.
Hypoalbuminemia	• Markers of severe disease.
Abnormal plasma lipid profile	• Triglycerides are usually elevated during the acute phase.
Sterile pyuria	• An important clue for diagnosis in incomplete KD. This is due to urethritis.
CSF pleocytosis	• Mainly seen in infants. Lymphocytic predominance.

(Contd.)

Table 12.1.4: Laboratory findings in KD *(Contd.)*

Laboratory abnormalities	*Comments*
Platelet counts	• Thrombocytosis, often in excess of 500–1,000 × 10^9/L, is seen by end of second week of illness. • Thrombocytosis is one of the surrogate markers for the KD in subacute phase of disease; however, it is usually not there to help the clinician in the crucial period of the first 7–10 days of fever. • Platelet counts are usually normal during the acute phase. • Thrombocytopenia during acute phase of illness is a marker of severe disease and may herald macrophage activation syndrome.

KD: Kawasaki disease; *CRP:* C-reactive protein; *CSF:* Cerebrospinal fluid

Table 12.1.5: Imaging in Kawasaki disease for cardiovascular assessment

Imaging modality	*Comments*
2D-echocardiography (2DE)	• 2DE is essential for detailed cardiovascular assessment in patients with KD. • It is important to highlight that diagnosis of KD is clinical, and normal 2DE examination can never rule out diagnosis of KD. • During the acute phase of illness frequent 2DE examinations are essential to recognize the coronary artery involvement. • Normal 2DE during the first week of illness does not exclude the possibility of later development of CAAs. • 2DE should be repeated at the time of discharge, at 2 weeks, and 6–8 weeks from the onset of disease. • Body surface area based 'Z' scores should be used to grade the severity of CAAs. • Apart from CAAs, children with KD can have cardiac dysfunction, mild pericardial effusion, valvular regurgitation, and aortic root dilatation. • CAAs can be seen in form of coronary artery dilation, aneurysms, coronary artery thrombosis, absence of normal distal tapering and increased brightness of coronary artery wall.
Computed tomography coronary angiography (CTCA)	• Due to the availability of higher slice CT (128, 256, and 320 slice) platforms and dual source (DS) CT scanners and radiation optimized technologies, detailed coronary artery evaluation is now possible in patients with KD. • CTCA is especially useful to evaluate the distal coronary artery segments, left circumflex coronary artery, and older children and adolescents where 2DE often have poor acoustic window. • CTCA provides information about coronary arteries and the major branches with exquisite details of both luminal caliber and intramural changes. • CT calcium scoring provided additional information
Magnetic resonance coronary angiography (MRCA)	• MRCA is still under evaluation for assessment of CAAs in children with KD • MRCA has lower spatial (related to image accuracy that measures the fineness of image) and temporal (scanning speed) resolution and poorer image quality compared to CTCA.

CAAs: Coronary artery abnormalities; *KD:* Kawasaki disease

CT Coronary Angiography and Cardiac MR Angiography are being increasingly used for evaluation and follow-up (Table 12.1.5).

MANAGEMENT

Table 12.1.6 summarizes the treatment option in children with KD.

Table 12.1.6: Treatment options in Kawasaki disease

	Treatment details	*Comments*
Standard therapy	Single-dose IVIg 2 g/kg administered over 8–12 hours AND Aspirin 30 mg/kg/day (anti-inflammatory dose) given every 6 hours during febrile phase followed by 3–5 mg/kg/day (antiplatelet dose) once the fever has resolved	**IVIg** • IVIg is the drug of choice as first line therapy and should be given in first 10 days of illness. **Aspirin** • Aspirin can be discontinued once follow-up 2DE at 6–8 weeks are normal and platelet counts have normalized. • Children with KD who develop CAAs are kept on long term aspirin.
Treatment for IVIg resistant KD	Second dose of IVIg OR IV pulse methylprednisolone (30 mg/kg for 3 days) followed by oral prednisolone in tapering doses over 2–3 weeks OR Infliximab (5–10 mg/kg IV single dose)	• In 10–15% patients, fever may persist even after 36–48 hours of IVIg administration or may recur after initial subsidence. Such patients are said to have IVIg resistant KD.
Preemptive intensification of therapy	Along with standard therapy, use of corticosteroids, infliximab and oral cyclosporine may be considered	• Preemptive intensification of therapy is necessary in the following situations: i. in infants ii. with CAAs at presentation iii. with evolving CAAs iv. in shock syndrome v. with macrophage activation syndrome vi. with severe myocarditis
Anticoagulants, antiplatelet agents, and statins	No CAAs	• Aspirin can be discontinued once platelet counts have normalized and follow-up 2DE at 6–8 weeks are normal.
	Coronary artery dilation (Z score: >2 to <2.5) and small CAAs (Z score: 2.5–5)	• Aspirin needs to be continued till normalization • Statins may be considered
	Medium-sized CAAs (Z score: 5–10)	• Aspirin needs to be continued until the CAAs persists • Statins can be considered
	Multiple complex aneurysm/large/giant aneurysms (Z score>10; absolute diameter >8mm)	• Patients with large/giant/multiple aneurysms need intensification of therapy • Therapeutic anticoagulation is required • Aspirin is usually continued for several years • Statins should be considered

2DE: 2D-echocardiography; *CAAs:* Coronary artery abnormalities; *IVIg:* Intravenous immunoglobulin; *KD:* Kawasaki disease

PROGNOSIS

Recurrences of KD can occur in 1–3% of cases. Mortality rates in KD were 1–2% in pre-IVIG era. With timely recognition and early institution of treatment during the acute phase of disease, mortality rates in KD in the developed world are presently 0.08%. At Chandigarh, the mortality rate in KD is 0.8%. Delays in diagnosis and institution of appropriate therapy are responsible for the majority of deaths.

SUMMARY

KD is a common childhood medium vessel vasculitis presenting as acute febrile illness in children. It is the most common cause of acquired heart disease in children in the developed world. Diagnosis of KD is clinical and there are no pathognomonic laboratory tests for confirmation. Etiology of KD is considered to be due to infectious and/or environmental trigger in a genetically predisposed individual. KD can result in CAAs which is responsible for significant long term morbidity and mortality. Timely diagnosis and early institution of appropriate therapy is crucial for prevention of development of cardiac complications. Children with KD requires long-term follow-up, irrespective of their cardiac status in the initial attack.

LEARNING POINTS

1. KD should be a differential diagnosis of fever in all infants and young children, when it persists beyond 5 days and there is no reasonable explanation for the continuing fever.
2. Diagnosis is clinical, though laboratory parameters can help in reaching at a diagnosis.
3. KD can results in coronary artery abnormalities.
4. The risk of coronary abnormalities can be decreased if intravenous immunoglobulin is given early, preferably within 10 days of onset of illness.
5. Being a systemic vasculitis, KD can involve other systems (e.g. hepatic, pulmonary, gastrointestinal, and central nervous systems).
6. Early recognition can prevent delays in diagnosis and allow the institution of appropriate therapy.

FURTHER READING

1. Jindal AK, Pilania RK, Prithvi A, et al. Kawasaki disease: characteristics, diagnosis, and unusual presentations. Expert Rev Clin Immunol. 2019; 15(10): 1089–104.
2. McCrindle BW, Rowley AH, Newburger JW, et al. Diagnosis, Treatment, and Long-Term Management of Kawasaki Disease: A Scientific Statement for Health Professionals From the American Heart Association. Circulation. 2017;135:e927–99.
3. Pilania RK, Bhattarai D, Singh S. Controversies in diagnosis and management of Kawasaki disease. World J Clin Pediatr. 2018; 7:27–35.
4. Pilania RK, Jindal AK, Bhattarai D, et al. Cardiovascular Involvement in Kawasaki Disease Is Much More Than Mere Coronary Arteritis. Front Pediatr. 2020; 8:526969.
5. Singh S, Vignesh P, Burgner D. The epidemiology of Kawasaki disease: a global update. Arch Dis Child. 2015; 100(11):1084–1088.

Chapter 12.2

Soft Tissue Rheumatism

BG Dharmanand

INTRODUCTION

Soft tissue rheumatism (STR) is a term used to describe pain and dysfunction arising from the soft tissues, namely tendons, ligaments, and muscles rather than from joints or bones, the "hard tissues". As a syndrome, it is much more common than inflammatory conditions arising from joints and bones in clinical practice. Soft tissue rheumatism *excludes* soft tissue lesions such as enthesitis of spondyloarthritis, myositis of dermatomyositis, and myalgia of polymyalgia rheumatica.

STR could be diffuse, regional, or localized. Fibromyalgia is the most common diffuse STR. Widespread aches along with multiple somatic symptoms characterize fibromyalgia. A patient with too many symptoms along with widespread pain and tenderness is likely to have fibromyalgia, that is further discussed separately. Somatoform disorders and multisite regional pain syndromes also fit into the concept of diffuse STR.

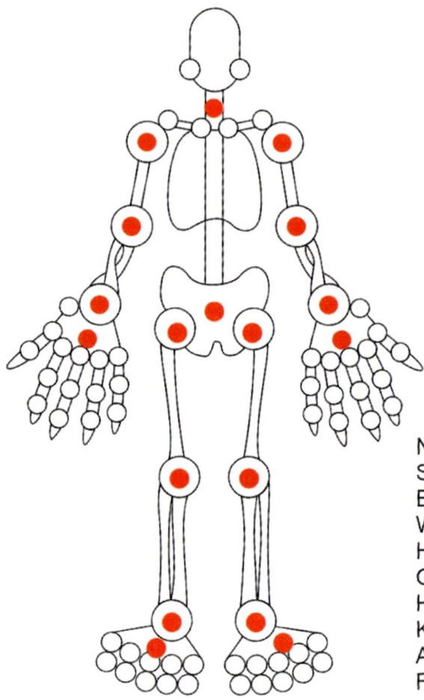

Fig. 12.2.1: Regional pain is classified based on which region it arises from. Regional pain can arise from neck, shoulder, elbow, wrist, hand regions in the upper limb, and pelvis, hip, knee, ankle or foot regions.

REGIONAL SOFT TISSUE RHEUMATISM

Patients with pain and dysfunction arising from a single musculoskeletal region, for example, the shoulder region or the hip region are considered as having regional pain. They are grouped depending on the anatomical region the pain is arising from (Fig. 12.1.1), for example, shoulder, hip, or neck. The risk factors for regional pain include performing unaccustomed activities, work-related strain, or poor posture, among others (Table 12.1.1).

APPROACH TO A PATIENT WITH REGIONAL PAIN SYNDROME

When a patient is evaluated for pain, a regional approach is more rational. For example, in the case of shoulder pain, consider the problem as *shoulder regional* pain rather than as *shoulder joint* pain. This is because pain may be arising from the shoulder joint complex or from the structures around the shoulder (Table 12.2.2). This approach would widen the differential diagnosis with different diagnostic possibilities.

Table 12.2.1: Risk factors for regional pain and soft tissue rheumatism
Unaccustomed activities
Work-related strain
Poor posture
Obesity
Sports related injuries
Hypermobile joint syndrome
Flat feet/hyperpronated feet
Poor footwear
Poor job satisfaction
Red flags
• Trauma
• Surgery
• Systemic rheumatic diseases
• Infections
• Malignancy

Table 12.2.2: Causes to consider when evaluating regional pain
The following conditions serve as a differential diagnosis when evaluating a patient who presents with regional pain
• Arthritis or intraarticular pathology
• Periarticular structures pathology
• Neurogenic pain
• Referred pain including myofascial pain syndrome (MFPS)

History: While evaluating regional pain, history taking must include:

- The **o**nset of pain
- Presence of any **p**rovoking factor or relieving factor
- **Q**uality of pain
- Whether there is any **r**adiation of pain or related symptoms
- **S**everity of pain
- **T**ime of pain

The mnemonic "OPQRST" is helpful to remember all the points to note down in the history. Other important points to note in the history are whether there was any occurence of trauma, surgery, or any unaccustomed activity (Table 12.2.1). Occupational history is important in understanding the potential predisposing factors. Poor job satisfaction is another risk factor for persistent regional pain syndromes like back ache. In some, regional pain syndromes may be a result of distress and predicament of life.

A constant and severe pain, without any variation with activity, is more likely to be of neuropathic or psychogenic origin and not of nociceptive origin. Neuropathic quality of the symptoms (paresthesia and tingling) would suggest entrapment neuropathy.

Physical examination: It includes musculoskeletal and neurological examinations.

Skin color changes along with allodynia and hyperesthesia point toward complex regional pain syndromes (CRPS). Passive and active movements should be checked along with resisted active movements. Pain arising mainly from resisted movements suggests periarthritis like enthesitis or tendon pathology.

If the regional examination is normal, an examination of the immediate proximal joint should be performed. As an example, hip osteoarthritis can present with knee pain. If the palpation of the region of pain does not elicit a nociceptive response, consider either neuropathic pain or pain arising from a different region that is referred to as the area of complaint.

Muscles around the region of pain have to be palpated for trigger points. Myofascial pain syndrome (MFS) can mimic neuropathic and arthritic conditions. Knowledge about trigger points and radiation patterns would be useful when evaluating regional pain. Joint hypermobility predisposes one to soft tissue rheumatism and thus should be a part of the evaluation.

LOCALIZED SOFT TISSUE RHEUMATISM

Some conditions are localized and present with typical symptoms and localized pathology. Some examples of localized soft tissue rheumatism are:

- deQuervain's tenosynovitis presents with lateral wrist and distal forearm pain. On examination, there is localized tenderness and a positive Finkelstein test. Diagnosis in this type of soft tissue rheumatism is straightforward.
- Plantar fasciitis presents with heel pain at the insertion of the plantar fascia with the calcaneus. Tenderness is elicited on palpation of the tendon at the insertion site.
- Tennis elbow or lateral epicondylitis. Tenderness is elicited on pressing the site and on resisting the supination of the forearm.

- Golfer's elbow or medial epicondylitis. Clinically diagnosed on eliciting tenderness on resisted pronation of the forearm.
- Trigger finger as the name suggests, finger movement gets restricted while flexing or extending due to the thickening of the retinacular sheath that encompasses the tendons. It is frequently seen in diabetics.
- Painful arc syndrome or shoulder impingement syndrome. The patient presents with shoulder pain. The rotator cuff tendons are impinged by the acromion within the subacromial space when the arm is abducted. The pain is reproduced at 60–120° of arm abduction (painful arc) or when lifting the arm over the head.
- Carpal tunnel syndrome is due to median nerve entrapment in the carpal tunnel space. The patient presents with pain at the wrist with tingling and numbness along the distribution of the median nerve.

When the symptoms and clinical signs are atypical, the approach suggested for regional pain would help in the correct diagnosis. If a patient with lateral elbow pain has much more diffuse pain and more widespread tenderness along the muscle bellies of extensor muscles, look for trigger points. If the resisted extension of the wrist is normal but there are trigger points on palpation of which pain is reproduced, a diagnosis of MFS is likely. The treatment approach would be different.

MANAGEMENT

Correct diagnosis usually leads to appropriate management strategies for regional and localized STR. Particular attention needs to be given to correctable or modifiable etiological factors. Ergonomic advice, correct sports techniques and footwear may prevent recurrences of symptoms.

Most acute STRs are self-limiting. Rest, ice, compression, and elevation (RICE) is sufficient. Splinting may be needed in some. NSAIDs are used for a brief period. But some can become chronic and may cause significant functional limitations. Physical therapy using local heat, therapeutic massage, exercises, and stretching are the mainstay of treatment. Eccentric loading exercises may be more effective for tendinopathies such as lateral epicondylitis than conventional exercises like stretching and strengthening exercises. Local steroid injection promptly provides short-term relief. Trigger point injections with local anesthetics or dry needling of trigger points are an effective treatment for MFS.

LEARNING POINTS

1. Soft tissue rheumatism is generalized (fibromyalgia), regional, and localized.
2. When a patient is evaluated for pain, a regional approach is more rational. For example, in the case of shoulder pain, consider the problem as *shoulder regional* pain rather than as *shoulder joint* pain.
3. Localized soft tissue rheumatism includes trigger finger, deQuervain's tenosynovitis, tennis elbow, golfer's elbow and carpal tunnel syndrome. In localized STR always consider myofascial syndrome in the differential diagnosis if the pain is more widespread and if there are trigger points on muscle examination.

FURTHER READING

1. Couppé C, Svensson RB, Silbernagel KG, et al. Eccentric or Concentric Exercises for the Treatment of Tendinopathies? J Orthop Sports Phys Ther. 2015; 45:853–63.
2. Dharmanand BG, Yathish GC. Regional pain. In: Wagh S, Ravindran V, editors. Rheumatology in primary care. First edition. Mumbai: National Book Depot; 2021. pp 32–43.
3. Hazleman B, Riley G, Speed C, editors. Soft tissue rheumatology. Oxford: Oxford University Press; 2004.
4. Hutson M, Dharmanand B. Soft tissue Rheumatism. Indian J Rheumatol 2014; 9 Suppl 2:S1–S70
5. Latt LD, Jaffe DE, Tang Y, et al. Evaluation and treatment of chronic plantar fasciitis. Foot Ankle Orthop. 2020; 5:2473011419896763.

Fibromyalgia

Sakir Ahmed, Able Lawrence

INTRODUCTION

Fibromyalgia (FM) is a chronic disease of widespread pain with fatigue, non-restorative sleep and various degrees of other overlapping symptoms. It is characterised by central sensitization. It is supposed to have a prevalence of 1–2% in the general population although community-based surveys have estimated around 5%. It predominantly affects women and incurs considerable distress at the personal level and economic and social burdens at the societal level.

CLINICAL FEATURES

The main complaint is persistent and widespread pain, often rated more severe than that of inflammatory arthritis. It may start regionally and then spread. Patients complain of morning stiffness or "swelling" but objective swelling is rare. Diverse sleep abnormalities and sleep disorders are common. Patients have non-restorative sleep that may worsen pain perception.

Patients have fatigue and poor tolerance to physical activities including exercise. Pathologic fatigue can be distinguished from sleep deprivation by sleep latency which is decreased in the latter and increased in patients with chronic fatigue syndrome (Table 12.3.1).

Table 12.3.1: Features of fibromyalgia

1. Generalized body pain
2. Allodynia
3. Sleep disturbance
4. Fatigue
5. Distress
6. 'Fibrofog'
7. Dysesthesia
8. Complaint of "swelling"
9. Change in skin color and temperature*
10. Dermatographism*
11. Raynaud's phenomenon*

*Rare in the Indian population

DIAGNOSIS

The use of a diagnostic criteria should be used to valid a FM diagnosis. The AAPT criteria is simple and easy to use for beginners. However, they may not be sensitive enough to capture all patients with FM. Thus, the use of tender points (ACR1990 criteria) or the more comprehensive ACR2016 criteria may be preferred by rheumatologists more attuned to FM.

Fibromyalgia should be considered in patients with persistent widespread pain for at least 3 months. Widespread is defined as pain in at least 4/5 areas (4 limbs plus axial). The **ACR 1990 criteria**: Require at least 11 out of 18 tender points. Certain physicians were often unwilling or untrained to look for tender points which made the diagnosis "physician centric". This led to the development of preliminary diagnostic criteria of 2010 which was further modified in 2016. The **ACR 2016 criteria** depend on two scales, (a) Widespread pain index (WPI) and (b) Symptoms severity scale (SS). A minimum WPI of 7 with SS of 5, or a WPI of 3–6 with SS of at least 9 are required for diagnosis (Fig. 12.3.1). Polysymptomatic distress scale (=WPI

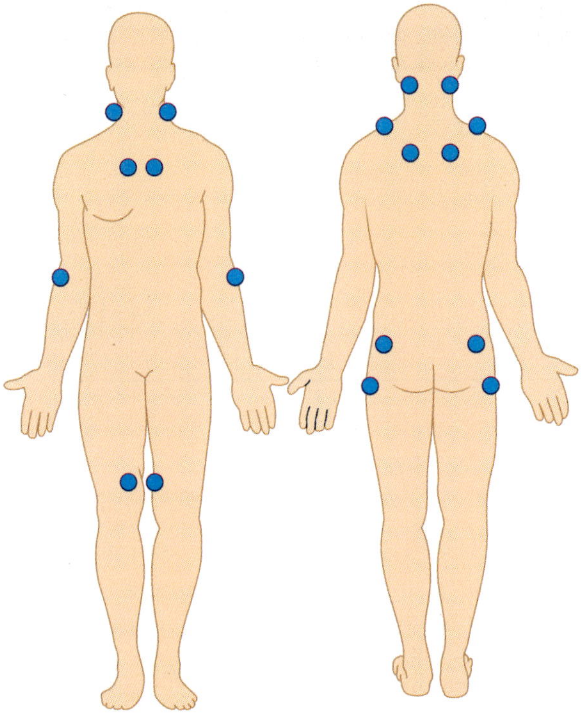

Fig. 12.3.1a: Tender points required for 1990 classification criteria

Widespread pain (in last 7 days) (√)					*Symptom severity*	
R Jaw		L Jaw			Severity of each symptom during the last 7 days	Score*
R shoulder		L shoulder			Fatigue	
R upper arm		L upper arm			Trouble thinking or remembering	
R lower arm		L lower arm			Waking up tired	
	Neck				* Scoring: 0 no problem; 1 slight problem; 2 moderate problem; 3 severe Problem	
	Chest					
	Abdomen				Tick (√) if present in last 6 months	
	Upper back					
	Lower back					
R hip or buttock		L hip or buttock			Pain or abdominal crap	
R upper leg		L upper leg			Depression	
R lower leg		L lower leg			Headache	
WPI = (Total no of ticks)					SS = (sum of symptom severity plus no of ticks)	

Fig. 12.3.1b: 2016 modified 2010 ACR diagnostic criteria for FM: WPI and SS

+ SS) gives an index of fibromyalgia severity, i.e. "fibromyalgianess".

The **AAPT** [The Analgesic, Anesthetic, and Addiction Clinical Trial Translations Innovations Opportunities and Networks (ACTTION) and the American Pain Society (APS) initiated ACTTION-APS Pain Taxonomy (AAPT)] criteria for FM are simple and easy to use in day-to-day practice. It requires ≥6 pain sites out of 9 defined sites [head, left arm, right arm, chest, abdomen, upper back and spine, lower back and spine (including buttocks), left leg, and right leg]; and Moderate-to-severe sleep

Table 12.3.2: Functional somatic syndromes

Conditions mimicking and/or overlapping fibromyalgia	
Inflammatory conditions 1. Seronegative spondyloarthropathy 2. Inflammatory myositis 3. Rheumatoid arthritis 4. Sjögren's syndrome 5. Lupus	**Medications** 1. Statins 2. Bisphosphonates 3. Opioids (opioid-induced hyperalgesia) 4. Aromatase inhibitors
Mechanical syndromes 1. Hypermobility syndrome 2. Degenerative disk disease 3. Myofascial pain 4. Osteoarthritis 5. Temporomandibular joint syndrome 6. Facet arthropathy **Psychiatric disorders** 1. Mood disorders 2. Stress disorders (including PTSD) 3. Anxiety Disorders	**Functional disorders** 1. Dysmenorrhea 2. Chronic fatigue syndrome 3. Functional bowel disorder syndrome 4. Hyperventilation syndrome 5. Interstitial cystitis 6. Irritable bowel syndrome 7. Migraine headache 8. Periodical limb movement syndrome (PLMS) 9. Vestibular disorders
Endocrine 1. Hypothyroidism 2. Hyperparathyroidism 3. Cushing syndrome 4. Addison disease **Osteomalacia**	**Miscellaneous** 1. Long COVID 2. Mitochondrial disease 3. Metabolic myopathies 4. Magnesium deficiency

problems OR fatigue; and both of the previous must be there for at least 3 months.

Physicians treating FM must be able to recognise the spectrum of overlapping disorders that can both mimic FM as well as coexist with it. Some have been grouped as "functional somatic syndromes (FSS)" or "central sensitization syndrome". Thus, it is important for the physician diagnosing FM to be familiar with and screen for these disorders (Table 12.3.2).

INVESTIGATIONS

The minimum investigations suggested are hemoglobin, acute phase reactants (ESR, CRP), serum calcium and phosphate, alkaline phosphatase and thyroid function tests. Depending on clinical presentation, creatinine kinase (CPK), X-ray or MRI of sacroiliac joints, HIV, etc may also be required. Polysomnography may be done in selected patients to diagnose sleep disorders. Ultrasound is an important tool to pick up inflammatory arthritis or Sjogren syndrome in doubtful cases.

MANAGEMENT

Patients with fibromyalgia require multidisciplinary care. Patient education and reassurance are cornerstones. Cognitive behavioural therapy and mindfulness meditation would help reduce maladaptive behavioural patterns. Patients should be encouraged to increase physical activity and aerobic exercise and obese patients should reduce weight.

There is considerable patient heterogeneity to different drugs and different patients may respond to one or the other (Table 12.3.3). Patients not responding one to one drug may be switched to the other or initiated combination therapy. The presence of comorbidities should guide initial therapy. Patients with clinically significant depression may be initiated on serotonin and norepinephrine reuptake inhibitors (SNRIs) while pure fibromyalgia without depression or those with features of restless legs syndrome should be initiated on pregabalin as the latter would worsen with antidepressant drugs. While highly selective serotonin reuptake inhibitors

Table 12.3.3: Management of fibromyalgia

A. Nonpharmacological
1. Patient education
2. Exercise and physiotherapy
3. Cognitive behavior therapy
B. Pharmacological
1. Anticonvulsants: Pregabalin, gabapentin
2. TCA: Amitriptyline, cyclobenzaprine
3. SNRIs: Duloxetine, milnacipran, mirtazapine
4. 5HT3 antagonist: Tropisetron
C. Others
1. Mindfulness techniques
2. Tai chi
3. Yoga
4. Acupuncture

(SSRIs) like citalopram and sertraline are effective and safe in depression, they do not relieve pain. Low-dose amitriptyline is also effective especially for those with difficulty sleeping. However, anticholinergic side effects may preclude use at higher doses.

Nonsteroidal anti-inflammatory drugs do not improve the pain of patients with fibromyalgia, and should not be used in those without inflammatory arthritis. Opioid analgesics should not be used as well as they worsen chronic pain and are ineffective due to overactive endogenous opioid pathways.

The successful treatment of fibromyalgia is highly dependent on the physician understanding the disease and prevalent comorbidities and conveying a proper management plan to the patient. It requires patience, communication skills, and ultimately expertise in the "Art of medicine".

LEARNING POINTS

- Establish the diagnosis: ACR1990 criteria (based on tender points) and the ACR2010/2016 modification criteria (based on widespread pain score and symptoms severity score) may be used complementarily (Table 12.3.1).
- The AAPT criteria may be more suited for general practice.
- Presence of FM does not exclude any other diagnosis: look for mimics as well as known comorbid conditions in FM. The 2016 criteria have not superseded or invalidated the 1990 criteria.
- Plan of therapy should incorporate the associated/comorbid conditions. Physical therapies, mindfulness techniques and cognitive behavioural therapies should supplement pharmacological therapies.

FURTHER READING

1. Ahmed S, Aggarwal A, Lawrence A. Performance of the American College of Rheumatology 2016 criteria for fibromyalgia in a referral care setting. Rheumatol Int. 2019; 39:1397–403.
2. Jones GT, Atzeni F, Beasley M, Flüß E, Sarzi-Puttini P, Macfarlane GJ. The prevalence of fibromyalgia in the general population: a comparison of the American College of Rheumatology 1990, 2010, and modified 2010 classification criteria. Arthritis Rheumatol. 2015; 67:568–75.
3. Katz RS, Wolfe F, Michaud K. Fibromyalgia diagnosis: a comparison of a clinical, survey, and American College of Rheumatology criteria. Arthritis Rheum. 2006; 54:169–76.
4. Wolfe F, Clauw DJ, Fitzcharles MA et al. The American College of Rheumatology preliminary diagnostic criteria for fibromyalgia and measurement of symptom severity. Arthritis Care Res (Hoboken). 2010; 62:600–10.
5. Wolfe F, Clauw DJ, Fitzcharles MA et al. 2016 Revisions to the 2010/2011 fibromyalgia diagnostic criteria. Semin Arthritis Rheum. 2016; 46:319–29.
6. Wolfe F, Smythe HA, Yunus MB, Bennett RM, Bombardier C, Goldenberg DL, Tugwell P, Campbell SM, Abeles M, Clark P, et al. The American College of Rheumatology 1990 Criteria for the Classification of Fibromyalgia. Report of the Multicenter Criteria Committee. Arthritis Rheum. 1990; 33:160–72.

Chapter 12.4

Primary Immunodeficiency Diseases: A Rheumatologist's Perspective

Aaqib Zaffar Banday, Dharmagat Bhattarai, Anju Gupta

INTRODUCTION

As primary immunodeficiency diseases (PIDs) are a vast group of disorders (Box 12.4.1) with varying pathophysiology, clinical manifestations and treatment, a comprehensive overview of all these disorders is well beyond the scope of a single write-up. In this chapter, therefore, we have included a brief overview of a few common PIDs. Though core symptoms of PID relate to predisposition to infections, other manifestations such as autoimmunity and malignancy are not uncommon. Recognition of PIDs in a setting of autoimmune/rheumatological manifestations is necessary since immunosuppressive therapy for autoimmunity may further aggravate the risk of infection in these individuals.

Box 12.4.1: Basic overview of primary immunodeficiency diseases (PIDs)

- The immune system is a coordinated network of blood cells and lymphoid tissues that, in addition to the well-known function of warding off pathogens, plays a crucial role in normal tissue healing and remodeling.
- Acquired abnormalities in the immune system have been noted in a majority of autoimmune diseases (including rheumatological or collagen vascular diseases), viral infections like HIV, malnutrition, antibodies against immune components, and cytotoxic therapies.
- Similarly, inherited abnormalities of the immune system can also lead to the development of immunodeficiency and immune-dysregulation (for example, autoimmunity). These disorders, more aptly termed inborn errors of immunity (IEIs), comprise an intricate group of close to 500 genetic disorders, which have been classified into 9 groups in the recent International Union of Immunological Societies (IUIS, 2019) classification.
- Although each PID may be rare individually, the frequency of all PIDs combined may be as high as 0.1% of the general population.
- In a majority of cases, PIDs present with infectious illnesses which are often recurrent, persistent, unusually complicated, or due to unusual and less pathogenic organisms.
- The infection profile usually provides vital clues towards the arm of the immune system affected by the underlying genetic defect. Aberrations in cell-mediated immunity predispose to viral, bacterial, fungal, and even parasitic infections; whereas, defects in humoral immunity result in mucosal (including respiratory and gastrointestinal tracts) and cutaneous infections primarily from encapsulated bacteria. Viral (except enteroviruses), fungal, and parasitic (except *Giardia* sp.) infections are rare in patients with humoral immunodeficiency.
- Features of immune dysregulation, including autoimmunity, malignancy, and rheumatological illnesses, can also be an important accompaniment in many PIDs. In such cases, especially in presence of other clues (for example family history, failure to thrive, etc.), consideration of an underlying PID seems prudent.
- A basic idea of the clinical features, a high index of suspicion, and expert guidance are necessary for diagnosis. Most often, these disorders are suspected by nonimmunologists who then seek diagnostic confirmation for such patients.

X-LINKED AGAMMAGLOBULINEMIA (XLA)

XLA is the prototype of humoral immunodeficiency (Fig.12.4.1) that presents with recurrent respiratory tract infections, diarrhea, skin/soft-tissue infections, and CNS infections. These children are predisposed to severe and sometimes life-threatening infections with enteroviruses including the oral (live) polio vaccine (OPV). Such is the sensitivity to OPV in XLA that the vaccine is not only contraindicated in children with XLA but also in close contacts of children with XLA. In fact, vaccine-associated paralytic poliomyelitis may be the presenting manifestation of XLA in some cases.

In addition to infections, arthritis may be seen in up to one-fourth of children with XLA. Large joint monoarthritis caused by *Mycoplasma* sp. is the most frequent musculoskeletal manifestation. Diagnosis is based on polymerase chain reaction for *Mycoplasma* sp. from the synovial fluid as serological tests are negative because of defects in antibody production. A prolonged course of azithromycin (often 2–3 weeks) is usually employed for its treatment. Additionally, children with XLA may rarely present with non-infective oligo- or polyarthritis which may mimic juvenile idiopathic arthritis (JIA).

COMMON VARIABLE IMMUNE DEFICIENCY (CVID)

CVID is the most common symptomatic PID in adults. The clinical profile is dominated by recurrent/persistent infections of respiratory and gastrointestinal tracts similar to XLA. Additionally, enteroviral infections may be problematic in CVID as well. Clinical presentation is in older children, adolescents and adults unlike in XLA where children can present with infection after the first 6 months of age.

CVID is notorious for its autoimmune manifestations which often lead to diagnostic delays and dilemmas. Autoimmune cytopenia, enteropathy, hepatitis, benign and malignant lymphoproliferation, arthritis, and vasculitis have been reported. It can also exhibit sarcoidosis-like manifestations with noncaseating granulomatous lesions in the skin, lungs, and lymph nodes.

CHRONIC GRANULOMATOUS DISEASE (CGD)

CGD is characterized by repeated deep-seated infections like recurrent or persistent pneumonia, liver abscess, lymphadenitis, and skin and musculoskeletal infections including osteomyelitis (Fig. 12.4.2). Inflammatory (noninfective) manifestations are an integral part of the clinical spectrum of CGD. These include inflammatory fevers, oral ulcers/stomatitis, inflammatory bowel disease like manifestations, vasculitis, and granulomatous inflammation in various organs such as liver, lung, gastrointestinal, and genitourinary tracts. Granulomatous inflammation may lead to obstructive symptoms such as ureteral/urethral stenosis and gastric outlet obstruction. Patients with

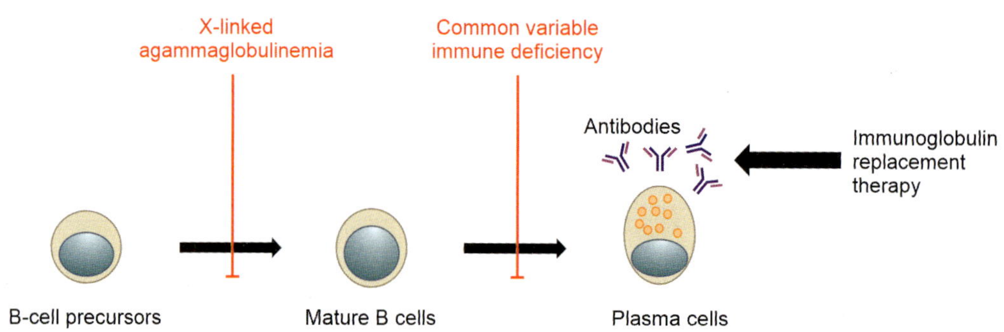

Fig. 12.4.1: A simplified summary of B-cell development and antibody production. XLA is caused by defects in BTK gene [encoding for Bruton tyrosine kinase (Btk) enzyme] which is critical for B cell development. Therefore, patients with XLA have pan-hypogammaglobulinemia and absent B cells. Maternally derived IgG antibodies often protect young infants (up to initial 4–6 months) from infections. In CVID, the maturation of B cells is defective. Hence, hypogammaglobulinemia and decreased switched memory B cells (and normal B cell counts) are characteristic immunological abnormalities. Since antibody production is defective, periodic replacement of the antibodies is the mainstay of treatment.

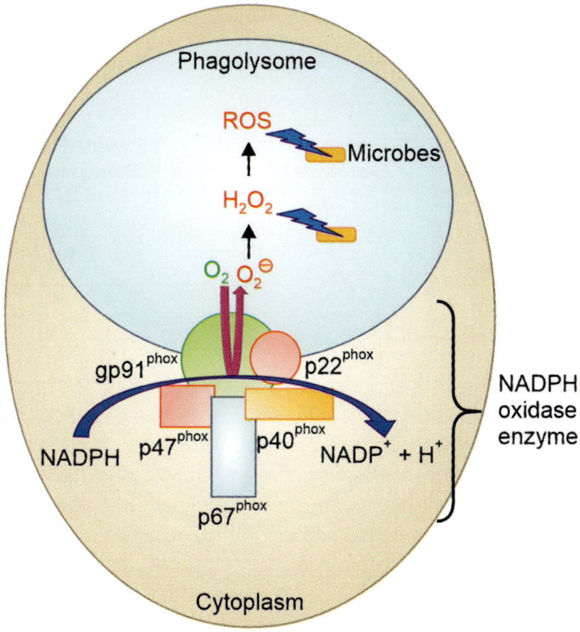

Fig. 12.4.2: Schematic representation of the role of phagocyte nicotinamide adenine dinucleotide phosphate (NADPH) oxidase enzyme in the generation of reactive oxygen species (ROS) utilized in the killing of phagocytosed bacteria. CGD can be caused by defects in any of the 5 main subunits of NADPH oxidase enzyme (gp91^{phox}, p22^{phox}, p47^{phox}, p67^{phox}, and p40^{phox}) resulting in the defective generation of reactive oxygen species (ROS). NADPH catalyzes the first and the most important step in the generation of ROS in the phagolysosome whereby superoxide ions are generated from oxygen. Hence, the signature organisms causing infections in CGD include catalase-positive organisms (*Staphylococcus aureus, Aspergillus* sp., *Candida* sp., *Pseudomonas* sp., *Burkholderia* sp., mycobacteria, and members of the Enterobacteriaceae family) which can degrade the small amounts of hydrogen peroxide formed in the phagolysosome.

CGD can also have sarcoidosis-like manifestations. Not only patients with CGD, but X-linked carriers (females) of CGD are also predisposed to autoimmune manifestations which notably include lupus-like disease.

WISKOTT ALDRICH SYNDROME (WAS)

WAS is one of the earliest PIDs to be described, named eponymously after Alfred Wiskott and Robert Aldrich who reported the clinical features of the illness in 1937 and 1954 respectively. WAS manifests as microthrombocytopenia, eczema, recurrent sinopulmonary infections, and bloody diarrhea. In addition to encapsulated bacterial infections, fungal and viral infections may also dominate the clinical picture.

WAS may present with a multitude of autoimmune and rheumatological manifestations. As isolated thrombocytopenia (and bleeding diathesis) may be the only or predominant manifestation (Fig.12.4.3), WAS is often misdiagnosed as immune thrombocytopenic purpura (ITP). Nonetheless, autoimmune cytopenias including thrombocytopenia may occur in addition to microthrombocytopenia. Vasculitis, IgA nephropathy, arthritis, and benign and malignant lymphoproliferation have been reported.

COMPLEMENT DEFICIENCY

The complement system (Fig.12.4.4) is a group of nearly four dozen soluble factors present in human plasma. These proteins play a crucial role in immunity against encapsulated bacteria and facilitate the clearance of immune complexes and apoptotic cells. Patients with complement deficiency present with bacterial infections; *meningococcus* in terminal complement deficiency, and pneumococcus and *H. influenzae* type B when other complements are deficient (Fig. 12.4.4).

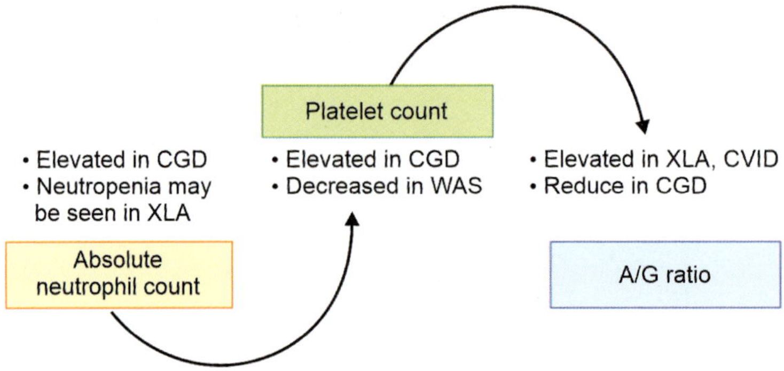

Fig. 12.4.3: Clues on basic laboratory investigations for diagnosis of important PIDs mentioned in the text. In patients with XLA and CVID who present with autoimmune/rheumatological manifestations, measurement of albumin to globulin (A/G) ratio and, more specifically, serum immunoglobulins provide crucial clues for diagnosis. Patients with autoimmune/rheumatological manifestations in absence of XLA and CVID often have hyperglobulinemia (with a low A/G ratio, often less than 1.0–1.2) resulting from hypergammaglobulinemia. In contrast, patients with CVID and XLA have hypoglobulinemia (elevated A/G ratio, often more than 1.5–1.8) resulting from less amount of immunoglobulin. In patients with WAS who present with rheumatological manifestations, a simple measurement of platelet count and mean platelet volume may help clinch the diagnosis. Patients with rheumatological manifestations in absence of WAS often have thrombocytosis or high-normal platelet counts (as platelets are the acute phase reactants). In contrast, patients with WAS have low (or mildly low) platelet counts even in presence of severe inflammation. Patients with CGD often have thrombocytosis and a low A/G ratio (due to hypergammaglobulinemia) resulting from chronic inflammation.

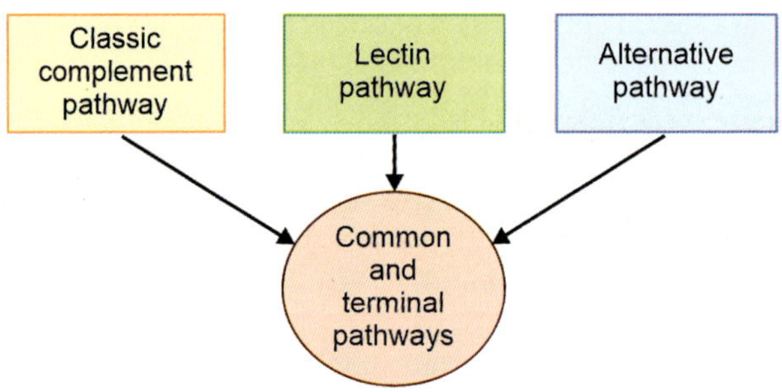

Fig. 12.4.4: The complement cascade is often subdivided into classical, alternate, mannose-binding lectin pathway, and finally terminal pathway. The classical pathway includes C1q/r/s, C2, and C4; and the alternate pathway comprises factors B, D, and properdin. The lectin pathway comprises mannose-binding lectins (MBL) and MBL-associated serine proteases. These pathways converge at C3 which sequentially activates C5–C9 (common and terminal pathways).

Patients with deficiency of early complement defects (of the classical pathway) also present with lupus-like manifestations including glomerulonephritis and discoid lupus (Table 12.4.1). Patients with mutations in alternate complement pathway may present with atypical hemolytic uremic syndrome (aHUS). Additionally, patients with loss of function (or autoantibodies) of complement regulating factors (factor I, H) may also present with aHUS. Besides, loss of other complement regulating factors (decay accelerating factor, CD59) presents with paroxysmal nocturnal hemoglobinuria.

Interferonopathies

Monogenic interferonopathies often refer to genetic defects leading to elevated type I interferon response (Interferon-α/β). In summary, these include loss-of-function defects in nucleic acid metabolizing enzymes, or interferon regulators; or

Table 12.4.1: Clinical features suggestive of early complement deficiency lupus as compared to the usual presentation of pediatric lupus

Feature	*Complement deficiency*	*Non-complement deficiency*
Age of onset	<7 years	Late 1st decade of life or adolescence
Gender predilection	Males	Females
History of infections	Before initiation of immunosuppressive therapy	Usually after initiation of immunosuppressive therapy
Family history	If present, suggests an autosomal recessive mode of inheritance	Lack of an obvious family history
Pattern of ANA positivity	Speckled, due to anti-Ro/SSA antibodies	Homogeneous with rim enhancement
Anti-ds-DNA	Negative or very low titers	Positive, often in high titers during active disease
Pattern of organ involvement	Predominance of CNS disease, chronic skin lesions	Predominance of renal disease, acute skins lesions, hematological involvement

gain-of-function variants in nucleic acid sensors or molecules downstream of type I interferon receptors. These intriguing disorders present with multisystem involvement and pattern recognition of clinical features often facilitates diagnosis (Table 12.4.2).

INFLAMMASOMOPATHIES

These are a group of autoinflammatory disorders similar to interferonopathies. As a group, these disorders present with recurrent fevers, which may have a striking periodicity, and prominent cutaneous manifestations. Similar to monogenic interferonopathies, pattern recognition of clinical features and clinical response to therapeutic drugs is the key for diagnosis (Table 12.4.3).

CONCLUSION

PIDs are a fascinating yet intriguing group of disorders that present with a myriad of clinical manifestations of immunodeficiencies and immune dysregulation. Although diagnostic confirmation and validation may require very specialized

Table 12.4.2: Pattern of the clinical features that can facilitate the diagnosis of monogenic interferonopathies

Disorder	*Clinical features*
Stimulator of interferon genes (STING)-associated vasculopathy of infancy	Fever, arthritis, severe cutaneous manifestations including gangrene, interstitial lung disease (ILD).
Aicardi-Goutières syndrome	Neurological involvement (including CNS calcifications), chilblain lupus-like lesions
Deficiency of adenosine deaminase 2	Polyarteritis nodosa like manifestations, CNS vasculopathy, hematological and immune manifestations (lymphopenia, low IgM)
COPA (Coatomer protein subunit α) syndrome	Early-onset deforming rheumatoid factor positive JIA-like manifestations, ILD, pulmonary hemorrhage, kidney disease
Haploinsufficiency of A20	Behçet disease-like manifestations (severe)
Spondyloenchondrodysplasia	Skeletal dysplasias, SLE-like manifestations, developmental delay, spastic diplegia
Proteasomopathies (like PSMB8 deficiency)	Fever, chronic dermatosis, lipoatrophy

laboratory facilities, meticulous documentation and in-depth analysis of history, examination, and basic laboratory features prove fruitful in the journey to pick up these diseases. An overview of the treatment of primary PIDs is presented in Table 12.4.4.

Table 12.4.3: Pattern of the clinicolaboratory features and response to therapeutic agents that can facilitate the diagnosis of inflammasomopathies

Disorder	*Clinical, laboratory features, and response to therapy*
Cryopyrin associated periodic syndrome	Caused by gain of function mutations in the NLRP3 inflammasome (involved in the production of IL-1β and IL-18). Episodes of inflammation are often triggered by exposure to cold. Sensorineural hearing loss and amyloidosis may occur in a subset.
Neonatal onset multisystem inflammatory disease	The most severe form of NLRP3 inflammasomopathy. Also called chronic infantile, neurological, cutaneous, and articular syndrome. Presents in early infancy with frequent fever episodes (the parents may complain that the child is almost always having disease episodes) that show a dramatic response to anti-IL-1 therapy.
Hyper IgD syndrome (mevalonate kinase deficiency)	Presents with fever, rash, abdominal pain, vomiting, and/or enlargement of lymph nodes, liver, spleen. Present in early childhood, duration of fever episodes is 3–7 days which may be characteristically triggered by vaccines, intervening asymptomatic period lasts for 3-6 weeks, and a partial response to anti-IL-1, steroid, or colchicine therapy. Elevated urinary excretion of mevalonic acid, especially during fever spikes, and elevated IgD levels are vital clues.
TNF-receptor associated periodic syndrome	Fever, painful rash which may be migratory, musculoskeletal pain, and periorbital swelling. Presents in older children and adults, duration of fever episodes is often more than a week, intervening afebrile period often lasts >6 weeks, and usually these patients respond to anti-IL-1 therapy.
Familial mediterranean fever (FMF)	Recurrent fevers, erysipelas like rash, and abdominal/chest pain due to serositis. Splenic enlargement, joint symptoms, and the risk of amyloidosis are other crucial manifestations. It is present at variable ages, fever episodes last for 1–3 days, the interval between afebrile episodes is variable, and usually respond to anti-IL-1 and colchicine therapy.

Table 12.4.4: An overview of the treatment of primary immunodeficiency diseases in resource-poor settings

XLA, CVID	• Immunoglobulin replacement therapy is the treatment of choice • Dosed at 400–600 mg/kg every 3–4 weeks • Further titration is based on trough IgG levels and clinical response • Cotrimoxazole prophylaxis can also be added • Immunomodulatory therapy may be needed for autoimmune manifestations
CGD	• Cotrimoxazole and itraconazole prophylaxis. • Hematopoietic stem cell transplantation (HSCT) is usually employed in children with a complicated clinical course. • Immunomodulators (especially steroids) for inflammatory manifestations.
WAS	• HSCT is the treatment of choice • In absence of HSCT, antimicrobial prophylaxis should be given.
Complement deficiency	• Fresh frozen plasma replacement • Antimicrobial prophylaxis • Immunomodulators for treatment of autoimmune manifestations
Interferonopathies	• Janus kinase inhibitors are emerging as the treatment of choice
Inflammasomopathies	• *See* Table 12.4.3

LEARNING POINTS

- PIDs present with infectious illnesses which are often recurrent, persistent, unusually complicated, or due to unusual and less pathogenic organisms.
- Infection profile usually provides vital clues towards the arm of the immune system affected by the underlying genetic defect.
- Immune dysregulation including autoimmunity, malignancy and rheumatological illness can be important accompaniment in many PIDs.

FURTHER READING

1. Bonilla FA, Khan DA, Ballas ZK, et al. Practice parameter for the diagnosis and management of primary immunodeficiency. J Allergy Clin Immunol. 2015;136:1186-205.e2078.
2. Bousfiha A, Jeddane L, Picard C, et al. Human Inborn Errors of Immunity: 2019 Update of the IUIS Phenotypical Classification. J Clin Immunol. 2020;40: 66–81.
3. McCusker C, Upton J, Warrington R. Primary immunodeficiency. Allergy Asthma Clin Immunol. 2018;14(Suppl 2):61.
4. Tangye SG, Al-Herz W, Bousfiha A, et al. Human Inborn Errors of Immunity: 2022 Update on the Classification from the International Union of Immunological Societies Expert Committee. J Clin Immunol. 2022;42: 1473–507.
5. Vignesh P, Rawat A, Singh S. An Update on the Use of Immunomodulators in Primary Immunodeficiencies. Clin Rev Allergy Immunol. 2017;52:287–303.

Chapter 12.5

Autoinflammatory Syndromes

Suma Balan

INTRODUCTION

Autoinflammatory syndromes are a heterogeneous group of rare disorders presenting with fever due to spontaneous onset of exuberant inflammation as a result of defects in the innate immune system. Clinical manifestations include recurrent or persistent episodes of fever, skin rashes, and systemic inflammation without evidence of infection or autoimmune disease or allergy.

In 1997 the MEFV gene mutation was found to be responsible for familial mediterranean fever (FMF). With progress in genomics in the past two decades, more than 50 autoinflammatory syndromes with a genetic basis have been newly described.

The innate immune system comprising of macrophages, natural killer cells, dendritic cells, mast cells, neutrophils, basophils, and eosinophils is the first line of defence against many infections and tissue damage. Once exposed to an infectious agent, the immune effector cells are activated and leads to the production of proinflammatory cytokines interleukin-1 beta (IL1β), tumor necrosis factor-alpha (TNFα), IL-6, and interferons (IFN) that enables clearance of infection. In inborn errors of innate immunity, a minor trigger leads to unresolved dysregulated production of proinflammatory cytokines, persistent effector cell stimulation and activation, resulting in autoinflammatory syndromes.

CLASSIFICATION

An improved understanding of basic immunological mechanisms of inflammation and advances in genetic diagnosis have led to the identification of the gene involved in various autoinflammatory syndromes, they can be classified as monogenic or polygenic, that is inherited or non-inherited.

Monogenic Autoinflammatory Syndromes

These disorders arise due to mutation of specific genes. The list below is not exhaustive and there are many other disorders newly described.

1. **Inflammasomopathies:** Disorders that are due to innate defects in the inflammasome. They are characterized by **periodic fevers** and a wide variety of **cutaneous manifestations** like urticarial, pustular, erysipelas-like erythema, or plaques. These cutaneous lesions can become necrotic and ulcerate. Systemic organ involvement is also present. Some inflammasomopathies are:
   a. Familial mediterranean fever (FMF).
   b. Cryopyrin-associated periodic fever syndromes (CAPS).
   c. Mevalonate kinase deficiency (MKD) or hyper-IgD syndrome.
   d. TNF receptor-associated periodic fever syndrome (TRAPS).
   e. Pyogenic arthritis, pyoderma gangrenosum, and arthritis (PAPA).
2. **Type1 interferonopathies:** There is an overlap of **neurological** and **cutaneous manifestations** among disorders in the group, caused by the upregulation of IFN-1 signaling. Some examples are:
   a. Aicardi-Goutières syndrome (AGS).
   b. STING-associated vasculopathy with onset in infancy (SAVI).

c. Chronic neutrophilic dermatosis panniculitis with lipodystrophy (CANDLE).
d. Spondyloenchondrodysplasia (SPENCD).
e. COPA (coatomer subunit-α) syndrome.

3. **Relopathies:** They are autoinflammatory syndromes due to inappropriate activation of nuclear factor kappa-light-chain-enhancer of activated B cells. Examples are:
 a. Haploinsufficiency of A20 (HA 20).
 b. LUBAC (Linear ubiquitin chain assembly complex) deficiency.
4. **Others:** Deficiency of adenosine deaminase 2(DADA 2) syndrome, deficiency of IL-1 receptor antagonist (DIRA), Majeed syndrome.

Polygenic Autoinflammatory Syndromes

Typical examples are:

a. Systemic onset juvenile idiopathic arthritis (SoJIA)
b. Chronic recurrent multifocal osteomyelitis (CRMO)
c. SAPHO syndrome
d. PFAPA syndrome

CLINICAL PRESENTATION

Given the large number of autoinflammatory diseases, each having multiple varied manifestations, it is important to make a clinical diagnosis so that investigations can be planned. On the basis of clinical presentation, we can group them as follows:

Syndromes presenting with recurrent fever, and systemic inflammation with urticarial rash are summarised in Table 12.5.1. Under this group are the iinflammasomopathies and haploinsufficiency A20.

Syndromes with sterile inflammation affecting skin, bone or joints are summarized in Table 12.5.2. Examples under this group are PAPA and deficiency of the interleukin 1 receptor antagonist (DIRA).

Type I interferonopathies are manifested by involvement of brain (intracranial calcifications), and skin vasculitis (Table 12.5.3). Another distinct feature of type 1 inferenopathies is presence of features of autoimmunity. Lupus like features seen in AGS and SPENCD, while interstitial lung disease is seen in SAVI and COPA.

DADA2 syndrome (Table 12.5.4) resembles polyarteritis nodosa (PAN). Therefore, clinical features suggestive of PAN in childhood should warrant evaluation for DADA2.

Periodic Fever with Aphthous Stomatitis, Pharyngitis, and Adenitis (PFAPA)

Of all the autoinflammatory syndromes whether monogenic and polygenic, this is perhaps the most common condition of autoinflammatory syndromes in children. The clinical features of PFAPA are self-explanatory from the name given to it. Episodes usually last 3–6 weeks and are unresponsive to antibiotics. A single dose of oral corticosteroid can abort the attack but can sometimes hasten the next episode. Colchicine is often useful in the prevention of episodes. This condition is different from others in that the genetic basis is as yet unknown and that most children are seen to resolve completely after primary school age.

When to Suspect Autoinflammatory Syndromes?

The first step is an awareness of what autoinflammatory syndromes are. One should suspect an autoinflammatory disorder in certain situations, like recurrent fevers with a asymptomatic phase in-between episodes, and onset usually in the first two years of life (Table 12.5.5).

APPROACH TO DIAGNOSIS

A detailed history, including duration of fever, the interval between episodes, presence of rashes, oral ulcers, joint swellings, abdominal pain and consanguinity, is essential. A fever diary should be advised to document the episodes. Observing the child during an acute episode and comparing the markers of inflammation during and after the episode can be helpful. However, the clinical pattern alone cannot completely predict which autoinflammatory syndrome the child might have.

The clinical workup of systemic inflammation should include CRP, ESR and CBC with differential counts. Patients should undergo a basic immunodeficiency workup that includes a history of infections, lymphocyte subsets and immunoglobulin levels according to their clinical presentation. Supportive investigations like skin biopsies show the pattern of inflammation. For example, neutrophilic and granulomatous infiltrations are suggestive of CAPS and Blau syndrome, respectively. Plasma level of ADA2 helps

Table 12.5.1: Syndromes presenting with recurrent fever, and syndromes with systemic inflammation with cutaneous manifestations

Condition	*Gene*	*Inheritance*	*Protein*	*Age of onset*	*Fever*	*Clinical features*	*Treatment*	*Amyloidosis*
Syndromes with recurrent fever								
FMF	MEFV	AR	Pyrin	10–20 years	1–3 days	Fever, erysipeloid rash, arthritis, pleuritis, peritonitis	Colchicine	Yes
TRAPS	TNFRSF1A	AD	TNF	median age 3 years	7–14 days	Fever, rash (urticarial), migrating erythema, periorbital edema, localized myalgia, arthralgia, abdominal pain and serositis, positive family history	Etanercept, anakinra	Yes
MKD	MVK	AR	Mevalonate Kinase	<1 year	3–7 days	Fever, rash, aphthous ulcers, cervical lymphadenopathy, GI (abdominal pain, hepatosplenomegaly) manifestation, arthralgia, elevated IgD, and urinary mevalonate levels	Simvastatin, etanercept, anakinra	Rare
Syndromes with systemic inflammation and urticarial rash								
FCAS*	CIAS1	AD	Cryopyrin	<6 months	6–24 hours	Fever, urticarial rash triggered by cold, conjunctivitis	Rilonacept	Yes, low
MWS*	CIAS1	AD	Cryopyrin	<1 year	1–2 days	Urticarial-like rash, sensorineural hearing loss,, conjunctivitis, arthralgia, arthritis	Anakinra, canakinumab	Yes
NOMID*	CIAS1	AD	Cryopyrin	At birth	Continuous	Urticarial-like rashes, developmental delay, aseptic meningitis, hearing loss, papilledema, epiphyseal overgrowth, arthropathy, distinctive facial appearance	Anakinra, thalidomide	Yes
HA 20	TNFAIP3	AD, LOF	—	1–10 years	—	Early onset systemic inflammation, arthralgia, orogenital ulcer, and ocular inflammation	csDMARDs, TNF inhibitors	Rare

*cryopyrin associated periodic fever syndromes (CAPS)

FMF: Familial Mediterranean fever; *TRAPS:* TNF receptor-associated periodic syndrome; *FCAS:* Familial cold autoinflammatory syndrome; *MWS:* Muckle wells syndrome; *NOMID:* Neonatal onset multisystem inflammatory disease; *MKD:* Mevalonate kinase deficiency; *HA 20:* Haploinsufficiency of A20; *LOF:* Loss-of-function; *AR:* Autosomal recessive; *AD:* Autosomal dominant *TNF:* Tumor necrosis factor; *DMARD:* Disease modifying antirheumatic drug

Table 12.5.2: Syndromes with sterile inflammation affecting skin, bone or joints

Condition	*Gene*	*Inheritance*	*Age of onset*	*Clinical features*
Predominantly bone/joints				
PAPA	PSTPIP1	AD	1–15 years	Pyoderma gangrenosum, pyogenic aseptic arthritis, acne
Majeed syndrome	LPIN2	AR	<10 years	CRMO, severe pain, tender soft tissue swelling, congenital dyserythropoietic anemia
DIRA	IL1RN	AR	<1-year	Neonatal onset of chronic multifocal osteomyelitis, pustulosis, and periostitis
Cherubism	SH3BP2	AR	2–7 years	Bone degeneration in jaws
Predominantly skin				
Blau syndrome	NOD2	AD	<5 years	Granulomatous dermatitis, arthritis, and uveitis (early onset sarcoidosis)
DITRA	IL-36RN	AR	<2 years	Pustular psoriasis (widespread and episodic), malaise, and leukocytosis. It is a life-threatening, multisystemic inflammatory disease
Otulipenia	OTULIN	AR	<1 year	Neonatal onset of recurrent fever, arthralgia, lipodystrophy, dermatitis, diarrhea, neutrophilia
CAMPS	CARD14	AD	<1 year	Psoriasis

PAPA: Pyogenic sterile arthritis, pyoderma gangrenosum, acne; *CRMO:* Chronic recurrent multifocal osteomyelitis; *DIRA:* Deficiency of the interleukin 1 receptor antagonist; *DITRA:* Deficiency of interleukin 36 receptor antagonist; *AD:* autosomal dominant; *AR:* Autosomal recessive, CAMPS, CARD14-mediated psoriasis.

Table 12.5.3: Type I interferonopathies

Name	*Gene*	*Inheritance*	*Age of onset*	*Clinical features*
Aicardi-Goutières syndromes (AGS) AGS1 AGS2 AGS3 AGS4 AGS5 AGS6 AGS7	 TREX1 RNASEH2B RNASEH2C RNASEH2A SAMDH1 ADAR IFIH1	 AR or AD AR AR AR AR AR or AD AD	<6 months	Progressive encephalopathy Intracerebral calcifications, cerebral atrophy, thrombocytopenia, elevated hepatic enzymes, lupus-like features
Spondyloendrodysplasia (SPENCD) with immune dysregulation	ACP5	AR	<5 years	Lupus-like autoimmunity, recurrent bacterial and viral infections, hemolytic anemia, thrombocytopenia, skeletal dysplasia.
STING-associated vasculopathy, infantile onset (SAVI)	TMEM173 or STING	AD	<1 year	Skin vasculopathy, intracerebral calcification, interstitial lung disease, arthritis
CANDLE	PSMB8	AR or AD	<1 year	Contractures, panniculitis, intracranial calcifications, fever
COPA syndrome	COPA	AD	<5 years	Interstitial lung disease, lung hemorrhage, arthropathy, glomerulonephritis

AR: Autosomal recessive; *AD:* Autosomal dominant; *CANDLE:* Chronic atypical neutrophilic dermatosis with lipodystrophy. *STING:* Stimulator of interferon genes

Table 12.5.4: Other autoinflammatory syndromes

AIDs	*Gene*	*Inheritance*	*Age of onset*	*Clinical features*	*Treatment*
DADA2	ADA2	AR	<10 years	Recurrent deep brain strokes Vasculitic skin lesions Livedo reticularis Hypogammaglobulinemia Pure red cell aplasia	TNF inhibitors

DADA: Deficiency of ADA 2; *AR:* Autosomal recessive; *TNF:* Tumor necrosis factor

Table 12.5.5: When to suspect autoinflammatory syndrome

Suspect autoinflammatory syndromes in the following situations

- Recurrent fever with a specific symptom complex with a normal general condition in between episodes.
- Onset at a young age, usually in the first two years of life.
- Persistent early onset fever with rashes, joint symptoms, and no evidence of infection or malignancy.
- History of similar illness patterns in the family.
- Evidence of systemic inflammation on investigations during the acute episode.
- Younger children who present with manifestations of acquired immunological disorders.

Autoinflammatory syndromes that phenotypically resemble acquired immunological disorders	**Acquired immunological disorders**
Blau syndrome	Sarcoidosis, JIA-uveitis
Hereditary complement deficiencies	SLE
Aicardi Goutier's syndrome	SLE
CANDLE	JDM
Deficiency of adenosine deaminase 2 (DADA-2) syndrome	Polyarteritis nodosa
Haploinsufficiency of A20	Behçet's disease, JIA, SLE

CANDLE: Chronic atypical neutrophilic dermatosis with lipodystrophy; *SLE:* Systemic lupus erythematosus; *JIA:* Juvenile idiopathic arthritis; *JDM:* Juvenile dermatomyositis

in diagnosing DADA2. Neuroimaging in suspected type 1 interferonopathies helps in identifying intracerebral calcification and cerebral atrophy.

However, final confirmation is by identifying the gene involved. In cases where the diagnosis can be ascertained by clinical features, a targeted sequencing will suffice. However, in the majority of patients, a whole exome sequencing may be required. Genetic testing on parents and other family members to detect carrier states is necessary following confirmation of disease in the proband so that parents are aware of the risk when planning the next child. Despite the typical nature of the disease, however, gene isolation is not always possible in all cases and a significant percentage could remain unproven.

MANAGEMENT

Targeted treatments are available for most autoinflammatory syndromes, which have made a significant difference in the outcomes. Colchicine is helpful in FMF, HA 20, etc. TNF inhibitors are effective in DADA2 syndrome and HA 20. Glucocorticoids and Janus Kinase inhibitors are of benefit in the control of type 1 interferonopathies.

The role of stem cell transplant is an emerging area, and gene therapy could also be a key player in the future. Patient support groups need to be formed and these conditions need to be entered into the rare diseases program to make the treatment within reach of those affected.

LEARNING POINTS

- Autoinflammatory disorders are inherited disorders of the innate immune system.
- They present as periodic fever syndromes in young children.
- Awareness of these disorders and referral for early diagnosis is recommended.
- Treatments are available for these disorders, albeit lifelong, which significantly mitigate the complications and improve quality of life.

FURTHER READING

1. Borst C, Symmank D, Drach M, Weninger W. Cutaneous signs and mechanisms of inflammasomopathies. Ann Rheum Dis. 2022; 81:454–65.
2. Crow YJ, Stetson DB. The type I interferonopathies: 10 years on. Nat Rev Immunol. 2022; 22:471–83.
3. Gedik KC, Lamot L, Romano M, et al. The 2021 European Alliance of Associations for Rheumatology/American College of Rheumatology points to consider for diagnosis and management of autoinflammatory type I interferonopathies: CANDLE/PRAAS, SAVI and AGS. Annals Rheum Dis. 2022; 81:601–13.
4. Romano M, Arici ZS, Piskin D, et al. The 2021 EULAR/American College of Rheumatology points to consider for diagnosis, management and monitoring of the interleukin-1 mediated autoinflammatory diseases: cryopyrin-associated periodic syndromes, tumour necrosis factor receptor-associated periodic syndrome, mevalonate kinase deficiency, and deficiency of the interleukin-1 receptor antagonist. Annals Rheum Dis. 2022; 81:907–21.
5. Sönmez HE, Özen S. A clinical update on inflammasomopathies. Int Immunol. 2017; 29: 393-400.
6. Stojanov S, Lapidus S, Chitkara P, et al. Periodic fever, aphthous stomatitis, pharyngitis, and adenitis (PFAPA) is a disorder of innate immunity and Th1 activation responsive to IL-1 blockade. Proc Natl Acad Sci U S A. 2011; 108:7148–53.

Primary Amyloidosis

Rajkiran Dudam, Prajakta Dekate

INTRODUCTION

Amyloid is a misfolded protein which accumulates as insoluble fibrils in various organs and tissue resulting in a clinical syndrome known as amyloidosis. Amyloids appear as amorphous fibrils under the electron microscope, appearing red in histopathological specimens stained with Congo red dye. When viewed in polarised light, these red deposits have an apple green birefringence.

CLASSIFICATION OF AMYLOIDOSIS

Primary amyloidosis is associated with paraproteinemia, plasma-cell dyscrasia or multiple myeloma. Secondary amyloidosis is secondary to chronic inflammatory or infectious conditions. Currently there are almost 36 different reported amyloid proteins and amyloidosis is named based on the fibril-forming protein (Table 12.6.1). The three most common types of amyloidosis are AL, AA, and ATTR amyloidosis.

AL amyloidosis (localised or systemic) is due to the accumulation of AL protein that is derived from the immunoglobulin (Ig) light chain. The protein in AA amyloidosis is derived from serum amyloid A (SAA) protein. ATTR amyloid is derived from transthyretin (TTR) protein, the accumulation of which is either wild type (wt) ATTR amyloidosis or hereditary ATTRV30M amyloidosis. It is important to use this nomenclature in diagnosis as the treatment plans for chemically distinct forms considerably differ.

CLINICAL MANIFESTATIONS

The clinical manifestations of AL amyloidosis are caused by an amyloidogenic Ig light chain secreted by a low proliferating bone marrow plasma cell

Table 12.6.1: Amyloidosis classified on the basis of amyloid protein

Amyloid	*Precursor*	*Systemic/local*	*Organ involvement*
AL	Monoclonal Ig light chains	Systemic, localised	Primary amyloidosis, associated with plasma dyscrasias Kidneys, heart, nerve, GI, liver, and soft tissue
AH	Monoclonal Ig heavy chains	Systemic	Kidneys, heart, liver
AA	Serum amyloid A	Systemic	AA amyloidosis is secondary to chronic inflammatory or infectious conditions. Kidneys, liver, GIT, heart, and spleen are involved
ATTR	Transthyretin -wild type	Systemic	Older age Heart, nerve, and soft tissue

(Contd.)

Table 12.6.1: Other autoinflammatory syndromes *(Contd.)*			
Amyloid protein	*Precursor*	*Systemic or localised form*	*Syndrome and organ involved*
ATTR	Genetic variants of Transthyretin	Systemic	Amyloid cardiomyopathy (hereditary) Amyloid polyneuropathy (familial)
Aβ2M	β2 – microglobulin	Systemic	Dialysis
ACys	Cystatin C	Systemic	—
AApoAI	Apolipoprotoien AI	Systemic, localised	Familial type has systemic with visceral involvement Localised type involves the aorta
AApoAII	Apolipoprotien AII	Systemic	Familial amyloidosis. Kidneys and heart are involved
AAPOAIV	Apolipoprotien AIV– Wild type	Systemic	Sporadic systemic amyloidosis associated with age

clone. AL amyloidosis is perhaps the most common and most severe form of systemic amyloidosis. AL amyloid light chain protein infiltrates peripheral nerves, connective tissues, blood vessels, smooth muscles, striated muscles etc causing organ dysfunction. This light chain is unique in that they undergo partial lysosomal proteolysis within macrophages. They are deposited extracellularly as insoluble amyloid filaments attached to a polysaccharide which makes them different from the normal light chain and that seen in myeloma.

People above 65 years are at the highest risk of AL amyloidosis. Organ infiltration occurs in the kidneys (75%), heart (60%), skin and soft tissue (30–40%), gastrointestinal tract (GIT) (20%), liver (27%), and peripheral nerves (18%). In the majority of patients there is more than one affected organ at diagnosis. AL amyloidosis is associated with monoclonal gammopathy of undetermined significance (MGUS) and most patients do not develop malignant disease or multiple myeloma.

The presenting symptoms are non-specific, because of which it is often undiagnosed/misdiagnosed. Fatigue, weight loss, edema, paraesthesia, carpal tunnel syndrome, macroglossia, and skin lesions are usual symptoms. Patients are referred to rheumatology due to arthralgia, and multisystem involvement.

Skin and Soft Tissue

Petechiae, periorbital purpura, and spontaneous or trauma-induced ecchymoses are the most common skin manifestations. Purpuric lesions in flexural regions such as the neck, axillae, nasolabial folds are also signs of amyloidosis. Waxy papules, nodules, or plaques over the eyelids, behind the ears, neck, or inguinal and anogenital regions are the most characteristic skin lesions. Diffuse infiltrates may mimic scleredema. Scalp involvements can cause patchy or diffuse alopecia, and dystrophic nail changes are observed in few.

Macroglossia is reported in about 20% cases of primary systemic amyloidosis. Macroglossia and periorbital purpura are highly specific for AL amyloidosis. Macroglossia is also seen in hypothyroidism, tongue cancer and acromegaly; hence alone is not pathognomonic of amyloidosis. Infiltration of the salivary glands may lead to xerostomia.

Heart

Cardiac involvement may cause angina, infarction, orthostatic hypotension, or arrhythmias. Cardiac involvement accounts for almost 40% deaths. Echocardiography usually reveals restrictive cardiomyopathy patterns. The left ventricle (LV) is concentrically thickened with a normal to small cavity, and granular sparkled appearance. LV ejection fraction can be normal.

Clinically cardiac AL amyloidosis and wt ATTR amyloidosis are indistinguishable. However, a technetium pyrophosphate scan can distinguish these two conditions, with a high uptake in ATTR versus no uptake in AL amyloid.

Cardiac MRI is used for the diagnosis of cardiac amyloidosis. Serum troponin T and N-terminal pro-brain natriuretic peptide (NT-proBNP) are used to assess prognosis.

Kidneys

Kidneys are frequently involved in AL amyloidosis, and manifests with nephrotic syndrome. Proteinuria is present in more than 90% of the cases. Often this is accompanied by elevated cholesterol levels. Enlarged kidneys are not routinely seen in ultrasound and CT.

Gastrointestinal Tract (GIT) and Liver

GI haemorrhage (that can be fatal) and malabsorption may result from infiltration of the GIT. GI amyloidosis is one differential diagnosis of coexistence of GI bleeding and pseudo-obstruction of the small intestine. Deposits can present in the stomach or colon as polyps. About 50% primary systemic amyloidosis have hepatomegaly, but splenomegaly is uncommon (<10%).

Peripheral Nerves

The manifestations are symmetrical peripheral neuropathy and carpal tunnel syndrome (CTS). These patterns of peripheral nerve involvement are common in diabetes too therefore if the patient is a diabetic both these manifestations could be attributed to diabetes per se, and amyloid can be missed. When only small fibres are involved, electrophysiological studies can miss amyloid-induced neuropathy. In such cases a skin biopsy with quantification of intraepidermal nerve fibres can help with the diagnosis.

CTS can be a presenting symptom in both ATTR and AL amyloid. If CTS is bilateral and doesn't improve after release surgery amyloid must be considered in the differential diagnosis.

Autonomic neuropathy can occur independent of peripheral neuropathy, and present as orthostatic hypotension, bowel dysmotility, erectile dysfunction (older adults).

Musculoskeletal System

Amyloid arthropathy can mimic gout or rheumatoid muscular system arthritis with bilateral arthritis of the hand joints and wrists. One should suspect amyloid if there is no response to disease modifying anti-rheumatic drugs (DMARDs), negative serology, and inflammatory markers. Shoulders and knees are other joints involved. The shoulder pad sign is a classic of amyloidosis.

Typically radiological findings of amyloid arthropathy are soft tissue swelling around the joint (juxta articular). An important radiological finding is subchondral cystic lesions with well-defined sclerotic and cortical margins. Periarticular osteoporosis is also seen.

Other systems

Easy bruising and severe bleeding diathesis due to acquired factor X deficiency is specific for AL amyloidosis. In this condition both activated partial thromboplastin time (APTT) and prothrombin time (PT) are prolonged. Low factor X levels are confirmed by a mixing study.

Vascular involvement leads to claudication of the jaw, calf, or buttock. Localized amyloidosis can occur in the renal collecting system, bladder, and urethra. In the lungs, localized AL deposits can present as pulmonary nodules.

INVESTIGATIONS AND DIAGNOSIS

AL amyloidosis should be suspected in any patient with unexplained peripheral neuropathy, nephrotic syndrome, cardiomyopathy with hypertrophy on echocardiography, chronic inflammatory demyelinating polyneuropathy with a monoclonal protein, and in those with unexplained fatigue, edema, and weight loss.

Tissue diagnosis is a must. The involved organ kidney, sural nerve, and myocardial tissue should be sampled in the absence of contraindications. The yield from cutaneous lesion is 50%, abdominal subcutaneous fat aspiration and rectal biopsy 80%, minor salivary gland is 68% and combined abdominal fat aspiration with bone marrow biopsy is 85%. On hematoxylin-eosin staining the features indicating amyloidosis are presence of a homogenous, faintly eosinophilic mass. Inflammatory infiltrates are usually absent. Congo red stain under polarised light will elicit an apple-green birefringence which is diagnostic of amyloid. The type of amyloid protein needs to be identified.

Demonstration of plasma dyscrasia on the bone marrow with predominance of λ- or κ-producing plasma cells or monoclonal light chain κ and λ in serum or urine confirms the diagnosis of AL amyloidosis. Simple protein electrophoresis will miss low levels of monoclonal light chains, so immunofixation immunoelectrophoresis (serum or urine) is the method of choice to detect monoclonal light chains.

A nephelometry based quantification of serum free light chains (FLC) is a prognostic marker. High FLC precedes AL amyloidosis by years, and is a marker for response to treatment. Because FLC are filtered by the kidneys, the κ:λ ratio, rather than the absolute level, is the relevant measurement in the patient with renal insufficiency. The normal κ:λ ratio is between 0.26 to 1.65. A ratio <0.26 indicates the presence of plasma cells that are producing clonal λ free light chains. A hallmark feature of AL amyloidosis is high frequency of λ light chain.

When routine immunofluorescence or immunohistochemical testing cannot type the amyloid deposits, laser microdissection and mass spectrometry-based proteomic analysis are useful. It identifies light chain and heavy chain amyloidosis and can be applied to many types of tissue sources. High levels of growth differentiation factor15 (GDF-15) is a serum biomarker associated with mortality and poor overall survival in AL amyloidosis.

MANAGEMENT OF AL AMYLOIDOSIS

Melphalan and prednisolone used to be the standard treatment. Current standards of treatment are with bortezomib based regimes. Bortezomib a proteasome inhibitor induces a rapid decrease in serum free light chain concentration in AL amyloidosis. Bortezomib is effective in achieving both a hematologic and organ response in AL amyloidosis, but having a neurotoxic potential it is avoided in severe peripheral neuropathy.

Cyclophosphamide, bortezomib, dexamethasone regime achieves a higher hematologic response than bortezomib alone or other combinations including bortezomib and melphalan and dexamethasone, or bortezomib and dexamethasone. Other agents tried are daratumumab, thalidomide, lenalidomide, and pomalidomide.

With advances in treatment the overall survival has improved, but those with advanced cardiac dysfunction at presentation are still at risk of early death with a median survival of 3–6 months.

Autologous Stem Cell Transplant (ASCT)

Treatment algorithms are based on patients' eligibility for ASCT. Induction treatment with bortezomib renders one-third of initially transplant ineligible patients capable of undergoing ASCT. Cardiac amyloidosis (before the onset of advanced congestive heart failure) carries a better outcome with ASCT. The 10-year survival after ASCT is up to 43%.

PROGNOSIS

The major cause of death are heart and kidney failure. If diagnosis is made before advanced cardiomyopathy has developed, then there is a better organ response with chemotherapy.

LEARNING POINTS

- AL amyloidosis is the most common amyloidosis syndrome.
- Kidney involvement presents with nephrotic syndrome, and less frequently as unexplained azotemia.
- Cardiac involvement present as restrictive cardiomyopathy.
- Patients with MGUS should be routinely screened for AL amyloidosis.
- One should consider amyloidosis in patients having unexplained fatigue, nephrotic syndrome, neuropathy, cardiomyopathy, arthropathy, etc.
- The echocardiographic features of advanced cardiac amyloid are pretty distinctive.
- Amyloid arthropathy can mimic gout or rheumatoid arthritis. Radiographic manifestations are soft tissue swelling and presence of subchondral bone cysts.

FURTHER READING

1. Bowie D, Bardi M, Hemmati I. Amyloid Arthropathy: A Rare Mimic of Rheumatic Disease. J Rheumatol. 2019;46:1540–1541.
2. Gertz, MA. Immunoglobulin light chain amyloidosis: 2020 update on diagnosis, prognosis, and treatment. Am J Hematol. 2020;95:848–860.
3. Vaxman I, Gertz M. When to Suspect a Diagnosis of Amyloidosis. Acta Haematol 2020;143:304–311.

Panniculitis

Vikas Gupta

INTRODUCTION

Panniculitis is inflammation of subcutaneous fat. The underlying cause for panniculitis varies widely and includes various systemic disorders, infections, malignancies and drugs. The subcutaneous fat is organized as a primary microlobule that aggregates to form secondary lobules that are surrounded by thin septa of connective tissue. Inflammation can predominantly involve the lobule (lobular panniculitis) or septa (septal panniculitis). The blood vessel may or may not be involved with inflammation (vasculitis).

All panniculitis present almost the same way, i.e. with a skin nodule on the lower limbs. Based on the size, distribution, presence of systemic symptoms, and other clinical features, one can narrow down the differential diagnosis. But a scalpel biopsy of the nodule in the active stage (that must include the deep subcutaneous fat) is essential to make a reliable clinicopathologic conclusion. In clinical practice, it is more common to get a picture of mixed inflammatory infiltrates in the septae as well as the lobule. Hence panniculitis is classified as predominantly as septal panniculitis with or without vasculitis (Table 12.7.1) and predominantly lobular with or without vasculitis (Table 12.7.2).

CLINICAL MANIFESTATION

Panniculitis which is encountered in clinical practice is discussed below.

I. Predominantly Septal Panniculitis without Vasculitis

'Mostly septal' group of panniculitis represents actually a primary dermis inflammation (for example deep morphoea, necrobiosis lipoidica profunda) with secondary inflammation of the subcutaneous fat.

Deep morphea, a form of localized scleroderma, is characterised by the deposition of inflammatory infiltrate and collagen-rich extracellular matrix in the subcutaneous tissue. It presents as indurated plaques or nodules on the trunk or lower limbs.

Whereas in erythema nodosum (EN) the inflammation begins in the septae primarily, as a late hypersensitivity reaction to various antigens (Table 12.7.3). The nodules of EN are multiple, painful, and located subcutaneously over the legs, though forearms and trunk are involved

Table 12.7.1: Predominantly septal panniculitis

Without vasculitis	*With vasculitis*
• Erythema nodosum • Rheumatoid nodule • Deep morphea • Necrobiosis lipoidica • Subcutaneous granuloma annulare • Necrobiosis xanthogranuloma	• Cutaneous polyarteritis nodosa (PAN) • Superficial thrombophlebitis

Table 12.7.2: Predominantly lobular panniculitis

Without vasculitis	*With vasculitis*
• Lupus panniculitis • Gouty panniculitis • Panniculitis in dermatomyositis • Post-steroid panniculitis • Infective panniculitis	• Erythema nodosum leprosum (ENL) • Erythema induratum of Bazin or nodular vasculitis • Panniculitis with crystals following etanercept injection
• Pancreatic panniculitis • Alpha-1 antitrypsin deficiency panniculitis • Traumatic panniculitis – Blunt trauma, cold, heat or electrical injury, chemical injury • Factitious panniculitis • Subcutaneous sarcoidosis • Sclerosing panniculitis (lipodermatosclerosis)	

Table 12.7.3: Conditions associated with erythema nodosum

Infections		
• *Bacterial/mycobacterial* Streptococcal infection Tuberculosis Leprosy *Yersinia*, *Salmonella*, *Campylobacter gastroenteritis*, brucellosis • *Fungal* Coccidiomycosis, blastomycosis, histoplasmosis • *Viral* Cytomegalovirus, Ebstein Barr virus, hepatitis B, hepatitis C		
Underlying systemic disease	**Malignancy**	**Drugs**
Crohn's disease Ulcerative colitis Behçet's disease Sarcoidosis Sweet syndrome	Hodgkin's lymphoma Acute myeloid leukemia Carcinoid tumor	Oral contraceptive pills Penicillin Sulfonamides Minocycline Phenytoin Thalidomide

occasionally. Another example in this category is rheumatoid nodules, they occur over extensor surfaces and pressure areas. These areas include the forearm, proximal ulna and olecranon process, the metacarpophalangeal and proximal interphalangeal joints. Other sites of involvement by rheumatoid nodules are the sacrum, occiput, palms, and soles.

II. Predominantly Septal Panniculitis with Vasculitis

As the name suggests cutaneous polyarteritis nodosa (PAN) is characterized by septal panniculitis and inflammation of small and medium arteries (arteritis) of the subcutaneous tissue, giving rise to painful skin nodules that ulcerate. A livedo rash also occurs. Unlike classical PAN there are no systemic features. Cutaneous PAN characteristically spares the venules and runs a chronic course. Since inflammation can involve the vessels in the local muscle and epineurium, patients may have myalgia and peripheral neuropathy.

The second example of this is superficial thrombophlebitis and cutaneous leukocytoclastic vasculitis.

III. Predominantly Lobular Panniculitis without Vasculitis

Nonvasculitic lobular panniculitis arises due to trauma or injury. Examples are factitious panniculitis, due to heat or cold or electrical injury (traumatic panniculitis), post-steroid injection, infective panniculitis. The second group is related to enzymatic disorders. Examples are pancreatic panniculitis and alpha-1 antitrypsin deficiency. The third group of diseases is rheumatology related: lupus panniculitis, gouty panniculitis, dermatomyositis, sarcoidosis, and lipodermatosclerosis.

Lupus Panniculitis

This is a manifestation of chronic cutaneous lupus. It presents as subcutaneous nodules or plaques which resolve to leave depressed, sunken areas. There is a predilection for the scalp, head, face, back, and proximal extremities (lateral arms, buttocks, and thighs). Lupus profundus is said to occur when a cutaneous discoid lesion overlies the area of panniculitis. A differential diagnosis of lupus panniculitis is subcutaneous panniculitis-like T cell lymphoma. Hence biopsy of nodules is essential to differentiate between the two.

Panniculitis in Dermatomyositis

Panniculitis in dermatomyositis is rare, histopathologically resembles lupus panniculitis with lobular panniculitis and predominance of lymphocytes in the inflammatory infiltrate. It presents as tender erythematous subcutaneous nodules on upper or lower limbs.

Gouty Panniculitis

Deposition of monosodium urate (MSU) crystals in the subcutaneous fat can occur in gout. Patients present with erythematous subcutaneous nodules or plaques which are frequently painful and can ulcerate discharging fluid. Nodules are distributed over the lower extremities, though upper extremities and trunk may also be involved. Histopathologic examination reveals granulomatous inflammatory infiltrate and MSU crystals.

Subcutaneous sarcoidosis or Darier-Roussy sarcoidosis is a form of nodular sarcoidosis that involves subcutaneous tissue in middle-aged females. It presents as erythematous or flesh-coloured nodules, usually over the upper extremities that are usually non-tender or only mildly tender. This is in contrast to the erythema nodosum lesions of sarcoidosis which have predilection for the lower limbs and are tender.

IV. Predominantly Lobular Panniculitis with Vasculitis

There are two important conditions in this group. One is erythema nodosum leprosum (ENL) an immune reaction to leprosy and the second is erythema induratum of Bazin, an immune reaction to mycobacteria tuberculosis.

ENL is an immune-mediated reaction (type 2 lepra reaction) seen in lepromatous leprosy and borderline leprosy, characterized by an eruption of multiple painful nodules on extensor surfaces of limbs and face. The lesions may form pustules and ulcerate discharging pus. Systemic symptoms like fever, headache, arthralgia or arthritis may accompany the skin manifestation. Histopathology of the nodules shows neutrophilic infiltrate against a background of chronic inflammation, with acid fast bacilli.

Erythema induratum of bazin is mostly lobular panniculitis, and vasculitis is present in most but not all lesions. The type of vessels inflamed are venules, veins, and arteries of the lobule and connective tissue septae. The tuberculin test is strongly positive, and the skin lesions respond very well to anti-tuberculous therapy. A non-tuberculous variant of erythema induratum is referred to as nodular vasculitis or erythema induratum of Whitfield.

LEARNING POINTS

- Panniculitis is inflammation of subcutaneous fat and can occur as a result of various systemic inflammatory disorders, infections, drugs or malignancies.
- Patients present with erythematous nodules or plaques and it may be difficult to reach a diagnosis based on clinical features alone.
- A scalpel skin biopsy is helpful in reaching the diagnosis and the histopathological examination often helps in categorising the panniculitis as septal or lobular with or without associated vasculitis.

FURTHER READING

1. Rangel LK, Villa-Ruiz C, Lo K, et al. Clinical Characteristics of Lupus Erythematosus Panniculitis/Profundus: A Retrospective Review of 61 Patients. JAMA Dermatol. 2020;156:1264–6.
2. Requena L, Sánchez Yus E. Panniculitis. Part II. Mostly lobular panniculitis. J Am Acad Dermatol. 2001;45:325–61.
3. Requena L, Yus ES. Panniculitis. Part I. Mostly septal panniculitis. J Am Acad Dermatol. 2001;45:163–83.
4. Segura S, Pujol RM, Trindade F, et al. Vasculitis in erythema induratum of Bazin: a histopathologic study of 101 biopsy specimens from 86 patients. J Am Acad Dermatol. 2008;59:839–51.
5. Wick MR. Panniculitis: A summary. Semin Diagn Pathol. 2017;34:261–72.

Index